Biomedical and Demographic Determinants of Reproduction

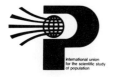

International union
for the scientific study
of population

The International Union for the Scientific Study of Population Problems was set up in 1928, with Dr Raymond Pearl as President. At that time the Union's main purpose was to promote international scientific co-operation to study the various aspects of population problems, through national committees and through its members themselves. In 1947 the International Union for the Scientific Study of Population (IUSSP) was reconstituted into its present form.

It expanded its activities to:
- stimulate research on population
- develop interest in demographic matters among governments, national and international organizations, scientific bodies, and the general public
- foster relations between people involved in population studies
- disseminate scientific knowledge on population

The principal ways through which the IUSSP currently achieves its aims are:
- organization of worldwide or regional conferences
- operations of Scientific Committees under the auspices of the Council
- organization of training courses
- publication of conference proceedings and committee reports.

Demography can be defined by its field of study and its analytical methods. Accordingly, it can be regarded as the scientific study of human populations primarily with respect to their size, their structure, and their development. For reasons which are related to the history of the discipline, the demographic method is essentially inductive: progress in knowledge results from the improvement of observation, the sophistication of measurement methods, and the search for regularities and stable factors leading to the formulation of explanatory models. In conclusion, the three objectives of demographic analysis are to describe, measure, and analyse.

International Studies in Demography is the outcome of an agreement concluded by the IUSSP and the Oxford University Press. The joint series is expected to reflect the broad range of the Union's activities and, in the first instance, will be based on the seminars organized by the Union. The Editorial Board of the series is comprised of:

John Cleland, UK   Henri Leridon, France
John Hobcraft, UK   Richard Smith, UK
Georges Tapinos, France

Biomedical and Demographic Determinants of Reproduction

Edited by
Ronald Gray
with
Henri Leridon and Alfred Spira

CLARENDON PRESS · OXFORD
1993

Oxford University Press, Walton Street, Oxford OX2 6DP

Oxford New York Toronto
Delhi Bombay Calcutta Madras Karachi
Petaling Jaya Singapore Hong Kong Tokyo
Nairobi Dar es Salaam Cape Town
Melbourne Auckland

and associated companies in
Berlin Ibadan

Oxford is a trade mark of Oxford University Press

Published in the United States
by Oxford University Press, New York

© *IUSSP 1993*

British Library Cataloguing in Publication Data
Data available

Library of Congress Cataloging in Publication Data
Biological and demographic determinants of reproduction / edited by
Ronald Gray with Henri Leridon and Alfred Spira.
(International studies in demography)
Includes bibliographical references and index.
1. Human reproduction—Regulation. I. Gray, Ronald H.
II. Leridon, Henri. III. Spira, Alfred. IV. Series.
[DNLM: 1. Demography—congresses. 2. Fertility—congresses.
3. Reproduction—congresses. WQ 205 B6 15]
QP251.B5627 1992 304.6'3—dc20 92–11491
ISBN 0–19–828371–7

Phototypeset by Alliance Phototypesetters Pondicherry
Printed in Great Britain by
Bookcraft (Bath) Ltd., Midsomer Norton

Preface

In 1986 the International Union for the Scientific Study of Population (IUSSP) established a Working Group on Biomedical Demography to encourage the integration of biology and medicine into demographic concerns. A particular focus of the Working Group was to foster seminars and other meetings in which biomedical and demographic scientists could exchange information on topics of common interest. The members of the Working Group were Dr John Bongaarts from the Population Council, Dr Lincoln Chen from Harvard University, and Dr Ronald Gray from Johns Hopkins University, who acted as chair.

From the perspective of research on reproduction, the Working Group built upon the efforts of other IUSSP Committees, particularly the Committee on Comparative Analysis of Fertility which held a Seminar on Natural Fertility in Paris in March, 1977. The proceedings were published by Ordina Editions of Liege in 1979 under the title *Natural Fertility* edited by Henri Leridon and Jane Menken. This previous seminar provided an excellent integration of knowledge on the concept of natural fertility and the factors affecting fertility in the absence of deliberate control of reproduction.

The Seminar on the Biomedical and Demographic Determinants of Human Reproduction was held at the Johns Hopkins University, School of Hygiene and Public Health in Baltimore, Maryland from 4–8 January 1988. It was organized jointly by the Working Group on Biomedical Demography and the IUSSP Committee on Comparative Analysis of Fertility and Family Planning. Funding support was provided by the IUSSP and the Institute for International Programs (IIP) at Johns Hopkins University. This volume presents the papers prepared for the seminar.

Contents

List of Contributors   x

List of Figures   xii

List of Tables   xvii

List of Abbreviations   xxii

Part I: Introduction and Overview

1   Introduction   3
    Ronald H. Gray

2   The Relative Contributions of Biological and Behavioural
    Factors in Determining Natural Fertility: A Demographer's
    Perspective   9
    John Bongaarts

Part II: Demographic and Behavioural Determinants of Reproduction

3   The Determinants of Adolescent Fertility with Special
    Reference to Biological Variables   21
    Stan Becker

4   The Relationship of Age at Menarche and Fertility in
    Undernourished Adolescents   50
    Ann P. Riley, Julia L. Samuelson, and Sandra L. Huffman

5   Age at Menopause and Fecundity Preceding Menopause   65
    Omar Rahman and Jane Menken

6   Coitus as Demographic Behaviour   85
    J. Richard Udry

Part III: Biomedical Determinants of Reproduction

7   The Pathophysiology and Epidemiology of Sexually
    Transmitted Diseases in Relation to Pelvic Inflammatory
    Disease and Infertility   101
    Willard Cates Jr., Robert T. Rolfs Jr., and Sevgi O. Aral

8   A Descriptive Epidemiology of Infertility in Costa Rica 126
    Mark W. Oberle, Luis Rosero-Bixby, and Pat Whitaker

9   The Effects of Exercise and Nutrition on the Menstrual Cycle 132
    David C. Cumming

10   Fertility Following Contraceptive Use   157
     George R. Huggins

11   Toxic Substances, Conception, and Pregnancy Outcome   170
     Michael J. Rosenberg

                    Part IV: Fecundability

12   Models of Fecundability   183
     Meredith L. Golden and Sara R. Millman

13   Age Patterns of Fecundability   209
     Maxine Weinstein, James Wood, and Chang Ming-Cheng

             Part V: Infertility and Assisted Conception

14   Artificial Insemination with Frozen Donor Semen: A Model to
     Appreciate Human Fecundity   231
     CECOS Fédération and J. Lansac

15   Hormonal Regulation in *in Vitro* Fertilization   243
     Gary D. Hodgen

16   Conception Probability and Pregnancy Outcome in Relation to
     Age, Cycle Regularity, and Timing of Intercourse   271
     A. Spira, B. Ducot, M. L. Guihard-Moscato, N. Job-Spira,
     M. J. Mayaux, J. Ménétrier, J. Wattiaux

            Part VI: Causes and Frequency of Foetal Loss

17   Biological Causes of Foetal Loss   287
     Joe Leigh Simpson and Sandra Carson

18   Endocrine Detection of Conception and Early Foetal Loss   316
     Allen J. Wilcox, Clarice R. Weinberg, Donna D. Baird, and
     Robert E. Canfield

19   The Relationship between Reduced Fecundability and
     Subsequent Foetal Loss   329
     Donna D. Baird, N. Beth Ragan, Allen J. Wilcox,
     and Clarice R. Weinberg

     Part VII: Post-Partum Infecundability and the Role of Lactation

20   Fecundability and Post-Partum Sterility:
     An Insuperable Interaction?   345
     Henri Leridon

21   Demographic Research on Lactational Amenorrhoea   359
     Kathleen Ford and Young J. Kim

22 Statistical Evidence of Links between Maternal Nutrition and
   Post-Partum Infertility   372
   A. Meredith John

23 Maternal Nutrition, Infant Feeding, and Post-Partum
   Amenorrhoea: Recent Evidence from Bangladesh   383
   Kathleen Ford and Sandra Huffman

24 Breastfeeding and Fertility   391
   A. S. McNeilly

25 Breastfeeding and the Length of Post-Partum Amenorrhoea:
   A Hazards Model Approach   413
   Germán Rodriguez and Soledad Diaz

26 The Return of Ovarian Function during Lactation:
   Results of Studies from the United States and the Philippines   428
   Ronald H. Gray, Ruben Apelo, Oona Campbell,
   Susan Eslami, Howard Zacur, and Miriam Labbok

27 Post-Partum Sexual Abstinence in Tropical Africa   446
   Etienne van de Walle and Francine van de Walle

Index of Names   461
Index of Subjects   469

List of Contributors

RUBEN APELO, Dr Jose Fabella Memorial Hospital, Manila

SEVGI O. ARAL, Division of Sexually Transmitted Diseases, Centers for Disease Control, Atlanta

DONNA D. BAIRD, Epidemiology Branch, National Institute of Environmental Health Sciences, North Carolina

STAN BECKER, Johns Hopkins University

JOHN BONGAARTS, The Population Council, New York

OONA CAMPBELL, School of Hygiene and Public Health, Johns Hopkins University

ROBERT E. CANFIELD, College of Physicians and Surgeons, Columbia University

SANDRA CARSON, Department of Obstetrics and Gynecology, University of Tennessee, Memphis

WILLARD CATES JR, Division of Sexually Transmitted Diseases, Centers for Disease Control, Atlanta

DAVID C. CUMMING, Departments of Obstetrics and Gynecology, and Medicine, Division of Endocrinology, University of Alberta, Edmonton

SOLEDAD DIAZ, Facultad de Ciencias Biológicas, Pontificia Universidad Católica de Chile, Santiago

BEATRICE DUCOT, Institut National de la Santé et de la Recherche Médicale (INSERM), Kremlin-Bicetre

SUSAL ESLAMI, School of Hygiene and Public Health, Johns Hopkins University

KATHLEEN FORD, Department of Population Planning and International Health, School of Public Health, University of Michigan

MEREDITH L. GOLDEN, Departments of Geography and Epidemiology, University of North Carolina

RONALD H. GRAY, School of Hygiene and Public Health, Johns Hopkins University

MARIE-LUCE GUIHARD-MOSCATO, INSERM

GARY D. HODGEN, Jones Institute for Reproductive Medicine, Department of Obstetrics and Gynecology, Eastern Virginia Medical School

SANDRA L. HUFFMAN, Center to Prevent Childhood Malnutrition, Bethesda

GEORGE R. HUGGINS, Department of Obstetrics and Gynecology, Francis Scott Key Medical Center, Baltimore

NADINE JOB-SPIRA, INSERM

A. MEREDITH JOHN, Office of Population Research, Princeton University

YOUNG J. KIM, Department of Population Dynamics, School of Hygiene and Public Health, Johns Hopkins University

MIRIAM LABBOK, School of Hygiene and Public Health, Johns Hopkins University

J. LANSAC, CHU Bretonneau, Tours

HENRI LERIDON, Institut National d'Études Demographiques, Paris

A.S. MCNEILLY, MRC Reproductive Biology Unit, University of Edinburgh

MARIE-JEANNE MAYAUX, INSERM

JACQUES MENETRIER, INSERM

JANE MENKEN, Princeton University and University of Pennsylvania

SARAH R. MILLMAN, World Hunger Program, and Population Studies and Training Center, Brown University

CHANG MING-CHENG, Taiwan Provincial Institute of Family Planning, Taichung, China

MARK W. OBERLE, Institute for Health Research (INISA), University of Costa Rica, San Jose

N. BETH RAGAN, Division of Biometry and Risk Assessment, National Institute of Environmental Health Sciences, North Carolina

OMAR RAHMAN, Harvard School of Public Health

ANN P. RILEY, University of Michigan Population Studies Center

GERMAN RODRIQUEZ, Office of Population Research, Princeton University

ROBERT T. ROLFS JR, Division of Sexually Transmitted Diseases, Centers for Disease Control, Atlanta

MICHAEL J. ROSENBERG, Department of Epidemiology and Obstetrics-Gynecology, University of North Carolina

LUIS ROSERO-BIXBY, Public Healthy Practice Program Office, Centers for Disease Control, Atlanta

JULIA L. SAMUELSON, Tulane University School of Public Health and Tropical Medicine

JOE LEIGH SIMPSON, Department of Obstetrics and Gynecology, University of Tennessee, Memphis

ALFRED SPIRA, INSERM

RICHARD UDRY, Carolina Population Center, University of North Carolina

ETIENNE VAN DE WALLE, University of Pennsylvania

FRANCINE VAN DE WALLE, University of Pennsylvania

J. WATTIAUX, INSERM

CLARICE R. WEINBERG, Statistics and Biomathematics Branch, National Institute of Environmental Health Sciences, North Carolina

MAXINE WEINSTEIN, Department of Demography, Georgetown University

PAT WHITAKER, Division of Reproductive Health, Center for Chronic Disease Prevention and Health Promotion, Centers for Disease Control, Atlanta

ALLEN J. WILCOX, Epidemiology Branch, National Institute of Environmental Health Sciences, North Carolina

JAMES WOOD, Department of Anthropology, University of Wisconsin at Madison

HOWARD ZACUR, School of Hygiene and Public Health, Johns Hopkins University

List of Figures

2.1   The rise in natural fertility associated with the removal of
      the fertility-inhibiting effects of behavioural and biological
      proximate determinants   13
2.2   The distribution of children ever born among ever-married
      women aged 45–9 in Bangladesh and Mexico   16
2.3   The timing of key events in the reproductive histories of
      rural Philippines women   17

3.1   Levels of adolescent fertility reported in recent years, by
      continent   22
3.2   Adolescent fertility levels since 1978, various nations   24
3.3   Median age at menarche, by region   30
3.4   Percentage of ovulatory cycles, by gynaecological age in two
      studies   34
3.5   Adolescent fertility and percentage of women 15–19 years
      old who are married   36

4.1   One-year rates of growth in height and weight by age,
      rural Bangladeshi adolescents compared to British
      standards   58
4.2   One-year rates of growth in weight and height by age and
      menarche status in rural Bangladeshi girls   59

5.1   Marital fertility rates by 5-year age-groups in ten historical
      populations   68

6.1   Frequency of intercourse for married women   87
6.2   The distribution of coitus during the follicular and luteal
      phases of the female cycle   93

7.1   Polymicrobial pathogenesis of sexually transmitted PID   105

9.1   Exercise and age at menarche   133
9.2   The effect of weekly training mileage on the prevalence of
      oligomenorrhoea   146
9.3   LH pulse frequency and amplitude in normally sedentary
      women, runners at rest, and runners following 60 minutes of
      running at 60 per cent of maximal aerobic capacity   147
9.4   The peripheral levels of B-endorphin/B-LPH and catechol
      oestrogens in sedentary women and swimmers during
      moderate or strenuous training   212

13.1   The age pattern of embryonic and foetal loss in women from
       populations in which induced abortion is not a competing risk   212
13.2   Age patterns of marital and non-marital coital frequency,
       US males and females 1938–47   212
13.3   The relationship between daily coital frequency and the
       duration of marriage in 1430 currently married US women   213
13.4   An idealized representation of the distribution of conception
       waits under homogeneous fecundability and heterogeneous
       fecundability   214
13.5   Model predictions of age-specific total and apparent
       fecundability when coital frequency is held constant and
       female reproductive physiology is allowed to vary   218
13.6   Model predictions of age-specific apparent fecundability
       when female reproductive physiology is held constant and
       coital frequency is allowed to vary   219
13.7   A comparison of two sets of model prediction of age-specific
       apparent fecundability and the fraction of age-related decline
       in apparent fecundability attributable to changes in female
       reproductive physiology   221
13.8   Fit of the negative binomial distribution to coital data
       reported by Taiwanese women aged 20–4   224

14.1   Cumulative success rate for 2872 women undergoing AID   234
14.2   AID success rate according to cycle day among 821 cycles
       with a single insemination   235
14.3   Success rate according to cycle day, with artificial and
       natural insemination   236

15.1   The five principal steps of *in vitro* fertilization and embryo
       transfer procedure   252
15.2   A woman with a high response to hMG stimulation   255
15.3   A woman with a low response to hMG stimulation   256
15.4   The patterns of steroidogenesis in the follicular phase after
       hMG stimulation   257
15.5   Comparison of women who received pre-treatment with
       GnRH antagonist with those who did not   258
15.6   Representative serum hormone values in a typical group III
       subject   259
15.7   A comparison of serum hormone levels in spontaneous and
       hMG/hCG-stimulated cycles   262
15.8   A comparison of serum progesterone values in pregnant and
       non-pregnant women after hMG/hCG-stimulated cycles   265
15.9   A comparison of cumulative pregnancy rates of *in vivo*, *in
       vitro*, and AID fertilization   266
15.10 The process of *in vitro* fertilization   268

15.11 A series of possible methods of egg or embryo donation   268

17.1   Relative timing for loss of murine autosomal monosomy and
       murine autosomal trisomy   289
17.2   Diagram of possible gametes and progeny of a
       phenotypically normal individual heterozygous for a
       Robertsonian translocation between chromosomes 14 and 21   296
17.3   Diagram illustrating the breakpoints leading to an inversion
       in chromosome 18   297
17.4   Diagrammatic representation of some mullerian fusion
       anomalies   301
17.5   Schematic diagram of the immunological responses operating
       in normal pregnancies   304

18.1   Three hormones measured in daily urines from a woman
       with two early pregnancy losses followed by a clinically
       recognized pregnancy   319
18.2   Luteinizing hormone and hCG measurements for a woman
       with an early pregnancy loss followed by a clinically
       recognized pregnancy   323
18.3   Urinary hCG concentrations for five typical examples of
       early pregnancy loss from five different women   325

19.1   Comparison of data on time to pregnancy collected
       prospectively and retrospectively on current and past
       pregnancies   331
19.2   Time-line of reproductive loss   333
19.3   Measured rate of pregnancy loss as a function of gestational
       age at time of pregnancy detection   334

20.1   Rate of conception, by months since return of menses,
       Matlab, Bangladesh   354
20.2   Time to conception, by duration of amenorrhoea, Matlab,
       Bangladesh   356
20.3   Crude distribution of duration of amenorrhoea, Matlab,
       Bangladesh   356

21.1   Empirical density and model estimate for all births,
       Bangladesh   365
21.2   Empirical density and model estimate for surviving births
       only, Bangladesh   365
21.3   Empirical density and model estimate for all births,
       Narangwal   366
21.4   Empirical density and model estimate for surviving births
       only, Narangwal   366
21.5   Model density functions for age-groups, Bangladesh   367

21.6   Model density functions for parity groups, Bangladesh   367

24.1   Infant feeding patterns, basal prolactin levels, menstruation,
       and suppression of urinary steroid excretion in a
       breastfeeding mother with amenorrhoea during lactation and
       ovulation before first menses   392
24.2   Infant feeding patterns, basal prolactin levels, menstruation,
       and suppression of urinary steroid excretion in a
       breastfeeding mother with menses during lactation and
       ovulation before first menses   393
24.3   Comparison of suckling episodes, suckling duration,
       supplementary feeds, and basal prolactin in breastfeeding
       mothers who did or did not ovulate after the introduction of
       supplementary feeds   395
24.4   Changes in urinary levels of pregnanediol glucuronide and
       menses prior to conception in seven breastfeeding women   396
24.5   Changes in the pulsatile secretion of LH in relation to the
       return of ovarian activity   399
24.6   Diagrammatic representation of the control of
       gonadotrophin secretion and its interaction with prolactin
       during lactational amenorrhoea and the resumption of
       follicle growth and ovulation in breastfeeding women   400
24.7   Induction of ovulation in a breastfeeding woman by the
       pulsatile infusion of LHRH (GnRH)   401
24.8   Changes in urinary oestrogen, pregnanediol, LH, and FSH
       in early morning specimens collected during the transition
       from lactational amenorrhoea to normal luteal function   402
24.9   Changes in suckling frequency, basal prolactin levels, and
       the prolactin response to suckling with time post partum   403

26.1   Mean daily luteal phase urinary Pd-G excretion comparing
       cycles with normal and abnormal luteal phases   431
26.2   Average daily breast, bottle, and other feeding episodes by
       week post partum, Manila   434
26.3   Average daily breast, bottle, and other feeding episodes by
       week post partum, Baltimore   435
26.4   Relationship between breastfeeding frequency and the use of
       solid feeds in Baltimore women   435
26.5   Relationship between breastfeeding frequency and the use of
       bottle feeds in Baltimore women   436
26.6   Timing of first menses and ovulation in Manila women   437
26.7   Timing of first menses and ovulation in Baltimore women   438
26.8   Feeding frequency and resumption of ovulation for subject
       A, who gave early supplementary feeds   439

26.9   Feeding frequency and resumption of ovulation for subject
       B, who maintained a high frequency of breastfeeding with
       only modest supplementation   439

27.1   Relationship between breastfeeding and amenorrhoea   455
27.2   Effect of abstinence on the non-susceptible period   456

List of Tables

2.1 Values of proximate determinants for a typical traditional developing country and for theoretical maximum biological fertility 12

2.2 Estimates of total fertility rates for contemporary developing countries and historical societies with natural fertility 14

2.3 Analysis of determinants of variability in natural fertility 15

3.1 Reports of median (or mean) age at menarche for various populations, by world region 25

3.2 Percentage of females 15–19 years of age who are married at two points in time, various nations 35

3.3 Mean frequency of sexual intercourse in a 4-week period for women aged 15–19 and 20–4 37

3.4 Legal abortion ratios by age of woman at conception for 13 nations (abortions per 100 known pregnancies) 39

3.5 Summary of biological and behavioural determinants of adolescent fertility 41

3.6 Available data for application of model of adolescent fertility to the USA 42

3.7 Contraceptive use and monthly failure rates in the USA 43

5.1 Estimates of age at menopause from selected studies 66

5.2 Marital age-specific fertility rates in populations of west European descent with no evidence of fertility limitation 68

5.3 Relative fertility rates according to the age of wife and husband, controlling for the effects of marriage duration and age of spouse 69

5.4 Relative fertility rates by marriage duration, controlling for the effects of the age of husband and wife 70

5.5 Estimates of the percentage of women sterile by age, comparing 17th- and 18th-century French women and early 20th-century Hutterites 71

5.6 Proportions infecund among currently married non-contracepting women, by age 72

5.7 The proportion infecund estimated for Cameroon, Ghana, Kenya, Lesotho, and Sudan (all women and women who had never used contraception) and for historical England 74

5.8   Rates of pregnancy, loss to follow-up, and drop-out by age, following artificial insemination in France   74

5.9   Estimated percentages of women who are sterile by age and age at marriage   76

5.10 Mean weekly coital frequency of married women by age in selected populations   77

5.11 Mean weekly coital frequency of married women by age, comparing data from Bangladesh and West Bengal   78

5.12 The potential impact of terminal abstinence on the age pattern of natural fertility, when the proportion of grandmothers and mothers-in-law practise abstinence as in Nigeria   79

5.13 Model estimates of fecundability and conception wait for different coital frequencies   80

6.1   Mean monthly frequency of marital intercourse by age of respondent for married women   86

6.2   Multiple regression of frequency of intercourse per month against selected social variables   89

7.1   Accuracy of clinical diagnosis of PID, by presence of visually confirmed salpingitis and other pathology, selected studies   102

7.2   Detection of *Chlamydia trachomatis* and *Neisseria gonorrhoeae* among women with acute PID, selected studies   104

7.3   Prevalence of history of infertility by five definitions, adjusted for age   108

7.4   Studies of *Chlamydia trachomatis* infection and subsequent tubal infertility   109

7.5   Estimated incidence of tubal infertility, USA   115

7.6   Estimated prevalence of tubal infertility, USA   116

8.1   The prevalence of a history of infecundity by selected variables, Costa Rican women aged 25–59, 1984   128

8.2   The prevalence of a history of infecundity by number of lifetime sexual partners and age at first coitus, Costa Rican women aged 25–59, 1984   129

8.3   The prevalence of a history of infecundity by serological status for three sexually transmitted diseases, Costa Rican women aged 25–59, 1984   129

10.1 Selected results of nine studies describing the impact of first-trimester induced abortion of a woman's first pregnancy on the rate of low birth-weight in the second pregnancy   158

10.2 Selected results of six studies describing the impact of first-trimester induced abortion of a woman's first pregnancy on the rate of premature delivery in the second pregnancy   159

10.3 Selected results of five studies describing the impact of
      first-trimester induced abortion of a woman's first pregnancy
      on the rate of mid-trimester spontaneous abortion of the
      second pregnancy   159
10.4 IUD use in women with primary tubal infertility and in
      controls, according to type of IUD   165
10.5 Relation of IUD use to the risk of primary tubal infertility   166
10.6 Relation of number of sexual partners and IUD use to the
      risk of primary tubal infertility   166

11.1 Sample size required to detect doubling in adverse
      reproductive outcomes   172
11.2 Occupational agents with reproductive toxicity in man or
      animal   174

12.1 Summary of fecundability estimated by type and model
      classification   202

13.1 Reported coital frequency in the last month, women aged
      20–49 in first marriages, Taiwan 1986   222
13.2 Expected waiting times to conception by age under three
      assumptions about variability in coital rates   223
13.3 Expected waiting times to conception under varying
      assumptions about heterogeneity in coital frequency, women
      aged 20–4   225

14.1 AID success rate by cervical score among 821 cycles with a
      single insemination   236
14.2 AID success rate according to quality of husband's semen   236
14.3 Mean success rates for AID according to characteristics of
      donor semen   237
14.4 AID success rates for first and succeeding pregnancies   238
14.5 AID success rates by age of woman among 2193 nulliparous
      women with azoospermic husbands   239
14.6 Results of *in vitro* fertilization using donor semen   240
14.7 Pregnancy rates after IVF-D and AID using the same
      ejaculates   240
14.8 Life-table cumulative pregnancy success rates for AID and
      IVF-D by treatment years   241

15.1 IVF results by category of infertility, Norfolk, 1981–4   246
15.2 IVF results for couples with male factor infertility, Norfolk,
      1981–4   247
15.3 IVF results of women with endometriosis, Norfolk, 1981–4   247
15.4 IVF results by woman's age, Norfolk, 1981–4   251
15.5 Multiple pregnancy rates rise along with the pregnancy rate
      as the number of embryos transferred increases   252

15.6 Hormonal parameters in IVF/ET patients relating oocyte
      yield to plasma steroid levels   260
15.7 Results of attempt to mature and fertilize human oocytes *in
      vitro* as compared to attempts to fertilize pre-ovulatory
      oocytes during the same period   261
15.8 Serum progesterone levels at the time of the endometrial
      biopsy   264

16.1 Conception probability and pregnancy outcome according to
      male age   274
16.2 Conception probability and pregnancy outcome according to
      female age   275
16.3 Conception probability and pregnancy outcome according to
      cycle regularity   276
16.4 Conception probability and pregnancy outcome according to
      the time of insemination   277

17.1 Chromosomal complements in spontaneous abortions
      recognized clinically in the first trimester   292
17.2 Balanced translocations in couples experiencing repeated
      abortions   296

19.1 Descriptive characteristics of the 1701 women of the
      Collaborative Perinatal Project   337
19.2 Relationship between fecundability and spontaneous
      abortion among women in the Collaborative Perinatal
      Project   338
19.3 Frequency of foetal loss in relation to fecundability among
      participants in the Early Pregnancy Study   339

20.1 Monthly conception rates for the first 3 years following a
      live birth   350
20.2 Monthly conception rates for the first 3 years following a
      live birth, by period   350
20.3 Time to conception, by duration of previous amenorrhoea,
      Matlab Study, 1975–9   355

21.1 Duration of breastfeeding and post-partum amenorrhoea in
      selected populations   360
21.2 Parameter estimates for the mixed distribution of Type I
      distributions   364

23.1 Median duration of total and full breastfeeding and
      amenorrhoea by maternal and infant characteristics   387
23.2 Estimates from hazard models of the relative risk of
      resuming menstruation   388

25.1   First menstrual events and woman days of exposure for the total sample and estimated risk of first menses and survival in amenorrhoeic state   418

25.2   Tabulation of menstrual events and woman days of exposure by duration post-partum and breastfeeding status   419

25.3   Goodness of fit statistics for models involving breastfeeding status   420

25.4   Parameter estimates for model with proportional effect of breastfeeding status   421

25.5   Goodness of fit statistics for models with frequency of suckling during the day and night   422

25.6   Parameter estimates for model with a proportional effect of frequency of suckling during the day   423

25.7   Parameter estimates for model with a proportional effect of frequency of suckling during the night   423

25.8   Parameter estimates for model with a proportional effect of the combination of daytime and night-time suckling   424

25.9   Parameter estimates for model with a combined frequency of suckling of at least seven daytime and three night-time episodes   424

25.10 Parameter estimates for proportional hazards model with an interaction effect of supplementation and frequency of suckling   425

26.1   Characteristics of the study populations in Baltimore and Manila   432

26.2   Number of women experiencing events during the study   433

26.3   Number and percentage of women who ovulated prior to first menses, by time post partum   436

26.4   Characteristics of first menstrual episode   437

26.5   Relative risk of ovulation in relation to breastfeeding frequency, Baltimore   440

26.6   Relative risk of ovulation in relation to the percentage of all feeds contributed by breast feeds, Manila   441

26.7   Percentage of anovulatory cycles in first menstrual episodes and percentage of ovulatory cycles which are normal among breastfeeders in 12 studies   442

27.1   Duration of post-partum abstinence, breastfeeding, and amenorrhoea: mean, minimum, and maximum by region of residence   449

List of Abbreviations

AID	artificial insemination by a donor
BBT	basal body temperature
BV	bacterial vaginosis
CNS	central nervous system
CVS	chorion villus sampling
EPF	early pregnancy factor
FSH	follicle-stimulating hormone
GnRH	gonadotrophin-releasing hormone
hCG	human chorionic gonadotrophin
hMG	human menopausal gonadotrophin
HPG axis	hypothalamic–pituitary–gonadal axis
IRMA	Immuno-radiometric assay
IUD	intra-uterine device
IUSSP	International Union for the Scientific Study of Population
IVF	*In vitro* fertilization
LH	luteinizing hormone
LH-RH	LH-releasing hormone
LPD	luteal phase deficiency
NFS	National Fertility Survey
NICHD	National Institutes for Child Health and Development
NSFG	National Survey of Family Growth
OC	oral contraceptive
PID	pelvic inflammatory disease
PRL	prolactin
RIA	radio immunoassay
SHBG	serum hormone binding globulin
STD	sexually transmitted disease
TFR	total fertility rate
WFS	World Fertility Survey
WHO	World Health Organization

Part I

Introduction and Overview

1 Introduction

RONALD H. GRAY

The Seminar on the Demographic and Biomedical Determinants of Human Reproduction, held in January 1988 at the Johns Hopkins University, was intended to be a sequel to a 1977 meeting on Natural Fertility, with particular emphasis on new biomedical developments of relevance to demographers. The objective of the seminar was an interdisciplinary exchange: contributors both examined the complementarity between population-based demographic and epidemiological studies and provided information on biological mechanisms derived from clinical or endocrinological investigations.

John Bongaarts provided an overview of the relative contributions of biological and social factors in determining natural fertility. In Chapter 2 below, Bongaarts presents a model suggesting that behavioural factors, such as age at marriage, coital frequency, and particularly the duration of breastfeeding, exert the greatest effect on fertility, whereas biological factors, such as sterility, intra-uterine mortality, and conception failure, play a less important role, though they are by no means insignificant.

Part II of this volume considers the demographic determinants of reproduction, particularly the determinants of the reproductive life-span. Stan Becker reviews the demographic determinants of menarche and adolescent sterility in Chapter 3. He shows that there are large variations in the age at menarche, with late menarche reported in several developing countries, particularly in Africa and Melanesia. However, variations in the level of adolescent fertility are more closely related to differences in the proportions married and the prevalence of contraceptive use at younger ages. In the developed countries, although there have been secular trends of declining age at menarche and increased sexual activity among unmarried adolescents, these changes have been counterbalanced by the increasing use of contraception and abortion. As a consequence of these complex changes, adolescent fertility has generally declined or remained constant over the past decade.

In Chapter 4, Ann Riley and her colleagues show that poor nutrition slows and delays growth and is associated with later ages at menarche. However, later menarche does not necessarily result in lower fertility. In some societies age at menarche is closely tied with age at marriage, and endocrinological studies suggest that late menarche coincides with a longer period of adolescent sterility. Overall the evidence that poor nutrition has a significant impact on fertility is equivocal. However, early childbearing during the period of adolescent growth may impair long-term growth, resulting in small adult stature and small pelvic diameter, which, in turn, are associated with a higher risk of morbidity and mortality among mothers and their offspring.

Age at menopause and fertility prior to menopause are reviewed by Omar Rahman and Jane Menken in Chapter 5. The age at menopause is much less variable than the age at menarche; it generally falls between 47 and 50 years in most populations. Recent studies have shown that reduced body fat and smoking are associated with earlier onset of menopause. Fertility declines from the mid-30s, and there is a growing concern about infecundity at later ages in industrialized countries where women frequently delay childbearing. The definition of infecundity is difficult, but recent reanalyses of WFS (World Fertility Survey) data using either a history of diagnosed infertility or the absence of a birth over five years as a definition of infecundity, show a much greater variation in the level of apparent sterility by age than was previously recognized.

Coital frequency is a major determinant of conception. In Chapter 6, Richard Udry reviews the literature on coital frequency, which shows clear declines with age and duration of marriage in all populations, as well as culturally determined variations in levels between populations. Contraceptors, particularly users of oral contraceptives, have a higher frequency of intercourse, but this appears to be due to behavioural self-selection. Udry shows that there is no simple relationship between hormone levels and coital frequency, except among adolescents in whom sexual activity is related to androgen levels. However, recent data suggest that the distribution of coital acts during the menstrual cycle may be related to endocrine changes, with a higher frequency of intercourse around the time of the mid-cycle luteinizing hormone (LH) surge.

Part III of the volume considers major biomedical determinants of reproduction. In Chapter 7, Willard Cates and colleagues review the aetiology and epidemiology of sexually transmitted diseases (STDs), pelvic inflammatory disease (PID), and infertility. PID is primarily caused by two sexually transmitted organisms, gonorrhoea and chlamydia, with secondary infections by a variety of other bacteria. Untreated or poorly treated PID damages the fallopian tubes, which leads to sterility. The risk of PID is increased during menstruation and in the presence of uterine instrumentation, as with IUDs, abortion, or delivery, but PID risk can be reduced by the use of barrier contraceptives. Recent studies by World Health Organization (WHO) have shown that infertility in African populations is largely due to tubal occlusion probably resulting from sexually transmitted diseases (STDs) or infections following childbirth and abortion. Surveys in Costa Rica presented by Mark Oberle and colleagues in Chapter 8 show that women with infertility have a higher number of sexual partners, earlier age at first intercourse, and serological evidence of prior STD infections.

The effects on reproduction of nutritional status, stress, and exercise are reviewed by David Cumming in Chapter 9. Vigorous physical exercise is associated with delayed menarche and with reversible endocrine disturbances such as anovulation or luteal phase defects in post-menarcheal women. These later disturbances result from reduced pulsatile LH release due to hypothalamic abnormalities which result from changes in neurotransmitters. The effects of exercise are potentiated in marginally nourished women or in the presence of weight loss, but studies linking specific anthropometric indices to delayed menarche or amenorrhoea are inconclusive because of conflicting results and the use of imprecise measures.

The effect of contraceptive use on subsequent fertility and pregnancy outcome is reviewed by George Huggins in Chapter 10. Extensive studies suggest only slight delays in the return of fertility following oral contraceptive use, a slight risk of infection and impaired fertility following first trimester therapeutic abortion, and an increased risk of tubal infertility among IUD users, primarily in women with multiple sexual partners. The effect of environmental and occupational hazards on reproduction has been an area of concern, but as discussed by Michael Rosenberg in Chapter 11, methodological problems hinder adequate studies. At present, only a small number of chemical and physical agents have been shown to be toxic to human reproduction.

Fecundability is a basic concept in demography summarized in Part IV of the volume. In Chapter 12 Meredith Golden and Sara Millman provide a summary of fecundability models based on waiting times to conception or the timing and frequency of intercourse during the cycle. Modelling has become more complex mathematically, but future progress is largely dependent on a better estimation of the biological variables and their distribution in populations. Maxine Weinstein and her colleagues present models in Chapter 13 which suggest that the decline in fecundability with age cannot be explained by a reduction in coital frequency and probably results from biological changes in older women.

Assisted conception provides insights into physiological process, and is considered in Part V. The results of artificial insemination by donor (AID) provide biological measures of fecundability. Extensive experience in France is summarized by Jaques Lansac and his colleagues in Chapter 14. Success rates with artificial insemination are greater with women under 30 years of age, especially if they have previously borne children and if the couple has a shorter history of infertility. Pregnancy is most common when inseminations take place during the three days before the nadir of the basal body temperature curve.

In vitro fertilization (IVF) also provides insight into the biological determinants of fecundability, and in Chapter 15 Gary Hodgen reviews the experience of one of the largest IVF programmes. The overall pregnancy rate with IVF is around 22 per 100 treatment cycles, and the pregnancy rate in relation to the number of embryos transferred is around 31 per cent. Approximately 12 per cent of fertilized eggs fail to develop, 30 per cent have chromosomal abnormalities, and 19 per cent of successfully transferred embryos are lost before term. The pregnancy rates are similar for all women under 37, but older women experience much higher rates of spontaneous abortion. Similar results from

French studies of IVF are reported by Alfred Spira and his colleagues in Chapter 16, who also describe a series of studies on conception probabilities and pregnancy outcome. Fecundability is highest around the time of ovulation. Spontaneous abortion rates in natural conceptions are highest with post-mature ova; in artificial insemination by donor (AID) they are highest with aged sperm due to pre-ovulatory inseminations.

Part VI discusses the frequency and the causes of foetal loss. The reduction in fertility prior to menopause is probably of biological origin, and Joe Leigh Simpson and Sandra Carson review the biomedical evidence on foetal loss including uterine/endocrine factors in Chapter 17. It is well known that the risk of spontaneous abortion increases with maternal age and that this is related to a higher frequency of trisomic abnormalities, particularly affecting the smaller chromosomes. However, there is also an age-related increase in the incidence of chromosomally normal spontaneous abortions, and chromosomal disorders play only a modest role in the overall increase in the rates of miscarriage. Animal studies using ovum transfer suggest that implantation failures are more common with either an older uterus (and a young ovum) or an older ovum (and a younger uterus), thus suggesting that both uterine and oocyte abnormalities play a significant role in reduced fertility with increasing age.

At least half of first trimester spontaneous abortions are chromosomally abnormal, and of these, 53 per cent have trisomic abnormalities largely of maternal origin. Polyploidy due to extra haploid chromosome complements is relatively uncommon and largely of paternal origin. Among other causes of spontaneous abortion, the most important preventable factors are genital tract infections, smoking, and alcohol consumption during pregnancy. The authors also show that the timing of clinically recognized losses is misleading since foetal death diagnosed by sonography occurs some 3–4 weeks prior to the expulsion of the conceptus. In Chapter 18, Allen Wilcox presents new data on the detection of early foetal loss prior to the first missed menstrual period using a sensitive assay for human chorionic gonadotrophin hormone (hCG) excreted in the urine. In a cohort of 221 women, the frequency of unrecognized early losses detected by hCG assay was 22 per cent; the rates were 19 per cent for women under 30 and 25 per cent for women over 30 years of age. Total pregnancy losses (recognized and unrecognized) were 31 per cent of conceptions. In Chapter 19, Donna Baird shows that subfecundity, as measured by delays in conception, is not associated with an increased risk of foetal loss in the absence of other factors such as higher maternal age or cigarette smoking.

The final section of the book (Part VII) focuses on post-partum infecundability and the role of lactation. In Chapter 20, Henri Leridon shows that there are inconsistencies in the data relating the duration of amenorrhoea to the waiting time to conception which suggests bias, particularly affecting the estimates for women with an early resumption of menstruation. In Chapter 21 Kathleen Ford and Young Kim analyse three prospective and two retrospective studies of the distribution of post-partum menses. In data from the Punjab, Bangladesh,

Philippines, and Mali, there is evidence of a bimodal distribution of menses, whereas in Guatemala and other populations the distribution is unimodal. It is not possible, however, to determine whether the differences in the shape of the distributions reflect data reporting errors or variation in the patterns of breastfeeding.

Meredith John reviews the evidence linking maternal nutrition and post-partum infertility in Chapter 22. Several studies have shown an association between maternal nutritional status and duration of amenorrhoea, but in general the effects are small, and in most investigations there was no considera-tion of breastfeeding behaviour which might be related both to fertility return and to maternal nutrition. In Chapter 23 Kathleen Ford and Sandra Huffman report results from prospective studies in Bangladesh which show that lower maternal nutrition is associated with delayed resumption of menses even after adjustment for some breastfeeding parameters. But the maximum difference in amenorrhoea between poorly nourished and well nourished women is 4 months in a population where the mean duration of amenorrhoea is 15.5 months.

The findings from endocrinological studies of breastfeeding and the post-partum return of pituitary/ovarian function are reviewed by Alan McNeilly in Chapter 24. It is clear that suckling stimulates the secretion of prolactin from the pituitary, and that the main role of prolactin is to maintain milk production. Suckling is also associated with suppression of ovarian activity and infertility due to inhibition of LH release from the pituitary as a consequence of inhibition of pulsatile LH-releasing hormone (LHRH) release from the hypo-thalamus. However, the role of prolactin as a cause of lactational infertility is unclear, and probably of minor significance. The suckling stimulus is critical to the maintenance of lactational infecundity, but there are no reliable and broadly applicable guidelines for the frequency or duration of suckling required to maintain infertility. Dr McNeilly also presents data from Scottish studies which show that the introduction of supplementary foods is associated with a reduction in suckling and the resumption of ovarian activity.

In Chapter 25 Germán Rodriguez and Soledad Diaz analyse Chilean data on breastfeeding in relation to the duration of amenorrhoea using a proportional hazards model. Partial breastfeeding increases the risk of menstruation, but this can be offset by maintaining a high frequency of suckling. Ronald Gray and colleagues present the results of studies of 100 women from the United States and the Philippines in Chapter 26. The Filipino women breastfed more fre-quently and had more protracted amenorrhoea than the American women. In the USA, supplements given by bottle but not by other means were associated with marked reductions of suckling frequency. A high proportion of first post-partum menses were anovulatory or had inadequate luteal phases in both populations, but this was more marked in the Filipino women. For those women with anovulatory first menses, the average time from first menses to first ovulation was around 80 days, suggesting that the duration of amenorrhoea used in demographic studies is an inaccurate and potentially biased marker of ovulation return. Proportional hazards analyses show that the patterns or levels of breastfeeding associated with ovulation return differ between the two populations and that it is not possible to predict ovulation reliably in individual women.

The importance of post-partum sexual abstinence and lactational amenorrhoea as determinants of the birth interval is examined by Etienne and Francine van de Walle in Chapter 27. In most tropical African countries the duration of abstinence is shorter than the duration of amenorrhoea, and the duration of abstinence has been declining with increasing modernization, urbanization, and the spread of Islamic influence.

The seminar provided a constructive interdisciplinary exchange and showed that technological advances, particularly in the use of urinary assays to monitor endocrine function, conception, and early pregnancy loss, provide important new tools for population-based research in both the demographic and biomedical sciences. We hope that this collection of contributions from the seminar will spread more widely the valuable insights gained there.

2 The Relative Contributions of Biological and Behavioural Factors in Determining Natural Fertility: A Demographer's Perspective

JOHN BONGAARTS

Although natural fertility has become a fundamental concept in demographic analysis, its definition is still frequently misunderstood. Some of this confusion stems from the fairly widespread but mistaken notion that natural fertility is solely or largely determined by biological factors. While biological factors are indeed crucial determinants of natural fertility, a number of behaviours are also very important (Leridon, 1977). Louis Henry (1972) identified the key role of breastfeeding and post-partum abstinence in lengthening birth intervals and reducing the rate of reproduction. And, of course, the frequency of intercourse affects natural fertility. If one considers overall natural fertility as measured by the total fertility rate, then age at marriage, marital disruption, and remarriage also become non-biological determinants. Behaviour clearly matters, and this paper will examine its role by discussing the relative contributions of biological and behavioural factors affecting natural fertility. More specifically, it will apply a simple reproductive model to quantify the relative effects of biological and behavioural determinants of levels and differentials in natural fertility.

A Model of Natural Reproduction

A model that quantifies the relationships between natural fertility and its proximate determinants is presented in this section. To make later analyses with this model manageable, a number of simplifying assumptions are made (e.g. a fixed rate of reproduction throughout the reproductive years). However, all key aspects of the natural reproductive process are included. The average number of children born per woman at the end of the reproductive years, TFR, which equals the total natural fertility rate, is estimated as the duration of the actual reproductive span, R, divided by the duration of the average birth interval, B:

$$TFR = R/B. \tag{1}$$

The reproductive span equals the difference between the age at onset of sterility, S, and the age at marriage, M (for simplicity, marital disruption, remarriage, and celibacy are ignored):

$$R = S - M. \tag{2}$$

The average birth interval equals the sum of its four component parts: (1) the post-partum infecundable interval, P, (2) the waiting time to conception, W, (3) time added by intra-uterine mortality, A, and (4) a full-term gestation, G:

$$B = P + W + A + G. \tag{3}$$

Substitution of equations (3) and (2) in (1) (and multiplication by 12 because S, M, B, and R are expressed in years, while P, W, A, and G are given in months) yields:

$$TFR = \frac{12\ (S - M)}{P + W + A + G}. \tag{4}$$

This simple reproductive model is essentially the same as the one used by Bongaarts and Menken (1983). For present purposes this model is extended by introducing the determinants of the conception wait, W. As shown by Bongaarts and Potter (1983), W is inversely related to fecundability, F:

$$W = \frac{1.5}{F}. \tag{5}$$

The factor 1.5 provides a rough adjustment for the effect of heterogeneity in fecundability. Fecundability is in turn related to several biological factors as well as to frequency of intercourse. Although more detailed models are available (see Bongaarts and Potter 1983 and Chapter 7, below), we will introduce here an aggregate equation for fecundability:

$$F = (1 - C)\ I. \tag{6}$$

where C equals the monthly risk of biological failure to conceive (e.g. due to failure to implant or early embryonic mortality) and I is a multiplier with values between 0 and 1 depending on the coital rate. With a high coital rate (e.g. once a day) $I = 1.0$, while $I = 0$ when the coital rate is zero. The relationship between the coital rate and I is not a linear one, but this issue need not be discussed further here. Equation (6) implies that the biological maximum fecundability is $1 - C$, which is attained with a high frequency of intercourse ($I = 1.0$).

Substitution of equations (6) in (5) and (5) in (4) now yields the overall model:

$$TFR = \frac{12\ (S - M)}{P + A + G + 1.5/[(1 - C)\ I]}. \tag{7}$$

This brief derivation of equation (7) has identified the following six proximate determinants of natural fertility:

Behavioural factors:
1. Age at marriage
2. Duration of post-partum infecundability (due to breastfeeding and abstinence)
3. Frequency of intercourse

Biological factors:
4. Age at onset of sterility
5. Intra-uterine mortality
6. Biological risk of conception failure

The quantitative relationship between these variables and natural fertility that is summarized in equation (7) will be used in the following sections to examine the relative effects of the different proximate determinants on natural fertility.

The Proximate Determinants of Natural Fertility

In a fairly typical society with natural fertility the average number of births per woman at the end of the reproductive span is about six or seven. While this level of fertility is high compared with populations in which contraceptive use is widespread, it is low compared with the biological, potential rate of human reproduction. Since a full gestation takes only nine months, women are, at least theoretically, capable of bearing children at a rate of 1 per year. If that rate of childbearing were to be maintained from age 15 to age 50 (the approximate limits of the reproductive life-span), then a woman would bear 35 children over the course of her lifetime. Although there are rare examples of women who have approached this rate of reproduction, observed natural fertility is only a fraction of this theoretical maximum.

The discrepancy between observed and theoretically feasible natural fertility rates is due to the fertility-inhibiting effects of both behavioural and biological factors. To estimate the extent to which each of these variables lowers natural fertility, a simple exercise will be undertaken using equation (7). The first column of Table 2.1 lists typical values for the six proximate variables for a population with a total natural fertility rate of 7 births per woman. These values can be contrasted with the levels needed to produce theoretical maximum biological fertility listed in the second column of Table 2.1. Fig. 2.1 illustrates the extent to which fertility would increase if the value of each of the proximate determinants were shifted from its natural level to its theoretical extreme. By comparing the results for the different behavioural and biological factors, their relative contribution in determining the level of natural fertility can be assessed. Fig. 2.1 clearly shows that, while biological and behavioural factors are both important, the effect of the three behavioural factors combined is about twice the total biological effect.

The ranking from most to least important proximate determinant is as follows:

1. post-partum infecundability
2. permanent sterility
3. coital rate
4. age at marriage
5. biological risk of conception failure
6. intra-uterine mortality

It should be noted that this ranking depends in large part on the values chosen to represent the standard natural fertility population. The estimates in Table 2.1 are typical for a traditional developing country. Somewhat different results would have been obtained if values typical of a historical European population had been used: with a higher age at marriage and a shorter duration of post-partum infecundability, the role of the former would be more important and the latter less so. However, behavioural factors would still account for most of the difference between natural and biological maximum fertility.

Proximate Determinants of Variation in Natural Fertility

While most of the variance in the fertility levels of contemporary populations is due to differences in contraceptive use and induced abortion, the absence of

TABLE 2.1. *Values of proximate determinants for a typical traditional developing country and for theoretical maximum biological fertility*

Proximate determinants	Typical traditional developing country	Theoretical maximum biological fertility
Age at marriage (M)	19	15
Duration of postpartum infecundability (P)	16	1.5
Coital rate multiplier (I)	0.4	1.0
Age at onset of sterility (S)	40	50
Time added by intra-uterine mortality (A)	2.7	0
Biological risk of conception failure (C)	0.55	0
Duration of gestation (G)	9.0	9.0
Total fertility rate (TFR)[a]	7	35

[a] Total fertility rate is calculated with equation (7).

Sources: The value of (C) is consistent with the maximum biological fecundability estimate of 0.45 obtained by Bongaarts and Potter (1983). The coital rate multiplier of 0.4, together with (C) = 0.45, yields a waiting time to conception of 8.33 months. The time added by intra-uterine mortality is estimated by $a(W + L)/(1 - a)$, where a is the probability of intra-uterine mortality, W the average conception wait, and L the average time lost to an aborted gestation and post-partum infecundability. With $a = 0.2$, $W = 8.3$, and $I = 2.5$, A equals 2.7 months. Values for the other proximate determinants are based on a review of available evidence in Bongaarts and Potter (1983) except for age at marriage which is based on MacDonald (1984).

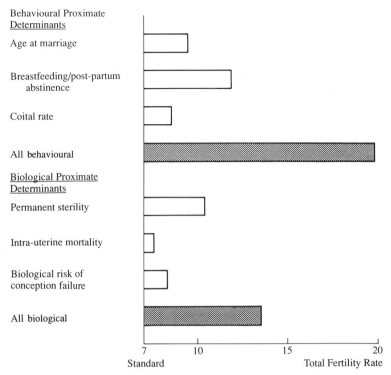

Fig. 2.1 The rise in natural fertility associated with the removal of the fertility-
inhibiting effects of behavioural and biological proximate determinants

such deliberate fertility control does not imply a fixed or nearly invariant level
of natural fertility. In fact, there is wide variation in natural fertility rates.
Table 2.2 lists estimates of total fertility rates in contemporary developing
countries with contraceptive prevalence levels below 5 per cent and in presumably non-contracepting historical populations. In the former, the total fertility
ranges from 8.5 in Yemen to 5.8 in Lesotho. The differences among the historical populations are even larger. Fertility of the Hutterites with a TFR of 9.5
is more than twice that estimated for Thezels Saint Sernin (TFR = 3.7).

Determining which proximate determinants are responsible for this variability in natural fertility would be a simple matter if there were estimates available
of the behavioural and biological factors for each of the populations listed in
Table 2.2. Unfortunately this is not the case, so an indirect procedure must be
used to explore the role played by each of the different proximate variables.
This procedure assumes that the extent to which a proximate determinant
causes variation in natural fertility depends on two factors: the variability in
the proximate determinant, and the sensitivity of natural fertility to variation
in the proximate variable. Proximate determinants with a wide range are
more likely to produce variation in fertility than determinants with a narrow

TABLE 2.2. *Estimates of total fertility rates for contemporary developing countries and historical societies with natural fertility*

Total fertility rate	Contemporary developing countries		Historical societies	
<5			Thezels Saint Sernin	3.7
5–6	Lesotho	5.8	Crulai	5.6
6–7	Nepal	6.3	Tourouvre	6.0
	Pakistan	6.3	Île de France	6.1
	Mauritania	6.3	Amish	6.3
	Cameroon	6.4		
	Ghana	6.5		
7–8	Senegal	7.2		
	Ivory Coast	7.4		
8–9	Kenya	8.2	Canada	8.0
	Yemen	8.5		
9–10			Hutterites	9.5

Sources: Leridon, 1977; Cleland and Hobcraft, 1984.

range. However, the degree of variability in a proximate determinant is not by itself an accurate indicator of how much fertility variation it produces, because natural fertility is not equally sensitive to all proximate factors. Sensitivity must therefore also be taken into account.

Table 2.3 presents the results of this analysis. The first column lists the approximate, observed ranges of the proximate determinants in a variety of natural fertility populations, including both contemporary developing populations and historical populations. The large majority of natural fertility populations can be expected to have values within the ranges given. (Exceptional cases, such as some African populations with high levels of sterility due to venereal disease, are not included; nor are populations in which spousal separation is unusually frequent.) The index of variability, estimated as the range divided by the median, is given in the second column. According to this index, post-partum infecundability has the highest variability, while the age of onset of sterility has the lowest. The third column gives the sensitivity index for each variable. This index equals the percentage change in natural fertility that occurs when there is a 1 per cent change in the proximate variable (all other variables are kept constant at their median values). The most sensitive variable is onset of sterility, while the risk of intra-uterine mortality is the least sensitive. The last column sums up the exercise by multiplying columns 2 and 3 to produce an overall index of the contribution to variability in marital fertility. A comparison of these indices suggests that the behavioural factors, in particular age at marriage and post-partum infecundability, are far more important determinants of variation in natural fertility than are the biological factors.

TABLE 2.3. *Analysis of determinants of variability in natural fertility*

Proximate determinants	Range of population averages	Variability index	Sensitivity index	Index of contribution to variability in natural fertility
Age at marriage (years)	16–28	0.55	−1.19	0.65
Post-partum infecundability (months)	4–24	1.43	−0.42	0.60
Coital rate multiplier	0.3–0.6	0.67	0.28	0.19
Onset of sterility (years)	39–42	0.074	2.19	0.16
Time added by intra-uterine mortality (months)	2–3	0.40	−0.08	0.03
Biological risk of conception failure	0.5–0.6	0.18	−0.35	0.06

Sources: Reviews of estimates of proximate determinants of natural marital fertility societies are provided in Bongaarts and Potter (1983) and Leridon (1977). The range for the coital rate multiplier is derived by assuming that the average conception wait ranges from about 5 to 12.5 months and by taking into account the (rather arbitrary) range of 0.5–0.6 for C.

Intra-uterine mortality and the biological risk of conception failure appear to be less important by more than an order of magnitude than the principal behavioural factors.

Determinants of Individual Natural Fertility

Differences in the natural fertility of individuals in a given population are even larger than the differences between societies. In contemporary as well as in historical societies, more than a quarter of ever-married women at the end of the reproductive span have had fewer than three or more than nine live births. Fig. 2.2 gives examples of the distributions of the number of children ever born in Bangladesh and Mexico.

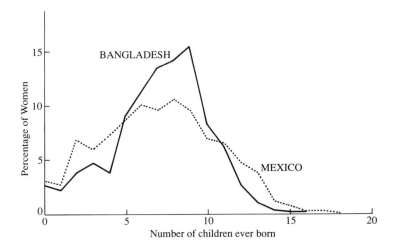

Source: Hodgson and Gibbs, 1980.
Fig. 2.2   Distribution of children ever born among ever-married women aged 45–9 in Bangladesh and Mexico

The causes of this heterogeneity in individual fertility have not received much attention in the literature on natural fertility. Some insight can be gained by examining the timing of key events in the reproductive histories of women with different completed family sizes. Fig. 2.3 illustrates a typical result from such an exercise. Not surprisingly, women with few children tend to marry late, terminate childbearing early (presumably due to an early onset of sterility), and have birth intervals that are longer than average. An examination of the birth-interval components would show that long post-partum infecundability intervals, long waiting times to conception, and intra-uterine mortality are more common among women with small family sizes. Variation in fertility is therefore in part attributable to variation in behavioural variables (e.g. age at marriage, frequency of intercourse, pattern and duration of breastfeeding) and biological determinants (risk of intra-uterine mortality, risk of conception failure, and onset of sterility). However, these factors do not provide a complete explanation because random variation and chance also play a crucial role. For example, in a group of couples who all have the same frequency of intercourse and the same biological endowment, some would conceive in the first month after return of fecundability while others would have conception delays of a year or more. Random variation is important in determining the timing of all events in the reproductive histories of individual women. Unfortunately, since the necessary measurements are lacking, it is not possible to partition the individual variation in natural fertility into the three classes of determinants: behaviour, biology, and chance.

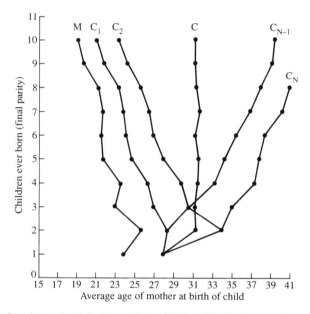

Average age of mother at the birth of her children [C(1) to C(N)] and at marriage (M), by number of children ever born (N); C̄ is the average for all women.

Source: Edlefsen, 1981.

Fig. 2.3 The timing of key events in the reproductive histories of rural Philippines women

Conclusion

The preceding analysis has demonstrated the significance of behaviour as a determinant of natural fertility. In fact, the behavioural factors (age at marriage, breastfeeding and post-partum abstinence, and frequency of intercourse) were demonstrated to be more important determinants of levels and differentials of natural fertility than the biological factors (onset of sterility, intra-uterine mortality, and the risk of conception failure). The crucial role of behaviour should not be interpreted as indicating the presence of deliberate individual decision-making regarding family size. By definition, natural fertility implies the absence of such deliberate control of fertility. Instead, variation between societies in these behaviours is largely caused by differences in social, economic, and environmental factors which, in turn, determine the social norms and customs that regulate reproductive behaviours. In natural fertility societies reproductive behaviour is largely under normative control, leaving little room for individual decision-making.

References

Bongaarts, J., and Menken, J. (1983), 'The Supply of Children: A Critical Essay', in R. Lee *et al.* (eds.), *Determinants of Fertility in Developing Countries*, Academic Press, New York.

—— and Potter, R. (1983), *Fertility, Biology and Behavior*, Academic Press, New York.

Cleland, J., and Hobcraft, J. (1984), *Reproductive Change in Developing Countries*, Oxford University Press, Oxford.

Edlefsen, L. (1981), 'The Timing Pattern of Childbearing', *Population Studies* 35(3): 375–86.

Henry, L. (1972), 'On the Measurement of Human Fertility', M. Sheps and E. Lapierre-Adamcyk (eds.), *Selected Writings of Louis Henry*, Elsevier, New York.

Hodgson, M., and Gibbs, J. (1980), *Children Ever Born*, WFS Comparative Studies, no. 12, International Statistical Institute, Voorburg, the Netherlands.

Leridon, H. (1977), *Human Fertility: The Basic Components*, University of Chicago Press, Chicago.

MacDonald, P. (1984), 'Nuptiality and Completed Fertility: A Study of Starting, Stopping and Spacing Behavior', *Comparative Studies* 35, International Statistical Institute, Voorburg, the Netherlands.

Part II

Demographic and Behavioural Determinants of Reproduction

3 The Determinants of Adolescent Fertility with Special Reference to Biological Variables

STAN BECKER

Introduction

The initiation of reproductive capacity in humans typically occurs in the second decade of life. Because menarche is a clearly defined event and pregnancy occurs to women, while the onset of male reproductive capacity is less clear and paternity is sometimes unknown, the human female is usually the focus of study for both the timing of entry into reproductivity and for adolescent fertility. Adolescence is usually defined as covering the period from puberty to age 20. The age of puberty itself will be considered in this paper, but for fertility statistics, the 15–19 year age-group is used. Thus, the term adolescence is used in a general sense.

There is variation in the age at menarche around the globe. After menarche, there is also wide variation among societies in the intermediate fertility variables (Davis and Blake, 1956), particularly in the age at entry into sexual union and the use of contraception and abortion. Observed fertility levels of adolescents reflect combinations of values of all the intermediate variables. After a brief overview of levels and trends of adolescent fertility, this paper examines the evidence on the age of menarche and its secular trend, fecundability after menarche, as well as observed spontaneous loss rates in the early reproductive years. Age at entry into sexual union and use of contraception and abortion within sexual unions are also considered, but in a perfunctory manner. To structure the discussion on fertility after menarche, the framework of the intermediate fertility variables is utilized.

Overview of Levels and Trends of Adolescent Fertility

Fig. 3.1 shows the levels of fertility of 15–19-year-olds for the most recent year for which data are available since 1977 (United Nations, 1980, 1981, 1982, 1983, 1984, 1985). Rates above 100 per 1000 have been reported for Malawi in Africa, for Bangladesh in Asia, for Honduras and several Caribbean islands in North America, and for Venezuela in South America. At the other extreme, rates below 20 have been reported for most nations of Northern and Western

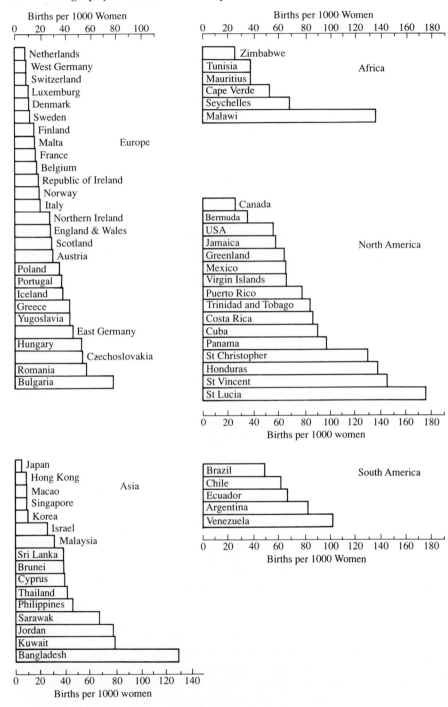

Sources: United Nations, 1980, 1981, 1982, 1983, 1984, 1985.

Fig. 3.1   Levels of adolescent fertility reported in recent years, by continent

Europe, for Japan, Hong Kong, Singapore, Malaysia, and Korea in Asia, but for no nation in North or South America.

Regarding trends in fertility, of the 63 nations reporting at least one rate to the United Nations since 1980 and three or more rates since 1975, 50 nations show declines in adolescent fertility over the period. Of the 13 nations remaining, nine have relatively constant levels. Small increases are found only in Poland, the Cook Islands, Puerto Rico, and Cyprus. Fig. 3.2 presents the results for a selection of the 63 nations.

Westoff *et al.* (1983) have recently analysed trends during the 1970s in teenage fertility in developed nations. They found that it has declined substantially in Western Europe, the USA, Canada, New Zealand, and Australia, but has increased in Eastern and Southern Europe. A study of determinants of teenage fertility in 37 developed nations found, as expected, high correlations between fertility and the intermediate variables, i.e. proportion married among 15–19-year-olds (positive), abortions per woman (positive), and proportion of currently married women using condoms (negative).

Age at Menarche

Menarche is defined as the initiation of uterine bleeding. It is one of several sexual characteristics which develop at about the same time in the human female (Lee, 1980; Hafez, 1978). Studies to determine age at menarche are of two basic types: prospective and cross-sectional. Prospective studies are rare due to their relatively long time-frame and higher cost, but they avoid some of the biases of retrospective studies. In cross-sectional retrospective studies, women of a given age-group are asked whether they have reached menarche or not and, if so, at what age or how long ago. Such data can be used to estimate the mean age at menarche for cohorts of any current age, but recall errors increase as the time since the event increases. Several validation studies—comparing actual ages of menarche with ages reported many years later—have found that the recall errors are fairly random, i.e. there does not appear to be a systematic bias in retrospective reports (Damon *et al.*, 1969; Livson and McNeill, 1962). 'Current status' data, i.e. a woman's current age and whether she has attained menarche or not, have the advantage of not being susceptible to recall bias. The techniques of probit and logit analysis can be used with these data to estimate median and mean ages at menarche, and a non-parametric estimate of the median can be obtained since the proportion of women at a given age that have not reached menarche estimates the survival curve at that age.

Table 3.1, drawn largely from Table 15 of Eveleth and Tanner (1976), gives the median age of menarche for various populations, ranked from the lowest to highest age within regions. Where multiple estimates are available for the same population over time, the latest is given. Fig. 3.3 shows box plots of the median ages for groups by continents. The 25th, 50th, and 75th percentiles are shown

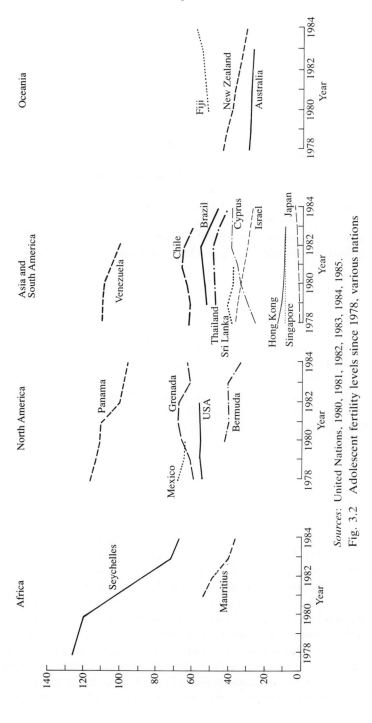

Sources: United Nations, 1980, 1981, 1982, 1983, 1984, 1985.

Fig. 3.2   Adolescent fertility levels since 1978, various nations

TABLE 3.1. *Reports of median (or mean) age at menarche for various populations, by world region*

Median age at menarche (* = mean)	Nation and area or sub-population	Year of study	Source
Europe			
12.3*	Italy, Naples (high economic class)	1969–70	Carfagna, et al., 1972
12.5*	Italy, Naples (middle economic class)	1969–70	Carfagna, et al., 1972
12.6	Italy, Carrara	1968	Eveleth and Tanner, 1976
12.6	Greece, Athens	1979	Dacou-Voutetakis, 1983
12.7*	Italy, Veneto	1975–6	Gallo, 1977
12.7*	Poland, Warsaw	1976	Laska-Mierzejewska, 1982
12.8	Spain, Madrid (high economic class)	1968	Eveleth and Tanner, 1976
12.8	Hungary, Budapest	1959	Eveleth and Tanner, 1976
12.9	United Kingdom, Warwick	1981	Dann and Roberts, 1984
12.9	Italy, Naples (low economic class)	1969–70	Carfagna, et al., 1972
13.0	Denmark, Copenhagen	1982–3	Helm and Helm, 1984
13.0	United Kingdom, London	1966	Eveleth and Tanner, 1976
13.0	Belgium	1965	Eveleth and Tanner, 1976
13.0	USSR, Moscow	1970	Eveleth and Tanner, 1976
13.0	Yugoslavia, Lipik	1972a	Eveleth and Tanner, 1976
13.1	Switzerland, Zurich	—	Eveleth and Tanner, 1976
13.1	Hungary (west)	1965	Eveleth and Tanner, 1976
13.1	Iceland	1970–3	Helm and Helm, 1984
13.2	Norway, Oslo	1970	Eveleth and Tanner, 1976
13.2	France, Paris	1966–8	Eveleth and Tanner, 1976
13.2	Hungary, Szeged	1958–9	Eveleth and Tanner, 1976
13.2	Finland, Helsinki	1965–9	Helm and Helm, 1984
13.3*	United Kingdom	1982	Mascie-Taylor, 1986
13.3	Romania (urban)	1963–6	Eveleth and Tanner, 1976
13.3	Sweden, Stockholm	1980s	WHO, 1986
13.4	Netherlands	1965	Eveleth and Tanner, 1976
13.4*	Poland (rural)	1976–8	Laska-Mierzejewska, 1982

TABLE 3.1. (*cont.*)

Median age at menarche (* = mean)	Nation and area or sub-population	Year of study	Source
13.4	United Kingdom, north-east England	1967	Eveleth and Tanner, 1976
13.4	Czechoslovakia, Bratislava	1960–2	Eveleth and Tanner, 1976
13.6	Yugoslavia (Gypsies)	1961–6	Eveleth and Tanner, 1976
14.2	Romania (rural)	1963–6	Eveleth and Tanner, 1976
14.4	USSR, Kirghiz (700 maltitude)	1968	Eveleth and Tanner, 1976
15.2	USSR, Kirghiz (2500 maltitude)	1968	Eveleth and Tanner, 1976
North America			
12.4*	USA	1980	Wyshak, 1983
12.5	USA (blacks)	1960–70	Eveleth and Tanner, 1976
12.5	Mexico, Yucutan	—	Eveleth and Tanner, 1976
12.8	Mexico, Xochimilco	1966	Eveleth and Tanner, 1976
12.8*	USA, Massachusetts	1965+	Zacharias and Wurtman, 1969
12.8	USA (whites)	1960–70	Eveleth and Tanner, 1976
12.8	USA, California	1950s	Zacharias and Wurtman, 1969
12.9	Cuba (whites)	1973	Eveleth and Tanner, 1976
13.0	Cuba (mixed race)	1973	Eveleth and Tanner, 1976
13.1	Canada, Montreal	1969–70	Eveleth and Tanner, 1976
13.2	USA, California (Japanese)	1971	Eveleth and Tanner, 1976
13.3	Guatemala, Guatemala City	1965	Eveleth and Tanner, 1976
13.8	USA, Alaska (Eskimos)	1968	Eveleth and Tanner, 1976
14.1	Martinique (African descendants)	—	Eveleth and Tanner, 1976
14.5*	Mexico (Zapotec-speaking in Oaxaca)	1978	Mascie-Taylor, 1986
15.1	Guatemala (Maya)	—	Eveleth and Tanner, 1976
South America			
12.3	Chile, Santiago (middle economic class)	1971	Eveleth and Tanner, 1976
12.6	Brazil, Recife	—	Linhares, *et al.*, 1986

12.7	Argentina, La Plata	1978	Lejarraga, 1980
12.7	Venezuela, Carabobo	1978	Farid-Coupal et al., 1981
12.9	Brazil (Japanese)	1965	Eveleth and Tanner, 1976
13.0	Chile, Santiago (high economic class)	1971	Eveleth and Tanner, 1976
Oceania			
13.0	New Zealand (Maori)	1970	Gray, 1977
13.0	Australia, Sydney	1970	Eveleth and Tanner, 1976
13.0	New Zealand of European descent	1970	Eveleth and Tanner, 1976
13.2	Australia (rural)	1970	Eveleth and Tanner, 1976
15.5	New Guinea, Megiar	1967	Eveleth and Tanner, 1976
15.6	New Guinea, Kaiapit	1967	Eveleth and Tanner, 1976
15.6	New Guinea, Karkar Island	1971	Eveleth and Tanner, 1976
16.5	New Guinea, Lufa	1971	Eveleth and Tanner, 1976
17.5	New Guinea, Chimbu	1965	Eveleth and Tanner, 1976
18.0	New Guinea, Bundi	1967	Eveleth and Tanner, 1976
18.4	New Guinea, Lumi	1967	Eveleth and Tanner, 1976
Africa			
12.6	Egypt, Cairo (high economic class)	—	Attallah, 1978
13.1*	S. Africa, Johannesburg (whites)	1976–7	Chaning-Pearce, 1987
13.2	Seychelles, Mahe	1978	Grainger, 1980
13.2*	Sudan (north)	1979	WFS
13.4*	Egypt	1980	WFS
13.4	Uganda, Baganda (high economic class)	1959–62	Eveleth and Tanner, 1976
13.4	Nigeria (high economic class)	—	Gray, 1977
13.4*	Sudan, Khartoum (high economic class)	1980	Attallah, et al., 1982
13.5*	Nigeria, Enugu (urban)	1978	Uche and Okorafar, 1970
13.6*	Nigeria, Ilorin	1983	Fakeye, 1985
13.8	Nigeria, Ife-Ife	1980s	WHO, 1986
13.9*	Sudan, Khartoum (middle economic class)	1980	Attallah, et al., 1982
13.9	Egypt (rural)	—	Attallah, 1978
13.9*	S. Africa, Johannesburg (blacks)	1976–7	Chaning-Pearce, 1987

TABLE 3.1. (*cont.*)

Median age at menarche (* = mean)	Nation and area or sub-population	Year of study	Source
14.0*	Tunisia	1978	WFS
14.0*	Nigeria	1981–2	WFS
14.1*	Sudan, Khartoum (low economic class)	1980	Attallah, et al., 1982
14.1	Nigeria, Ibo (high economic class)	—	Gray, 1977
14.4*	Yemen	1979	WFS
14.4*	Kenya	1977–8	WFS
14.6*	Lesotho	1977	WFS
14.6	Senegal, Dakar	1970	Eveleth and Tanner, 1976
14.8	S. Africa (Bantu, low economic class)	—	Eveleth and Tanner, 1976
14.8*	Cameroon	1978	WFS
14.9	Ghana	1979	WFS
14.9	S. Africa (Bantu, urban, low economic class)	—	Eveleth and Tanner, 1976
14.9	Tanzania, Nyakyusa	1969	Eveleth and Tanner, 1976
15.0	S. Africa (Bantu, middle economic class)	—	Eveleth and Tanner, 1976
15.2	Egypt (Nubians)	1966	Eveleth and Tanner, 1976
15.4	S. Africa, Transkei (Bantu, low economic class)	—	Eveleth and Tanner, 1976
16.5	Rwanda (Tutsi)	1957–8	Eveleth and Tanner, 1976
16.6	S. Africa (Dobe Kung)	1963–9	Howell, 1979
17.0	Rwanda (Hutu)	1957–8	Eveleth and Tanner, 1976
Near East and Asia			
12.4*	Japan	1979–80	Hoshi and Kouchi, 1981
12.4*	Hong Kong (high economic class)	1977–9	Leridon, 1977
12.4*	Turkey, Istanbul (high economic class)	1965	Neyzi, et al., 1975
12.7*	Hong Kong (low economic class)	1977–9	Low, et al., 1982
12.7	Singapore (middle economic class)	1968	Eveleth and Tanner, 1976
12.8	Hong Kong	1980s	WHO, 1986
12.9	India, Madras (urban)	1974–5	Dryfoos, et al., 1981

13.0	Singapore (low economic class)	1968	Eveleth and Tanner, 1976
13.2	India, Assam (urban)	1957	Eveleth and Tanner, 1976
13.2	India, Kerala (urban)	—	Eveleth and Tanner, 1976
13.2	Burma (urban)	1957	Eveleth and Tanner, 1976
13.2*	Turkey, Istanbul (low economic class)	1965	Eveleth and Tanner, 1976
13.2	Israel, Tel Aviv	1959–60	Eveleth and Tanner, 1976
13.3	Iran (urban)	1963	Eveleth and Tanner, 1976
13.4	Tunisia, Tunis (high economic class)	1970	Eveleth and Tanner, 1976
13.4	India, Andra Pradesh (low economic class)	1971–2	Gray, 1977
13.5	Sri Lanka, Colombo	1980s	WHO, 1986
13.6	Iran, Baghdad (high economic class)	1969	Eveleth and Tanner, 1976
13.7	Malaysia	1976–7	Ann, et al., 1983
13.7	India (urban)	1956–65	Eveleth and Tanner, 1976
13.8	Sri Lanka, Jaffna	1981	Prakash, et al., 1984
13.8*	Sri Lanka, Kandy	1971	Balasuriya, et al., 1983
14.0	Iraq, Baghdad (low economic class)	1969	Eveleth and Tanner, 1976
14.0	Tunisia, Tunis (low economic class)	1970	Eveleth and Tanner, 1976
14.2	India, Madras (rural)	1960	Eveleth and Tanner, 1976
14.4	Sri Lanka, Peradeniya	1980s	WHO, 1986
14.4	India, Kerala (rural)	—	Eveleth and Tanner, 1976
14.4	India (rural)	1956–65	Eveleth and Tanner, 1976
14.4*	Sri Lanka, Nuwara Eliya (low economic class)	1971	Balasuriya, 1983
15.0	USSR (rural Buriats)	—	Gray, 1977
15.4*	Nepal, Kagate	1978	Bangham and Sacherer, 1980
15.8	Bangladesh, Matlab (Muslims)	1976	Chowdhury, et al., 1977
15.9*	Nepal (Sherpas)	1978	Bangham and Sacherer, 1980
16.0	Bangladesh, Matlab (Hindus)	1976	Chowdhury, et al., 1977
16.2	Nepal (rural)	1981	Beal, 1983
17.0*	Nepal, Helambu	1978	Bangham and Sacherer, 1980
17.1	Philippines (Agta foragers)	1980–82	Goodman, et al., 1983

Note: Some of the studies are undated.

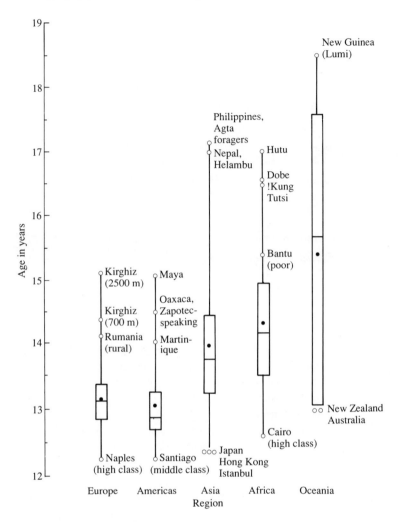

Source: Based on data presented in Table 2.1

Fig. 3.3   Median age at menarche, by region

by the box, with some outliers designated and the arithmetic mean given by a dot. There is considerable variation both within and between continents. Differences between developed, nutritionally well-off populations and less developed populations are apparent. For example, the highest ages are found among the New Guinea tribes, rural Bangladeshis and Nepalis, rural Rwandans, and the nomadic Dobe !Kung. The lowest ages are typically found among well-off urban populations. In Europe the lowest values are generally from the south, and all of the values above 13.5 are in the east. The ranges are largest in Oceania, Africa, and Asia. Numerous investigations have found a secular decline in the mean or median age at menarche. Tanner (1973) and Wyshak and Frisch (1982) used both historical data and more recent studies from Europe and the USA to document the decline in those regions. Helm and Helm (1984) review the declines in Scandinavia, and Prado (1984) documents the decline in Spain. The average decrease has been about two months per decade.

It has also been observed that the decline is slackening or coming to a halt, at least in England (Roberts and Dann, 1975; Dann and Roberts, 1984), Norway (Helm and Helm, 1984; Brundtland *et al.*, 1980), the USA (Zacharias *et al.*, 1976), and Japan (Hoshi and Kouchi, 1981). These are all nations with quite a low median age: England, 12.9; Norway, 13.2; USA, 12.8; Japan, 12.4. It seems clear that a biological minimum age at menarche exists and the distributions of age at menarche in some developed nations are pushing up against this limit.

In the case of secular change outside Europe, North America, and Japan the results are mixed. In South Africa a decline was found for black girls from 14.8 in the 1960s to 13.9 in the late 1970s (Chaning-Pearce and Solomon, 1987). In Hong Kong, Low *et al.* (1982) found a significant decline in the mean age of menarche from 13.3 in 1961 to 12.7 in 1977–9 for women at lower socio-economic levels but a non-significant change for women at higher socio-economic levels. In Venezuela, using data from all available studies, a downward trend is seen, but, if one discards early studies which used the recall method, not much change is seen from 1957 to 1978 (Farid-Coupal *et al.*, 1981). The same lack of trend has been documented for the Zapotec-speaking communities in Oaxaca, Mexico (Malina *et al.*, 1983). In Matlab, Bangladesh, the age at menarche actually increased from 12.9 in 1961 to 17.4 (for Muslims) in 1977 (Chowdhury *et al.*, 1977). This increase was ascribed to worsening nutritional conditions because of the war in 1971 and famine in 1974.

Therefore, to predict changes in the age at menarche, it is important to know both its current level and changes in variables which are known to be related to it, specifically socio-economic status and nutrition. A review of the various determinants of age at menarche is beyond the scope of this paper; suffice it to note that using individual data, none of the measures (genetic or environmental) alone or together have very high explanatory power (Johnston, 1974).

Intermediate Fertility Variables

Taking the age at menarche as given, a model of the reproductive process provides a framework for discussion of the intermediate fertility variables. For this purpose the model presented originally by James (1979) is used. F is used to denote the probability that a recognizable conception occurs during a menstrual cycle; F is also called recognized fecundability.

$$\text{Let } F = p_1 \, p_2 \, p_3 \, p_4 \qquad (1)$$

where p represents the following probabilities

p_1 = Pr(a menstrual cycle is ovulatory)
p_2 = Pr(insemination occurs during the fertile period | ovulation occurs)
p_3 = Pr(insemination leads to fertilization | it occurs during the fertile period)
p_4 = Pr(conception is recognizable | fertilization occurs)

Also, to distinguish pregnancies that result in live births, define:

F' = Pr(a live birth conception occurs during a menstrual cycle). F' is also
called effective fecundability. Thus $F' = p_5 F$ where p_5 = Pr(live
birth | conception is recognized).

To compare estimates of F or F' with observed fertility, the results of Sheps and
Menken (1973) are used. Specifically, under stationary conditions, the monthly
birth-rate is given by:

$$b = p_5 F/[F G + (1 - F)]$$ (2)

where $G = p_5 m + (1 - p_5) w$; m is equal to the mean duration of the non-
susceptible period associated with a live birth; and w is the corresponding mean
associated with a non-live birth. Finally, the yearly birth-rate can be estimated
from b as $b^* 12$. To simplify, one can categorize p_1 and p_4 as basically biological
quantities, while p_2, p_3, and p_5 are subject to human volition: p_2 via the timing
and frequency of sexual intercourse, p_3 via the use of contraception, and p_5 via
the use of induced abortion. p_3 and p_5 also have biological components. This is
a simplification because hormonal contraception (e.g. oral pills) affects p_1 by
suppressing ovulation, the use of the rhythm method of contraception affects
p_2, barrier methods affect p_3, and the IUD affects p_4 through early losses of the
embryo. However, since contraceptive failure is typically measured in terms of
detected pregnancy rates with use, in this simplified model all contraception is
assumed to act through p_3. A separate section is devoted to evidence on each of
the probabilities (p_1, p_2, p_3, p_4, and p_5) for adolescents.

Probability of Ovulation (p_1)

The direct determination of ovulation involves invasive techniques. However,
ovulation can be inferred from a sustained rise in serum levels of pregnanediol,
which is reflected in increased excretion of pregnanediol in the urine. In earlier
studies ovulation was inferred from the mid-cycle rise in basal body temperature
(BBT) and a normal time (12–13 days) from then to the next menstrual cycle. It
can be deduced that ovulation is infrequent if cycle lengths are very variable,
though regular cycles do not necessarily imply that ovulation is occurring, i.e.
regular cycle lengths are a necessary but not a sufficient condition for ovulation.

In an early study of a group of German women with the BBT method, Doring
(1969) estimated the proportion of anovular cycles to be 60 per cent for girls
12–14 years of age, 43 per cent for girls aged 15–17, and 27 per cent for women
aged 18–20, and 13 per cent for women aged 21–5, with a further decline to 5
per cent for women 26–30 years of age. In addition, a high proportion of cycles

among teenage women had a short luteal phase which will not support pregnancy. Doring estimated the proportion of such cycles to be .39 for women 15–19 years of age. With a prospective design and using the pregnanediol assays, Brown *et al.* (1978) found that the interval from menarche to ovulation was very variable among 38 Australian girls. In this context a woman's gynaecological or menarcheal age is often used; it is defined as the time since menarche.

Metcalf and Mackenzie (1980) also measured pregnanediol levels in urine samples from 254 women in New Zealand over a three month interval. From these data, estimates of percentages of ovulatory cycles by age-group were 68 ± 14 for women aged 15–19, 62 ± 9 for women aged 20–4, and 88 ± 8 for women aged 25–9. These percentages agree closely with those of Doring. In a subsequent study of 622 women, Metcalf (1983) found 48 per cent of cycles ovulatory in women aged 10–14, 65 per cent for women aged 15–19, 72 per cent for women aged 20–24, and 98 per cent for women 30–39 years of age (standard errors not available).

Talbert *et al.* (1985) conducted a similar study in a sample of 100 girls from the southern part of the United States. A comparison of these results with those from the New Zealand study is shown in Fig. 3.4. In summary, the percentage of ovulatory cycles is low right after menarche and increases slowly to reach a maximum in the mid- to late-twenties. For women 15–19 years of age, only 60–70 per cent of cycles are ovulatory. However, all these results are from developed nations; it is unclear to what extent this pattern holds for developing nations. There is evidence of a greater variability in cycle length among women of all reproductive ages in Bangladesh than among women in developed nations (Menken, 1975); this could indicate lower proportions of ovulatory cycles or possibly higher rates of unrecognized foetal losses.

Probability of Coitus in the Fertile Period (p_2)

The second factor affecting fertility is the probability of coitus during the fertile period. In most societies coitus is still quite rare outside marital unions; therefore, age at entry into such unions is an important factor in the determination of adolescent fertility. Table 3.2 shows the percentage of married women in the 15–19 year age-group in 25 countries at two points in time: a year in the 1970s and a year in the 1980s. The percentage declined in all the nations except the Philippines, and many of the declines were of substantial magnitude. In Europe 9 of the 15 nations had reductions of more than 50 per cent. In Asia the reductions were less great. The direct relation between proportion married and fertility among adolescents is illustrated with data from the World Fertility Survey (Fig. 3.5). The correlation between the two variables in these data is .84. Thus the declining proportion of adolescents who are married is an important factor in explaining the declines in adolescent fertility.

In some societies however, coitus outside marriage is quite common among

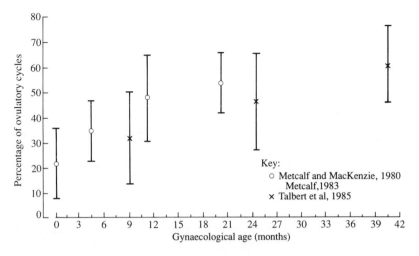

Sources: Metcalf and Mackenzie, 1980; Metcalf, 1983; Talbert *et al.*, 1985.

Fig. 3.4   Percentage of ovulatory cycles by gynaecological age in two studies

teenagers. Indeed, with low marriage rates for adolescents in the United States, for example, the evidence of pre-marital intercourse is clear: non-marital births outnumber marital births for women under 19 years of age (NCHS, 1987). A recent study documented the levels of sexual intercourse among teenagers in Sweden, the USA, the UK, France, the Netherlands, and Canada (Jones *et al.*, 1986). By 18 years of age, the percentages of women who had ever had intercourse were estimated as 79, 58, 55, 49, 48, and 30 in the respective nations. Comparison with the data from Table 3.2 clearly indicates that most of these sexual encounters occur outside marriage. Recent fertility surveys in Latin America have also included a module on sexual intercourse (Morris, 1987). The percentage of 15–19-year-olds reporting pre-marital coitus ranged from 12 per cent in Guatemala City to 55 per cent in Jamaica. Thus, there is significant pre-marital exposure to coitus during the fertile period in some nations.

Age at first coitus and age at marriage have been found to depend on the age of menarche in many societies. In particular, menarche must precede marriage and/or coitus in most societies. In addition, among post-menarcheal women at a given age, the risks of coitus and marriage are greater for women with earlier menarche. An early documentation of this relationship was from the US National Fertility Survey of 1965 (Ryder and Westoff, 1971). Udry and Cliquet (1982) have shown these relationships for samples from Belgium, Pakistan, and Malaysia in addition to the USA. Zabin *et al.* (1986) have documented the same pattern of earlier coitus for those with earlier menarche among a group of inner city adolescents in the USA, and they speculate about the inter-action of the biological and normative determinants of coital behaviour according to age.

TABLE 3.2. *Percentage of females 15–19 years of age who are married
at two points in time, various nations*

Region and nation	Year 1	Percent Married (p1)	Year 2	Percent Married (p2)	Percent change 100*(p2 − p1)/p1
Europe					
Austria	1972	7.4	1980	4.5	−39
Denmark	1972	3.2	1982	0.9	−72
Finland	1972	4.8	1981	2.0	−58
France	1972	4.7	1980	4.6	−1
East Germany	1972	6.5	1980	4.9	−25
West Germany	1972	8.0	1981	3.1	−61
Hungary	1972	12.4	1981	4.3	−65
Iceland	1974	3.8	1980	1.9	−50
Italy	1972	11.7	1980	1.9	−84
Netherlands	1972	5.3	1982	2.2	−58
Norway	1972	5.5	1981	2.1	−62
Poland	1972	4.6	1980	4.5	−2
Sweden	1972	1.6	1981	0.7	−56
England and Wales	1972	8.7	1981	4.5	−48
Scotland	1972	8.4	1981	5.0	−40
Oceania					
New Zealand	1976	10.4	1981	6.6	−37
North America					
Canada	1972	11.0	1980	4.4	−60
Greenland	1974	1.5	1982	0.3	−80
USA	1972	9.2	1982	8.0	−13
Asia					
Hong Kong	1976	3.9	1981	3.4	−13
Israel	1972	8.7	1980	7.5	−9
Japan	1975	1.4	1980	1.0	−29
South Korea	1975	2.6	1980	1.8	−31
Philippines	1975	12.4	1980	14.3	+15
Turkey	1975	21.9	1980	21.7	−1

Source: United Nations, 1982, Table 24, pp. 623–33.

Within marriage, coital frequency by duration of marriage has also been studied. In the USA, Kinsey *et al.* (1953) found a median weekly frequency of 2.8 for married women 16–20 years of age and 2.5 for women aged 21–5. Table 3.3 summarizes data on the frequency of sexual intercourse from more recent studies in several nations. The frequencies for 15–19-year-olds are clearly higher than those for women 20–4 years of age in all the populations studied except El Salvador. Within marriage, the probability of coitus during the fertile period is thus at its highest for adolescents.

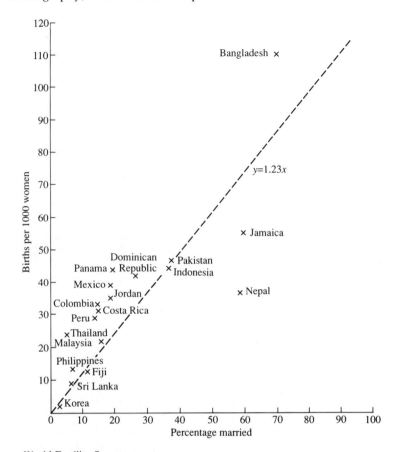

Source: World Fertility Survey reports.

Fig. 3.5   Adolescent fertility and percentage of women 15–19 years old who are married

The possibility that a biological variable (hormone levels) affects the probability of coitus after menarche had been explored by Udry *et al.* (1986), using blood samples and questionnaires on sexual behaviour and motivation from 78 post-menarcheal girls. While they found a positive association between sexual motivation and androgen levels, no association was found with coitus. However, the proportion with sexual experience was low (two had intercourse in a one-month period), and there was an association between testosterone levels and masturbation.

Probability of Fertilization given Coitus in the Fertile Period (p_3)

In modern societies this probability is largely determined by the level and effectiveness of contraceptive use. The World Fertility Survey has documented the proportion of married teenagers using contraception in over 40 countries.

TABLE 3.3. *Mean frequency of sexual intercourse in a 4-week period for women aged 15–19 and 20–4.*

| Nation and study site | Year of study | Age-group | | (2)/(3) |
| | | < 20 | 20–4 | |
	(1)	(2)	(3)	(2)/(3)
Colombia	1976	8.48	7.84	1.08
Bangladesh (Matlab)	1978	9.2	6.8	1.35
India (Bombay)	1970–7	10.0	9.6	1.04
Ghana	1979	10.0	9.32	1.07
Philippines	1978	10.72	9.52	1.13
Ivory Coast	1980	11.92	11.32	1.05
USA	1975	12.1	10.0	1.21
Guatemala	1981	12.8	11.2	1.14
El Salvador	1981	15.6	15.6	1.00
Dominican Republic	1981	16.4	13.6	1.21
Honduras	1981	18.0	16.0	1.13

Note: The results from studies reporting figures in a week period have been multiplied by four for comparative purposes.

Sources: Kapoor and Aravindakshan, 1980; Ruzicka and Bhatia, 1982; Pineda *et al.*, 1984; Udry, 1980; Trussel and Westoff, 1980; Cleland and Kabule-Sabiti, 1984.

Use rates range from a low of 1 per cent in Nepal and Pakistan to a high of 45 per cent in Colombia and 62 per cent in Jamaica (Carrasco, 1981). Data for some developed countries are found in Jones *et al.* (1986). They found that contraceptive use was relatively low among both the married and unmarried. For the former, the reason is often desire for pregnancy; for the latter, reasons include lack of knowledge and lack of easy access (Zelnik and Kantner, 1979).

When there is no use of contraception, what is the probability of conception following coitus during the fertile period? It is very difficult to obtain evidence on this probability for women of any age. Data on coitus from women studied by Hertig (1967), combined with data from endometrial biopsies done on the same women near the time of ovulation, yield an estimate of .85 for women who had intercourse within 24 hours of the time of ovulation. Bongaarts and Potter (1983) argue that this is an underestimate because of errors in the timing of ovulation relative to coitus and propose a value of .95. James (1979) hypothesizes that p_3 varies little by age.

Probability a Conception is Recognized given Fertilization Occurs (p_4)

Early foetal loss is also difficult to study. Women recognize that they are pregnant at varying lengths of time after the first missed menses, which is already 2 weeks after conception. In an early study, Hertig (1967), estimated from biopsy results that the probability a conception is recognized is in the order of .5, i.e. half of all fertilized ova abort before the conception is recognized.

Recent advances in assays of human chorionic gonadotrophin (hCG) have allowed less invasive measurement of very early foetal loss. Miller *et al.* (1980), using urine samples every other day for 197 women, estimated the spontaneous abortion rate to be 43 per cent. Edmonds *et al.* (1982) with similar techniques for 82 women, estimated embryonic loss before 12 weeks' gestation at 62 per cent. A study with daily samples found four losses among 17 clinical pregnancies (Wilcox *et al.*, 1985). The wide differences in estimates from these studies are probably due to differences in procedures or to sampling error. Wilcox, using a much better technique (see Chapter 18, below), observed that 22 per cent of embryos aborted between implantation and recognition of pregnancy, and 9 per cent aborted thereafter. Assuming an exponential distribution for the pattern of abortion by gestational age and given these values, an estimate of the proportion of fertilized embryos which abort between fertilization and implantation can be made by extrapolation and thereby an estimate of p_4. The value of p_4 so determined is .39. Whether p_4 varies with age is unknown. However, in the absence of data, one hypothesis is that the pattern by age would be similar to that of later pregnancy loss, which is discussed in the next section.

Probability of Live Birth given that Conception is Recognized (p_5)

This probability is affected by two competing risks: the risk of spontaneous abortion and the risk of induced abortion. Regarding induced abortion, Tietze (1983) compiled the ratio of pregnancies ending in legal abortion to the total of known pregnancies for 13 nations (this data is reproduced in Table 3.4). Eight of the nations have abortion ratios which are twice as high for adolescents as for women 20–4 years of age. With abortions per 100 pregnancies reaching levels above 40 in five of the nations, it is obvious that the probability of induced abortion is substantial in some adolescent populations.

With respect to recognized spontaneous abortion, in a review of the literature Leridon (1977) found six studies which reported a higher rate for women under 20 years compared with those of 20–4 years of age and six studies which found a lower rate for the younger group. However, the grouping of women aged 15–19 may be the problem, since the age distributions of pregnant women below age 20 were probably quite different in the various studies. Thus, a later review concludes 'it is generally agreed that very young women . . . are at increased risk of spontaneous abortion' (Roman and Stevenson, 1983).

Recently several authors have explored the possible relation between menarcheal age and foetal loss rates. Liestol (1980) found that Norwegian women with menarcheal age below 12 had an abortion rate 1.7 times greater than that of women who had menarcheal ages of 14 or later. Three other studies in the United States reported similar patterns: Wyshak (1983*a*) with data for 8853

TABLE 3.4. *Legal abortion ratios by age of women at conception for
13 nations (abortions per 100 known pregnancies)*

Nation	Year	Age-group		Ratio
		< 20	20–4	
	(1)	(2)	(3)	(2)/(3)
Norway	1979	40.3	16.4	2.45
New Zealand	1979	11.7	4.8	2.44
England and Wales	1979	30.0	12.3	2.44
Finland	1978	40.9	17.1	2.39
Scotland	1980	22.7	9.7	2.34
Sweden	1979	47.8	20.6	2.32
Denmark	1979	46.8	20.6	2.27
Canada	1980	32.2	14.2	2.27
USA	1980	40.0	29.9	1.35
Singapore	1979	36.4	28.5	1.28
Hungary	1979	23.4	20.3	1.15
East Germany	1975	18.8	17.5	1.07
Czechoslovakia	1980	14.3	16.6	0.86

Source: Tietze, 1983, Table 6, p. 49.

women; Casagrande *et al.* (1981) with data from Los Angeles County; and
Sandler *et al.* (1984) with data for 2000 college freshmen. However, there has
been one study with a negative finding. Bracken *et al.* (1985), with data from
about 4000 subjects in New Haven, USA found no significant association
between menarcheal age and first miscarriage rate. This literature is reviewed
in more detail in Chapter 4, below.

Discussion

The age when reproduction becomes possible in the human female varies
between populations; the difference between the highest and lowest median
age is about four years. The documented decline in age at menarche in many
populations of the world implies greater reproductive potential for adolescents.
Populations in Africa and Asia, where the median age is relatively high, would
be expected to experience a decline if socio-economic conditions improve. On
the other hand, with deteriorating socio-economic conditions, the opposite can
happen.

An increase in the age at marriage has offset the effect of declining age of
menarche on adolescent fertility, higher proportions of adolescents being
outside marital union today than in previous decades. The trend toward higher
age at marriage appears to be worldwide.

However, in some nations, the level of pre-marital sexual activity is signific-ant. The proportions of adolescents with marital or pre-marital sexual activity combined with the frequency of coitus, the use of contraception (given coitus), and the use of abortion (given conception), act together in producing observed fertility rates. The observed downward trends in adolescent fertility imply that the delayed entry into marital union has probably been the predominant factor influencing recent changes in fertility.

Besides and behind these behavioural variables are the biological variables affecting adolescent fertility among post-menarcheal girls: the probability of non-ovulatory cycles and the probability of foetal loss. These probabilities are higher among adolescents than among women in their twenties. Table 3.5 summarizes the biological and behavioural factors affecting adolescent fertility. As an application of the model, estimates of p_1 to p_5 were made for the USA. Tables 3.6 and 3.7 show the data available, which were chosen to represent the situation in 1976 as closely as possible. The estimation of fertility in this age-group in the USA is conducted as follows:

p_1 = Pr(cycle ovulatory and can support a pregnancy) = .45

For pill users this is estimated from Grady's results as .0099 for married and .0260 for unmarried.

p_2 = Pr(coitus in fertile period)
   Pr(coitus in fertile period $\mid$ x acts of coitus in 4 weeks)
   = 1 − Pr(no act of coitus occurs in fertile period)
   = 1 − $(1 - 2/28)^x$

Substituting for married,

$$p_2\,m = 1 - (1 - 2/28)^{12.1} = .592$$

and for unmarried sexually active,

$$p_2\,u = 1 - (1 - 2/28)^{1.92} = .133$$

p_3 = Pr(fertilization $\mid$ coitus in fertile period)

Since most contraceptive methods affect p_3 but the pill affects p_1, we estimate the product $p_1\,p_3$ for the married and unmarried populations by summing across methods (from data in Table 3.7) as

$p_1,\,m\,p_3,\,m$ = .45[(.065)(.023) + (.047)(.067) + (.081)(.09) + (.306)(.850)]
     + (.0099) [(.493)(.850)] = .1224 + .0041 = .1266
$p_1,\,u\,p_3,\,u$ = .45[(.022)(.036) + (.126)(.084) + (.174)(.133) + (.366)(.850)]
     + (.0260) [(.312)(.850)] = .1555 + .0069 = .1624
p_4 = .61
p_5 = [1 − Pr(spontaneous abortion after recognized pregnancy)] ×
   [1 − Pr(induced abortion)]

TABLE 3.5. *Summary of biological and behavioural determinants of adolescent fertility*

Probability of interest	Biological variables	Behavioural variables
Pr(ovulation)	age of menarche ovulatory function after menarche	entry into marriage proportion of females with pre-marital intercourse frequency of intercourse
Pr(coitus|ovulation)		
Pr(fertilization|coitus)	exact timing of coitus relative to ovulation	contraception
Pr(recognized conception| fertilization)	very early foetal loss	
Pr(live birth|recognized conception)	late spontaneous loss rates	induced abortion

TABLE 3.6. *Available data for application of model of adolescent fertility to USA*

Item	Value	Year	Source
Proportion of cycles ovulatory and able to support a pregnancy	0.45	—	Metcalf and McKenzie, 1980; Doring, 1969
Proportion of adolescents married	0.084	1976	United Nations Demographic Yearbook
Proportion who are unmarried and sexually active	0.37	1978	Dryfoos and Bourque-School, 1981
Mean acts of intercourse per 4 weeks for married	12.1	1975	Trussel and Westoff, 1980
Mean acts of intercourse per 4 weeks for never married	1.92	1976	Zelnik and Kantner, 1977
Length of fertile period (days)	2.0	—	Bongaarts and Potter, 1983
Pr(fertilization|coitus in fertile period)	0.85	—	Hertig, 1967
Proportion of embryos aborting before pregnancy recognized	0.39	1988	Wilcox, 1988; author's calculation
Proportion of spontaneous abortions after recognized pregnancy	0.232	—	Leridon, 1977
Abortion rate for unmarried women	0.346	1976	Tietze, 1979
Abortion rate for married women	0.083	1976	Tietze, 1979
Mean months of pregnancy at loss	3.0	1979	Tietze, 1979; Leridon, 1977
Mean months of post-partum sterility associated with foetal losses	1.0	—	Gray (personal communication)
Mean months of pregnancy for a live birth	9.0	—	
Mean months of post-partum sterility associated with a live birth	2.0	—	Bongaarts and Potter, 1983, formula using mean derived from data in Pratt *et al.* 1984

for married p_5, $m = (1 - .232)(1 - .083) = .704$
for unmarried sexually active p_5, $u = (1 - .232)(1 - .346) = .502$

$F_m = p_2\, p_1,\, m\, p_3,\, m\, p_4 = (.592)(.1266)(.61) = .0457$
$F_u = p_2\, p_1,\, u\, p_3,\, u\, p_4 = (.133)(.1624)(.61) = .0132$
$G_m = (.704)(11) + (.296)(4) = 8.9$

and

$G_u = (.502)(11) + (.498)(4) = 7.5$

and

$b_m = (.704)(.0457)/[(.0457)(8.9) + (1 - .0457)] = .0337$
$b_u = (.502)(.0132)/[(.0132)(7.5) + (1 - .0132)] = .0061$

so, weighting these by the proportions of the teenage population married and unmarried but sexually active, the monthly birth-rate for the total population is

$b = (.084)(.0337) + (.37)(.0061) = .00509$

and the estimated yearly birth-rate would be $12 \times .00509 = .061$
The observed birth-rate in this group is .055

For p_1, since it is unknown to what extent cycles with a short luteal phase are incompatible with pregnancy, all the anovular cycles and half of the short luteal phase cycles reported by Doring (1969) were combined, giving an estimate of p_1 of .45. To estimate p_2, data on numbers of coital acts in a 4-week period were used for the married and unmarried populations. Assuming that acts of coitus are independently distributed and are independent of cycle day, these data can be converted into an estimate of p_2. For p_3, data from the 1976 National Survey of Family Growth (NSFG; Zelnik and Kantner 1979) were used to estimate the proportion of women using contraceptive methods. Contraceptive failure rates in a 12-month period were available for the married and single populations from the 1982 NSFG (Jones and Darroch-Forrest 1989). These were adjusted to monthly rates and the result was divided by the product of the weighted average of p_1, p_2, and p_4 (across age) for the NSFG population to isolate an estimate of p_3 for each method. For those using no contraception, the value of .85 from Hertig (1967) was used for p_3. For p_4 the estimate of .61, derived from

TABLE 3.7. *Contraceptive use and monthly failure rates in the USA*

Method	Use among 15–19 age-group (%)		Monthly pregnancy rate[a] (per 1000)		Estimated value of p_3 (per 1000)	
	married	unmarried	married	unmarried	married	unmarried
Pill	49.3	31.2	2.4	4.8	10[b]	26[b]
IUD	6.5	2.2	5.1	4.6	23	32
Condom	4.7	12.6	12.6	9.5	67	81
Other	8.1	17.4	18.4	18.4	90	117
None	30.6	36.6	43.3[c]	48.2[c]	850[d]	850[d]

[a] Estimated from the 12-month rate X as $1 - (1 - X)^{1/12}$
[b] Since the pill acts on ovulation, these are values of p_1
[c] Not used in the calculations
[d] Taken from Hertig

Sources: Table 3 in NCHS, 1981; Table 10 in NCHS, 1982; Tables 2 and 4 in Grady *et al.*, 1986; Table 12 in Zelnik and Kantner, 1977.

the data of Wilcox (1988), is used. For p_5, the estimate of spontaneous abortion from Leridon (1977) is combined with the estimate of induced abortion from Tietze (1979). Since these estimates are net risks (i.e. estimated in the absence of the other risk), they must be combined by multiplication.

The mean non-susceptible period associated with live births is estimated as nine months for gestation plus two months of post-partum non-susceptibility. For spontaneous and induced abortions, an average of four months for the nonsusceptible period is assumed. With these values, the estimated monthly live birth conception rates for married and unmarried sexually active 15–19-year-olds are .0236 and .0061 respectively. Combining these with the proportions married and unmarried sexually active, and multiplying by 12, the estimated yearly birth rate is 51 per 1000. This estimate is only 4 per cent below the observed fertility rate of 55 per 1000 in 1976. Given the variety of data sources and assumptions underlying the estimation procedures, the closeness of these values is surprising. Either errors in estimation of one parameter are offset by errors in approximation of another parameter, or the values of the parameters are reasonably accurate.

References

Ann, T. B., Othman, R., Butz, W. P., and DaVanzo, J. (1983), 'Age at Menarche in Peninsular Malaysia: Time Trends, Ethnic Differentials and Association with Ages at Marriage and First Birth', *Malaysian Journal of Reproductive Health* 1(2): 91–108.

Attallah, N. L. (1978), 'Age at Menarche of Schoolgirls in Egypt', *Annals of Human Biology* 5(2): 185–9.

—— Matta, W. M., and El-Mankoushi, M. (1982), 'Age at Menarche of Schoolgirls in Khartoum', *Annals of Human Biology* 10(2): 185–8.

Balasuriya, S., and Fernando, M. A. (1983), 'Age at Menarche in Three Districts in Sri Lanka', *Ceylon Medical Journal* 28: 227–31.

Bangham, C. R. M., and Sacherer, J. M. (1980), 'Fertility of Nepalese Sherpas at Moderate Altitudes: Comparison with High-Altitude Data', *Annals of Human Biology* 7(4): 323–30.

Beal, C. M. (1983), 'Ages at Menopause and Menarche in a High-Altitude Himalayan Population', *Annals of Human Biology* 10(4): 365–70.

Bongaarts, J., and Potter, R. G. (1983), *Fertility, Biology and Behaviour*, Academic Press, New York.

Bracken, M. B., Bryce-Buchanan, C., Stilten, R., and Holford, T. (1985), 'Menarcheal Age and Habitual Miscarriage: Evidence for an Association', *Annals of Human Biology* 12(6): 525–31.

Brown, J. B., Harisson, P., and Smith, M. (1978), 'Oestrogen and Pregnanediol Excretion through Childhood, Menarche and First Ovulation', *Journal of Biosocial Science*, supplement 5: 43–62.

Brundtland, G. H., Liestol, K., and Walloe, L. (1980), 'Height, Weight and Menarcheal Age of Oslo Schoolchildren during the Last 60 Years', *Annals of Human Biology* 7(4): 307–22.

Carfagna, M., Figuerelli, E., Matarese, G., and Matarese, S. (1972), 'Menarcheal Age of Schoolgirls in the District of Naples, Italy in 1969–1970', *Human Biology* 44(1): 117–25.

Carrasco, E. (1981), *Contraceptive Practice*, World Fertility Survey Cross National Studies no. 9, International Statistical Institute, London.

Casagrande, J. T., Pike, M. C., and Henderson, B. E. (1981), 'Menarcheal Age and Spontaneous Abortion', letter to the editor, *American Journal of Epidemiology* 115: 481–3.

Chaning-Pearce, S. M., and Solomon, L. (1987), 'Pubertal Development in Black and White Johannesburg Girls', *South African Medical Journal* 71: 22–4.

Chowdhury, A. K. M. A., Huffman, S. L., and Curlin, G. T. (1977), 'Malnutrition, Menarche and Marriage in Rural Bangladesh', *Social Biology* 24: 316–25.

Cleland, J. G., and Kabule-Sabiti, I. (1984), 'Sexual Activity within Marriage: The Analytic Utility of World Fertility Survey Data', WFS Technical Paper no. 2265.

Dacou-Voutetakis, C., Klontza, D., Lagos, P., Tzonou, A., Katsarou, E., Antoniadis, S., Papazisis, G., Papadopoulos, G., and Matsaniotis, N. (1983), 'Age of Pubertal Stages including Menarche in Greek Girls', *Annals of Human Biology* 10(6): 557–63.

Damon, A., Damon, S. T., Reed, R. B., and Valadian, I. (1969), 'Age at Menarche of Mothers and Daughters with a Note on Accuracy of Recall', *Human Biology* 41: 161–75.

Dann, T. C., and Roberts, D. F. (1984), Menarcheal Age in University of Warwick Students, *Journal of Biosocial Science* 16: 511–19.

Davis, K. J., and Blake, J. (1956), 'Social Structure and Fertility: An Analytic Framework', *Economic Development and Cultural Change* 4(4): 211–35.

Doring, G. K. (1969), 'The Incidence of Anovular Cycles in Women', *Journal of Reproductive Fertility*, supplement 6: 77–81.

Dryfoos, J. G., and Bourque-Scholl, N. (1981), *Factbook on Teenage Pregnancy*, Alan Guttmacher Institute, New York.

Edmonds, D. K., Lindsay, K. S., Miller, J. F., Williamson, E., and Wood, P. J. (1982), 'Early Embryonic Mortality in Women', *Fertility and Sterility* 38: 447–53.

Eveleth, P. B., and Tanner, J. M. (1976), *Worldwide Variation in Human Growth*, Cambridge University Press, London.

Fakeye, O. (1985), 'The Interrelationships between Age, Physical Measurements, and Body Composition at Menarche in Schoolgirls at Ilorin, Nigeria', *International Journal of Gynaecological Obstetrics*, 23: 55–8.

Farid-Coupal, N., Contreras, M. L., and Castellano, H. M. (1981), 'The Age at Menarche in Carabobo, Venezuela with a Note on the Secular Trend', *Annals of Human Biology* 8(3): 283–8.

Gallo, P. G. (1977), 'The Age at Menarche in Some Populations of Veneto, North Italy', *Annals of Human Biology* 4(2): 179–81.

Goodman, M., Estioko-Griffin, P. B., and Grove, J. S. (1983), 'Menarche, Pregnancy, Birth Spacing and Menopause among the Agta Women Foragers of Cagayan Province, Luzon, the Phillipines', *Annals of Human Biology* 12(2): 169–77.

Grady, W. R., Hayward, M. D., and Yagi, J. (1986), 'Contraceptive Failure in the United States: Estimates from the 1982 National Survey of Family Growth', *Family Planning Perspectives* 18(5): 200–9.

—— Hirsch, M. B., Keen, N., and Vaughan, B. (1988), 'Contraceptive Failure and

Continuation among Married Women in the United States, 1970–75', *Studies in Family Planning* 14(1): 9–19.

Grainger, C. R. (1980), 'The Age of Menarche in Schoolgirls in Mahe, Seychelles', *Transactions of the Royal Society of Tropical Medicine and Hygiene* 74(1): 123–4.

Gray, R. (1977), 'Biological Factors other than Nutrition and Lactation which may Influence Natural Fertility: A Review', in H. Leridon and J. Menken (eds.) *Natural Fertility Ordina*, Liège, Belgium.

Hafez, E. S. E. (1978), *Human Reproductive Physiology*, Ann Arbor Science, Ann Arbor, Mich.

Helm, P., and Helm, S. (1984), 'Decrease in Menarcheal Age from 1966 to 1983 in Denmark', *Acta Obstetricia et Gynecologica Scandinavica* 63: 633–5.

Hertig, A. T. (1967), 'The Overall Problem in Man', in K. Benirschke (ed.), *Comparative Aspects of Reproductive Failure*, Springer-Verlag, New York.

Hoshi, H., and Kouchi, M. (1981), 'Secular Trend of the Age at Menarche of Japanese Girls with Special Regard to the Secular Acceleration of the Age at Peak Height Velocity', *Human Biology* 53(4): 593–8.

Howell, N. (1979), *Demography of the Dobe !Kung*, Academic Press, London.

Jain, A. K. (1969), 'Fecundability and its Relation to Age in a Sample of Taiwanese Women', *Population Studies* 23(1): 69–85.

James, W. H. (1979), 'The Causes of the Decline in Fecundability with Age', *Social Biology* 26(4): 330–4.

Johnston, F. E. (1974), 'Control of Age at Menarche', *Human Biology* 46(1): 159–71.

Jones, E. F., and Darroch-Forrest, J. (1989), 'Contraceptive Failure in the United States: Revised Estimates from the 1982 NSFG', *Family Planning Perspectives* 21: 103–9.

—— Forrest, J. D., Goldman, N., Henshaw, S. K., Lincoln, R., Rosoff, J., Westoff, C. F., and Wulf, D. (1985), 'Teenage Pregnancy in Developed Countries: Determinants and Policy Implications', *Family Planning Perspectives* 17(2): 53–62.

—— —— —— —— —— —— —— —— (1986), *Teenage Pregnancy in Industrialized Countries*, Yale University Press, New Haven, Conn.

Kapoor, I., and Aravindakshan, S. T. K. (1980), 'Coital Frequency of Urban Couples Attending Family Planning Clinic at Bombay', *Journal of Family Welfare* 26(4): 50–63.

Kinsey, A. C., Pomeroy, W. B., Martin, C. E., and Gebhard, P. H. (1953), *Sexual Behaviour in the Human Female*, Saunders, Philadelphia, Pa.

Laska-Mierzejewska, T., Milicer, H., and Piechaczek, H. (1982), 'Age at Menarche and its Secular Trend in Urban and Rural Girls in Poland', *Annals of Human Biology* 9(3): 227–33.

Lee, P. A. (1980), 'Normal Ages of Pubertal Events among American Males and Females', *Journal of Adolescent Health Care* 1: 26–9.

Lejarraga, H. (1980), 'Age at Menarche in Urban Argentinian Girls', *Annals of Human Biology* 7(6): 579–81.

Leridon, H. (1977), *Human Fertility: The Basic Components*, University of Chicago Press, Chicago.

Liestol, K. (1980), 'Menarcheal Age and Spontaneous Abortion: A Causal Connection?', *American Journal of Epidemiology* 111(6): 753–8.

Linhares, E. D. R., Round, J. J., and Jones, D. A. (1986), 'Growth, Bone Maturation, and Biochemical Changes in Brazilian Children from Two Different Socioeconomic Groups', *American Journal of Clinical Nutrition* 44: 552–8.

Livson, N. and McNeill, D. (1962), 'The Accuracy of Recalled Age at Menarche', *Human Biology* 34: 218–21.

Low, W. D., Kung, L. S., and Leong, J. C. Y. (1982), 'Secular Trend in the Sexual Maturation of Chinese Girls', *Human Biology* 54(3): 539–51.

Malina, R., Selby, H. A., Buschang, P. H., Aronson, W. L., and Wilkinson, R. G. (1983), 'Adult Stature and Age at Menarche in Zapotec-Speaking Communities in the Valley of Oaxaca, Mexico, in a Secular Perspective', *American Journal of Physical Anthropology*, 60: 437–49.

Mascie-Taylor, C. G. N., and Boldsen, J. L. (1986), 'Recalled Age of Menarche in Britain', *Annals of Human Biology* 13(3): 253–7.

Menken, J. (1975), 'Estimating Fecundability', Ph.D. dissertation, Princeton University, Princeton, NJ.

Metcalf, M. G. (1983), 'Incidence of Ovulation from the Menarche to the Menopause: Observations of 622 New Zealand Women', *The New Zealand Medical Journal* 96: 645–48.

—— and Mackenzie, J. A. (1980), 'Incidence of Ovulation in Young Women', *Journal of Biosocial Science* 12: 345–352.

—— Skidmore, D. S., Lowry, G. F., and Mackenzie, J. A. (1983), 'Incidence of Ovulation in the Years after Menarche', *Journal of Endocrinology* 97: 213–19.

Miller, J. F., Williamson, E., Blue, J., Gordon, Y. B., Grudzinskas, J. G., and Sykes, A. (1980), 'Fetal Loss after Implantation: A Prospective Study', *Lancet* 2: 554–6.

Morris, L. (1987), 'Premarital Sexual Experience and Use of Contraception among Young Adults in Latin America', paper presented at American Public Health Association, New Orleans, La.

National Center for Health Statistics (1981), *Contraceptive Utilization, U.S. 1976*, series 23, no. 7, US Government Printing Office, Washington, DC.

—— (1982), *Trends in Contraceptive Practice: U.S. 1965–1976*, series 23, no. 10, US Government Printing Office, Washington, DC.

—— *Vital Statistics of the United States*, ii. *Mortality Part A*, vols. for 1980, 1981, 1982, and 1983, US Government Printing Office, Washington, DC.

—— (1987), *Vital Statistics of the United States—1983*, i. *Natality*, US Government Printing Office, Washington, DC.

Neyzi, O., Alp, H., and Orlon, A. (1975), 'Sexual Maturation in Turkish Girls', *Annals of Human Biology* 2(1): 45–9.

Pineda, M. A., Araya, J. D., Bertrand, J. T., Cuervo, L. I., Espino, E. E., Infante, X., Liriano, R. L., Grijalva, A. R., Bixby, L. R., and Suazo, M. (1984), 'Coital Frequency and the Calculation of Couple-Months-of-Protection in Eight Latin American Countries' (unpublished manuscript).

Prado, C. (1984), 'Secular Change in Menarche in Women in Madrid', *Annals of Human Biology* 11(2): 165–6.

Prakash, S., and Pathmanathan, G. (1984), 'Age at Menarche in Sri Lankan Tamil Girls in Jaffna', *Annals of Human Biology* 11(5): 463–6.

Pratt, W., Mosher, W., Bachrach, C., and Horn, M. (1984), 'Understanding U.S. Fertility: Findings from the National Survey of Family Growth, Cycle III', *Population Bulletin* 39(5): 1–42.

Roberts, D. F., and Dann, T. C. (1975), 'A 12-year Study of Menarcheal Age', *British Journal of Preventive and Social Medicine* 29: 31–9.

Roman, E., and Stevenson, A. C. (1983), 'Spontaneous Abortion', in S. L. Barron and A. M. Thomson (eds.), *Obstetrical Epidemiology*: 63–88, Academic Press, London.

Ruzicka, L. T., and Bhatia, S. (1982), 'Coital Frequency and Sexual Abstinence in Rural Bangladesh', *Journal of Biosocial Science* 14: 397–420.

Ryder, N. B., and Westoff, C. F. (1971), *Reproduction in the United States 1965*, Princeton University Press, Princeton, NJ.

Sandler, D. P., Wilcox, A. J., and Horney, L. F. (1984), 'Age at Menarche and Subsequent Reproductive Events', *American Journal of Epidemiology* 119(5): 765–74.

Sheps, M. C., and Menken, J. (1973), *Mathematical Models of Conception and Birth*, University of Chicago Press, Chicago.

Talbert, L. M., Hammond, M. G., Groff, T., and Udry, R. J. (1985), 'Relationship of Age and Pubertal Development for Ovulation in Adolescent Girls', *Obstetrics and Gynecology* 66(4): 542–4.

Tanner, J. M. (1973), 'Trend towards Earlier Menarche in London, Oslo, Copenhagen, the Netherlands and Hungary', *Nature* 243: 95–6.

Tietze, C. (1979), *Induced Abortion: 1979*, 3rd edn., the Population Council, New York.

—— (1983), *Induced Abortion: A World Review, 1983* 5th edn., the Population Council, New York.

Trussel, J., and Westoff, C. F. (1980), 'Contraceptive Practice and Trends in Coital Frequency', *Family Planning Perspectives* 12(5): 146–249.

Uche, G. O., and Okorafar, A. E. (1970), 'The Age of Menarche in Nigerian Urban School Girls', *Annals of Human Biology* 6(4): 395–8.

Udry, J. R. (1980), 'Changes in the Frequency of Marital Intercourse from Panel Data', *Archives of Sexual Behaviour* 9(4): 319–25.

—— and Cliquet, R. L. (1982), 'A Cross-Cultural Examination of the Relationship between Ages at Menarche, Marriage and First Birth', *Demography* 19(1): 53–63.

—— Talbert, L. M., and Morris, N. M. (1986), 'Biosocial Foundations for Adolescent Female Sexuality', *Demography* 23(2): 217–30.

United Nations, *Demographic Yearbook*, vols. for 1980, 1981, 1982, 1983, 1984, and 1985, United Nations, New York.

Westoff, C. F., Calot, G., and Foster, A. D. (1983), 'Teenage Fertility in Developed Nations 1971–1980', *Family Planning Perspectives* 9(2): 45–9.

Wilcox, A. (1988), 'Endocrine Detection of Conception and Early Fetal Loss', paper presented at a Seminar on Biomedicine and Demographic Determinants of Human Reproduction, Baltimore, Md.

—— Weinberg, C. R., Wehmann, R. E., Armstrong, E. G., Canfield, R. E., and Nisula, B. C. (1985), 'Measuring Early Pregnancy Loss: Laboratory and Field Methods', *Fertility and Sterility* 44(3): 366–73.

World Fertility Survey, First Country Reports for Sudan, Egypt, Tunisia, Nigeria, Yemen, Kenya, Lesotho, Cameroon, and Ghana, International Statistical Institute, London.

World Health Organization (1986), 'World Health Organization Multicenter Study on Menstrual and Ovulatory Patterns in Adolescent Girls, I: A Multicenter Cross-Sectional Study of Menarche', *Journal of Adolescent Health Care* 7: 229–35.

—— (1986), 'World Health Organization Multicenter Study on Menstrual and Ovulatory Patterns in Adolescent Girls, II: Longitudinal Study of Menstrual Patterns in the

Early Postmenarcheal Period, Duration of Bleeding Episodes and Menstrual Cycles', *Journal of Adolescent Health Care* 7: 236–44.

Wyshak, G. (1983*a*), 'Age at Menarche and Unsuccessful Pregnancy Outcome', *Annals of Human Biology* 10(1): 69–73.

—— (1983*b*), 'Secular Changes in Age at Menarche in a Sample of US Women', *Annals of Human Biology* 10(1): 75–7.

—— and Frisch, R. E. (1982), 'Evidence for a Secular Trend in Age of Menarche', *New England Journal of Medicine* 306(17): 1033–5.

Zabin, L. S., Smith, E. S., Hirsch, M. B., and Hardy, J. B. (1986), 'Ages of Physical Maturation and First Intercourse in Black Teenage Males and Females', *Demography* 23(4): 595–605.

Zacharias, L., and Wurtman, R. J. (1969), 'Age at Menarche: Genetic and Environmental Influences', *New England Journal of Medicine*, 280(16): 868–73.

—— Rand, W. M., and Wurtman, R. J. (1976), 'A Prospective Study of Sexual Development and Growth in American Girls: The Statistics of Menarche', *Obstetrical and Gynelogical Survey* 31(4): 325–36.

Zelnik, M. (1979), 'Reasons for Nonuse of Contraception by Sexually Active Women aged 15–19', *Family Planning Perspectives* 11(5): 289–96.

—— and Kantner, J. F. (1977), 'Sexual and Contraceptive Experience of Young Unmarried Women in the United States, 1976 and 1971', *Family Planning Perspectives* 9(2): 55–71.

4 The Relationship of Age at Menarche and Fertility in Undernourished Adolescents

ANN P. RILEY

JULIA L. SAMUELSON

SANDRA L. HUFFMAN

Introduction

The relationship of age at menarche to fertility is important in developing countries, where the average age at menarche is sometimes two or three years later than in developed countries. The average age at menarche is between 12.5 and 13 years in most contemporary US and European populations (Marshall and Tanner, 1986). In addition, marriage occurs soon after menarche in many developing countries, and there is virtually no use of effective contraception between marriage and first birth. Thus, the interval between menarche and first birth may be only a few years or less.

Nutritional status is widely recognized as one of the most important non-genetic determinants of the onset of menstruation. Evidence to support this hypothesis comes from three principal sources:

(1) historical and retrospective studies that suggest a secular decline in age at menarche in industrialized countries (Tanner, 1978; Wyshak and Frisch, 1982; Wyshak, 1983);

(2) socio-economic differentials in age at menarche within countries and ethnic groups; and

(3) inter-country differences among developed and developing countries that coincide with differences in both socio-economic and nutritional status (Eveleth and Tanner, 1976; Marshall and Tanner, 1986; Rana et al., 1986; Nakamura et al., 1986; Chowdhury et al., 1977). A direct relationship between diet and menarche has been observed in the United States (Dreizen et al., 1967) and in India (Bhalla and Shrivatava, 1974).

A number of studies have also found that strenuous exercise is associated with later menarche and attribute this to lower body weight and lower proportion of body fat in athletes (Frisch et al., 1980; Frisch et al., 1981; Malina et al., 1978). However, these studies do not adequately adjust for potential confounding with diet or with physical and psychological stress, which may also affect menarche and amenorrhoea.

Warren (1980) addressed directly the impact of stress compared to controls on delayed menarche in ballet dancers, and to musicians seeking professional careers. Age at menarche and breast development occurred later in the dancers, although pubic hair development was the same in all three groups. Since musicians and dancers had similar ages at menarche, it is suggested that stress does not influence age at menarche. However, decreasing or stopping exercise for at least two months was associated with earlier pubertal progression and onset of menarche, despite no significant changes in weight or body composition during this time period, thus, weight change alone cannot explain the delay.

It is unclear whether high energy expenditure activities, other than those associated with athletics, are also related to menarcheal age. Of particular interest is the daily activity of adolescent females in developing countries, such as carrying wood and water, harvesting, and pounding grain. These activities require considerable energy expenditure and strength, but do not place the same demands on the cardiovascular and muscular skeletal systems as do the athletic activities assessed in these studies.

An important aspect of the nutrition–menarche relationship is whether nutritionally induced changes in age at menarche influence fertility. It has been suggested that improvements in nutrition and adolescent health would decrease age at menarche and lead to younger age at first birth and even higher fertility in developing countries (Van der Spuy and Jacobs, 1983). However, malnutrition does not have an isolated influence on the onset of menstrual cycles. Under-nutrition can also delay and slow the entire adolescent growth spurt and result in smaller adult body size. While the notion that stunting is an adaptive mechanism has been debated, there is no evidence that lower maternal height or weight have any benefit in terms of reproduction. In fact, maternal weight and height are both positively associated with birth-weight (Raman, 1981; Scott *et al.*, 1981) and may be important factors influencing infant mortality.

There are several mechanisms through which the age at menarche could affect fertility, including the length of the reproductive period (primarily through its influence on age at marriage and first birth), adolescent subfecundity, and foetal wastage. Menarche may also be a marker of reproductive fitness and some anthropological works suggest that women with early menarche have shorter birth intervals and greater lifetime fertility (Borgerhoff-Mulder, 1989). However, these findings are based on a small, select sample and all data on menarche and births are based on recalled self reports. An additional consideration is the relationship of age at menarche to adolescent growth and reproductive development in chronically undernourished populations. These issues are of particular concern in populations where the interval between menarche and first birth is short, because pregnancy may occur before the growth spurt is complete. The following discussion will focus on these issues and is primarily limited to the more recent literature. Extensive reviews of the nutritional determinants of age at menarche are presented elsewhere (see Marshall and Tanner, 1986; Eveleth and Tanner, 1976; Frisch, 1985; Ellison, 1981). Becker describes worldwide patterns in age at menarche and adolescent fertility and discusses a structural framework to explain their variability in Chapter 3, above.

Length of the Reproductive Period

A direct link between earlier menarche and increased fertility assumes that marriage is so closely tied to menarche that a decrease in the age at menarche would invoke a similar decline in age of exposure to unprotected intercourse that is independent of age at menarche. Since the risk of pregnancy begins with marriage, rather than menarche, the effect of declining age at menarche on fertility is likely to be small (Gray, 1983; Bongaarts, 1980).

In some traditional societies, however, menarche is an important marker of maturity and readiness for marriage. Women may even marry before menarche in some cases, although cohabitation might not occur until after menses has begun. Age at marriage in Bangladesh, for example, is closely tied to age at menarche for both Hindu and Muslim women (Chowdhury *et al.*, 1977). The Gainj population of Highland New Guinea has an average interval between menarche and marriage of about one year that is fairly constant across age at menarche. However, couples do not cohabit during the first year even though some sexual activity takes place (Wood *et al.*, 1985).

Even in populations with long intervals between menarche and marriage, an association between age at menarche and age at marriage has been observed (Udry and Cliquet, 1982; Sandler *et al.*, 1984). Udry and Cliquet (1982) studied the relationship between age at menarche and age at marriage in several diverse countries and ethnic groups. The populations examined varied widely in ages at menarche and marriage, as well as in the interval between the two events. These findings show a strong correlation between age at menarche and age at marriage, even when the interval between them is large. A similar relationship between menarche and first birth was also observed. Biological differences between early and late maturers, and social interpretations of readiness for reproduction are cited as possible mechanisms for the observed trends. In a prospective study of US women, Sandler *et al.* (1984) also found a positive relationship between age at menarche and ages at marriage and first conception. However, this research does not address the issue of how changes in menarcheal age affect age at marriage within any given level, and similar correlations could be maintained between the two events even if the interval between them were to be lengthened.

Adolescent Subfecundity

The effects of malnutrition and delayed menarche on adolescent subfecundity are not well understood. Although a number of researchers have examined this issue, methodological problems and conflicting results leave many unanswered questions. In a longitudinal study of over 200 healthy 7–17-year-old school girls in Helsinki, Apter and Vihko (1983) and Vihko and Apter (1984) found that early menarche is followed by a rapid onset of ovulatory cycles compared to later maturing girls. Subjects were examined at three 1.5-year intervals, followed by one 5-year interval. Attrition rates were high, with 50 per cent (118) of the original sample remaining at the third examination and only 25 per cent (50) by the final stage of data collection. Blood specimens were drawn twice per cycle: once at 6–9 days and once at 17–30 days since last menstruation. These investigators found that early menarche is characterized by a faster growth spurt (Vihko and Apter, 1984) and a shorter period between menarche and the onset of ovulatory cycles (Apter and Vihko, 1983) compared to girls with later ages at menarche. The latter conclusion may be biased by the use of infrequent sample collection and counting forward from the first day of the menstrual cycle to collect samples. Menstrual cycles shortly following menarche are longer than cycles of women who are more mature (Treloar *et al.*, 1967). Whether these are differences in cycle length by menarcheal age is unknown. However, since the follicular phase is more variable than the luteal phase, attempting to measure ovulation with 6–9-day and 17–30-day samples is likely to miss ovulatory cycles when the length of the follicular phase is extended.

Using urinary assays, Borsos *et al.* (1986) found that ovarian function immediately following menarche (within 100 days) is unpredictable. However, they do not conclude that menarche is always followed by a period of infertility. While anovulatory and aluteal cycles are more frequent shortly after the onset of menstruation, ovulatory menstruation can occur at menarche. Unfortunately these investigators did not examine differences associated with age at menarche or nutritional status, so it is unclear what factors underlie the observed variability. Their findings are, however, important as they suggest that the period of adolescent subfecundity is highly variable and may not occur in all women.

Wood *et al.* (1985) report that adolescent sterility is the dominant factor responsible for an interval of at least three years between marriage and conception in the Gainj population of New Guinea. However, non-cohabitation during the first year of marriage is an important social factor. A single cross-sectional blood sample was used to estimate average age at menarche (20.9 years). This estimate, however, is likely to be greater than the true mean, because the investigators were actually measuring luteal function and not the presence of menstrual cycles. Further, this method would underestimate the number of women with luteal function, since blood specimens were drawn cross-sectionally with no reference within the menstrual cycle. The authors have since recognized this problem and have reappraised the evidence in a forthcoming paper, where the mean age at menarche is estimated at around 18.6 years (personal communication, James Wood). This figure corresponds with other findings in another nearby highland population, where the mean age at menarche was estimated at 18.8 years (Malcolm, 1970).

Foetal Wastage

Foetal wastage is another mechanism through which age at menarche could affect fertility. The uterus in young women may be structurally or functionally less able to carry a foetus to term than in older women, even though conception may occur. This question has been difficult to study since many spontaneous abortions take place in the first few months of pregnancy and are undetected or unreported. Improved radio-immunoassay techniques, such as those described by Wilcox in Chapter 18 below, will allow for more accurate investigation of this question.

Liestol (1980) studied the relationship between age at menarche and spontaneous abortion retrospectively in a sample of more than 1000 middle-class Norwegian women. The risk of spontaneous abortion was 1.5–2 times greater in women with menarcheal ages of 12 years or less or 14 years or greater compared to women with intermediate ages at menarche. Social factors were examined, but no significant differences were detected. Age at first pregnancy had no statistically significant influence on the risk of spontaneous abortion. Liestol noted that nearly all women who reported spontaneous abortions at five or more months gestation were repeat aborters. These results suggest that an increased risk of spontaneous abortion may explain the lower fertility of earlier maturers.

Casagrande *et al.* (1981) confirm some of these findings in data combined from three case-control studies (n = 706) of breast cancer in Los Angeles County. They observed a similar, but not statistically significant, pattern for first pregnancies. Higher rates of spontaneous abortions were observed in women with menarcheal ages less than 13 years, with consistently decreasing rates as age at menarche increased. Their results, however, failed to replicate the finding that women with late age at menarche also experience higher risks of spontaneous abortion. Further, they found that age at first pregnancy was an important factor, younger age being associated with higher risks.

Wyshak (1983) also reports a higher risk of poor pregnancy outcome in women with both early age (under 12 years) and late age (14 and older) at menarche compared to girls in the intermediate range of 12 to 13 years of age. Pregnancy outcome, in this instance, includes both spontaneous abortion and stillbirths. The sample comprised of about 4000 white, middle-class US women, less than 40 years of age at the time of interview. Although this sample is presumably homogeneous, no social or economic factors were examined. Additionally, no information on previous induced abortions was collected.

Bracken *et al.* (1985) also reported an increased risk of spontaneous abortion for young ages at menarche (especially 11 years and under) and older ages (16 years and over). These results differed somewhat from previous studies, in that the increased risk associated with age at menarche was only present in habitual aborters. In contrast, no relationship was found for women who experienced only one miscarriage. Liestol's (1980) findings were also suggestive of this, at least for late abortions. Further, Bracken *et al.* (1985) found a significant difference in the rate of spontaneous abortion by age at first pregnancy, with younger women experiencing higher risks.

The Menstrual and Reproductive Survey provides a prospective look at reproductive outcomes by age at menarche (Sandler *et al.*, 1984). Although only about 16 per cent of the women in this sample contributed prospective data on age at menarche, 74 per cent of the women reported their age at menarche within ten years of the event, and all reproductive events were observed prospectively. The original sample is biased, however, in terms of social and demographic characteristics, and further selection accumulates as women drop out of the study during the lengthy follow-up period that averages 20 years over all participants.

A non-significant negative relationship between the risk of spontaneous abortion and age at menarche is present when no control is made for age at conception. When age at conception is controlled, women with very early menarche (less than 11 years) have a 1.5 times greater risk of spontaneous abortion over all pregnancies, although no such relationship was observed for first pregnancies. Thus, it appears that the relationship between age at menarche and spontaneous abortion is due to factors other than some underlying risk associated with age at menarche *per se*. These data suggest that the increased risk of spontaneous abortion associated with women with an early age at menarche may be caused by a few women that experience repeat abortions.

Data on foetal wastage in developing countries are rare and generally less complete than those from developed countries. In Bangladesh, poor nutritional status of mothers influences the risk of stillbirths and abortions (Pebley *et al.*, 1985). Pre-pregnancy weight and weight gain during pregnancy were positively associated with higher risks of foetal loss, although no such relationship was observed for maternal height. Unfortunately, data did not permit any adjustment for age at menarche.

Interval from Menarche to First Birth

The timing of the first birth relative to menarche is perhaps the most interesting issue from a demographic perspective. Populations where marriage (and cohabitation) precede menarche are few in number and selective in terms of social and ethnic composition. Therefore, they are unlikely to have any notable demographic impact or to provide biological implications that can be generalized to other populations. On the other hand, societies where marriage follows menarche by a period of less than three years are more common. However, there is little evidence for a period of adolescent subfecundity that extends significantly beyond this period.

Nair (1983) suggests that adolescent subfertility persists in Indian women until the age of 19 or 20 years, but the possibility that menarcheal age is also a determinant of adolescent subfertility is not considered. A mean waiting time to conception of 3.2 years was estimated for women married at the age of 15, compared to a waiting time of 2.7 years in women with regular cycles. Both of these waiting times are high for non-contracepting populations. The comparison population is not described, nor are the criteria for normal cycles defined.

Few prospective studies have addressed the relationship of age at menarche to age at first birth, while adjusting for age at marriage. In the United States, Sandler *et al.* (1984) found no association between the interval from marriage to first birth and age at menarche. In this population, however, average age at menarche is about 13 years while first marriage was usually in the early 20s.

Foster *et al.* (1986) conducted a hazard-model analysis of reproductive outcomes of over 1500 Bangladeshi adolescents aged 10–20 years. In a sub-sample of girls who were married before menarche, the median interval between menarche and conception of a live birth was 1.5 years. The same interval for better nourished women who married in their twenties was 0.75 years.

A second, and possibly more important, finding in the Foster research is that the period of adolescent sterility is significantly shorter in women with late age at menarche compared to earlier maturers, even when age at marriage is controlled. This contrasts with the Apter and Vihko studies based on endocrinological data. Aside from the very different analytical techniques and outcomes studied in these papers, differences in nutritional status between the two populations may partially explain the disagreement in their findings.

Age at Menarche and Adolescent Growth

In developed countries, adolescent pregnancy has been associated with low birth-weight (Stanley and Mauger 1986, Zlatnick and Burmeister 1976, Erkan, Rimer, and Stine 1971), infant mortality (Menken 1980, Naeye 1981) and complications of pregnancy (Duenhoelter, Jiminez and Baumann 1975; Battaglia, Frazier and Hellighers 1963; McAnarney 1981, and Menken 1980). Recent discussions have focused on the impact of biological immaturity of adolescent mothers on birth-outcome in the US. However, social and economic factors appear to explain most of the higher risk of neonatal mortality and pregnancy complications observed in teenage mothers in the United States (Mangold, 1983; Makinson, 1985; Geronimus, 1987).

Two important issues concerning adolescent pregnancy and growth remain unresolved. First, it is unclear whether age at menarche is related to the length or magnitude of post-menarcheal growth in either well- or under-nourished adolescents. Second, early pregnancy may interfere with the completion of growth in some women. In well-nourished populations, menarche occurs after the peak in height velocity in some 99 per cent of girls (Marshall and Tanner,

1986). Tanner (1978) and Zacharias and Rand (1983) report that girls grow an average of 6 cm following menarche, although Roche and Davila (1972) estimate an average increase of nearly 8 cm following the onset of menstrual cycles. Some researchers have found that age at menarche has a negative relationship with the magnitude of post-menarcheal growth in height (Roche and Davila, 1972). However, Tanner (1978) and Marshall and Tanner (1986) assert that post-menarcheal growth is independent of age at menarche. Dreizen *et al.* (1967) found that age at menarche is not an important determinant of post-menarcheal growth, although nutritional status does have a significant influence. The length of the post-menarcheal growth period has been reported to be as short as 1.4 years (Zacharias and Rand, 1983) and as long as 5 years (Roche and Davila, 1972).

Additionally, there is some discussion over the long-term effects of age at menarche on adult height and weight. Marshall and Tanner (1986) assert that there is no difference in stature between early and late maturers, while girls with early menarche tend to be fatter as adults than girls with late menarche. Other research finds that early maturers are both shorter and fatter than later maturing girls, both at menarche and as adults (Garn *et al.*, 1986). The relationship in under-nourished adolescents remains unclear, although Dreizen *et al.* (1967) found that under-nutrition leads to greater and longer growth in stature when age at menarche is held constant.

Kulin *et al.* (1982) studied height, weight, arm circumference, and stages of pubertal development in middle-class urban, and lower-class rural children in Kenya. Rural children have later menarche and are less advanced in their development of secondary sex characteristics. Marked differences in anthropometric indices at the onset of puberty and during the early stages of adolescent development were also reported. These differences, however, do not persist into the advanced stages of puberty. Results from this study suggest that considerable catch-up growth occurs in under-nourished children during adolescence.

A recent analysis of adolescent growth in rural Bangladeshi girls provides additional insights into the relationship between menarche and growth in under-nourished adolescents (Riley *et al.*, 1989; Riley, 1990). Monthly measurements of height and weight were taken over the course of one year on 1069 adolescents aged 10–20 years. Data on time since menarche was collected on 290 girls who were post-menarcheal at the start of the study. Menarche was attained during the follow-up period for 118 girls, and 656 girls were pre-menarcheal throughout the period of observation.

Bangladeshi adolescents are short and light for their age compared to US National Center for Health Statistics standards, and age at menarche is nearly 16 years. Post-menarcheal girls in the sample are taller and heavier than pre-menarcheal girls at every age. For the subsample of girls who reached menarche during the period of observation, there was a non-significant increasing trend in weight with age at menarche. No such pattern was observed for height at menarche (Riley, 1990).

Fig. 4.1 illustrates that the growth spurt in height and weight is spread out in Bangladeshi girls compared to British standards (Tanner *et al.*, 1966). Additionally, the rate of growth is lower throughout the adolescent spurt. The time between the peak in height and weight velocity also appears to be greater in Bangladeshi girls than in British girls. Since the study used a mixed cross-sectional and longitudinal design, no distinct beginning or end point in the spurt in height or weight could be identified; thus, the magnitude of the growth spurt could not be examined.

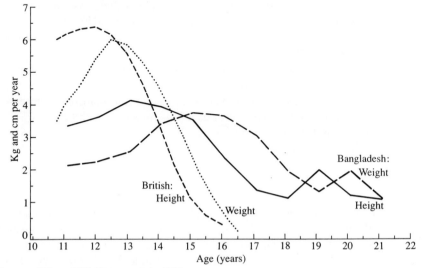

Sources: Riley, 1990; Tanner *et al.*, 1966.

Fig. 4.1   One-year rates of growth in height and weight by age: rural Bangladeshi adolescents compared to British standards

Growth-rates were also compared among pre-menarcheal, post-menarcheal, and transitional girls (Fig. 4.2). Growth-rates in height are higher for pre-menarcheal girls at virtually every age. Transitional girls (those who reached menarche during the follow-up period) have intermediate rates, and post-menarcheal girls have the slowest rates. This suggests that, as in well-nourished populations, menarche occurs after the peak in height velocity has passed. Growth-rates for weight behave somewhat differently since the peak in weight gain occurs later than the peak in height. Transitional girls experience the most rapid rates of growth in weight, followed by pre-menarcheal and post-menarcheal girls.

Multivariate analysis was employed to study differences in growth-rates by chronological age and time since menarche, while controlling for socio-economic factors and seasonal variation in growth. Time since menarche is a more important determinant of post-menarcheal growth in height and weight than is chronological age. However, chronological age does have an independent

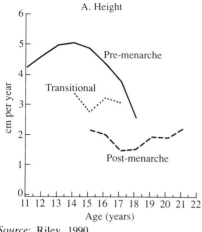

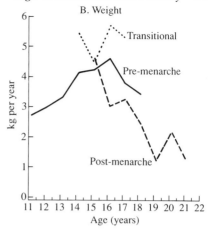

Source: Riley, 1990.

Fig. 4.2　One-year growth-rates in weight and height by age and menarche status in rural Bangladeshi girls

effect, especially for growth in stature. An interaction between age and time since menarche indicates that time since menarche does not have the same implications for biological maturity for girls with early and late age at menarche (Riley *et al.*, 1989).

These findings are important because they strongly suggest that adolescent growth extends past the age of first conception in some women. Mean age at first birth is estimated to be 18.8 years in Matlab (personal communication, A. K. M. A. Chowdhury). Thus, some young women may become pregnant before their adolescent growth is complete. In Bangladesh, as in many developing countries, early childbearing coincides with late menarche. If delays in menarche correspond to an extended adolescent growth then young mothers may experience higher risks of poor pregnancy outcome. More important, perhaps, is the possibility that pregnancy may interfere with continued growth of the mother and result in smaller adult stature, lower body weight, and smaller pelvic diameter. These outcomes would continue to affect maternal and infant health adversely throughout the reproductive period.

It has been hypothesized that the competing growth needs of the mother and foetus may contribute to poor pregnancy outcomes and explain lower birth-weight relative to weight gain during pregnancy in adolescents (Naeye, 1981; Zlatnick and Burmeister, 1977). However, few studies have directly attempted to study growth in pregnant adolescents (Frisancho *et al.*, 1984a; Frisancho *et al.*, 1984b; Frisancho *et al.*, 1983; Garn *et al.*, 1984).

Research on US adolescents shows that the higher weight gain observed in pregnant adolescents compared to adults cannot be attributed to continued statural growth in young mothers (Garn *et al.*, 1984). These investigators found that pregnant teenagers are no longer undergoing rapid growth in height or weight during, or subsequent to, their first pregnancy. However, it is unclear whether the young women under study had completed their adolescent spurt before conception occurred or if early pregnancy interfered with the normal course of growth.

Frisancho *et al.* (1984*a*, 1984*b*, 1983) found that teenagers in Peru who are still growing have a higher rate of low birth-weight than girls of the same age who have completed their growth. The mechanism responsible for this difference is cited as a decreased availability of nutrients to the foetus or inadequate placental function (Frisancho *et al.*, 1984*a*). However the criterion used to identify girls who were still growing was inappropriate. Growth status was determined by height of the pregnant teenager's mother. If the adolescent's height was less than her mother's height she was classified as still growing. 59 per cent of pregnant teenagers were classified as having completed their growth by this criterion. This assumes that growth is the same for all adolescents regardless of age at menarche.

Given the young age of this sample, it is highly unlikely that over 50 per cent had completed their adolescent growth, especially if menarche and growth are delayed. Thus, many girls who were classified as mature were probably still in active growth. Likewise, some of the adolescents who were classified as still growing may have reached their adult height since not every woman achieves her mother's height. An additional consideration is whether or not these teenagers would have continued to grow had they not become pregnant. The possibility that pregnancy may arrest growth in adolescents was not specifically addressed.

Conclusion

In this review, the effects of under-nutrition on age at menarche and reproductive development and their implications for fertility are discussed. It is widely accepted that nutritional status, particularly weight, is associated with age at menarche and that poor nutrition slows or delays growth throughout infancy and childhood. Whether or not delays in menarche and growth *per se* translate into lower fertility in chronically under-nourished women is debatable.

While age at marriage is closely tied to age at menarche in populations with late age at menarche (Chowdhury *et al.*, 1977; Udry and Cliquet, 1982; Wood *et al.*, 1985), the relationship has also been observed in populations with early menarche and relatively late age at marriage (Udry and Cliquet, 1982; Sandler *et al.*, 1984). There is no evidence to suggest that a downward shift in the age at menarche will cause a similar decline in age at marriage or age at first birth.

Endocrinological research in developed countries suggests that late age at menarche coincides with a longer period of adolescent subfecundity (Apter and Vihko, 1983; Vihko and Apter, 1984). However, demographic data from Bangladesh shows that the interval between marriage and first birth is, in fact, shorter in women with late age at menarche compared to earlier maturing girls (Foster *et al.*, 1986).

The evidence for a relationship of age at menarche to foetal wastage is also mixed. There is some evidence for an increased risk of abortion and possibly stillbirth, among women with very early (less than 12 years) and late (at least 16 years) ages at menarche, compared to girls who reach menarche between 12 and 16 years of age (Liestol, 1980; Casagrande *et al.*, 1981; Wyshak, 1982). However, more recent work suggests that this may hold only for women who experience more than one abortion (Sandler *et al.*, 1984; Bracken *et al.*, 1985).

This review finds no strong evidence in the literature to support the hypothesis that nutritional status has a significant impact on fertility. However, there are other considerations of demographic importance. Since delayed menarche is accompanied by delayed growth and reproductive development, there arises the possibility that pregnancy may occur before full growth potential is reached. While several attempts have been made to assess the effects of continued growth in pregnant adolescents on birth outcome, the impact of pregnancy on continued maternal growth and its implications for reproductive health have not been investigated. Further research in this area is indicated. Specifically, studies of the effect of menarche and the interval to first birth on maternal height and weight and on pregnancy outcome are needed to determine whether early pregnancy interferes with adolescent growth or influences reproductive outcomes.

If, in fact, adult height and weight are compromised by pregnancy in undernourished girls, the demographic impact may be far-reaching in terms of morbidity and mortality of mothers and children. Maternal height, weight, and pelvic size are associated with birth-weight and pregnancy complications, and both of these factors are, in turn, associated with higher risks of morbidity and mortality in mothers and their offspring. It is important to consider that these effects would persist throughout reproductive life.

Nutritional programmes could help to assure that young women achieve their growth potential and full reproductive maturity before first conception occurs. The benefits of better nutritional status for women's health and possible improvements in the survival of their future offspring outweigh the risk of minimally higher fertility.

References

Apter, D., and Vihko, R. (1983), 'Early Menarche, a Risk Factor for Breast Cancer, Indicates Early Onset of Ovulatory Cycles', *Journal of Clinical Endocrinology and Metabolism* 57(1): 82–6.

Battaglia, F. C., Frazier, T. M., and Hellegers, A. E. (1963), 'Obstetric and Pediatric Complications of Juvenile Pregnancy', *Pediatrics* 902–10.

Bhalla, M., and Shrivatava, J. R. (1974), 'A Prospective Study of the Age of Menarche in Kampur Girls', *Indian Pediatrics* 11(7): 487–93.

Bongaarts, J. (1980), 'Does Malnutrition Affect Fecundity? A Summary of Evidence', *Science* 208: 564–69.

Borgerhoff-Mulder, M. B. (1989), 'Menarche, Menopause and Reproduction in the Kipsigis of Kenya', *Journal of Biosocial Science* 21: 179–92.

Borsos, A., Lampe, L. G., Balogh, A., Csoknyay, J., and Ditroi, F. (1986), 'Ovarian Function Immediately after the Menarche', *International Journal of Gynaecology and Obstetrics* 24: 239–42.

Bracken, M. B., Bryce-Buchanan, C., Stilten, R., and Holford, T. (1985), 'Menarcheal Age and Habitual Miscarriage: Evidence for an Association', *Annals of Human Biology* 12(6): 525–31.

Casagrande, J. T., Pike, M. C., and Henderson, B. E. (1981), 'Menarcheal Age and Spontaneous Abortion: A Causal Connection?' *American Journal of Epidemiology* 115: 481–3.

Chowdhury, A. K. M. A., Huffman, S. L., and Curlin, G. T. (1977), 'Malnutrition, Menarche and Age at Marriage in Bangladesh', *Social Biology* 24: 316–25.

Dreizen, S., Spirakis, C. N., and Stone, R. E. (1967), 'A Comparison of Skeletal Growth and Maturation in Undernourished and Well-Nourished Girls before and after Menarche', *The Journal of Pediatrics* 70(2): 256–63.

Duenhoelter, J. H., Jimenez, J. M., and Baumann, G. (1975), 'Pregnancy Performance of Patients under Fifteen Years of Age', *Obstetrics and Gynecology* 46(1): 49–52.

Ellison, P. T. (1981), 'Threshold Hypotheses, Developmental Age, and Menstrual Function', *American Journal of Physical Anthropology* 54: 337–40.

Erkan, K. A., Rimer, B. A., and Stine, O. C. (1971), 'Juvenile Pregnancy: Role of Physiologic Maturity', *Maryland State Medical Journal* 20: 50–52.

Eveleth, P. B., and Tanner, J. M. (1976), *World Wide Variations in Human Growth*, Cambridge University Press, Cambridge.

Foster, A., Menken, J., Chowdhury, A. K. M. A., and Trussell, J. (1986), 'Female Reproductive Development: A Hazards Model Analysis', *Social Biology* 33(3–4), 183–99.

Frisancho, A. R., Matos, J., and Flegel, P. (1983), 'Maternal Nutritional Status and Adolescent Pregnancy Outcome', *American Journal of Clinical Nutrition* 38: 739–46.

—— —— and Bollettino, L. A. (1984a), 'Influence of Growth Status and Placental Function on Birth Weight of Infants Born to Young Still-Growing Teenagers', *American Journal of Clinical Nutrition* 40: 801–7.

—— —— —— (1984b), 'Role of Gynecological Age and Growth Maturity Status in Fetal Maturation and Prenatal Growth of Infants Born to Young Still-Growing Adolescent Mothers', *Human Biology* 56(3): 583–93.

Frisch, R. E. (1985), 'Demographic Implications of the Biological Determinants of Female Fecundity', *Social Biology* 22(1): 17–22.

—— Wyshak, G., and Vincent, L. (1980), 'Delayed Menarche and Amenorrhea in Ballet Dancers', *New England Journal of Medicine* 303(1): 17–19.

—— Gotz-Welbergen, A. V., McArthur, J. W., Albright, T. T., Witschi, J., Bullen, B., Birnholz, I., Reed, R. B., and Herman, H. (1981), 'Delayed Menarche and Amenorrhea of College Athletes in Relation to Age of Onset of Training', *Journal of the American Medical Association* 246(14): 1559–63.

Garn, S. M., LaVelle, M., Pesick, S. D., and Ridella, S. A. (1984), 'Are Pregnant Teenagers Still in Rapid Growth?' *American Journal of Diseases in Childhood* 138: 32–4.

—— —— Rosenberg, K. R., and Hawthorne, V. M. (1986), 'Maturational Timing as a Factor in Female Fatness and Obesity', *American Journal of Clinical Nutrition* 43: 879–83.

Geronimus, A. T. (1987), 'On Teenage Childbearing and Neonatal Mortality in the United States', *Population and Development Review* 13(2): 245–79.

Gray, R. H. (1983), 'The Impact of Health and Nutrition on Natural Fertility', in R. Bulatao and R. Lee (eds.), *Determinants of Fertility in Developing Countries* ii. 139–62.

Kulin, H. E., Bwibo, N., Mutie, D., and Santner, S. J. (1982), 'The Effect of Chronic Childhood Malnutrition on Pubertal Growth and Development', *American Journal of Clinical Nutrition* 36: 527–36.

Liestol, K. (1980), 'Menarcheal Age and Spontaneous Abortion: A Causal Connection?' *American Journal of Epidemiology* 111(6): 753–8.

McAnarney, E. R. (1981), 'The Precious Dyad-Special Requirements of the Pregnant Adolescent and her Fetus', in J. T. Bond, L. J. Filer, G. A. Leveille, A. M. Thomson, and N. B. Neil (eds.), *Infant and Child Feeding*, Academic Press, 225–37.

Makinson, C. (1985), 'The Health Consequences of Teenage Fertility', *Family Planning Perspectives*, 17(3): 132–9.

Malcolm, L. A. (1970), 'Growth and Development of the Bundi Child of the New Guinea Highlands', *Human Biology* 42: 293–327.

Malina, R. M., Spirduso, W. W., Tate, C., and Baylor, A. M. (1978), 'Age at Menarche and Selected Menstrual Characteristics in Athletes at Different Competitive Levels and in Different Sports', *Medicine and Science in Sports* 10(3): 218–22.

Mangold, W. D. (1983), 'Age of Mother and Pregnancy Outcome in the 1981 Arkansas Birth Cohort', *Social Biology* 30(2): 205–10.

Marshall, W. A., and Tanner, J. M. (1986), 'Puberty' in W. A. Marshall and J. M. Tanner (eds.), *Human Growth* ii, 2nd edn., Plenum Press, London: 171–209.

Menken, J. (1980), 'The Health and Demographic Consequences of Teenage Pregnancy and Childbearing', in C. S. Chilman (ed.), *Adolescent Pregnancy and Childbearing*, National Institutes of Health Publications, Public Health Service, US Department of Health and Human Services: 157–205.

Naeye, R. L. (1981), 'Teenaged and Pre-Teenaged Pregnancies: Consequences of the Fetal–Maternal Competition for Nutrients', *Pediatrics* 67(1): 146–50.

Nair, N. (1983), 'On a Distribution of First Conception Delays in the Presence of Adolescent Sterility', *Demography India* 12(2): 269–75.

Nakamura, I., Shirmura, M., Nonakand, K., Miura, T. (1986), 'Changes of Recollected Menarcheal Age and Month among Women in Tokyo over a Period of 90 Years', *Annals of Human Biology* 13(6): 547–54.

Pebley, A. R., Huffman, S. L., Chowdhury, A. K. M. A., and Stupp, P. W. (1985), 'Intra-Uterine Mortality and Maternal Nutritional Status in Rural Bangladesh', *Population Studies* 393(3): 425–40.

Raman, L. (1981), 'Influence of Maternal Nutritional Factors Affecting Birthweight', *American Journal of Clinical Nutrition* 34: 775–83.

Rana, T., Raman, L., Rau, P., and Rao, K. V. (1986), 'Association of Growth Status and Age at Menarche in Urban Upper Middle Income Group Girls of Hyderabad', *Indian Journal of Medical Research* 84: 522–30.

Riley, A. P. (1989), 'Dynamic and Static Measures of Growth among Pre- and

Post-menarcheal Females in Rural Bangladesh', *American Journal of Human Biology* 2: 225–64.

Riley, A. P. (1990), 'Dynamic and Static Measures of Growth among Pre- and Post-Menarcheal Females in Rural Bangladesh', *American Journal of Human Biology* 2: 255–64.

—— Huffman, S. L., and Chowdhury, A. K. M. A. (1989), 'Age at Menarche and Postmenarcheal Growth in Rural Bangladeshi Females', *Annals of Human Biology* 16(4): 347–59.

Roche, A. F., and Davila, G. H. (1972), 'Late Adolescent Growth in Stature', *Pediatrics* 50(6): 874–80.

Sandler, D. P., Wilcox, A. J., and Horney, L. F. (1984), 'Age at Menarche and Subsequent Reproductive Events', *American Journal of Epidemiology* 119(5): 765–74.

Scott, A., Moar, V., and Ounsted, M. (1981), 'The Relative Contributions of Different Maternal Factors in Small-for-Gestational-Age Pregnancies', *European Journal of Obstetrics, Gynecology, and Reproductive Biology* 12: 157–65.

Stanley, F. J., and Mauger, S. (1986), 'Birth-Weight Patterns in Aboriginal and Non-Aboriginal Singleton Adolescent Births in Western Australia, 1979–83', *Australian and New Zealand Journal of Obstetrics and Gynaecology* 26: 49–54.

Tanner, J. M. (1978), *Physical Growth from Conception to Maturity*, Harvard University Press, Cambridge, Mass.

—— Whitehouse, R. H., and Takaish, M. (1966), 'Standards from Birth to Maturity for Height, Weight, Height Velocity, and Weight Velocity: British Children, 1965', *Archives Diseases of Childhood* 41: 613–35.

Treloar, A. E., Boynton, R. E., Behn, B. G., and Brown, B. W. (1967), 'Variation of the Human Menstrual Cycle through Reproductive Life', *International Journal of Fertility* 12(1): 77–126.

Udry, J. R., and Cliquet, R. L. (1982), 'A Cross-Cultural Examination of the Relationship between Ages at Menarche, Marriage, and First Birth', *Demography* 19(1): 53–63.

Van der Spuy, Z. M., and Jacobs, H. S. (1983), 'Weight Reduction, Fertility and Contraception', *IPPF Medical Bulletin* 17(5).

Vihko, R., and Apter, D. (1984), 'Endocrine Characteristics of Adolescent Menstrual Cycles: Impact of Early Menarche', *Journal of Steroid Biochemistry*, 20(1): 231–6.

Warren, M. P. (1980), 'The Effects of Exercise on Pubertal Progression and Reproductive Function in Girls', *Journal of Clinical Endocrinology and Metabolism* 51: 1150–7.

Wood, J. W., Johnson, P. L., and Campbell, K. L. (1985), 'Demographic and Endocrinological Aspects of Low Natural Fertility in Highland New Guinea', *Journal of Biosocial Science* 17: 57–79.

Wyshak, G. (1983), 'Age at Menarche and Unsuccessful Pregnancy Outcome', *Annals of Human Biology* 10(1): 69–73.

—— and Frisch, R. E. (1982), 'Evidence for a Secular Trend in Age of Menarche', *New England Journal of Medicine* 306(17): 1033–5.

Zacharias, L., and Rand, W. M. (1983), 'Adolescent Growth in Height and its Relation to Menarche in Contemporary American Girls', *Annals of Human Biology* 10(3): 209–22.

Zlatnik, F. J., and Burmeister, L. F. (1977), 'Low "Gynecologic Age": An Obstetric Risk Factor', *American Journal of Obstetrics and Gynecology* 128(2): 183–6.

5 Age at Menopause and Fecundity Preceding Menopause

OMAR RAHMAN

JANE MENKEN

Introduction

The reproductive life-span of a woman is delimited by menarche and menopause. In contrast to age at menarche and adolescent fertility, age at menopause and fertility preceding menopause have received relatively little attention in the scientific literature. Female fecundity does not decline precipitously; rather, menopause is the culmination of a gradual decline that results from both biological and socio-cultural factors (Gray, 1979a, 1979b). Recently, as more women in developed countries have chosen to delay first births, there has been increased interest in the availability of accurate information about fecundity in the period shortly preceding menopause and about factors affecting age at menopause. In developing countries, involuntary sterility due to disease remains an important concern. Additionally, the long life expectancy of women today means a significant proportion, especially in the developed world, can expect to live for two or three decades past the age of natural menopause. Post-menopausal women have a number of increased health risks: osteoporosis (Lindquist et al., 1981) and increased risk of cardiovascular disease (Kannel et al., 1976) are two of the more prominent. Thus, knowledge about factors affecting age at menopause and the consequent duration of exposure to post-menopausal health risks has become more crucial (McKinlay et al., 1985).

Age at Menopause

Menopause, defined as the cessation of menstruation, is intrinsically difficult to estimate because of the problem of distinguishing between complete cessation and temporary amenorrhoea. However, despite methodological problems (recall bias, digit clustering) in existing studies, there is a striking degree of consensus about the age at cessation of menstruation, at least among Caucasian women (see Table 5.1). The median is about 50 years, with reports ranging from 49.8 years to 51.4 years. Reported values for non-Caucasian women vary more, ranging from 43.4 years in Punjabi women to 49.7 years in South African Bantu women (Gray, 1979a). It is difficult to determine whether the generally

TABLE 5.1. *Estimates of the age at menopause from selected studies*

Country	Year of study	Race	Mean or median age at menopause in years		Study design
USA	1981–2	Caucasian	51.4	median	Cross-sectional
Scotland	1970	Caucasian	50.1	median	Cross-sectional
England	1965	Caucasian	50.8	median	Cross-sectional
			47.5	mean	
England	1951–61	Caucasian	49.8	median	Cross-sectional
USA	1934–74	Caucasian	49.8	median	Cohort
			49.5	mean	
USA	1966	Caucasian	50.0	median	Cross-sectional
		Negro	49.3	median	
		Both races	49.8	median	
Germany	1972	Caucasian	49.1	mean	Retrospective
Finland	1961	Caucasian	49.8	mean	Retrospective
Switzerland	1961	Caucasian	49.8	mean	Retrospective
Israel	1963	Caucasian	49.5	mean	Retrospective
Netherlands	1969	Caucasian	51.4	median	Cross-sectional
New Zealand	1967	Caucasian	50.7	median	Cross-sectional
South Africa	1971	Caucasian	50.4	median	Cross-sectional
		Negro	49.7	median	
South Africa	1960	Negro	48.1	median	Retrospective
			47.7	mean	
South Africa	1960	Caucasian	48.7	mean	Retrospective
Punjab, India	1966	Asian	44.0	median	Cohort and cross-sectional
New Guinea	1973	Melanesian			Cross-sectional
		non-malnourished	47.3	median	
		malnourished	43.6	median	

Sources: For the USA, McKinlay *et al.*, 1985; for the remaining countries, Gray, 1976.

lower age at menopause for non-Caucasian women and the wider variability reflect genetic or ethnic differences, or result from other biological factors such as nutrition, or are due to age mis-statement.

For the USA, there is evidence that thinner women reach menopause earlier than those who are heavier (MacMahon and Worcester, 1966). A recent study from Bangladesh (Karim *et al.*, 1985) also found slightly earlier menopause for thinner women; the investigators suggest that leanness is a marker for poorer nutritional status and that better nourished women continue menstruating longer than their poorly nourished sisters. Studies in two New Guinea populations that vary in nutritional statuses show that severe malnutrition may depress the age at menopause (Scragg, 1973). Some investigators have argued that there has been a secular trend in the age of menopause; they claim that this evidence, when combined with improvements in food supply over time, supports the hypothesis that nutritional status influences age at menopause. Recently others (e.g. McKinlay *et al.*, 1985; Gray, 1976) have demonstrated conclusively that there has been no significant trend in age of menopause, thus weakening the evidence for a link with chronic malnutrition. Thus, nutrition appears to play a role in determining age at menopause, but this relationship has not been clearly delineated.

Various factors, apart from nutrition, that may affect age at menopause have been considered (cf. Van Keep *et al.*, 1979; McKinlay *et al.*, 1985). Although suggestive trends have been observed (for example age at menarche and smoking status are negatively related to age at menopause, while number of children, marital status, duration of oral contraceptive use, and education are positively related), the only statistically significant relationship now established is with smoking status. According to a recent multivariate analysis (McKinlay *et al.*, 1985), smokers tend to reach menopause an average of 1.74 years earlier than non-smokers. The quantity smoked is not a significant variable. The associations between age at menopause and education, duration of oral contraceptive use, marital status, and parity were complex and difficult to unravel given the degree of confounding present in the McKinlay study, and they require additional prospective studies for clarification.

Decline of Fecundity Preceding Menopause

While it is true that post-menopausal women are infecund, sterility (defined as the inability to have a live birth) usually precedes menopause and marks the end of a gradual process of declining fecundity.

Age-specific marital fertility declines have been well documented in natural fertility populations (Coale and Trussell, 1974). While there are population-based differences in the levels of fertility, there is a surprisingly consistent pattern in the rate of fertility decline in historical populations of Western European descent, which is summarized in Table 5.2. There is a moderate drop from the age-groups 20–4 to 30–4 years and a much sharper downturn thereafter. Fertility for the 35–9 year age-group is about 31 per cent lower than the 20–4 year age-group and fertility for the 40–4 year age-group (the years preceding menopause) appears to be about 50 per cent lower than the 35–9 year age-group (Menken and Larsen, 1986).

Marital fertility is a complex function of the age of the wife, the age of the husband, and the duration of marriage. Marital fertility schedules such as the one illustrated in Table 5.2 do not allow us to disaggregate these competing effects. Recently, Mineau and Trussell (1982) developed a multiplicative model, $F(W, H, D) = B^*w(W)^*h(H)^*d(D)$, in which the fertility rate, F, for couples married D years and in which the wife was age W and the husband age H was the product of a baseline value B and the effects of female age, $w(W)$,

TABLE 5.2. *Marital age-specific fertility rates in populations of West European descent with no evidence of fertility limitation*

Age (years)	Decline (%)
20–4	0
25–9	6
30–4	14
35–9	31
40–4	64
45–9	95

Source: Menken and Larsen, 1986.

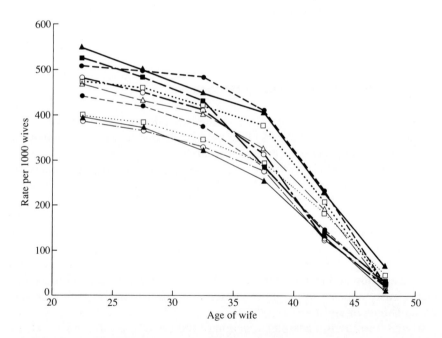

The ten populations (in descending order at age 20 to 24) are Hutterites, marriages 1921–30 (▲); Geneva bourgeoisie, husbands born 1600–49 (■); Canada, marriages 1700–30 (●); Normandy, marriages 1760–90 (○); Hutterites, marriages before 1921 (□); Tunis, marriages of Europeans 1840–59 (△); Normandy, marriages 1674–1742 (●); Norway, marriages 1874–76 (□); Iran, village marriages, 1940–50 (▲); Geneva bourgeoisie, husbands born before 1600 (○).

Source: Menken and Larsen, 1986.

Fig. 5.1   Marital fertility rates by 5-year age-groups in ten historical populations

male age, $h(H)$ and marriage duration, $d(D)$. Tables 5.3 and 5.4 show the resulting estimates for a Mormon group in which family limitation is unlikely to have been practised. The results indicate a very gradual decline in female fertility up to age 35 with a much sharper decline subsequently. Women aged 35 to 39, however, are still about 90 per cent as likely as those aged 20 to 24 to have a baby (assuming that the latter women's husbands were aged 20 to 24 and marriage duration was less than five years). The impact of marriage duration is also significant and is probably mediated through declining coital frequency and the cumulative negative effect of multiple pregnancies. Male ageing contributes relatively little to the decline in marital fertility with age. Thus, the declining fecundity of couples as they grow older is primarily due to changes associated with duration of marriage and the ageing of women. Although it seems likely that these effects are related to decreasing coital frequency, increasing reproductive impairment due to childbearing, and biological ageing, the contribution of each is impossible to assess from data of this type.

Termination of Reproductive Capacity

Two demographic measures have commonly been used to assess the termination of reproductive capability in a population: mean age at last birth and age-specific prevalence of sterility. Each of these measures is discussed in detail below.

TABLE 5.3. *Relative fertility rates according to the age of wife and husband, controlling for the effects of marriage duration and age of spouse*

Age (years)	Relative rate[a]	
	Wife	Husband
15–19	0.96	0.90
20–4	1.00	1.00
25–9	1.03	0.99
30–4	0.99	1.04
35–9	0.90	0.97
40–4	0.62	0.83
45–9	0.14	0.82
50–4	—	0.73
55–9	—	0.48

[a] Rates are relative to the base value 471 births per 1000 wives, estimated for couples married less than 5 years and in which both the husband and the wife are aged 20–4.

Source: Mormon genealogical data, wives born between 1840 and 1859 (Mineau and Trussell, 1982).

TABLE 5.4. *Relative fertility rates by marriage duration, controlling for the effects of the age of wife and husband*

Marriage duration (years)	Relative rate
0–4	1.00
5–9	0.84
10–14	0.77
15–19	0.79

Note: Data, underlying model, and base value are as described for Table 5.3.

Source: Mineau and Trussell, 1982.

Age at Last Birth

One measure used to approximate the average age of termination of reproduction is mean age at last birth. In natural fertility populations with no voluntary constraints on reproduction, this index should closely parallel age at onset of sterility. Mean age at last birth seems to be surprisingly consistent for a wide variety of natural fertility populations and is estimated to be approximately 40 years (Knodel, 1978). This is true even for populations with different ages at marriage, different rates of infant mortality, and differences in occupations of husbands. The uniformity of the estimate of the completion of childbearing suggests that, at least for natural fertility populations, mean age of sterility is relatively invariant except in populations with high rates of venereal disease.

For populations using contraception the relationships between age at last birth, age at onset of sterility, and age at menopause are more complex. However, it is clear that median age at last birth and at onset of sterility antedate median age at menopause by a significant margin in all populations.

Age-specific Prevalence of Sterility

Age at sterility is inherently impossible to measure accurately in most women because, unless there are observable defects of the reproductive system or unless it is certain that a woman has reached menopause, she may have very low fecundity, but still not be absolutely incapable of conceiving and bearing a child. Most studies of sterility focus on the capacity to bear a live infant, not just on fecundability, the capacity to conceive. In the discussion that follows, we will use this definition, but recognize that there will be some imprecision of concept, since we cannot distinguish between very low fecundity and true sterility.

Demographic methods based on the proportion of women bearing no more children after a particular age have been used to calculate estimates of the proportion of women of that age who are sterile. Bongaarts (1982) calculated age-specific sterility schedules using historic data from seventeenth- and eighteenth-century France and for early twentieth-century Hutterites. The proportion sterile increased only modestly from 4 per cent for the 20–24 age-group to 9 per cent for the 30–34 age-group and then sharply jumped to 20 per cent for the 35–39-year-olds (Table 5.5).

TABLE 5.5. *Estimates of percentage of women sterile by age, comparing 17th- and 18th-century French women and early 20th-century Hutterites*

Age (years)	Percent sterile		
	France	Hutterites	Average
20–4	5	3	4
25–9	6	3	5
30–4	10	9	9
35–9	18	22	20

Source: Bongaarts, 1982.

These estimates can be cross-checked to a certain extent by using data from the World Fertility Survey (WFS) (Table 5.6). In these calculations, a woman was considered infecund either if she reported that it was physically impossible for her and her husband to have a child (supposing they wanted one) or if she had not borne a child in the five years prior to the survey and had not used contraception in that period. One major problem in interpreting these figures is that all contraceptors were considered fecund. Especially in countries where fertility control is common, even results from women who have never used contraception must be viewed with caution due to the well-known selection biases whereby less fecund women are less likely to be contraceptive users. Thus, the survey data may be less biased for those countries where there is very little contraceptive use (e.g. Bangladesh), but since in many of these countries accuracy of age and date reporting is questionable, the data may still be problematic. A final problem is sample size: each woman contributes one observation, her fertility in the five years prior to the survey. Since the number of women in a particular age-group may be rather small, the estimates are subject to sampling variability. With all these caveats, the WFS data provide estimates of age-specific infecundity that are generally somewhat higher at the older ages than the Bongaarts data presented in Table 5.5 and than Henry's (1965) earlier estimates for European populations.

More complex measures of sterility have been developed. They are based on the proportion of women at a particular age who produce no more children until the end of their reproductive span, taken to be age 50 (Henry, 1965;

TABLE 5.6. *Proportions infecund in various countries among currently married non-contracepting women, by age*

Country	Age at survey				
	20–4	25–9	30–4	35–9	40–4
Kenya	5	9	18	28	42
Lesotho	6	16	27	44	63
Senegal	4	8	13	32	49
Sudan	7	13	22	30	58
Jordan	1	5	13	19	43
Syria	3	6	15	21	46
Bangladesh	8	9	19	32	55
Nepal	9	9	17	29	58
Pakistan	5	8	12	26	47
Sri Lanka	4	9	23	41	72
Indonesia	5	13	30	51	77
Korea	0	3	11	28	61
Malaysia	1	8	16	34	65
Philippines	1	5	11	22	52
Thailand	4	10	22	51	76
Colombia	2	9	13	23	47
Paraguay	6	11	18	31	45
Peru	2	6	14	19	49
Venezuela	3	8	18	31	51
Costa Rica	5	13	29	48	58
Dominican Republic	5	12	23	32	55
Mexico	2	8	15	25	56
Panama	2	12	28	40	57
Guyana	3	11	23	46	63
Haiti	7	9	17	24	44
Jamaica	4	13	27	39	54
Trinidad and Tobago	7	11	24	44	59

Note: A woman was considered infecund either if she reported that she and her husband were unable to have a child or if she had not given birth to a child in the five years preceding the survey and had not used contraception in that period.

Sources: Vaessen, 1984; data from the World Fertility Survey.

Leridon, 1977; Trussell and Wilson, 1985), or for some subsequent period, say five years (Larsen and Menken, 1989). These figures overestimate the true proportion of women sterile at that age since, clearly, not all women aged x who bear no more children in the defined subsequent period are already sterile at age x. Some are still fecund but simply fail to bear a(nother) child before they reach sterility; when they are followed only for five subsequent years, it is still possible for them to have another child later. However, since fertility decreases and conversely sterility increases with age monotonically, this estimate must equal the proportion sterile at some later age, usually called the reference age. Henry (1965) first suggested that these measures could be used to estimate the age-specific prevalence of sterility. He, however, assumed that the reference age was the midpoint of the age interval. Leridon (1977) refined the method, as did Trussell and Wilson (1985) who used computer simulations to test their procedures. These methods could be applied only when data for women who had completed their reproductive years were available. Larsen and Menken (1989) used the Trussell–Wilson approach through simulation models to adapt the methods for use when the data available are from younger women who may still bear additional children. They calculated the proportion of women who do not bear a child within 5 years subsequent to a particular age. This figure is an estimate of the proportion sterile at a reference age that is somewhat higher than when complete birth histories are available.

The results obtained by Trussell and Wilson and by Larsen and Menken are shown in Table 5.7. The estimates for Africa are based on World Fertility Data; the data-sets for Kenya and Sudan were also used by Vaessen (1984). The proportions sterile are quite similar for ages under 30 except for Cameroon. At ages over 30, they are higher for Lesotho and Sudan as compared to historic England; for Kenya and Ghana, they are systematically lower; and for Cameroon, higher. Where these estimates can be compared to the WFS results, they are generally somewhat higher, as is to be expected from the way they are calculated: the WFS results for a given age-group refer to past fertility, whereas those in Table 5.7 consider the woman's fertility after a particular age. Again, as expected, the prevalence of infecundity is almost always higher for women who have never used contraception.

The above estimates of age-specific sterility (Tables 5.5–5.7) are, with the exception of countries like Cameroon where early sterility due to venereal disease is suspected, considerably lower and in sharp contrast, especially at ages under 40, to estimates of age-specific sterility from a recent French study (Fédération CECOS *et al.*, 1982). This study employed the commonly used medical definition of infertility as the inability to conceive within a year (or twelve menstrual cycles), given optimal coital frequency. Looking at artificial insemination of women with azoospermic husbands, it found much higher estimates of infertility at all ages (Table 5.8). Approximately 74 per cent of women below age 30 conceived within 12 insemination cycles, with the figures falling to 61 per cent and 56 per cent for women aged 30–4 and 35–9 respectively. This study is considered to be especially important because it controls for two important confounding factors, male infertility and decreasing coital frequency with age, both of which contribute to the decline of female fertility with age.

The Fédération CECOS study has been criticized by Bongaarts (1982), however, who made the point that artificial insemination results in lower

TABLE 5.7. *The proportions infecund estimated for Cameroon, Ghana, Kenya, Lesotho, and Sudan (all women and women who had never used contraception) and for historical England*

Calculation age-group	Cameroon		Ghana		Kenya	
	All women	Never used	All women	Never used	All women	Never used
20–4	.17	.18	.05	.06	.05	.07
25–9	.26	.27	.08	.10	.08	.10
30–4	.38	.39	.16	.18	.14	.16
35–9	.51	.52	.30	.33	.26	.28
40–4	.69	.69	.52	.55	.52	.55
Sample size	4468	3212	2869	1769	4037	2731

Calculation age-group	Lesotho		Sudan		England 1550–1849[a]
	All women	Never used	All women	Never used	
20–4	.10	.13	.09	.09	.07
25–9	.10	.23	.14	.14	.13
30–4	.30	.35	.27	.27	.23
35–9	.47	.50	.46	.44	.35
40–4	.69	.72	.74	.71	.58
Sample size	2200	1614	2228	1859	1859

[a] Women married between ages of 15 and 19.

Note: The estimates for Africa are derived from incomplete birth histories, for England from complete histories.

Sources: For Africa, Larsen and Menken, 1989; for England, Trussell and Wilson, 1985.

TABLE 5.8. *Rates of pregnancy, loss to follow-up, and drop-out by age, following artificial insemination in France*

	Age-group				
	<25	26–30	31–5	>35	(36–40)
Mean rate/cycle					
Pregnancy	11.0	10.5	9.1	6.5	(6.5)
Losses to follow-up	2.8	2.5	2.4	2.4	
Drop-outs	4.0	4.0	4.7	4.9	
Cumulative pregnancy rate after 12 cycles	73.0	74.1	61.5	53.6	(55.8)

Source: Fédération CECOS *et al.*, 1982.

conception frequencies than natural insemination. He presented evidence from a British study that 80 to 89 per cent of women who stop using contraception other than the pill conceive within 12 cycles, depending on parity (Vessey *et al.*, 1978). He also pointed out that the arbitrary cut-off point of twelve menstrual cycles probably overestimates infertility. Historical evidence appears to indicate that a substantial proportion of couples take more than a year to conceive, and the inability of older women to conceive within twelve menstrual cycles should not be taken as evidence of permanent sterility (Trussell and Wilson, 1985). Another study in which artificial insemination was continued for 18 months found much higher conception rates (Kremer, 1982). It is interesting to note, however, that in the Fédération CECOS study fecundability among women aged 40–4 was 59 per cent of fecundability of women aged 20–4, a figure very close to the one reported in Table 5.3 for the same comparison.

The publication of the French study raised questions about whether women who were delaying childbearing into their 30s were taking undue risks that they could never have a child. When the disparity between these results and those from historical European populations was pointed out, the argument was made that the latter might be a more appropriate comparison group for modern women who were delaying childbearing. The counter-argument was made, however, that estimates derived from historical populations may not hold for nulliparous women, since most of the older women in the historical populations already had children. In response, Menken and Larsen (1986) examined the effect of biological ageing on reproductive capacity exclusively among women who delayed childbearing by postponing marriage. Using historical data from seven populations of Western European descent, they calculated the proportion of couples who remained childless, by the age of the bride. They derived a typical age-specific infertility schedule, based on women who married within an age interval, which estimates the proportion of women sterile when sterility is solely due to ageing. Also, Trussell and Wilson (1985) were able to estimate sterility by age and age at marriage (thereby including marriage duration in their results). Both sets of results (Table 5.9) show only a modest rise in infertility from the age of 20 to about the age of 35 (5 per cent to 16 per cent). After age 35 infertility increases sharply, but even in the age-group 40–5 only reaches a maximum of 62 per cent. The median age of onset of sterility, where sterility is only due to ageing, according to these schedules is about 44 years. The figures are quite consistent with Bongaarts' earlier estimates (Table 5.2).

Trussell and Wilson's (1985) work demonstrates conclusively that infecundity for any age is positively related to duration of marriage, probably reflecting decreases in frequency of intercourse and parity-specific decreases in fertility (due to the cumulative damage of multiple childbirths). No data-sets other than the English historical material have been analysed using their methods, but it is obvious that estimates of sterility in a specific population are affected by its distributions of duration of marriage, age of husband, and probably parity as

TABLE 5.9.   *Estimated percentages of women who are sterile by age and age at marriage*

Menken–Larsen (1986)		Trussell–Wilson (1985)	
Age at marriage	Risk of childlessness (%)	Reference age[a]	Percentage sterile
20–4	5.7	23.4	4.6
25–9	9.3	28.5	9.1
30–4	15.5	35.1	16.6
35–9	29.6	40.6	25.4
40–4	63.6	45.2	62.2

[a] An estimated 4.6 percent of women who were married at ages 20–4 were sterile when they were 23.4 years old (the reference age corresponding to age at marriage 20 to 24). See Trussell and Wilson, 1985 for the determination of reference ages.

Sources: Menken and Larsen, 1986; Trussell and Wilson, 1985.

well. Differentials among populations according to these factors may explain some of the variation in proportions sterile, especially among women in their thirties, seen in the data presented in Tables 5.6 and 5.7.

Factors Influencing the Decline in Fertility with Age

A variety of socio-cultural and biological factors may lead to reductions in fertility preceding menopause. In the following discussion we will first focus on the socio-cultural factors, which are mediated largely through decreases in frequency of intercourse.

Socio-cultural Factors

Post-partum abstinence.   One potential influence on fertility decline with age is post-partum abstinence that changes with age. However, there does not seem to be much evidence for any significant change in duration of abstention with age, so that this particular post-partum practice is unlikely to be a significant determinant of the decline in fertility preceding menopause (Knodel, 1983).

Coital frequency and terminal abstinence.   There is a fair amount of evidence that in most societies coital frequency diminishes markedly by age (see Table 5.10). Thus it is somewhat surprising that terminal abstinence as a factor in decreased old-age marital fertility has received relatively little attention. The demographic literature has largely ignored cultural norms regarding the age when childbearing should be completed, in contrast to the age when childbearing begins (Ware, 1979).

TABLE 5.10. *Mean weekly coital frequency of married women by age in selected populations*

Age	British	American White	Hindu	Sheikh Muslim	Non-Sheikh Muslim
19	2.47	3.7	1.5	1.7	2.3
20–4	2.10	3.0	1.9	2.4	2.6
25–9	1.72	2.6	1.8	2.4	2.7
30–4	1.33	2.3	1.1	1.8	2.1
35–9	1.37	2.0	0.7	1.4	1.5
40–4		1.7	0.2	1.0	0.8

Sources: For British and Americans, Cartwright, 1976, Table 58; for Hindus and Muslims, Nag, 1972, Table 4.

In contrast to European societies, where there are relatively few cultural proscriptions on changes in sexual activity with age, a number of non-Western societies have evolved fairly explicit norms about the termination of childbearing, usually mediated through abstinence. These norms are couched in terms of phases of the life-cycle (grandmotherhood, grandfatherhood, etc.) rather than chronological age *per se* (Ware, 1979).

Traditional Hindu society provides one of the few examples of explicit proscriptions on male sexual activity with age. According to Hindu religious custom, a person's life is divided into four phases or *ashrama*, and only the second phase, stretching approximately from the age of 25–50, should be devoted to childbearing. 'It is the general feeling that a man's sexual activity should cease by the time all his children are grown and he has a grandchild' (Opler, 1964). Adherence to this norm is attested to by the fact that the average age at which male participants in the Mysore Population Study stated that men should cease reproduction was 44.2 (urban) and 47.5 (rural) (United Nations, 1961).

In contrast to the relatively few instances of culturally sanctioned declines in sexual activity for males, many societies have some sort of norm indicating the appropriateness of decreasing sexual activity by age for females. In many non-Western cultures, expectations about the appropriate level of sexual activity are related to life-cycle events such as becoming a grandmother rather than chronological age. Although coital frequency rates decline for women by age in all cultures, the rate of decline is very variable.

Evidence from India for Hindu women indicates that there is a marked drop in coital frequency after the age of 35 (Nag, 1972). This closely parallels the ideal age for completion of childbirth reported by female participants in the Mysore Population Study, 35.7 (rural) and 36.0 (urban) (United Nations, 1961). In many parts of India, it is considered unseemly for women to procreate if they have adult children and especially if they have already become grandmothers. Adherence to old-age abstinence, however, is less rigid when it conflicts with other, competing norms such as having at least one male child (Ware, 1979).

In contrast to the Hindu data from West Bengal, a recent Bangladeshi survey reporting on both Hindu and Muslim women (Table 5.11) reports a very gradual rise in abstinence with age, ranging from 8 per cent to 13 per cent for younger women and rising to a maximum of 19 per cent for women aged 45 and above. Grandmotherhood and the presence of adult children were deemed important causes of abstinence in only a very small number of cases. Absence of the spouse due to migration patterns was the most common cause of marital abstinence (Ruzicka and Bhatia, 1982) and is the likely explanation for the surprising negative association found between duration of marriage and abstinence. The authors note, however, that the generally higher coital frequency rates and the lack of a grandmotherhood effect reported may be due in part to various selection biases: the study was restricted to women who had not abstained in the month prior to the survey and a non-random selection methodology may have favoured the inclusion of sexually active women.

TABLE 5.11. *Mean weekly coital frequency of married women by age,*
comparing data from Bangladesh and West Bengal

Age	India (W. Bengal)			Bangladesh	
	Hindu	Sheikh Muslim	Non-Sheikh Muslim	Hindu	Muslim
15–19	1.5	1.7	2.3	2.1	2.9
20–4	1.9	2.4	2.6	1.6	2.1
25–9	1.8	2.4	2.7	1.7	1.8
30–4	1.1	1.8	2.1	1.5	1.6
35–9	0.7	1.4	1.5	1.2	1.5
40–4	0.2	1.0	1.8	1.2	1.4
45+	0.3	0.4	0.4	1.3	1.0
N	167	204	395	1348	566

Sources: For India, Nag, 1972; for Bangladesh, Ruzicka and Bhatia, 1982.

African norms about terminal abstinence closely parallel the Indian Hindu experience, although there is wide variation. The most detailed information comes from studies of the Yoruba in Western Nigeria (Caldwell and Caldwell, 1977). Grandmothers were much more likely to abstain than their age peers regardless of parity. Of women aged 40–4 in the non-grandmother category, 75 per cent were sexually active compared to only 25 per cent of grandmothers.

A number of investigators have estimated the impact of terminal abstinence by grandmothers on fertility. It is determined to a large extent by age at first birth, as in most societies biological infertility sets in before women become grandmothers. Caldwell and Caldwell (1977) have calculated that the Yoruba custom results in a reduction in average completed family size of half a child.

Knodel (1983) demonstrated that grandmother abstinence can have a significant impact on fertility only if the age of first childbirth is very low (as in Nepal),
resulting in a high proportion of grandmothers at each age, and if abstinence
due to grandmotherhood status is high (as in Nigeria). Table 5.12 shows his
calculations of the impact of abstinence when the proportion of grandmothers
who adopt the practice is taken from the Nigerian data and the proportion of
women at each age are grandmothers is taken from Nigeria and Nepal. Even in
early-marrying populations, the effects are negligible until the late thirties,
when fertility can be reduced by as much as 20 per cent. Proportionally, the
potential effect is even greater in the early forties, but, since fertility is already
low at that age, there is less impact on lifetime fertility. Although these effects
are plausible, there is little empirical evidence to support an impact of this
magnitude either in Nepal (Knodel, 1983) or in Nigeria (Caldwell and Caldwell,
1977, Appendix B; Weiss and Udo, 1981).

TABLE 5.12. *The potential impact of terminal abstinence on the*
age pattern of natural fertility when the same proportion of
grandmothers practise abstinence as in Nigeria

	Index values of marital fertility (20–4 = 100)					
	Age-group					
	20–4	25–9	30–4	35–9	40–4	45–9
Coale–Trussell standard	100	94	86	70	36	5
Estimated impact of terminal abstinence when the proportion of grandmothers is as in Nigeria	100	94	86	66	27	2
Nepal[a]	100	94	83	56	20	1

[a] Nepal has much lower age at first birth and consequently a much higher
proportion of grandmothers at each age than Nigeria.

Source: Knodel, 1983, Table 5.

The data on coital frequency by age is clearly difficult to validate. Studies in
the literature report widely different rates, even in similar populations (e.g.
compare Nag, 1972 and Ruzicka and Bhatia, 1982). Despite the problems in
estimating the absolute levels for different ages, it is none the less clear that
there is a marked decline in coital frequency with age in all populations.
Terminal abstinence and post-partum abstinence *per se* do not appear to have a
significant impact on pre-menopausal fertility. Estimates of the importance of
coital frequency as a determinant of fertility come primarily from simulation or
probability models (cf. Barrett and Marshall, 1969). Bongaarts' (1983) estimates of fecundability according to frequency of coitus (Table 5.13) illustrate the
magnitude of this relationship.

TABLE 5.13. *Model estimates of fecundability and conception wait for different coital frequencies*

Average coital frequency per menstrual cycle[a]	Approximate number of coital acts per week	Fecundability	Duration of conception wait[b]
1	0.27	.035	43.8
2	0.54	.068	22.1
3	0.81	.100	15.0
4	1.08	.130	11.5
5	1.35	.159	9.4
6	1.62	.187	8.0
7	1.88	.213	7.0
8	2.15	.238	6.3
9	2.42	.262	5.7
10	2.69	.284	5.3
11	2.96	.305	4.9
12	3.23	.324	4.6
13	3.50	.342	4.4
14	3.77	.359	4.2
15	4.04	.374	4.0
20	5.38	.429	3.5

[a] All coital acts are assumed to take place during the inter-menstrual interval, estimated to average 26 days.

[b] Estimated as 1/fecundability.

Source: Bongaarts, 1983.

Biological Factors

Considerable evidence exists that there are biologically derived declines with age in the probability of conception (fecundability) and in the probability that conception leads to a live birth.

Decline in fecundability with age.   A number of investigators have documented a rise in the number of anovulatory cycles and cycles with short luteal phases in the peri-menopausal period leading to unsuccessful conceptions. Approximately 12 per cent of cycles among women aged 41–5 are anovular, and the proportion of cycles with short luteal phases rises significantly above the age of 40 (Doring, 1969). Chiazze *et al.* (1968) report that the proportion of cycles with short luteal phases (less than 25 days) increases progressively from a low of 7.3 per cent in the 20–9 year age-group to 19.6 per cent at ages 40–4. The relatively modest changes in anovulation and corpus luteum failure with age shown in the above physiological data contrasted with the major decline in fertility in pre-menopausal women indicate that only a small proportion of this decline can be explained on the basis of anovulation and cycles with short luteal phases.

Age-related declines in female fertility may in part reflect declines in male fertility. There is evidence of declining testicular androgen production after the age of 30 due to a deterioration of Leydig cells and decreases in spermatogenesis after maturity. The impact of these biological changes in male fertility and consequently on the reproductive potential of the female is difficult to quantify. Anderson (1975), however, was able to demonstrate a significant decline in fertility among Irish men over the age of 57, controlling for duration of marriage and the age of the spouse. This change was substantiated by Mineau and Trussell's (1982) model-derived estimates reported in Table 5.3.

Decline in likelihood of a foetus to live birth. Other biological factors causing age-related decreases in female fertility are mediated through increasing rates of spontaneous foetal wastage, which in turn are believed to be due largely to chromosomal abnormalities. Although there are recognized problems in estimating foetal wastage (early in gestation it is difficult to distinguish between menstrual irregularity and foetal wastage, and recall may be biased due to the stigma attached to induced abortions), at least 10 to 15 per cent of all pregnancies result in foetal wastage (Leridon, 1975). Foetal wastage increases with age at all levels of parity and gravidity in prospective studies (Shapiro *et al.*, 1970; Naylor, 1974; Leridon, 1975). 60 per cent of all spontaneous abortions at less than twelve weeks (which constitute the vast majority of abortions) have chromosomal abnormalities; it is well documented that the risk of chromosomal abnormalities increases with maternal age (Lazar *et al.*, 1973; Creasy *et al.*, 1976).

Other biological factors. A number of other factors have been suggested as causes of declines in age-specific fertility. Medical conditions which may lead to increased rates of spontaneous foetal wastage and premature sterility include venereal syphilis, malaria, and obstetrical and genital tract trauma in the case of spontaneous foetal loss, and gonorrhoea, genital tuberculosis and post-partum and post-abortal sepsis and obstetrical trauma in the case of premature sterility. Except in the case of specialized populations with high rates of the above medical conditions (e.g. in parts of Africa), these factors are unlikely to account for a large part of the decline in marital fertility with age. The increased delay between the deposition of sperm and ovulation due to the decline in coital frequency with age may lead to over-ripe gametes with a lower probability of conception. Uterine abnormalities (e.g. fibroids or carcinoma), which increase with age, may lead to an inhospitable uterine environment for implantation (Gray, 1979*a*). The latter two causes are theoretically plausible but no data exist documenting their contribution to declines in old-age fertility.

Conclusion

The decline in age-specific marital fertility results from a complex interaction of social and biological factors. For many societies, the social factors are primarily mediated through a decline in coital frequency with age, and the biological factors are largely due to increased foetal losses with age, which, in turn, are caused by increases in chromosomal abnormalities with age. Among healthy women who are postponing childbearing, the rise in infertility is gradual and modest until the late thirties. As yet, however, there is no satisfactory explanation for the wide variations in proportions of women who, in their thirties, are sterile and infecund. The extent to which disease and reproductive impairment contribute to these differentials is not known. This situation is not surprising when we consider three factors: the difficulty of measuring infertility, the fact that reasonable data for a full range of countries are only recently available, and the lack, until quite recently, of appropriate methods for analysing such data. The collection of data by the Demographic and Health Surveys which is now underway should improve the situation and make possible more extensive analysis of trends and differentials in sterility and infertility. One of the issues that must be addressed is the priority that should be attached to such an undertaking: why do we want to know what these levels and differentials are, and how would this information affect our recommendations for health and population policy?

References

Anderson, B. A. (1975), 'Male Age and Fertility: Results from Ireland prior to 1911', *Population Index* 41: 561–6.
Barrett, J. C., and Marshall, J. (1969), 'The Risk of Conception on Different Days of the Menstrual Cycle', *Population Studies* 23: 455.
Bongaarts, J. (1982), 'Infertility after Age 30: A False Alarm', *Family Planning Perspectives* 14(2): 75–8.
—— (1983), 'The Proximate Determinants of Natural Marital Fertility', in R. A. Bulatao and R. D. Lee (eds.), *Determinants of Fertility in Developing Countries: Supply and Demand for Children*: 103–38, Academic Press, New York.
Caldwell, J. C., and Caldwell, P. (1977), 'The Role of Marital Sexual Abstinence in Determining Fertility: A Study of the Yoruba in Nigeria', *Population Studies* 31: 193–218.
Cartwright, A. (1976), *How many Children?*, Routledge & Kegan Paul, London.
Chiazze, L., Brayer, F. T., Macisco, I. J., Parker, M. P., and Duffy, B. J. (1968), 'The Length and Variability of the Human Menstrual Cycle', *Journal of the American Medical Association* 20: 377–88.
Coale, A., and Trussell, J. (1974), 'Model Fertility Schedules: Variation in the Age Structure of Childbearing in Human Populations', *Population Index* 40: 185–201.
Creasy, M. R., Crolla, J. A., and Alberman, E. D. (1976), 'A Cytogenetic Study of Human Spontaneous Abortion Using Banding Techniques', *Human Genetics* 31: 177.
Doring, G. K. (1969), 'The Incidence of Anovular Cycles in Women', *Journal of Reproduction and Fertility* 6 (supplement): 256–63.
Fédération CECOS, Schwartz, D., Mayaux, M. J. (1982), 'Female Fecundity as a

Function of Age: Results of Artificial Insemination in 2193 Nulliparous Women with Azoospermic Husbands, *New England Journal of Medicine* 306: 404–6.

Gray, R. (1976), 'The Menopause: Epidemiological and Demographic Considerations, in R. J. Beard, (ed.), *The Menopause*: 25–40, MTP Press, London.

—— (1979*a*), 'Biological and Social Interactions in the Determination of Late Fertility', *Journal of Biosocial Sciences* 6 (supplement): 97–115.

—— (1979*b*), 'Biological Factors other than Nutrition and Lactation which may Influence Natural Fertility: A Review', in H. Leridon and J. Menken (eds.), *Natural Fertility*: 217–50, Ordina Editions, Liège, Belgium.

Henry, L. (1965), 'French Statistical Research in Natural Fertility', in M. Sheps and J. C. Ridley, (eds.), *Public Health and Population Changes*: 333–50, University of Pittsburgh Press, Pittsburgh.

Kannel, W. B., Hjortland, M. C., McNamara, P. M., and Gordon, T. (1976), 'Menopause and Risk of Cardiovascular Disease: The Framingham Study', *Annals of Internal Medicine* 85: 447–52.

Karim, A., Chowdhury, A. K. M. A., and Kabir, A. (1985), 'Nutritional Status and Age at Secondary Sterility in Rural Bangladesh', *Journal of Biosocial Sciences* 17: 497–502.

Knodel, J. (1978), 'Natural Fertility in Preindustrial Germany', *Population Studies* 32: 481–510.

—— (1983), 'Natural Fertility: Age Patterns, Levels, and Trends', in R. A. Bulatao and R. D. Lee (eds.), *Determinants of Fertility in Developing Countries: Supply and Demand for Children*: 61–102, Academic Press, New York.

Kremer, J. (1982), 'Factors Affecting Pregnancy Rate after AID', in E. S. E. Hafez and K. Semm (eds.), *Instrumental Insemination*: 193–6, Matinus Nijhoff, The Hague.

Larsen, U., and Menken, J. (1989), 'Measuring Sterility from Incomplete Birth Histories', *Demography* 26(2): 185–201.

Lazar, P., Gueguen, S., Boué, J., and Boué, A. (1973), 'Épidémiologie des avortements spontanés précoces: à propos de 1,409 avortements caryotypés', in A. Boué and C. Thibault (eds.), *Chromosomal Errors in Relation to Reproductive Failure*: 317, proceedings of the symposia sponsored by Institut National de la Recherche Médicale and Organization Mondiale de la Santé, Centre International de l'Enfance, Paris.

Leridon, H. (1975), 'Biostatistics of Human Reproduction', in C. Chandrasekaran, and A. I. Hermalin (eds.), *Measuring the Effects of Family Planning Programs on Fertility*: 93–131, Ordina Editions, Dolhain, Belgium.

—— (1977), 'Sur l'estimation de la stérilité', *Population* 32 (numéro special): 231–45.

Lindquist, O., Bengtsson, C., Hansson, T., and Roos, B. (1981), 'Bone Mineral Content in Relation to Age and Menopause in Middle-Aged Women', *Scandinavian Journal of Clinical Laboratory Investigation* 41: 215–23.

McKinlay, S. M., Bifano, N. L., and McKinlay, J. B. (1985), 'Smoking and Age at Menopause in Women', *Annals of Internal Medicine* 103: 350–6.

MacMahon, B., and Worcester, J. (1966), *Age at Menopause: United States 1960–61*, U.S. Vital and Health Statistics Monographs, series 11, no. 19, Government Printing Office, Washington.

Menken, J., and Larsen, U. (1986), 'Fertility Rates and Aging', in L. Mastroianni and C. A. Paulsen (eds.), *Ageing, Reproduction, and the Climacteric*: 147–66, Plenum Press, New York.

—— Trussell, J., and Larsen, U. (1986), 'Age and Infertility', *Science* 233: 1389–94.

Mineau G., and Trussell, J. (1982), 'A Specification of Marital Fertility by Parents' Age, Age at Marriage, and Marital Duration', *Demography* 19(3): 335–50.

Nag, M. (1972), 'Sex, Culture and Human Fertility: India and the United States', *Current Anthropology* 13: 231–41.

Naylor, A. F. (1974), 'Sequential Aspects of Spontaneous Abortions: Maternal Age, Parity and Pregnancy Compensation Artifact', *Social Biology* 21: 195–201.

Opler, J. (1964), 'Cultural Context and Population Control Programs in Village India', in E. Court and G. Bowles (eds.), *Fact and Theory in Social Science*, Syracuse University Press, Syracuse: 362–8.

Ruzicka, L. T., and Bhatia, S. (1982), 'Coital Frequency in Bangladesh', *Journal of Biosocial Sciences* 14: 401–20.

Scragg, R. F. R. (1973), 'Menopause and Reproductive Life Span in Rural New Guinea', paper presented at the Annual Symposium of the Papua/New Guinea Medical Society, Port Moresby.

Shapiro, S., Levine, H. S., and Abramowicz, Z. (1970), 'Factors Associated with Early and Late Foetal Loss', in *Advances in Planned Parenthood*, Proceedings of the VIIIth American Association of Planned Parenthood Physicians Meeting, vi: 45, Excerpta Medica, Amsterdam.

Trussell, J., and Wilson, C. (1985), 'Sterility in a Population with Natural Fertility', *Population Studies* 39: 269–86.

United Nations (1961), *The Mysore Population Study: A Co-operative Project of the United Nations and the Government of India*, United Nations, New York.

Vaessen, M. (1984), *Childlessness and Infecundity*, World Fertility Studies Comparative Studies no. 31, International Statistical Institute, Voorburg, the Netherlands.

Van Keep, P. A., Brand, P. C., and Lehert, P. (1979), 'Factors Affecting the Age at Menopause', *Journal of Biosocial Sciences* 6 (supplement): 37–55.

Vessey, M. P., Wright, N. H., McPherson, K., and Wiggins, P. (1978), 'Fertility after Stopping Different Methods of Contraception', *British Medical Journal* 1(4 Feb.), 6108: 265–7.

Ware, H. (1979), 'Social Influences on Fertility at Later Ages of Reproduction', *Journal of Biosocial Sciences* 6 (supplement): 75–96.

Weiss, E. and Udo, A. A. (1981), 'The Calabar Rural Maternal and Child Health/Family Planning Project', *Studies in Family Planning* 12: 47–57.

6 Coitus as Demographic Behaviour

J. RICHARD UDRY

The scientific study of coitus is not solely justified by its status as a demographic behaviour, that is, by the fact that it has relationships to reproduction. From the point of view of the participant, it has intrinsic interest. From the point of view of the biologist or sociologist, the determinants of coital behaviour may be just as interesting as the consequences. From the point of view of the social scientist, the import of coitus goes far beyond its reproductive consequences into fundamental dimensions of human relationships. As contraception becomes more nearly perfect and as other means of conception control are perfected, the significance of coitus as consummatory behaviour comes more and more to the forefront.

In this paper, I will discuss some basic dimensions of coitus which have been of interest to demographers and omit dimensions which are no less important sociologically, but whose demographic consequences are less easy to discuss. I will omit the question of who copulates with whom. I will focus on the frequency of coitus and its determinants, but defer to others concerning the consequences of frequency. I will discuss temporal and biological rhythms of coitus, but defer to others concerning the consequences of these rhythms. Finally, I will discuss the measurement of coitus and how measurement techniques depend on the purposes of the measurement.

Frequency of Coitus

Demographic interest in frequency of coitus is intuitively easy to comprehend. Since, from the behavioural perspective, coitus is the proximate cause of conception, the differences between some coitus and no coitus is related to the difference between some probability of conception and none.

Various models have been constructed of the relationship between coital frequency and probability of conception (Lachenbruch, 1967). These models generally agree that variance in the low frequencies (below 10 per cycle) are more important than variance in the high frequencies (above 10 per cycle). In real populations of copulating couples, the means and variances of frequencies vary by a few known factors, while between populations the variance in means is considerable. Anthropologists have informally reported coital frequencies averaging more than three times per day, but these reports are to be taken with some scepticism. Table 6.1 shows the frequency of marital coitus in two

TABLE 6.1. *Mean monthly frequency of marital intercourse by age of respondent for married women*

Age of respondent (years)	Thailand, 1969			Japan, 1975			Belgium, 1975		
	Mean	SD	No.	Mean	SD	No.	Mean	SD	No.
Total	6.42	6.48	795	8.3	4.8	617	10.03	5.52	3987
<25	7.97	7.30	173	10.5	5.0	110	12.48	6.46	911
25–34	6.11	5.64	377	8.2	4.7	390	10.45	5.16	1545
35–44	5.85	6.90	245	6.6	4.4	117	8.15	8.15	1531

United States

	NFS 1965			NFS 1970			FPEP 1974		
	Mean	SD	No.	Mean	SD	No.	Mean	SD	No.
Total	6.9	5.2	3512	8.5	7.0	4560	9.5	8.2	1633
<25	9.2	6.7	706	10.6	8.7	1093	11.6	9.1	565
25–34	7.2	4.9	1344	8.9	6.8	1935	9.2	7.7	781
35–44	5.5	4.0	1462	6.5	5.1	1532	5.9	5.8	287

Note: NFS: National Fertility Survey; FPEP: Family Planning Evaluation Project.
Source: Udry *et al.*, 1982.

Western and two Eastern countries, based on surveys in the last couple of decades, for couples at reproductive ages. The means per month range from 6 to 10, but the standard deviations are sometimes as large as the means and sometimes half the size of the means. One standard deviation below the mean puts us into the 'low' frequency range in nearly every sample. Thus, much of the variance in coital frequency is in the range which, according to demographic models, should have substantial effects on the probability of conception. However, it is also clear from Table 6.1 that the variance in frequency should have more effect in the older than the younger age groups. Fig. 6.1 compares frequencies of marital coitus by age for the Kinsey female sample (Kinsey *et al.*, 1953) and the 1982 National Study of Family Growth (Pratt *et al.*, 1984). This gives an interesting picture of the changes in coital frequencies reported over a half century. While the overall pattern is one of stability over time, there is a distinct shift from lower to higher coital frequencies in the 41–5 age-group.

Determinants of Frequency of Coitus

What determines the frequency of coitus? The best known determinants are age and duration of marriage. Cross-sectional studies of the effects of age are

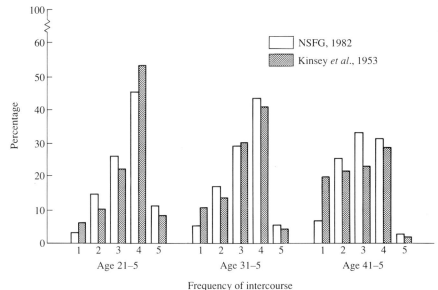

1 = once a month   2 = 2 or 3 times a month
3 = once a week   4 = several times a week
5 = almost every day or every other day

Fig. 6.1   Frequency of intercourse for married women, comparison of Kinsey *et al.*, 1953, with NFSG III, 1982

all congruent in their finding that frequency of coitus declines with age (see Table 6.1). During the reproductive years, this decline is associated with the age of the wife (Udry and Morris, 1979), while during the older years, it is associated with the age of the husband. This is probably primarily a biological phenomenon, since it occurs in all mammals, but it certainly has some social components.

One exception to this pattern of declining coital frequency with age is the anomalous finding of Jasso (1985) that male frequency declines with age, while female frequency increases with age. Since we are talking about the frequency of marital coitus, it would take a mathematical model of Ptolemaic complexity to reconcile the opposite effects among males and females. However, Kahn and I (1986) have shown this finding to be associated with data errors and misspecification and not to be taken seriously.

There are two panel-data studies which allow us to answer the question of whether the observed declines with age are true ageing effects of cohort effects. Jasso (1985) showed that between 1970 and 1975, among the couples of the NFS (National Fertility Survey) panel, copulations declined in frequency at a rate of .15 copulations per month per year. Udry and Morris (1979) showed that our panel of married couples under age 30 experienced a decline in frequency of copulations per month per year of .59.

It is somewhat difficult to separate the effects of age from the effects or duration of marriage. In the data-sets we have examined, coital frequency during the first year of marriage declines by 50 per cent and then enters a period of relative stability with only slight declines over the next decade, but with greater declines at durations of over 20 years (James, 1981). Whether the newly-wed phenomenon will survive the current trend towards couples establishing sexual relationships and cohabitation before marriage remains to be seen.

Data by Westoff *et al.* (1969) from the 1965 NFS suggests that use of the contraceptive pill increases coital frequency. In a double-blind controlled experiment with random assignment to treatment and control groups, Morris and I showed that, even with pills with much higher dosage than those used today, contraceptive pills have no effect on frequency of coitus (Morris and Udry, 1978). This experiment shows that there is no biological effect of pills on frequency. Thus, the relationship observed by Westoff and colleagues must be due either to selection or to psychological effects.

A considerable amount of research has examined the effect of steroid hormone levels on coital frequency and sexual interest levels (see Bancroft and Skakkebaek, 1978, for a review). Studies of normal populations show no effects of androgen levels on coital frequency for either men or women and ambiguous effects on sexual interest. However, this does not mean that androgens are irrelevant, but only that the influence of androgens on sexual behaviour is subject to ceiling effects. Almost all adult males have androgen levels higher than that required for normal sexual behaviour. Among adults of both sexes with abnormally low androgen levels, sexual interest and coital frequency are low. Among adolescents of both sexes, increasing androgen levels are associated with increased interest in sex and, for males, with increased probability of coitus (Udry *et al.*, 1985, 1986).

Several studies have examined sociological determinants of frequency of coitus in population samples, but a lack of theory to guide the search has resulted in non-comparable and inconsistent findings. Generally we must agree with Kinsey that the usual sociological categories of education, occupation, religion, and the like show no reliable relationships with frequency of coitus. In a sample of mine from the mid-1970s, I prepared the data shown in Table 6.2 predicting coital frequency as reported by women.

Among the more interesting observations on frequency of coitus in the US are secular trends. Kinsey's data shows that frequency of marital coitus declined substantially over the first decades of this century. Recent data from the National Fertility Surveys indicate increases in coital frequency from 1965 to 1970 in all age cohorts (Westoff, 1974). Kinsey *et al.* (1953) attribute the early declines to decreasing attentiveness on the part of males to female sexual interest. I attribute the increase since 1965 to the increasing sexualization of society. As increasingly positive value is placed on sex by the culture and sexual messages and stimulation become ubiquitous, everyone thinks about sex more.

TABLE 6.2. *Multiple regression of frequency of intercourse per month against selected social variables*

A. Married women aged 15–44, husband present

	b	Beta	F	Cumulative R^2
Whites (N = 1288)				
Age	−0.20	−0.17	34.55[a]	.05
IUD use	4.03	0.13	22.23[a]	.07
IQ	0.04	0.09	11.78[a]	.07
Age at first pregnancy	−0.23	−0.10	12.20[a]	.08
Pill use	1.82	0.11	13.82[a]	.09
Religious affiliation	−3.53	−0.07	7.56[a]	.10
Male sterilized	2.36	0.07	6.64[a]	.10
Lived with natural father while growing up	−0.86	−0.04	2.52	.10
Blacks (N = 598)				
Age	−0.15	−0.14	7.82[a]	.03
Religious participation	0.78	0.16	16.18[a]	.05
Protestant	−5.32	−0.19	16.80[a]	.07
Age of husband	−0.06	−0.08	2.53	.08
Farm birthplace	0.82	0.09	4.31[a]	.08
Other religious affiliation	−5.07	−0.08	3.47	.09
IQ	0.02	0.06	2.37	.09
Husband's education	0.18	0.06	2.02	.10

B. Ever-married women aged 15–44 without husbands

	b	Beta	F	Cumulative R^2
Whites (N = 243)				
Age	−0.17	−0.18	6.79[a]	.06
Pill use	2.29	0.16	6.40[a]	.08
IQ	0.04	0.12	3.92[a]	.10
Neat house interior	−1.24	−0.14	5.21[a]	.11
Religious affiliation	−4.41	−0.11	3.33	.12
Number of children	−0.43	−0.11	2.44	.13
Farm birthplace	0.77	0.09	2.00	.14
Blacks (N = 362)				
Age at first intercourse	−0.78	−0.26	15.08[a]	.03
Household income	0.41	0.14	7.26[a]	.06
Religiosity	−1.01	−0.11	4.45[a]	.07
Pill use	1.38	0.09	3.04	.07
Age at first pregnancy	0.26	0.12	3.43	.08
Prettiness	0.78	0.08	2.66	.09

[a] Significant beyond the .05 level.

Source: Udry, 1979.

Cycles of Coitus

Five rhythmic aspects of coitus have received attention in the literature:

(1) Distribution throughout the day
(2) Distribution by day of the week
(3) Distribution throughout the menstrual cycle
(4) Annual or seasonal cycles

We have examined the daily coital rhythm of several samples of married women with husbands present (Palmer *et al.*, 1982). The same pattern recurs in each sample, with about two-thirds of the copulations occurring between 10 pm and 1 am. This pattern is a little different on Saturday and Sunday, with a small increase also occurring about 7 am. It would be interesting to see what rhythms are shown by couples in which both spouses work, but on different shifts.

Weekly rhythms also occur in all the samples we have observed, with elevated rates on weekends, particularly Sunday (Palmer *et al.*, 1982). In a small sample of women who worked rotating days of the week, this pattern was obliterated (Udry and Morris, 1970). It would be interesting to compare coital rhythms by day of the week in countries where Christians and Muslims live in the same areas.

Speculation has appeared in the literature concerning possible seasonal rhythms of coitus which might drive the seasonal pattern of births found in all populations. In one small sample of married women, for which we had up to 2 years of daily reports, we found a seasonal coital pattern, but it could not be reconciled with seasonal patterns of birth in the US population (Udry and Morris, 1979). It is unlikely that anyone will try to replicate our findings, because of the enormous data-collection effort involved.

Demographers have been interested in the distribution of coitus throughout the menstrual cycle. The literature on this topic goes back more than fifty years. The empirical literature is difficult to interpret because of the differences in methods used to collect and analyse the data. The interest driving the research is twofold. First, there is the fact that only coitions around the time of ovulation can produce conceptions. However, it is still not possible, even with the most sophisticated methods, to determine with certainty when an ovulation has taken place. If there are five copulations per cycle and they are evenly or randomly distributed in the cycle, then the probability of conception is obviously going to be lower than if the five are grouped around the time of ovulation.

The second reason for interest in the menstrual distribution of coitus is that if there are distinct patterns of coitus, they may indicate a hormonal engine driving the coital rhythm, since each part of the menstrual cycle has its own distinctive hormonal composition.

For twenty years I have been tracking the distribution of coitus within the menstrual cycle. There is no easy way to summarize the findings of the studies that I and others have conducted on the topic. Progress has come slowly and is closely related to methodological developments. If women are asked retrospectively to report at what time of their cycle they have coitus most frequently they tell you before and after menses. Every sample that anyone has studied shows a substantial proportion avoiding or reducing frequency of coitus during menses, especially during the days of heavy flow. The reported pattern is easy to interpret as due to anticipation of and release from a period of abstinence. Morris and I have shown that the avoidance of coitus during menses is due to the woman's lack of interest rather than the man's avoidance (Morris and Udry, 1983). However, all scholars realize that retrospective reports covering even a week are highly unreliable for the purpose of delineating any of the cycles of coitus discussed in this paper. This is why, from the beginning, I and my colleagues have always used daily reports, collected daily to avoid backfilling. In some studies we have collected daily reports independently from both husband and wife. Comparison of husband and wife reports gives almost 100 per cent concordance.

If you want to look at the distribution of coitus in a single menstrual cycle of an individual woman, all you have to do is to collect daily reports of menses and coitus and make a graph. It would be easy to combine reports from the same woman for different cycles and to combine cyclic reports from many women, if all menstrual cycles were the same length. Alas, variation within and between women in cycle length is very great. This raises the problem of how to combine data for cycles of different lengths, when all you have is a marker for menstruation. Several different techniques have been reported. Forward cycle days is the most straightforward, but the short cycles start dropping out at about 22 days. It has long been believed, and subsequently corroborated, that the number of days from ovulation to menses is less variant than the number of days from menses to ovulation. If lining up ovulations is what you are interested in, then it would appear that reverse cycle days would be a better method. In this case, the early part of the cycle is dispersed as cycles of different length are combined. The Gold–Adams (1978) technique arbitrarily assigns days to groups representing parts of the cycle. The standardized cycle-day method compresses data from long cycles and stretches out data from short cycles. Morris and I have shown that if you take the same data and array it by each method, you can come up with just about whatever pattern you like (Udry and Morris, 1977).

At my first meeting of the Population Association of American in 1967, I reported data from a sample of women organized by reverse cycle days which showed a distinct mid-cycle peak and a luteal trough, with a recovery at the end of the cycle (Udry and Morris, 1968). Ever since then, the debate has been over whether or not there is a mid-cycle peak. After Morris and I published these data in *Nature*, James (1971) combined several data-sets—of varying quality and collected with different methods—into sets of cycles with equal length. He showed no mid-cycle peak. Since then he has held the high ground. He attributed our mid-cycle peak to a post-menstrual concentration after menstrual abstinence in short cycles. We have shown that this is not the case. Others have contributed to this debate. We have found similar patterns in other samples, but in some we have not found any cyclicity at all. In one of our most intriguing study results, we examined the effects of contraceptive pills on coital distribution, using a random assignment, double blind, controlled experiment, with an a–b–a design (Udry *et al.*, 1973). We found that in initial control cycles, women showed a mid-cycle peak and a luteal trough. When women went on the contraceptive pill, the luteal trough was weakened in its depth in the first cycle and obliterated in the second. We attributed the trough to the effects of endogenous progesterone and its obliteration to the suppression of ovulation (and therefore endogenous progesterone) by the pill.

I have long since held the conclusion that little can be learned beyond our present knowledge by organizing cycles around menstrual markers, if our interest is either in the timing of coitus with respect to ovulation or the relationship between hormones and behaviour. If you want to see how ovulation and coitus are related, you have to have a measurement for when ovulation occurs. The necessity for this was shown by Farris 30 years ago when he first showed the wide dispersal of days on which ovulation presumably occurred. If you want to study hormone–behaviour relationships, you must measure the hormones you think are causally related to the behaviour. Furthermore, you cannot rely on a method in which the timing of ovulation is only approximate if you expect to learn anything. You must know the exact day on which ovulation occurred.

Morris and I first approached this problem in the mid-1970s by taking daily blood samples from forward cycle day 10 to day 20 and assaying the serum for LH (luteinizing hormone) (Morris *et al.*, 1977). We assumed that ovulation occurred on the day of the LH peak. Even here we failed to identify some LH peaks, either because none occurred or because they occurred after day 20. Not many subjects will tolerate the daily venipuncture, and, besides, it is expensive and difficult to arrange for free-ranging humans to be venipunctured daily at a certain time. Some other method is needed. LH cannot be measured in saliva, but it can be measured in urine. Unfortunately, most other steroids of interest are only represented in urine by their metabolites. Even so, glucuronides and pregnanediol in urine give reliable substitutes for oestrogen and progesterone profiles, respectively. LH assays have been refined so that they can pick up the fragments of LH molecules in urine. Work today therefore should rely on one or more of these assays to identify the time of ovulation if one wants to study the distribution of coitus within the menstrual cycle.

In our most recent study, based on a sample of urban women in residential sexual relationships in Harare, Zimbabwe, we approached the coital cyclicity problem again, taking our own advice (Hedricks *et al.*, 1987). For these women, we collected daily urine samples at their homes each morning. On the urine container the woman marked whether or not she had menstruated and whether or not she had had coitus in the previous 24 hours. We assayed the urine for LH and plotted LH profiles for cycles. Inevitably, some days have missing urines. Inevitably, the cycles do not look as neat as the textbook examples. Unaccountably, some of the cycles have two LH peaks, and, predictably, some have no LH peak at all.

We now have the problem of determining when ovulation occurred and how we should relate coital events to the timing of ovulation. We identified the LH surge as the point of impending ovulation, instead of the peak. We organized the coital reports around the LH surge for the beginning of the cycle and around the LH peak for the end of the cycle. We obtained the graph shown in Fig. 6.2. You can see that there is almost a monotonic increase in the probability of coitus from menses to the day of the LH surge. After the LH peak, the probability drops off to below average for the cycle and stays there until near the end of the cycle.

I think the data in Fig. 6.2 make a convincing case for the fact that there is a distribution of coitus in the menstrual cycle which peaks just before ovulation, an ideal time for conception to occur, and declines thereafter. We also showed that the traditional methods of organizing the cycle using menstrual markers would have missed this pattern almost completely. We must therefore reinforce what we said a decade ago, that we must abandon the organization of menstrual

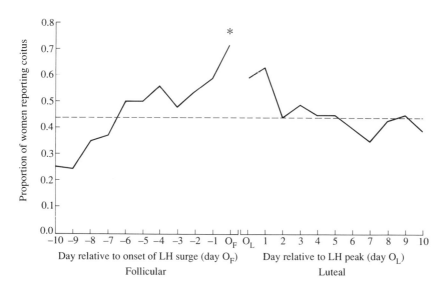

The distribution of coitus during the follicular phase of the cycle was organized around onset of LH surge day (day O_F); the distribution of coitus during the luteal phase of the cycle was organized around LH peak day (day O_L). The dashed horizontal line represents the mean coital rate (0.44 ± 0.06) across a menstrual cycle. The asterisk (*) is a value significantly different from the mean coital rate ($p < .05$).

Fig. 6.2 The distribution of coitus during the follicular and luteal phases of the female cycle

data by menstrual markers alone and use hormone measurements to get at the theoretical basis of the phenomenon of interest. Assuming that you are convinced that there is a non-linear rhythm of coitus in the menstrual cycle which increases the probability of conception beyond what one would obtain from a constant or random coital pattern, then what is the proximate mechanism which maintains the pattern?

Morris and I have devoted considerable attention to the proximate mechanisms of the mid-cycle peak and luteal trough. We do not believe that the peak in female testosterone at mid-cycle is a good explanation for the mid-cycle peak in coitus, because testosterone effects in other studies seem to have a considerable time-lag, with effects related to cumulative continuing levels of testosterone rather than to transitory changes. We conducted an intricate experiment (Morris and Udry, 1979) using a hypothesized sexual pheromone identified by Michael and Bonsall. In this double-blind, randomized treatment experiment, women anointed themselves nightly before retiring with one of four random treatments, one of which has the putative pheromone. Unfortunately the results of the experiment were ambiguous, since the sample turned out to be the only one we have studied which showed no cyclical pattern of coitus. We are inclined to believe that the luteal trough we have observed is a progesterone effect which works directly by reducing female sexual interest. Early work with high-progesterone contraceptive pills documented definite loss of sexual interest as one of the most common side-effects (Morris and Udry, 1971), not found in low-progesterone pills (Adams *et al.*, 1978). We are still inclined to believe that the rise in coital frequency in the follicular phase up to ovulation is a pheromone effect which is attributable to the effect on males of an oestrogen by-product, but we have not satisfactorily documented this.

Measurement of Coital Behaviour

The measurement of coitus is fraught with methodological problems. How to measure it is inextricably bound to the purpose of the measurement. When the exact placement of each coital episode on a particular day or time of day is important, there is no substitute for daily reporting. The validation of such reports requires an external criterion which is hard to come by. Morris and I did a validity study of daily reports (Udry and Morris, 1967*a*). It was based on examining daily urine specimens for sperm and therefore is only a one-way test (presence of sperm means coitus, but absence of sperm means nothing). This test showed that two women in a sample of 35 provided daily reports of coitus which were substantially inconsistent with sperm observations. Another test is comparison of husband and wife reports. This test has shown more than 99 per cent congruence in reports in our studies. However, Leridon (1986) obtained discrepant and paradoxical results from comparison of reports from spouses.

Measuring frequency of coitus can, of course, also be done from daily reports, but we often wish to obtain information on frequency of coitus where the specific timing of coitions is of no interest. We want to ask survey respondents to give us an estimate of their coital frequency over some period of weeks. Researchers have tried many different formats. The most common question asks frequency over the past 4 weeks. Since it is absurd to imagine that respondents are actually recalling and summing individual episodes, how do we think they arrive at an answer to such a question? From other studies of cognitive processes in arriving at answers to questions with a similar structure, we can imagine that they take some shorter time-period that they can remember, say a week, and multiply to arrive at a response. To avoid imposing this task, we have sometimes given the respondent a week's calendar, and ask them to indicate the days on which they have had coitus. Another technique we have used asks, 'Did you have sex today? Yesterday? The day before yesterday? And what about the day before that?' (Udry, 1968). These latter two techniques simplify the cognitive task at the cost of getting a measure which is sensitive to perturbations by day of interview, time of day, menstrual status, or passing whim.

No studies have been done which show the relative validity of various ways of asking frequency of coitus. Morris and I have compared the frequencies we compute from daily reports over 100 days with an estimate made at the end of the period by the respondents of average frequency during the same period. The two estimates produce distributions with the same mean and standard deviation, and the two estimates correlate well with one another. But this comparison was made in a situation which might strengthen recall and therefore exaggerates the validity estimate. Clark and Wallin (1964) found that husband and wife reports of frequency correlate rather well, but are subject to psychological responses to the frequency. Wives who state that they would prefer a lower coital frequency report frequencies higher than their husbands report; while wives who state they would prefer a higher coital frequency report frequencies that are the same as their husbands report.

Since coital frequency has become a routine question in fertility surveys, it would be worthwhile to build some validity checks into the questionnaire. At least, we might ask the question two ways in the same questionnaire to find out how the estimates differ and how they correlate with other variables. The Demographic and Health Surveys programme is fielding questionnaires in some countries using two different questions to measure coital frequency. Even better, we might profit from some exploration of the cognitive steps by which respondents answer such questions, to see if we like the way they are arriving at the answer. I suspect we will learn some things we don't want to know.

References

Adams, D. B., Gold, A. R., and Burt, A. D. (1978), 'Rise in Female Initiated Sexual Activity at Ovulation and its Suppression by Oral Contraceptives', *New England Journal of Medicine* 299: 1145–50.

Bancroft, J., and Skakkebaek, N. (1978), 'Androgens and Human Sexual Behavior', in *Ciba Foundation Symposium 62* (NS): 209–26, Exerpta Medica, Amsterdam.

Clark, A. L., and Wallin, P. (1964), 'The Accuracy of Husbands' and Wives' Reports of the Frequency of Marital Coitus', *Population Studies* 18: 165–73.

Gold, A. R., and Adams, D. B. (1978), 'Measuring the Cycles of Female Sexuality', *Contemporary Obstetrics and Gynecology* 12: 147–56.

Hedricks, C., Piccinino, L., Udry, J. R., and Chimbira, T. T. K. (1987), 'Peak Coital Rate Coincides with Onset of Luteinizing Hormone (LH) Surge', *Fertility and Sterility* 49(2): 235–56.

James, W. H. (1971), 'The Distribution of Coitus within the Human Intermenstrum', *Journal of Biosocial Science* 3: 159–71.

—— (1981), 'The Honeymoon Effect on Marital Coitus', *Journal of Sex Research* 17: 114–23.

Jasso, G. (1985), 'Marital Coital Frequency and the Passage of Time: Estimating the Separate Effects of Spouses' Ages and Marital Duration, Birth and Marriage Cohorts, and Period Influences', *American Sociological Review* 50: 224–41.

Kahn, J. R., and Udry, J. R. (1986), 'Marital Coital Frequency: Unnoticed Outliers and Unspecified Interactions Lead to Erroneous Conclusions', *American Sociological Review* 51: 734–7.

Kinsey, A. C., Pomeroy, W. B., Martin, C. E., and Gebhard, P. H. (1953), *Sexual Behavior in the Human Female*, Saunders, Philadelphia, Pa.

Lachenbruch, P. A. (1967), 'Frequency and Timing of Intercourse: Its Relation to the Probability of Conception', *Population Studies* 20: 23–31.

Leridon, H. (1986), 'La Comparison des réponses données par les deux conjoints d'un même couple: problèmes d'observation, de codage et de saisie', in *Demographie et Sociologie*: 147–66, Publications de la Sorbonne, Paris.

Morris, N. M., and Udry, J. R. (1971), 'Sexual Frequency and Contraceptive Pills', *Social Biology* 18: 40–5.

—— —— (1978), 'Pherhormonal Influences on Human Sexual Behavior: An Experiment Search', *Journal of Biosocial Science* 10: 147–57.

—— —— (1983), 'Menstruation and Marital Sex', *Journal of Biosocial Science* 15: 173–83.

—— Underwood, L., and Udry, J. R. (1977), 'A Study of the Relationship between Coitus and the Luteinizing Hormone Surge', *Fertility and Sterility* 28: 440–2.

Palmer, J. D., Morris, N. M., and Udry, J. R. (1982), 'Diurnal and Weekly but no Lunar rhythms in Marital Coitus', *Human Biology*, 54(1): 111–21.

Pratt, W. F., Mosher, W. D., Bachrach, C. A., and Horn, M. (1984), 'Understanding US Fertility: Findings from the National Survey of Family Growth, Cycle III', *Population Bulletin* 39: 3–42.

Udry, J. R. (1968), 'Coital Frequency, Delayed Fertilization, and outcome of Pregnancy', *Nature* 219: 618–19.

—— (1979), 'Changes in the Frequency of Marital Intercourse from Panel Data', *Archives of Sexual Behavior* 94: 319–25.

—— and Morris, N. M. (1967a), 'A Method for Validation of Reported Sexual Data', *Journal of Marriage and the Family* 29: 442–6.

—— —— (1967b), 'Seasonality of Coitus and Seasonality of Birth', *Demography* 4(2): 673–9.

—— —— (1968), 'Distribution of Coitus in the Menstrual Cycle', *Nature* 220: 593–6.

Udry, J. R., and Morris, N. M. (1970), 'Frequency of Intercourse by Day of the Week', *Journal of Sex Research* 6: 229–34.

—— —— (1977), 'The Distribution of Events in the Menstrual Cycle', *Journal of Reproduction and Fertility* 51: 419–25.

—— —— and Waller, L. (1973), 'Effect of Contraceptive Pills on Sexual Activity in the Luteal Phase of the Human Menstrual Cycle', *Archives of Sexual Behavior*, 2: 205–14.

—— Deven, F. R., and Coleman, S. (1982), 'A Cross-National Comparison of Marital Intercourse', *Journal of Biosocial Science* 14: 1–6.

—— Talbert, L. M., and Morris, N. M. (1986), 'Biosocial Foundations for Adolescent Female Sexuality', *Demography* 23(2): 217–30.

—— Billy, J. O. G., Morris, N. M., and Groff, T. R. (1985), 'Serum Androgenic Hormones Motivate Sexual Behavior in Adolescent Boys', *Fertility and Sterility* 43(1): 90–4.

Westoff, C. F. (1974), 'Coital Frequency and Contraception', *Family Planning Perspectives* 6: 136–41.

—— Bumpass, L., and Ryder, N. B. (1969), 'Oral Contraception, Coital Frequency, and Time Required to Conceive', *Social Biology* 16: 1–10.

Part III

Biomedical Determinants of Reproduction

7 The Pathophysiology and Epidemiology of Sexually Transmitted Diseases in Relation to Pelvic Inflammatory Disease and Infertility

WILLARD CATES, Jr.

ROBERT T. ROLFS, Jr.

SEVGI O. ARAL

Introduction

Unravelling the relationship among sexually transmitted diseases (STD), pelvic inflammatory disease (PID), and infertility is a complex exercise in aetiological reasoning. It involves examining correlations among conditions with varying definitions, imprecise diagnoses, and a two-phase temporal lag in clinical expression, first from STD to PID, and then from PID to infertility. Our discussion of the pathophysiology and epidemiology of these conditions will distinguish these two phases. In addition, we will draw on the existing imperfect evidence to estimate the current proportion of STD-related infertility in the United States.

Sexually Transmitted Diseases and Pelvic Inflammatory Disease

Diagnosis

The term pelvic inflammatory disease has come to represent clinically suspected endometritis and/or salpingitis that has not been objectively confirmed pathologically or visually (Hager *et al.*, 1983). This diagnosis is usually made in sexually active women who complain of lower abdominal pain and are found to have cervical, uterine, and adnexal tenderness. Although the range is wide, an average of two-thirds of women with this clinical diagnosis actually have laparoscopically-evident salpingitis (Table 7.1). Data indicate using laparoscopy in women with suspected PID to establish a more definitive diagnosis carries no additional economic burden (Method *et al.*, 1987). A higher percentage of visually confirmed salpingitis may be obtained among women with

TABLE 7.1. *Accuracy of clinical diagnosis of PID, by presence of visually confirmed salpingitis and other pathology, selected studies*

Author (Year)	Diagnosis (%)			
	Suspected PID cases	Acute salpingitis	Normal tubes	Other
Jacobson and Westrom (1969)	811	66	23	12
Chaparro *et al.* (1978)	223	46	23	31
Kolmorgen *et al.* (1978)	182	51	18	32
Wolner-Hanssen *et al.* (1983)	104	73	21	5
Allen and Shoon (1983)	103	61	13	26
Brunham *et al.* (1987*b*)	71	70	—30—	
Brihmer *et al.* (1987)	357	52	37	10

Source: Adapted from Table 7 of Eschenbach, 1986, with references updated.

cervical cultures positive for *Neisseria gonorrhoeae* or *Chlamydia trachomatis* or who manifest an elevation of temperature, white blood cells, C-reactive protein, or sedimentation rate (Hadgu *et al.*, 1986).

Other terms describing both lower and upper genital tract infection have been more objectively defied in the past several years. Cervicitis has been characterized by the presence of excessive white blood cells in the cervical mucus, evidenced by the appearance of yellow mucus or of ⩾10 WBC's per 1000 × microscopic field (Brunham *et al.*, 1984). Endometritis has been based on a pathologic diagnosis of plasma cells within the endometrium, which is highly correlated with the isolation of *C. trachomatis* (Paavonen *et al.*, 1985*a*). Salpingitis is diagnosed visually by the presence of erythema, oedema, and either pus or exudate in the tubal area (Jacobson and Westrom, 1969). Pathological and cytological criteria are less commonly used.

Chronic, subacute, and/or latent endometrial/tubal infection may be present in a large number of women, but a consensus definition of these clinically subtle infections is lacking. Endometritis leading to eventual salpingitis has been reported in women with symptoms of PID, but who had normal tubes by laparoscopy (Paavonen *et al.*, 1985*b*). Moreover, endometritis has been found in over one-quarter of women with cervicitis, but who had no PID symptoms (Paavonen *et al.*, 1985*a*). Diagnosing endometritis through objective histological measures may complement laparoscopy as a tool to increase the sensitivity of PID diagnosis.

Microbial Aetiology

Recent investigations have emphasized the polymicrobial nature of PID (Eschenbach *et al.*, 1975; Sweet *et al.*, 1980; Wasserheit *et al.*, 1985; Heinonen *et al.*, 1985). In general, three major groups of micro-organisms are recognized as playing an aetiologic role for PID in the United States: *N. gonorrhoeae*, *C. trachomatis*, and a wide variety of anaerobic and aerobic bacteria.

Genital mycoplasmas have also been recovered from a small number of women, but their role in PID is less clear (Eschenbach, 1986). Many feel *N. gonorrhoeae* and *C. trachomatis* initiate tubal infection, and that anaerobic and aerobic bacteria from the cervix and/or vagina are secondary invaders (Mardh, 1980; Wasserheit, 1987). Bacterial vaginosis (BV) may be a precursor for PID. The organisms involved in BV are similar to the non-gonococcal, non-chlamydial bacteria frequently isolated from the upper genital tract of women with acute PID (Eschenbach, 1980).

The rate at which these micro-organisms have been found in patients with symptomatic PID differs widely, probably because of variations among the populations studied, differences in the time interval during which the investigations took place, and variations in the severity of infection (Table 7.2). *Neisseria gonorrhoeae* has a particularly wide range of recovery rates among women with PID. Cervical *N. gonorrhoeae* has been cultured from 80 per cent of some urban American populations with PID (Thompson *et al.*, 1980). However, not all PID is caused by *N. gonorrhoeae*, and in some European locations the recovery rate of this micro-organism is less than 10 per cent (Henry-Suchet *et al.*, 1980; Moller *et al.*, 1981; Gjonnaess *et al.*, 1982; Moss and Hawkswell, 1986).

In both Europe and North America, more recent investigations have generally found a higher proportion of *C. trachomatis* than *N. gonorrhoeae* in women with symptomatic PID (Table 7.2). In Scandinavia, between one-quarter and one-half of PID was associated with culture and/or serological evidence of *C. trachomatis* infection. Chlamydia has also been isolated in up to 51 per cent of some North American populations suffering from PID (Bowie and Jones, 1981).

In nearly all studies where abdominal cultures were taken, both gonorrhoea and chlamydia were isolated at a lower rate from tubal compared to cervical specimens (Table 7.2). This is not unexpected since extraluminal tubal swabs may not be as efficient in obtaining organisms as endocervical techniques. Chlamydia antibodies, indicative of either present or past infection, were usually found in higher proportions than organisms isolated from the cervix or tubes.

Pathogenesis

The exact mechanism(s) by which micro-organisms reach the upper genital tract has not been elucidated. PID is usually an acute infection in which organisms ascend into the uterus and fallopian tubes from the cervix. Both *N. gonorrhoeae* and *C. trachomatis* commonly cause endocervicitis (Brunham *et al.*, 1984). Between 20 and 40 per cent of women with untreated gonococcal or chlamydia cervicitis develop acute PID (Platt *et al.*, 1983; Stamm *et al.*, 1984).

TABLE 7.2. *Detection of* Chlamydia trachomatis *and* Neisseria gonorrhoeae *among women with acute PID, selected studies*

Author (Year)	Neisseria gonorrhoeae (%)		Chlamydia trachomatis (%)		
	Cervix	Tubes	Cervix	Tubes	Antibody
Europe					
Henry-Suchet *et al.* (1980)	0	25	38	24	—
Moller *et al.* (1981)	5	—	22	—	20
Mardh *et al.* (1977, 1981)	17	7	38	30	37
Gjonnaess *et al.* (1982)	8	0	46	16	40
Adler *et al.* (1982)	18	—	5	—	31
Ripa *et al.* (1980)	19	—	33	—	46
Osser and Persson (1982)	20	—	47	—	51
Paavonen *et al.* (1979, 1980, 1981)	26	—	32	—	26
Moss and Hawkswell (1986)	9	—	41	—	—
Stacey *et al.* (1987)	27	—	44	—	—
Eilard *et al.* (1976)	32	5	27	9	—
North America					
Bowie and Jones (1981)	35	—	51	—	—
Eschenbach *et al.* (1975)	44	13	20	2	20
Sweet and Draper (1981)	46	23	5	0	23
Thompson *et al.* (1980)	80	33	10	10	—
Sweet *et al.* (1983)	40	—	27	—	—
Brunham *et al.* (1987*a*)	—	42	—	16	—
Cramer *et al.* (1987)	27	—	39	—	—

Source: Adapted from Tables 2 and 3 of Eschenbach (1986), with references updated.

A unifying concept to explain the pathogenesis of acute polymicrobial PID has recently been proposed (Wasserheit, 1987). Pelvic inflammatory disease usually starts as a cervical infection with *C. trachomatis* and/or *N. gonorrhoeae* (Fig. 7.1). The cervico-vaginal micro-environment becomes altered as the rapidly growing cervical pathogens consume nutrients and produce metabolic waste products. Changes in parameters such as the availability of oxygen and the pH of the vagina permit overgrowth of endogenous and anaerobic flora, which results in coexistent BV. When host defenses ebb, the original cervical pathogen and/or BV organisms ascend sequentially along contiguous mucosal surfaces into the endometrium, fallopian tubes, and peritoneal cavity (Wolner-Hanssen *et al.*, 1982). Prolonged inflammatory response in association with latent chlamydial infection of the endometrium and/or fallopian tube may further predispose to infection with aerobic and anaerobic bacteria that gain access to these sites (Cleary and Jones, 1985). Ciliary motion may also carry bacteria within the tubes.

The onset of PID symptoms within the first 7 days of the menstrual cycle in

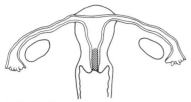

1. Cervical infection (C. trachomatis and/or N. gonorrhoeae).

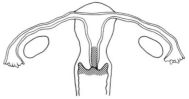

2. Alteration of cervicovaginal micro-environment.

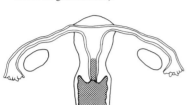

3. Overgrowth of vaginal and anaerobic flora, resulting in BV.

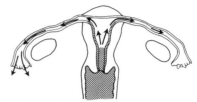

4. Progressive ascent of original cervical pathogen and/or BV anaerobes into the endometrium, fallopian tubes, and the peritoneal cavity.

1. Cervical infection (*Chlamydia trachomatis* and/or *Neisseria gonorrhoeae*.
3. Overgrowth of vaginal facultative and anaerobic flora, resulting in BV.

2. Alteration of cervico-vaginal micro-environment.
4. Progressive ascent of original cervical pathogens and/or BV anaerobes into the endometrium, fallopian tubes, and the peritoneal cavity.

Source: Wasserheit, 1987.

Fig. 7.1   Polymicrobial pathogenesis of sexually transmitted PID

the majority of women with gonococcal and/or chlamydial PID suggests that these organisms disseminate from the cervix to the upper genital tract at the time of menses (Sweet *et al.*, 1985). Cervical mucus appears to be a mechanical barrier preventing bacterial ascent, and its loss during menses may allow the spread of micro-organisms from the cervix into the endometrial cavity. In addition, the bacteriostatic effect of cervical mucus is lowest at the onset of menses (Sweet *et al.*, 1985). No such association with menses was found to exist for non-gonococcal, non-chlamydial PID.

In addition, individual organisms may have potential virulence factors associated with the pathogenesis of acute PID. Gonococcal virulence factors include (1) transparent colony phenotype (Draper *et al.*, 1980); (2) arginine, hypoxanthine, and uracil-requiring auxotype (Knapp *et al.*, 1978); and (3) bactericidal lipopolysaccharide (Gregg *et al.*, 1980). Certain chlamydial proteins, such as the 60kD and 75kD antigens, may be associated with salpingitis (Brunham *et al.*, 1987a) and tubal infertility (Brunham *et al.*, 1985). No specific virulence factors that facilitate the development of acute PID have been identified for the non-gonococcal, non-chlamydial bacteria, nor for the genital mycoplasmas.

Other factors could contribute to the ascent of these bacteria, causing upper genital tract infection. First, the insertion of an IUD or other uterine instrumentation facilitates the upward spread of vaginal and cervical bacteria (Mishell *et al.*, 1966). Second, spermatozoa or trichomonads may carry bacteria from the male urethra or vagina into the upper genital tract (Toth *et al.*, 1982; Keith *et al.*, 1984). Third, ascending infections with a sexually transmitted organism such as cytomegalovirus (CMV) could produce further immunosuppression either locally or systemically, thus facilitating establishment of upper genital tract infections (Hallberg *et al.*, 1985).

Risk Factors

Studies which have examined factors associated with PID have usually failed to distinguish the confounding influence of lower genital tract infections. Because of the role of STD in the pathogenesis of PID, any of the same risk factors/risk markers which are correlated with cervical gonococcal/chlamydial infections would be expected to show a similar association with PID. Moreover, the role of sexual behaviour (other than multiple male partners) as a correlate of PID has been inadequately addressed (Newton and Keith, 1985). Thus, potential risk factors such as frequency of intercourse, timing of coitus, practices of anal and oral sex, number of partners among the male partners of PID patients, age of onset of sexual activity, and douching practices all need to be properly assessed.

Certain variables have been strongly associated with PID. First, age is a risk marker. Sexually active teenagers are three times more likely to be diagnosed with PID than 25–9-year-old women (Bell and Holmes, 1984). Whether this is due to behavioural (O'Reilly and Aral, 1985) or biological (Washington *et al.*, 1985*b*) factors affecting these teenagers remains to be determined. Various interacting explanations have been offered: lower prevalence of protective antibodies, larger zones of cervical ectopy, greater penetrability of cervical mucus, more sexual partners, and higher prevalence of STDs in the partner pool (Wasserheit, 1987).

Second, contraceptive choice influences the occurrence of PID. The intrauterine device (IUD) is associated with an increased risk of developing PID, primarily in the first several months after insertion (Lee *et al.*, 1983; Vessey *et al.*, 1981). In contrast, most studies have shown that barrier methods reduce the risk for PID (Stone *et al.*, 1986).

Current literature raises paradoxical questions regarding the role of oral contraception and PID. Nearly all studies have found that use of such contraception is associated with increased detection of lower genital tract chlamydia (Washington *et al.*, 1985*a*). However, its use has also been associated with lower risks of both gonococcal and chlamydial PID (Senanayake and Kramer, 1980; Svensson *et al.*, 1985; Wolner-Hanssen *et al.*, 1987). In part, this paradox may be due either to undefined behavioural factors interacting with the different variables (Newton and Keith, 1985) or to a detection bias because users of oral contraception may have less severe symptoms of PID (Svensson *et al.*, 1984). Alternatively, the particular hormonal components of such contraceptives may play a role in producing these conflicting findings (Cramer *et al.*, 1987; Cates, 1987*b*).

Third, women who have had previous episodes of gonococcal PID are more likely to have recurrent infections (Holmes *et al.*, 1980). Biologically, it is difficult to distinguish between the flaring of inadequately treated earlier STD and the acquiring of new infections due to continued high risk sexual behaviour. A similar pattern probably exists for chlamydial PID and non-gonococcal, non-chlamydial PID.

STD/PID and Infertility

Definition

Studies relating STD/PID to infertility have used a variety of terms to define these conditions. STD has been measured by self-reports (Sherman *et al.*, 1987; WHO, 1987), cervical cultures (Henry-Suchet *et al.*, 1987), and serologic evidence of previous infection (Eschenbach, 1986; Cates, 1984). PID has been defined by self-reports (Aral *et al.*, 1987; WHO, 1987; Daling *et al.*, 1985; Cramer *et al.*, 1985), clinical symptoms or signs (Adler *et al.*, 1982), and laparoscopic verification (Westrom, 1975). Finally, infertility has been classified by measures of behaviour over time in a population-based sample (Mosher, 1985; Aral *et al.*, 1987) or by clinical evaluation in selected samples of couples requesting infertility services (WHO, 1987; Daling *et al.*, 1985; Cramer *et al.*, 1985). The less rigid the definition, the greater the potential for misclassification; thus, the less likely a given investigation will be able to determine a true aetiological association.

The definition of infertility also affects both the characteristics of the infertile population and the likelihood of future conception (Marchbanks, submitted). Women categorized as infertile using the definition of no pregnancy after unprotected intercourse for 12 and 24 months were more likely to be black and less educated than women categorized as infertile using stricter infertility definitions. This is not surprising, since those from lower socio-economic classes would be less likely to seek infertility evaluation (Hirsch and Mosher, 1987). Thus, they would be under-represented when more precise infertility categories are used. As expected, the more stringent the definition, the lower the true infertility prevalence (Table 7.3) and the greater the predictive value of the couple's being unable to get pregnant.

Aetiology

Regardless of the measures used, all studies to date have found a strong association between STD/PID and infertility, predominantly tubal infertility.

TABLE 7.3. *Prevalence of history of infertility by five definitions, adjusted for age*

Definition	Data source	Prevalence (%)
1. No conception after 12 months of unprotected intercourse	Life event	15.2
2. No conception after 24 months of unprotected intercourse	Life event	9.6
3. No conception after 2 years of trying to conceive	Questionnaire	5.8
4. Def. 3 and couple consulted a physician for the problem	Questionnaire	4.5
5. Defs. 3 and 4 and physician diagnosed infertility	Questionnaire	2.8

Source: Adapted from Marchbanks *et al.* (1989).

The classic cohort studies from Lund, Sweden remain the scientific cornerstone for the aetiological link between salpingitis and infertility (Westrom, 1987). In addition, women with a self-reported history of gonorrhoea (Sherman *et al.*, 1987) or non-specific STD/PID (WHO, 1987) were almost three times more likely to have tubal occlusion as a cause of their infertility. Similarly, among women with a PID history (Aral *et al.*, 1987), the proportion with fertility problems (44 per cent) was double that among women without such a history (21 per cent). This difference held for both nulliparous and multiparous women.

Salpingitis associated with either *N. gonorrhoeae* or *C. trachomatis* has been causally related to tubal infertility (Westrom, 1985). Current prospective data show the fertility prognosis of symptomatic PID caused by either gonococcal or chlamydial agents is poor (Westrom, 1985; Whittington *et al.*, 1987; Plummer *et al.*, 1987; Brunham *et al.*, 1987*b*). Gonorrhoea has been related to tubal infertility in studies using self-reported cervical infections (Sherman *et al.*, 1987), clinical diagnoses (Falk, 1965), laparoscopically-proven salpingitis (Westrom, 1975), and serological correlation (Mabey *et al.*, 1985; Tjiam *et al.*, 1985). However, other investigations from England and Denmark have not found gonococcal antibody to be as strongly associated with tubal occlusion as chlamydia antibody (Moller *et al.*, 1985; Robertson *et al.*, 1987).

The aetiological role of previous chlamydial infection in causing tubal infertility has been more exhaustively studied than that of gonococcal infection (Cates, 1984). At least 21 investigations have examined the relationship between serological evidence of past chlamydial infection and tubal infertility (Table 7.4). Despite wide variations in design, these results from 14 countries have uniformly documented that tubal occlusion is significantly associated with a greater percentage of women having chlamydial antibody.

Chlamydia trachomatis apparently causes more severe sub-clinical tubal inflammation—and ultimately tubal damage—than other agents, despite its

TABLE 7.4. *Studies of Chlamydia trachomatis infection and subsequent tubal infertility*

Study details	C. trachomatis antibody level	Diagnosis of women studied (all were infertile unless indicated otherwise)	Findings Antibody positive/tubal occlusion (%)	Relative risk
Punnonen et al., Turku, Finland (1979)	MIF ⩾ 1:16	Abnormal HSG Normal HSG	91 51	1.8
Henry-Suchet et al., Paris, France (1980)	MIF ⩾ 1:64	Tubal obstruction No tubal obstruction	26 4	2.8
Jones et al., Indianapolis, Ind. (1982)	MIF ⩾ 1:8	Chlamydia antibodies No chlamydia antibodies	75 28	2.9
Moore et al., Seattle, Wash. (1982)	MIF ⩾ 1:32	Tubal occlusion Adhesions No tubal conditions	75 21 0	n/a
Gump et al., Burlington, Vt. (1983)	MIF ⩾ 1:16	Abnormal HSG Normal HSG	64 28	2.3
Ballard et al., Johannesburg, South Africa (1981)	MIF ⩾ 1:8	Tubal pathology Pregnant women	87 38	2.3
Cevenini et al., Bologna, Italy (1982)	MIF ⩾ 1:8	Salpingitis No salpingitis	90 27	3.2

TABLE 7.4. (*cont.*)

Study details	*C. trachomatis* antibody level	Diagnosis of women studied (all were infertile unless indicated otherwise)	Findings — Antibody positive/tubal occlusion (%)	Relative risk
Padjen et al., Leyden, Netherlands (1984)	EIA	Inflammatory abnormalities No tubal abnormalities	83 16	5.2
Conway et al., Bristol, England (1984)	MIF ≥ 1:32	Tubal damage No tubal damage	75 31	2.4
Kane et al., London, England (1984)	MIF ≥ 1:8	Hydrosalpinx Normal tubes	41 12	3.4
Brunham et al., Winnipeg, Canada (1985)	MIF ≥ 1:32	Tubal damage No tubal damage	72 9	8.0
Mabey et al., Banjul, Gambia (1985)	EIA	Tubal damage Pregnant women	68 35	1.9
Battin et al., Los Angeles, Calif. (1984)	MIF ≥ 1:32	Tubal pathology No tubal pathology	94 86	1.1
Kelver et al., Galveston, Texas (1986)	MIF ≥ 1:16	Positive chlamydia serology Negative serology	77 35	2.2

Study	Test	Category		
Hawes and Gilbert, Melbourne, Australia (1986)	MIF ≥ 1:160	Tubal damage	67	6.9
		No tubal damage	7	
		Pregnant women	10	
Sellors et al., Hamilton, Canada (1988)	EIA	Undergoing tuboplasty	81	2.5
		Women having tubal ligation	37	
		Women having hysterectomy	33	
Quinn et al., Toronto, Canada (1987)	MIF ≥ 1:32	Tubal occlusion	71	4.4
		Ovulation defects	19	
		Normal women	16	
Anestad et al., Oslo, Norway (1987)	MIF ≥ 1:8	Tubal occlusion	91	1.7
		Normal tubes	55	
		Pregnant women	47	
Reniers et al., Franceville, Gabon (1989)	MIF ≥ 1:64	Tubal obstruction	n/a	9.7
		Normal tubes		1.4
		Pregnant women		1.0
Guderian and Trobough, Los Gatos, Calif. (1986)	MIF ≥ 1:32	Tubal pathology	83	5.2
		Normal tubes	16	
Moller et al.; Aarhus, Denmark (1985)	MIF ≥ 1:32	Abnormal HSG	33	2.5
		Normal HSG	13	

Note: MIF: Micro-immunofluorescence, EIA: Enzyme immunoassay, HSG: Hystero-salpingogram.

apparently more benign symptoms/signs (Gjonnaess *et al.*, 1982; Svensson *et al.*, 1980). That tubal damage can be severe despite mild clinical signs is probably due to chlamydia salpingitis being more chronic than salpingitis caused by other organisms. This hypothesis is supported by the low prevalence of immunoglobulin M antibody to chlamydia among women with acute salpingitis (Gjonnaess *et al.*, 1982).

Pathogenesis

PID creates havoc by causing post-infectious scarring that accompanies the healing process. Infertility occurs when bilateral intra-tubal adhesions interfere with the transit of sperm or ova either by damaging the mucosa and cilia or by occluding the fallopian tubes. Peri-tubal scarring may also limit tubal motility and compromise the fimbrial ostia, thereby interfering with ovum capture.

Recent animal studies have demonstrated that repeated chlamydial infection eventually produces tubal occlusion and infertility (Swenson and Schachter, 1984; Patton, 1985). Serial inoculations of chlamydia into the fallopian tube of pig-tailed monkeys result in intra-tubal adhesions, and distal tubal obstruction (Patton *et al.*, 1987). Untreated chlamydia salpingitis may show symptoms of resolution in the face of progressive tubal damage. Moreover, in mice, treatment with tetracycline had to be started early in the course of tubal infection to have any influence on reducing infertility (Swenson *et al.*, 1986).

Clinically 'silent' PID accounts for a sizeable portion of tubal infertility. A variety of investigations have found that more than half of women with documented tubal occlusion reported no history of previous PID (Gump *et al.*, 1983; Brunham *et al.*, 1985; Guderian and Trobough, 1986; Anestad *et al.*, 1987). Moreover, morphological and physiological analysis of tubal epithelium from women with distal tubal obstruction found extensive ultra-structural damage, even in those without knowledge of previous PID (Patton *et al.*, 1987). Thus, clinical evidence of symptomatic PID is not a necessary precursor for the eventual development of tubal infertility.

Risk Factors

Several factors affect the prognosis of whether PID will proceed to tubal occlusion. First, the most important variable is the number of previous PID episodes (Westrom, 1985). In general, each new salpingitis episode doubles the rate of post-salpingitis infertility. Approximately 12 per cent of women are infertile after a single episode of PID, almost 25 per cent after two episodes, and over half after three or more episodes (Westrom, 1985).

Second, a woman's age also affects her fertility prognosis (Westrom, 1985). Women who have salpingitis between the ages of 15 and 24 suffer less tubal damage than do older women. In addition, younger women have less infertility than older ones even when stratified by number of salpingitis episodes or by severity of inflammatory changes noted laparoscopically during acute salpingitis.

Third, the severity of the pelvic inflammation, judged by laparoscopy, influences the fertility outcome. Women with severe inflammatory changes had five-fold higher rates of tubal infertility than those with mild disease (Westrom, 1975); women with moderate changes were in between.

Fourth, contraceptive choice also affects infertility after PID. Women using IUDs were found to have a higher risk of tubal factor infertility, with the Dalkon Shield accounting for most of this risk. Copper-containing IUDs had much lower risks of tubal infertility (Daling *et al.*, 1985; Cramer *et al.*, 1985). Barrier methods of contraception—including both condoms and spermicides—provided protection against tubal infertility (Cramer *et al.*, 1987). While the mechanical benefits of condoms provided only marginal.protection, when coupled with the chemical benefits of spermicides these combination barrier methods provided a two-fold protection from tubal infertility. Finally, use of oral contraceptives did not protect against tubal infertility (Cramer *et al.*, 1987). In fact, use of contraceptives with higher levels of oestrogen appeared to have a harmful influence.

Unfortunately, our most sobering news regarding fertility prognosis after PID is that tertiary prevention has been disappointing: the treatment regimens recommended for symptomatic PID have had only a minimal impact on fertility outcome. This pessimistic picture is further aggravated by the prescription of inappropriate antibiotics by private physicians to treat PID (Grimes *et al.*, 1986; Gelphman *et al.*, 1987; Thompson *et al.*, 1985). However, while most currently recommended antibiotic regimes can cure symptoms of acute infection (Goodrich, 1982; Brunham, 1984), it appears that even these antibiotics probably have a limited effect on tubal damage that already existed before treatment was started (Plummer *et al.*, 1987). No available data suggest that infertility will be markedly influenced even by newer antibiotic regimens, including those active against *C. trachomatis* (Eschenbach, 1987; Teisala *et al.*, 1987).

Examining the Lund PID cohort, in women who were treated over a 10-year interval with a variety of antibiotics, tubal infertility occurred among 10 to 13 per cent regardless of the therapy used (Westrom *et al.*, 1979). Antibiotic regimes that inhibited *N. gonorrhoeae*, *C. trachomatis*, or predominantly facultative anaerobes were associated with virtually identical tubal infertility rates. It appears that if we wish to have a sizeable impact on STD-related tubal infertility, the infections will have to be prevented before they reach the fallopian tube.

Estimates of STD-related Infertility

A wide range of estimates has been proposed for the magnitude and proportion of infertility related to sexually transmitted diseases. While making this distinction may seem an academic exercise, in fact determining the level of STD-related infertility has public health importance since first, STD-related causes are the only causes of infertility which are preventable (Office of Technology Assessment, 1988); second, the prognosis for surgical management of distal tubal obstruction—the main type of infertility caused by STD—is dismal (Hull *et al.*, 1985; Bateman *et al.*, 1987); and third, STD-related causes of infertility have been associated with increased psychological reactions, especially guilt, in couples learning of this aetiology (Mahlstedt, 1985).

Methodological Considerations

The differences among estimates of STD-related infertility are primarily due to interaction among different databases used as a starting-point for the estimates; different assumptions applied to the databases to arrive at the final estimate; and whether the estimates are for incidence (the number of new cases of STD-related infertility per year) or prevalence (the total number of reproductive age individuals who are infertile due to STD-related causes at any point in time). Three different approaches can be used to estimate the magnitude of STD-related infertility. Each is marked by a distinct set of data requirements, strengths, and weaknesses.

1. *Estimates Based on STD Occurrence.* Estimates based on STD occurrence require data on gonorrhoea and chlamydia incidence and assumptions regarding the organism-specific probability first of lower genital tract infection ascending to PID and then of PID leading to infertility. This approach avoids problems in defining infertility (see above) and also minimizes the problem of undiagnosed PID. Its main weaknesses are the inadequacy of existing surveillance data on gonorrhoea and chlamydia incidence and the difficulty of accurately estimating probabilities of lower genital tract infection leading to PID and of PID leading to infertility.

2. *Estimates Based on PID Occurrence.* Estimates based on PID occurrence may focus on either the incidence or the prevalence of PID, yielding concomitant estimates of the incidence and prevalence of infertility, respectively. Incidence-focused estimates require data on PID incidence and assumptions regarding the probability of PID leading to infertility. Preferably both the incidence data and the probability assumptions should be organism-specific because STDs vary by time and place and the probabilities may vary by organism. This approach avoids problems in defining infertility and estimating the probability that lower genital tract infection leads to PID. However, its weaknesses are our inability to determine the magnitude of undiagnosed ('silent') PID, the inadequacy of available PID incidence data, and the difficulties involved in developing the probability assumptions. Prevalence-focused estimates require data on PID prevalence and assumptions regarding the probability of PID leading to infertility. This approach is simple, provides prevalence estimates, and avoids the problems of infertility ascertainment.

However, it is also directly affected by the magnitude of silent PID, is not organism-specific, and depends on the accuracy of health reports of PID history.

3. *Estimates Based on Infertility Occurrence.* Estimates based on infertility occurrence require data on the extent of infertility and make assumptions regarding both the percentage of ascertained infertility categorized as tubal factor and the proportion of tubal infertility that is STD-related. This approach avoids the difficulties of making assumptions regarding the probabilities of ascending infection related to specific organisms. Its major weaknesses include the problems of defining infertility and the unrepresentativeness of patients seeking infertility services compared to the general population.

Current Estimates of STD-related Infertility

Keeping in mind these methodological considerations, we provide estimates of the current level of STD-related infertility in Table 7.5. Looking first at incidence, estimates of STD-related infertility can be based on three data sources: (1) the number of annual infections of the lower genital tract in females caused by chlamydia and gonorrhoea (Cates, 1987*a*); (2) the annual number of PID cases (Washington *et al.*, 1984; Blount *et al.*, 1984); and (3) the annual number of infertility visits (Aral and Cates, 1983; CDC, 1985). Approximately 3 million lower genital tract infections with either chlamydia or gonorrhoea occur in women each year in the United States. Assuming 25 per cent of these ascend to pelvic inflammatory disease (Platt *et al.*, 1983; Stamm *et al.*, 1984) and 17 per cent of those lead to tubal occlusion (Westrom, 1985), an estimated annual incidence of 125 000 cases of STD-related infertility are occurring each year. Similarly, using published numbers of PID cases or infertility visits, a range of between 75 000 and 225 000 cases of STD-related infertility results (Table 7.5).

Turning next to prevalence (see Table 7.6), three databases are also available: (1) the cumulative annual incidence of STD-related infertility estimated above; (2) the cross-sectional prevalence of self-reported PID (Aral *et al.*, 1985); and

T ABLE 7.5. *Estimated incidence of tubal infertility, USA*

Basis	Number	Assumptions	Annual incidence
STD incidence	Gonorrhoea: 1 million Chlamydia: 2 million	25% PID 17% tubal occlusion	125 000
PID incidence	Ambulatory: 1 million (Hospitalized: 300 000)	17% tubal occlusion	170 000
Infertility incidence	MD visits: 1.5 million	50% evaluation 10–30% tubal occlusion	75 000– 225 000

Note: Figures refers to all women aged 15–44.

TABLE 7.6. *Estimated prevalence of tubal infertility, USA*

Basis	Number	Assumptions	Prevalence
Cumulative annual incidence of tubal infertility	125 000/year	15 years	1.9 million
Self-reported PID prevalence	10 million	17% tubal occlusion	1.7 million
Infertility prevalence	2–9 million	10%–20% tubal occlusion	200 000– 2.7 million

Note: Figures refer to all women aged 15–44.

(3) the cross-sectional amount of infertility in the most recent national population-based survey (Mosher, 1985). Applying reasonable assumptions to these three databases, we estimate that approximately 2 million women (range 200 000–2.7 million) currently suffer tubal occlusion in the United States. However, only about half may desire more children, and a smaller percentage will seek infertility services (Henshaw and Orr, 1987).

While the above estimates of the incidence and prevalence of STD-related infertility are crude, they are consistent with the best available evidence regarding the overlapping relationships of the number of sexually transmitted infections, the reported number of ambulatory and hospitalized PID cases, the number of infertility visits to private clinician's offices, and cross-sectional, self-reported levels of PID and infertility in the American population of reproductive-age women.

Conclusion

Data strongly implicate sexually transmitted infections as a primary aetiology of tubal infertility, acting largely through the intermediary of pelvic inflammatory disease. The key organisms implicated in tubal occlusion are *C. trachomatis*, *N. gonorrhoeae*, and anaerobic bacteria frequently associated with bacterial vaginosis. Many different estimates of the incidence and prevalence of STD-related infertility have appeared in the literature. Because of difficulties with definition, diagnosis, and selection (detection) bias, the magnitude of STD-related infertility can be either over- or understated. Our best estimates from the current review are in the range of 125 000 cases per year in the United States.

Growing evidence emphasizes that the focus for preventing STD-related infertility must be at the level of reducing lower genital tract infections. While we should make every effort to identify and treat pelvic inflammatory disease early in its natural history, this may have a relatively limited impact on subsequent infertility because of the role of silent PID, which accounts for more than half the tubal occlusion found in most clinical series of infertile couples and because of the lack of evidence that any current PID treatment regimen has a positive impact on future fertility. Thus, investments to prevent lower genital tract STD may pay dividends in reducing eventual upper genital tract PID and subsequent tubal infertility.

References

Adler, M. W., Belsey, E. H., and O'Connor, B. H. (1982), 'Morbidity Associated with Pelvic Inflammatory Disease', *British Journal of Venereal Disease* 58: 151–7.

Allen, I., and Schoon, M. G. (1983), 'Laparoscopic Diagnosis of Acute Pelvic Inflammatory Disease', *British Journal of Obstetrics and Gynaecology* 90: 966.

Anestad, G., Lunde, O., Moen, M., and Dalaker, K. (1987), 'Infertility and Chlamydial Infection', *Fertility and Sterility* 48: 787–90.

Aral, S. O., and Cates, W., Jr. (1983), 'The Increasing Concern with Infertility: Why Now?', *Journal of the American Medical Association* 250: 2327–31.

—— Mosher, W. D., and Cates, W., Jr. (1985), 'Self-Reported Pelvic Inflammatory Disease in the U.S.: A Common Occurrence', *American Journal of Public Health* 75: 1216–18.

—— —— —— (1987), 'Contraceptive Use, Pelvic Inflammatory Disease, and Fertility Problems among U.S. Women', *American Journal of Obstetrics and Gynecology* 157: 59–64.

Ballard, R. C., Fenler, H. G., and Duncan, M. O. (1981), 'Urethritis and Associated Infections in Johannesburg—the Role of Chlamydia trachomatis', *South African Journal of Sexually Transmitted Diseases* 1: 24–6 (cited in Mabey *et al.*, 1985).

Bateman, B. G., Nunley, W. C., Jr., and Kitchin, J. D. (1987), 'Surgical Management of Distal Tubal Obstruction—Are we Making Progress?', *Fertility and Sterility* 48: 523–42.

Battin, D. A., Barnes, R. B., Hoffman, D. I., Schachter, J., diZerega, G. S., and Yonekura, M. L. (1984), 'Chlamydia trachomatis is not an Important Cause of Abnormal Postcoital Tests in Ovulating Patients', *Fertility and Sterility* 42: 233–8.

Bell, T. A., and Holmes, K. K. (1984), 'Age-Specific Risks of Syphilis, Gonorrhea, and Hospitalized Pelvic Inflammatory Disease in Sexually Experienced U.S. Women', *Sexually Transmitted Diseases* 11: 291–5.

Blount, J. H., Reynolds, G. H., and Rice, R. J. (1984), 'Pelvic Inflammatory Disease: Incidence and Trends in Private Practice', *Morbidity and Mortality Weekly Report* 32(4SS): 27SS–34SS.

Bowie, W. R., and Jones, H. (1981), 'Acute Pelvic Inflammatory Disease in Outpatients and Associates with Chlamydia trachomatis and Neisseria gonorrhoeae', *Annals of Internal Medicine* 95: 685.

Brihmer, C., Kallings, I., Nord, C.-E., and Brundin, J. (1987), 'Salpingitis: Aspects of Diagnosis and Etiology: A 4-year Study from a Swedish Hospital', *European Journal of Obstetrics, Gynaecology and Reproductive Biology* 24: 211–20.

Brunham, R. C. (1984), 'Therapy for Acute Pelvic Inflammatory Disease: A Critique of Recent Treatment Trials', *American Journal of Obstetrics and Gynecology* 148: 235–40.

Brunham, R. C., Paavonen, J., Stevens, C. E., Kiviat, N., Kvo, C. C., Critchlow, C. W., and Holmes, K. K. (1984), 'Mucopurulent Cervicitis—The Ignored Counterpart in Women of Urethritis in Men', *New England Journal of Medicine* 311: 1–6.

—— Maclean, I. W., Binns, B., and Peeling, R. W. (1985), 'Chlamydia trachomatis: Its Role in Tubal Infertility', *Journal of Infectious Diseases* 152: 1275–82.

—— Peeling, R., Maclean, I., McDowell, J., Persson, K., and Osser, S. (1987a), 'Postabortal Chlamydia trachomatis Salpingitis: Correlating Risk with Antigen-Specific Serologic Responses and with Neutralization', *Journal of Infectious Diseases* 155: 749–55.

—— Binns, B., Guijon, F., and Danfoarth, D. (1987b), 'Etiology and Outcome of Acute Pelvic Inflammatory Disease (Abstract 180)', presented at the International Society for STD Research, Atlanta, Ga.

Cates, W., Jr. (1984), 'Sexually Transmitted Organisms and Infertility: The Proof of the Pudding', *Sexually Transmitted Diseases* 11: 113–16.

—— (1987a), 'Epidemiology and Control of Sexually Transmitted Diseases: Strategic Evolution', *Infectious Disease Clinics of North America* 1: 1–23.

—— (1987b), 'Tubal Infertility: An Ounce of (More Specific) Prevention', *Journal of the American Medical Association* 257: 2480.

—— Farley, T. M. M., Rowe, P. J., and the WHO Task Force on the Diagnosis and Treatment of Infertility (1985), 'Worldwide Patterns of Infertility: Is Africa Different?', *Lancet* 11: 596–8.

CDC (Centers for Disease Control) (1985), 'Infertility—United States, 1982', *Morbidity and Mortality Weekly Report* 34: 197–9.

Cevenini, R., Possati, G., and LaPlaca, M. (1982), 'Chlamydia trachomatis Infection in Infertile Women', in P.-A. Mardh, K. K. Holmes, D. J. Oriel, P. Piot, and J. Schachter (eds.), *Chlamydial infections*: 189–92, Elsevier Biomedical Press, Amsterdam.

Chaparro, M. V., Ghosh, S., Nashed, A., and Pollak, A. (1978), 'Laparoscopy for the Confirmation and Prognostic Evaluation of Pelvic Inflammatory Disease', *International Journal of Gynaecological Obstetrics* 15: 307.

Cleary, R. E., and Jones, R. B. (1985), 'Recovery of Chlamydia trachomatis from the Endometrium in Infertile Women with Serum Antichlamydial Antibodies', *Fertility and Sterility* 44: 233–5.

Conway, D., Glazener, C. M. A., Owen, C. E., Hodgson, J., Hull, M. G. R., Clarke, S. K. R., and Stirrat, G. M. (1984), 'Chlamydial Serology in Fertile and Infertile Women', *Lancet* 1: 191–3.

Cramer, D. W., Schiff, I., Schoenbaum, S. C., Gibson, M., Belisle, S., Albrecht, B., Stillman, R., Berger, M. J., Wilson, E., Stadel, B. V., and Seibel, M. (1985), 'Tubal Infertility and the Intrauterine Device', *New England Journal of Medicine* 312: 941–7.

—— Goldman, M. B., Schiff, I., Belisle, S., Albrecht, B., Stadel, B., Gibson, M., Wilson, E., Stillman, R., and Thompson, I. (1987), 'The Relationship of Tubal Infertility to Barrier Method and Oral Contraceptive Use', *Journal of the American Medical Association* 257: 2446–50.

Cromer, E. A., and Heald, F. P. (1957), 'Pelvic Inflammatory Disease Associated with Neisseria gonorrhoeae and Chlamydia trachomatis: Clinical Correlates', *Sexually Transmitted Diseases* 14: 125–9.

Cunningham, F. G., Hauth, J. C., and Gilstrap, L. C. (1978), 'The Bacterial Patho-genesis of Acute Pelvic Inflammatory Disease', *Obstetrics and Gynecology* 52: 161.

Daling, J. R., Weiss, N. S., Metch, D. J., Chow, W. H., Soderstrom, R. M., Moore, D. E., Spadoni, L. R., and Stadel, B. V. (1985), 'Primary Tubal Infertility in Relation to the Use of an Intrauterine Device', *New England Journal of Medicine* 312: 937–41.

Draper, D. L., James, J. F., Brooks, G. F., and Sweet, R. L. (1980), 'Comparison of Virulence Markers of Peritoneal–Fallopian Tube and Endocervical Neisseria gonor-rhoeae Isolates from Women with Acute Salpingitis', *Infect. Immun.*, 27: 882–6.

Eilard, T., Brorsson, J.-E., Hamark, B., and Forssman, L. (1976), 'Isolation of Chlamydia in Acute Salpingitis', *Scandinavian Journal of Infectious Diseases* 9 (supplement): 82.

Eschenbach, D. A. (1980), 'Epidemiology and Diagnosis of Acute Pelvic Inflammatory Disease', *Obstetrics and Gynecology*, 55(S), 142S–151S.

—— (1986), 'Acute Pelvic Inflammatory Disease', in J. Sciarra (ed.), *Gynecology and Obstetrics*, i ch. 44: pp. 1–20, Harper and Row, Philadelphia, Pa.

—— (1987), 'Infertility Caused by Infection', *Contemp Ob/Gyn* 16 (fertility supple-ment): 29–46.

—— Buchanan, T. M., Pollock, H. M., Forsyth, P. S., Alexander, E. R., Lin, J. S., Wang, S. P., Wentworth, B. B., McCormack, W. M., and Holmes, K. K. (1975), 'Polymicrobial aetiology of acute pelvic inflammatory disease', *New England Journal of Medicine* 293: 166–70.

Falk, V. (1965), 'Treatment of Acute Non-Tuberculous Salpingitis with Antibiotics alone and in Combination with Glucocorticoids', *Acta Obstetrica et Gyncologica Scandinavica*, 44 (supplement 6): 85–97.

Gelphman, K. A., Gale, J. L., Commons, M., Thapa, P. B., and Handsfield, H. H. (1987), 'Pelvic Inflammatory Disease: Diagnosis and Treatment Patterns as Reported by the Providers (Abstract 185)', presented at the International Society for STD Research, Atlanta, Ga.

Gjonnaess, H., Dalaker, K., Anestad, G., Mardh, P.-A., Kvile, G., and Bergan, T. (1982), 'Pelvic Inflammatory Disease: Etiologic Studies with Emphasis on Chlamydial Infection', *Obstetrics and Gynecology* 59: 550–5.

Goodrich, J. T. (1982), 'Pelvic Inflammatory Disease: Considerations Related to Therapy', *Review of Infectious Diseases* 4 (supplement): S778–S787.

Grayston, J. T., Wang, S.-P., Yeh, L.-J., and Kuo, C.-C. (1985), 'Importance of Reinfection in the Pathogenesis of Trachoma', *Review of Infectious Diseases* 7: 717–25.

Gregg, C. R., Melly, M. A., and McGee, Z. A. (1980), 'Gonococcal Lipopolysaccharide: A Toxin for Human Fallopian Tube Mucosa', *American Journal of Obstetrics and Gynecology* 138: 981–4.

Grimes, D. A., Blount, J. H., Patrick, J., and Washington, A. E. (1986), 'Antibiotic Treatment of Pelvic Inflammatory Disease, Trends Among Private Physicians in the United States, 1966–1982', *Journal of the American Medical Association* 256: 3223–6.

Guderian, A. M., and Trobough, G. E. (1986), 'Residues of Pelvic Inflammatory Disease in Intrauterine Device Users: A Result of Intrauterine Device or Chlamydia trachomatis Infection?', *American Journal of Obstetrics and Gynecology* 154: 497–503.

Gump, D. W., Gibson, M., and Ashikaga, T. (1983), 'Evidence of Prior Pelvic Inflammatory Disease and its Relationship to Chlamydia trachomatis Antibody and

Intrauterine Contraceptive Device Use in Infertile Women', *American Journal of Obstetrics and Gynecology* 146: 153–9.

Hadgu, A., Westrom, L., Brooks, C. A., Reynolds, G. H., and Thompson, S. E. (1986), 'Predicting Acute Pelvic Inflammatory Disease: A Multivariate Analysis', *American Journal of Obstetrics and Gynecology* 155: 954–60.

Hager, W. D., Eschenbach, D. A., Spence, M. R., and Sweet, R. L. (1983), 'Criteria for Diagnosis and Grading of Salpingitis', *Obstetrics and Gynecology* 61: 113–14.

Hallberg, T., Wolner-Hanssen, P., and Mardh, P.-A. (1985), 'Cell-Mediated Immune Response to Chlamydial Antigens in Patients with Pelvic Inflammatory Disease Infected with Chlamydia trachomatis', *British Journal of Venereal Disease* 61: 247–51.

Hawes, L. A., and Gilbert, G. L. (1986), 'Seroepidemiology of Chlamydia trachomatis Infection in Infertile Women in Melbourne', *Medical Journal of Australia* 45: 497–9.

Heinonen, P. K., Teisala, K., Punnonen, R., Miettinen, A., Lehtinen, M., and Paavonen, J. (1985), 'Anatomic Sites of Upper Genital Tract Infection', *Obstetrics and Gynecology* 66 (3): 384–8.

Henry-Suchet, J., Catalan, F., Loffredo, V., Serfaty, D., Siboulet, A., Perol, Y., Sanson, M. J., Debache, C., Pigeau, F., Coppin, R., de Brux, J., and Poynard, T. (1980), 'Microbiology of Specimens Obtained by Laparoscopy from Controls and from Patients with Pelvic Inflammatory Disease or Infertility with Tubal Obstruction: Chlamydia trachomatis and Ureaplasma urealyticum', *American Journal of Obstetrics and Gynecology* 138: 1022–5.

—— Utzmann, C., de Brux, J., Ardoin, P., and Catalan, F. (1987), 'Microbiologic Study of Chronic Inflammation Associated with Tubal Factor Infertility: Role of Chlamydia trachomatis', *Fertility and Sterility* 47: 274–7.

Henshaw, S. K., and Orr, M. T. (1987), 'The Need and Unmet Need for Infertility Services in the United States', *Family Planning Perspectives* 19: 180–6.

Hirsch, M. B., and Mosher, W. D. (1987), 'Characteristics of Infertile Women in the United States and their Use of Infertility Services', *Fertility and Sterility* 47: 618–25.

Holmes, K. K., Eschenbach, D. A., and Knapp, J. S. (1980), 'Salpingitis: Overview of Etiology and Epidemiology', *American Journal of Obstetrics and Gynecology* 138: 893–900.

Hull, M. G., Glazener, C. M., Kelly, N. J., Conway, D. I., Foster, P. A., Hinton, R. A., Coulson, C., Lambert, P. A., Watt, E. M., and Desai, K. M. (1985), 'Population Study of Causes, Treatment and Outcome of Infertility', *British Medical Journal* 291: 1693–7.

Jacobson, L., and Westrom, L. (1969), 'Objectivized Diagnosis of Acute Pelvic Inflammatory Disease', *American Journal of Obstetrics and Gynecology* 105: 1088–93.

Jones, R. B., Ardery, B. R., Hui, S. L., and Cleary, R. E. (1982), 'Correlation between Serum Antichlamydial Antibodies and Tubal Factor as a Cause of Infertility', *Fertility and Sterility* 38: 553–8.

Kane, J. L., Woodland, R. M., Forsey, T., Darougar, S., and Elder, M. G. (1984), 'Evidence of Chlamydial Infection in Infertile Women with and without Fallopian Tube Obstruction', *Fertility and Sterility* 42: 843–8.

Keith, L. G., Berger, G. S., Edelman, D. A., Newton, W., Fullan, N., Bailey, R., and Friberg, J. (1984), 'On the Causation of Pelvic Inflammatory Disease', *American Journal of Obstetrics and Gynecology* 149: 215–24.

Kelver, M. E., and Ngamani, M. (1986), 'Chlamydial Serology and Women with Tubal Infertility', paper presented at the Annual Meeting of the American College of Obstetricians and Gynecologists, New Orleans, La.

Kiviat, N. B., Wolner-Hanssen, P., Peterson, M., Wasserheit, J., Stamm, W. E., Eschenbach, D. A., Paavonen, J., Lingenfelter, J., Bell, T., Zabriski, V., Kirby, B., and Holmes, K. K. (1986), 'Localization of Chlamydia trachomatis Infection by Direct Immunofluorescence and Culture in Pelvic Inflammatory Disease', *American Journal of Obstetrics and Gynecology* 154: 865–73.

Knapp, J. S., Thornsberry, C., Schoolnik, G. A., Weisner, P. J., and Holmes, K. K. (1978), 'Phenotypic and Epidemiologic Correlates of Auxotype in Neisseria gonorrhoeae', *Journal of Infectious Diseases* 138: 160–5.

Kolmorgen, U. K., Seidenschnur, G., and Wergien, G. (1978), 'Diagnostik und Therapie des akuten Adnexprozesses beirn einsatz der Laparoskopie', *Zentralblatt für Gynakologie* 100: 1103.

Lee, N. C., Rubin, G. L., Ory, H. W., and Burkman, R. T. (1983), 'Type of Intrauterine Device and the Risk of Pelvic Inflammatory Disease', *Obstetrics and Gynecology* 62: 1–6.

Mabey, D. C. W., Ogbaselassie, G., Robertson, J. N., Heckels, J. E., and Ward, M. E. (1985), 'Tubal Infertility in the Gambia: Chlamydial and Gonococcal Serology in Women with Tubal Occlusion Compared to Pregnant Controls', *WHO Bulletin* 63: 1107–13.

McCormack, W. M., Strumacher, R. J., Johnson, K., Donner, A. (1977), Clinical spectrum of gonococcal infection in women, *Lancet*, 1: 1182–5.

Mahlstedt, P. T. (1985), 'The Psychological Component of Infertility', *Fertility and Sterility* 43: 335–46.

Marchbanks, P. A., Peterson, H. B., Rubin, G. L., Wingo, P. A., and The Cancer and Steroid Hormone Study Group (1989), 'Infertility: The Impact of Definition', *American Journal of Epidemiology* 130: 259–67.

Mardh, P.-A., (1980), 'An Overview of Infectious Agents of Salpingitis, their Biology, and Recent Advances in Methods of Detection', *American Journal of Obstetrics and Gynecology* 138: 933–51.

—— and Taylor-Robinson, D. (1984), 'Bacterial Vaginosis', *Scandanavian Journal of Urology and Nephrology* (supplement): 86–90.

—— Ripa, T., Svensson, L., and Westrom, L. (1977), 'Role of Chlamydia trachomatis Infection in Acute Salpingitis', *New England Journal of Medicine* 296: 1377.

—— Lind, I., Svensson, L., Westrom, L., Moller, B. R. (1981), 'Antibodies to Chlamydia trachomatis, Mycoplasma hominis, and Neisseria gonorrhoeae in Sera from Patients with Acute Salpingitis', *British Journal of Venereal Disease* 57: 125–9.

Method, M. W., Urnes, P. D., Nearing, R., Sciarra, J. J., and Keith, L. G. (1987), 'Economic Considerations in the Use of Laparoscopy for Diagnosing Pelvic Inflammatory Disease', *Journal of Reproductive Medicine* 32: 759–64.

Mishell, D. R., Jr., Bell, J. H., Good, R. G., Moyer, D. L. (1966), 'The Intrauterine Device: A Bacteriologic Study of the Endometrial Cavity', *American Journal of Obstetrics and Gynecology* 96: 119–26.

Moller, B. R., Mardh, P.-A., Ahrons, S., and Nussler, E. (1981), 'Infection with Chlamydia trachomatis, Mycoplasma hominis, and Neisseria gonorrhoeae in Patients with Acute Pelvic Inflammatory Disease', *Sexually Transmitted Diseases* 8: 198–202.

—— Taylor-Robinson, D., Furr, P. M., Toft, B., Allen, J. (1985), 'Serological

Evidence that Chlamydiae and Mycoplasmas are Involved in Infertility in Women', *Journal of Reproduction and Fertility* 73: 237–40.

Moore, D. E., Spadoni, L. R., Foy, H. M., Wang, S. P., Daling, J. R., Kvo, C. C., Grayston, J. T., Eschenbach, D. A. (1982), 'Increased Frequency of Serum Antibodies to Chlamydia trachomatis in Infertility due to Distal Tube Disease', *Lancet*, 2: 574–7.

Mosher, W. E. (1985), 'Reproductive Impairments in the United States, 1965–1972', *Demography* 22: 415–30.

Moss, T. R., and Hawkswell, J. (1986), 'Evidence of Infection with C. trachomatis in Patients with Pelvic Inflammatory Disease: Value of Partner Investigation', *Fertility and Sterility* 45: 429–30.

Newton, W., and Keith, L. G. (1985), 'Role of Behavior in the Development of Pelvic Inflammatory Disease', *Journal of Reproductive Medicine* 30: 82–8.

Office of Technology Assessment (1988), *Infertility Prevention and Treatment*, Office of Technology Assessment, Washington, DC.

O'Reilly, K. R., and Aral, S. O. (1985), 'Adolescents and Sexual Behavior: Trends and Implications for STD', *Journal of Adolescent Health Care* 6: 262–70.

Osser, S., and Persson, K. (1982), 'Epidemiologic Serodiagnostic Aspects of Chlamydial Salpingitis', *Obstetrics and Gynecology* 59: 206.

Paavonen, J. (1980), 'Chlamydia trachomatis in Acute Salpingitis', *American Journal of Obstetrics and Gynecology* 138: 957.

—— Saiku, P., and Vestermen, E. (1979), 'Chlamydia trachomatis in acute salpingitis', *British Journal of Venereal Disease* 55: 203.

—— Valtonen, V. V., and Kasper, D. C. (1981), 'Serologic Evidence for the Role of *Bacteroides fragilis* and Enterobacteriaceae in the Pathogenesis of Acute Pelvic Inflammatory Disease', *Lancet*, 1: 293.

—— Kiviat, N., Brunham, R. C., Stevens, C. E., Kvo, C. C., Stamm, W. E., Miettinen, A., Soules, M., Eschenbach, D. A., and Holmes, K. K. (1985a), 'Prevalence and Manifestations of Endometritis among Women with Cervicitis', *American Journal of Obstetrics and Gynecology* 152: 280–4.

—— Aine, R., Teisala, K., Heinonen, P. K., and Punnonen, R. (1985b), 'Comparison of Endometrial Biopsy and Peritoneal Fluid Cytologic Testing with Laparoscopy in the Diagnosis of Acute Pelvic Inflammatory Disease', *American Journal of Obstetrics and Gynecology* 151: 645–50.

Padjen, A., Nash, L. D., and Fiscelli, T. (1984), 'The Relationship between Chlamydia Antibodies and Involuntary Infertility', *Fertility and Sterility* 41 (supplement): 97S–98S.

Patton, D. L. (1985), 'Immunopathology and Histopathology of Experimental Chlamydial Salpingitis', *Review of Infectious Diseases* 7: 746–53.

—— Moore, D. E., Hicks, L. A., Soules, M. R., and Spadoni, L. R. (1987), 'Silent PID: A Morphological and Physiological Analysis of the Tubal Epithelium (Abstract 178)', paper presented at the International Society for STD Research, Atlanta, Ga.

Platt, R., Rice, P. A., and McCormack, W. M. (1983), 'Risk of Acquiring Gonorrhea and Prevalence of Abnormal Adnexal Findings among Women Recently Exposed to Gonorrhea', *Journal of the American Medical Association* 250: 3205–9.

Plummer, F., Simonsen, J. N., D'Costa, L. J., Gakinya, M., Ndinya-Achola, J. O., and Brunham, R. C. (1987), 'A Comparison of Doxycycline (DOX) and Metronidazole (MET) with Trimethaprim Sulfametrole (TMP/SMT) and Metronidazole for Treatment of Pelvic Inflammatory Disease (PID): Assessment of Effect on Infertility

(Abstract 65)', paper presented at the International Society for STD Research, Atlanta, Ga.

Punnonen, R., Terho, P., Nikkanen, V., and Meurman, O. (1979), 'Chlamydial Serology in Infertile Women by Immunofluorescence', *Fertility and Sterility* 31: 656–9.

Quinn, P. A., Petric, M., Barkin, M., Butany, J., Derzko, C., Gysler, M., Lie, K. I., Shewchuck, A. B., Shuber, J., Ryan, E., and Chapman, M. L. (1987), 'Prevalence of Antibody to Chlamydia trachomatis in Spontaneous Abortion and Infertility', *American Journal of Obstetrics and Gynecology* 156: 291–6.

Reniers, J., Collet, M., Frost, E., LeClerc, A., Ivanoff, B., and Meheus, A. (1989), 'Chlamydial Antibodies and Tubal Infertility', *International Journal of Epidemiology* 18: 261–3.

Ripa, K. T., Svensson, L., Treharne, J. D., Westrom, L., and Mardh, P.-A. (1980), 'Chlamydia trachomatis Infection in Patients with Laparoscopically Verified Acute Salpingitis', *American Journal of Obstetrics and Gynecology* 138: 960.

Robertson, J. N., Ward, M. E., Conway, D., and Caul, E. O. (1987), 'Chlamydial and Gonococcal Antibodies in Sera in Fertile Women with Tubal Obstruction', *Journal of Clinical Pathology* 40: 377–83.

Sellors, J. W., Mahony, J. B., Chernesky, M. A., and Rath, D. J. (1988), 'Tubal Factor Infertility: An Association with Prior Chlamydial Infection and Asymptomatic Salpingitis', *Fertility and Sterility* 49: 451–7.

Senanayake, P., and Kramer, D. G. (1980), 'Contraception and the Etiology of Pelvic Inflammatory Disease: New Perspectives', *American Journal of Obstetrics and Gynecology* 138: 852–60.

Sherman, K. J., Daling, J. R., and Weiss, N. S. (1987), 'Sexually Transmitted Diseases and Tubal Infertility', *Sexually Transmitted Diseases* 14: 12–16.

Stacey, C. M., Munday, P. E., Taylor-Robinson, D., Beard, R. W., Ison, C. A., and Thomas, B. J. (1987), 'A Clinical and Microbiological Study of Laparoscopically Confirmed Pelvic Inflammatory Disease in London (Abstract 181)', paper presented at the International Society for STD Research, Atlanta, Ga.

Stamm, W. E., Guinan, M. E., Johnson, C., Starcher, T., Holmes, K. K., and McCormack, W. M. (1984), 'Effect of Treatment Regimens for *N. gonorrhoeae* on Simultaneous Infection with *C. trachomatis*', *New England Journal of Medicine* 310: 545–49.

Stone, K. M., Grimes, D. A., and Magder, L. S. (1986), 'Personal Protection against Sexually Transmitted Diseases', *American Journal of Obstetrics and Gynecology* 155: 180–8.

Svensson, L., Westrom, L., Ripa, K. T., and Mardh, P.-A. (1980), 'Differences in some Clinical and Laboratory Parameters in Acute Salpingitis Related to Culture and Serologic Finding', *American Journal of Obstetrics and Gynecology* 138: 1017.

—— Westrom, L., and Mardh, P.-A. (1984), 'Contraceptives and Acute Salpingitis', *Journal of the American Medical Association* 251: 2553–5.

—— Mardh, P.-A., and Westrom, L. (1985), 'Infertility after Acute Salpingitis with Special Reference to Chlamydia trachomatis', *Fertility and Sterility* 40: 322–9.

Sweet, R. L. (1977), 'Acute Salpingitis: Diagnosis and Treatment', *Journal of Reproductive Medicine* 19: 21–30.

—— and Draper, D. L. (1981), 'Etiology of Acute Salpingitis: Influence of Episode Number and Duration of Symptoms', *Obstetrics and Gynecology* 58: 62.

Sweet, R. L., Mills, J., Hadley, K. W., Blumenstock, E., Schachter, J., Robbie, M. O., Draper, D. L. (1979), 'Use of laparoscopy to determine the microbiologic etiology of acute salpingitis', *American Journal Obstetrics and Gynecology* 134: 68–74.

—— Draper, D. L., Schachter, J., James, J., Hadley, W. K., and Brooks, G. F. (1980), 'Microbiology and Pathogenesis of Acute Salpingitis as Determined by Laparoscopy: What is the Appropriate Site to Sample?', *American Journal of Obstetrics and Gynecology* 138: 985–9.

—— Schachter, J., and Robbie, M. O. (1983), 'Failure of Beta-Lactam Antibiotics to Eradicate *Chlamydia trachomatis* from the Endometrium in Patients with Acute Salpingitis despite Apparent Clinical Cure', *Journal of the American Medical Association* 250: 2641–5.

—— Blankfort-Doyle, M., Robbie, M. O., and Schachter, J. (1985), 'The Occurrence of Chlamydial and Gonococcal Salpingitis during the Menstrual Cycle', *Journal of the American Medical Association* 255: 2062–4.

Swenson, C. E., and Schachter, J. (1984), 'Infertility as a Consequence of Chlamydial Infection of the Upper Genital Tract in Female Mice', *Sexually Transmitted Diseases* 11: 64–7.

—— Sung, M. L., and Schachter, J. (1986), 'The Effect of Tetracycline Treatment on Chlamydial Salpingitis and Subsequent Fertility in the Mouse', *Sexually Transmitted Diseases* 13: 40–4.

Teisala, K., Heinonen, P. K., Aine, R., Punnonen, R., and Paavonen, J. (1987), 'Second Laparoscopy after Treatment of Acute Pelvic Inflammatory Disease', *Obstetrics and Gynecology* 69: 343–6.

Thompson, S. E., Hagar, W. D., and Wong, K.-H. (1980), 'The Microbiology and Therapy of Acute Pelvic Inflammatory Disease in Hospitalized Patients', *American Journal of Obstetrics and Gynecology* 136: 1790.

—— Brooks, C. A., Eschenbach, D. A., Spence, M. R., Cheng, S., Sweet, R. L., and McCormack, W. M. (1985), 'High Failure Rates in Outpatient Treatment of Salpingitis with either Tetracycline Alone or Penicillin/Ampicillin Combination', *American Journal of Obstetrics and Gynecology* 152: 635–41.

Tjiam, K. H., Zeilmaker, G. H., Alberda, A. T., van Heijst, B. Y., de Roo, J. C., Polak-Vogelzang, A. A., van Joost, T., Stolz, E., and Michel, M. F. (1985), 'Prevalence of Antibodies to Chlamydia trachomatis, Neisseria gonorrhoeae, and *Mycoplasma hominis* in Infertile Women', *Genitourinary Medicine* 61: 175–8.

Toth, A., O'Leary, W. M., and Ledger, W. (1982), 'Evidence for Microbial Transfer by Spermatozoa', *Obstetrics and Gynecology* 59: 556–8.

Vessey, M. P., Yeates, D., Flavel, R., and McPherson, K. (1981), 'Pelvic Inflammatory Disease and the Intrauterine Device: Findings in a Large Cohort Study', *British Medical Journal* 282: 855–7.

Washington, A. E., Cates, W., Jr., Zaidi, A. A. (1984), 'Hospitalizations for Pelvic Inflammatory Disease: Epidemiology and Trends in the United States, 1975 to 1981', *Journal of the American Medical Association* 251: 2529–33.

—— Grove, S., Schachter, J., and Sweet, R. L. (1985a), 'Oral Contraceptives, Chlamydia trachomatis Infection, and Pelvic Inflammatory Disease: A Word of Caution about Protection', *Journal of the American Medical Association* 253: 2246–50.

—— Sweet, R. L., and Shafer, M.-A. B. (1985b), 'Pelvic Inflammatory Disease and its Sequelae in Adolescents', *Journal of Adolescent Health Care* 6: 298–310.

Wasserheit, J. N. (1987), 'Pelvic Inflammatory Disease and Infertility', *Maryland Medical Journal* 36: 58–63.

—— Bell, T. A., Kiviat, N. B., Wolner-Hanssen, P., Zabriskie, V., Kirby, B. D., Prince, E. C., Holmes, K. K., Stamm, W. E., and Eschenbach, D. A. (1985), 'Microbial Causes of Proven Pelvic Inflammatory Disease and Efficacy of Clindamycin and Tobramycin', *Annals of Internal Medicine* 104: 187–91.

L. Westrom (1975), 'Effect of Acute Pelvic Inflammatory Disease on Fertility', *American Journal of Obstetrics and Gynecology* 121: 707–13.

—— (1980), 'Incidence, Prevalence, and Trends of Acute Pelvic Inflammatory Disease and its Consequences in Industrialized Countries', *American Journal of Obstetrics and Gynecology* 138: 880–92.

—— (1985), 'Influence of Sexually Transmitted Diseases on Sterility and Ectopic Pregnancy', *Acta Europaea Fertilitatis* 16: 21–32.

—— (1987), 'Pelvic Inflammatory Disease: Bacteriology and Sequelae', *Contraception* 36: 111–28.

—— Iosif, S., Svensson, L., and Mardh, P.-A. (1979), 'Infertility after Acute Salpingitis: Results of Treatment with Different Antibiotics, *Current Therapeutic Research, Clinical and Experimental* 26: 752–9.

Whittington, W. L., Spence, M. R., Belsey, E., and Thompson, S. E. (1987), 'Infertility after Pelvic Inflammatory Disease: Report on American Inner City Women (Abstract 66)', paper presented at the International Society for STD Research, Atlanta, Ga.

Wolner-Hanssen, P., Mardh, P.-A., Moller, B., and Westrom, L. (1982), 'Endometrial Infection in Women with Chlamydial Salpingitis', *Sexually Transmitted Diseases* 9: 84–8.

—— —— Svensson, L., and Westrom, L. (1983), 'Laparoscopy in Women with Chlamydia Infections and Pelvic Pain: A Comparison of Patients with and without Salpingitis', *Obstetrics and Gynecology* 61: 299–303.

—— Paavonen, J., Stevens, C., Koutsky, L., Eschenbach, D., Kiviat, N., Crichlow, C., DeRouen, T., and Holmes, K. K. (1987), 'Pelvic Inflammatory Disease and Contraception: Multivariate Analysis of Cases and Controls Infected with *C. trachomatis*, *N. gonorrhoeae*, or Neither Organism (Abstract 182)', paper presented at the International Society for STD Research, Atlanta, Ga.

World Health Organization Task Force on the Diagnosis and Treatment of Infertility (1987), 'Infections, Pregnancies, and Infertility: Perspectives on Prevention', *Fertility and Sterility* 47: 964–8.

8 A Descriptive Epidemiology of Infertility in Costa Rica*

MARK W. OBERLE

LUIS ROSERO-BIXBY

PAT WHITAKER

Introduction

The prevalence of infecundity in many Latin American countries has been calculated primarily from World Fertility Survey (WFS) data and from clinic-based studies. Vaessen (1984) used the 1976 WFS data to produce the only published estimates of the prevalence of infecundity in Costa Rica. In that study, a woman was considered infecund either if she reported that she was unable to have a child or if she had not had a child in the five years before the interview and had not used contraception during that period. By this definition, the prevalence of infecundity ranged from 5 per cent of women 20–4 years of age to 58 per cent of women 40–4 years of age.

A national survey in Costa Rica in 1984 obtained information on infecundity, using questions that differed from those included in the WFS. This study allowed us to compile a population-based description of the characteristics of Costa Rican women with a history of infecundity. In addition, serum specimens obtained at the interviews were used to compare the respondents' history of infecundity to serological evidence of infection with three sexually transmitted diseases.

Methods

These data are derived from a case-control study of cervical and breast cancer that was conducted in 1984–5 by the Costa Rican Demographic Association and the Centers for Disease Control in collaboration with the Costa Rican Ministry of Health, the Costa Rican Social Security Administration, and Family Health International (Irwin *et al.*, 1988; Rosero-Bixby *et al.*, 1987; Oberle *et al.*, 1989). The purpose of the original study was to define the relationship between hormonal contraceptive use and cervical and breast cancer. Since the members of the control group are representative of the general population, we restricted

---

* Based on data provided by the Costa Rican Demographic Association and the Centers for Disease Control and Costa Rican National Tumor Registry.

our attention to this group for our secondary analysis of infecundity. The controls consisted of a nationally representative, household sample of 870 women aged 25–59 years. Details of sample selection, weighting procedures, and demographic characteristics have been published previously (Irwin *et al.*, 1988; Rosero-Bixby and Oberle, 1987; Oberle *et al.*, 1989). Confidence intervals, including design effect, ranged from ± 4–13 per cent for the total sample estimate and the smallest stratum presented, respectively.

The questionnaire contained three questions about infecundity modelled after questions used in the Centers for Disease Control's Cancer and Steroid Hormone Study (Irwin *et al.*, 1988; Marchbanks *et al.*, 1989). First, each woman was asked if she had ever tried for two consecutive years to become pregnant and failed to do so. Women who responded positively to the first question were asked whether they had consulted a physician about their fecundity problem, and those who did consult a physician were asked whether the doctor had made a diagnosis. Finally, those who had received a physician's diagnosis were asked at what age they had been diagnosed. These questions only measure infecundity as a perceived problem, so that an infecund woman who is not interested in becoming pregnant would not be classified as infecund. Thus these definitions depend on both physiological infecundity and a woman's desire for pregnancy.

Interviewers attempted to facilitate accurate recall by using a life-history calendar. For each interval of 12 months or longer with no pregnancy or contraceptive code, the interviewer asked whether the respondent was sexually active or not. On the basis of the calendar, 33.4 per cent of women had at least one interval of 24 months or longer during which they had unprotected sexual intercourse. However, because the original purpose of the calendar was not to measure infecundity, but rather to obtain accurate contraceptive histories, we do not know whether a woman had unprotected intercourse for each month of an unprotected interval. Thus the calendar information alone was of limited use in measuring infecundity.

At the time of the interview, a laboratory technician obtained a serum specimen from 88 per cent of the control women. Women who agreed to provide a serum specimen did not differ in demographic characteristics from those who did not provide a serum specimen (Ramirez *et al.*, 1987). These sera were analysed for antibodies to three sexually transmitted diseases as a measure of previous exposure: *Treponema pallidum*, *Herpes simplex* type 2 (HSV-2), and *Chlamydia trachomatis* (Oberle *et al.*, 1989; Larsen *et al.*, 1991; Vetter *et al.*, 1990). Differences between strata were tested by a test of proportions.

Results

Overall, 8.1 per cent of Costa Rican women in the national sample reported a history of difficulty in becoming pregnant at some point in their lives. However, only 3.2 per cent of all women reported having a physician's confirmation and diagnosis of a fertility problem. The characteristics of women with a history of difficulty in becoming pregnant differed minimally according to whether or not they had a physician's diagnosis, so the characteristics of all women with a history of infecundity are given in Table 8.1. The prevalence of a history of infecundity varied little by age-group, despite the presumption that older women would have a greater cumulative probability of developing secondary infecundity at some point in their lives (see Table 8.1). Minimal differences were also noted by region, education, and socio-economic status.

Women with two or more lifetime sex partners were more likely to report infecundity than women with only one sex partner ($p < 0.02$, see Table 8.2). Some 11.9 per cent of women with two or more sex partners reported a history of infecundity compared to 7.1 per cent of monogamous women. Women

TABLE 8.1. *The prevalence of a history of infecundity by selected variables, Costa Rican women aged 25–59, 1984*

Variable	% infecund	(N)
Age		
25–9	9.3	(129)
30–4	8.2	(159)
35–9	6.0	(151)
40–4	7.6	(105)
45–9	10.7	(122)
50–4	5.5	(109)
55–9	8.4	(95)
Region		
San José	8.4	(297)
Rest of urban valley	5.2	(151)
Rural valley	8.9	(140)
Urban, outside valley	6.7	(91)
Rural, outside valley	9.9	(191)
Education		
None	5.5	(93)
Primary, incomplete	9.4	(284)
Primary, complete	8.7	(214)
High school	7.8	(195)
University	5.8	(84)
Income Index		
Low	6.0	(308)
Middle	9.6	(342)
High	8.6	(220)
TOTAL	8.1	(870)

TABLE 8.2. *The prevalence of a history of infecundity by number of lifetime sexual partners and age at first coitus, Costa Rican women aged 25–59, 1984*

	Number of sexual partners			Age at first coitus			
	0	1	≥2	None	<16	16–19	≥20
% infecund	n/a	7.1	11.9	n/a	13.1	8.6	7.0
(N)	(45)	(573)	(250)	(45)	(123)	(314)	(384)

whose first coitus occurred when they were less than 16 years of age were more likely to report difficulty in becoming pregnant than women whose first intercourse occurred after age 19 ($p < 0.05$, see Table 8.2). These two variables are, however, closely correlated and difficult to dissociate from one another.

Overall, 39.4 per cent of women had antibodies to HSV-2; 6.4 per cent had serological evidence of previous syphilis infection; and 56.1 per cent had chlamydia antibodies (Oberle *et al.*, 1989; Vetter *et al.*, 1990; Larsen *et al.*, 1991). For each of these serological tests, sero-positive women were more likely than sero-negative women to report a history of infecundity, although these differences were of borderline statistical significance. However, there was the suggestion of a cohort effect: among older women only (age 40–59), those with a history of infecundity were more likely to be sero-positive to each of the three STDs ($p < .05$). Most infecund women (57.7 per cent) were diagnosed before the age of 30, although this estimate was based on only 26 women who reported having a physician's diagnosis.

The data presented here reflect a history of infecundity at any time rather than the prevalence of infecundity. An estimate of incidence or prevalence would be a much more useful public health measure of the potential demand for

TABLE 8.3. *The prevalence of a history of infecundity by serological status for three sexually transmitted diseases, Costa Rican women aged 25–59, 1984*

STD serological status	% infecund	(N)
Syphilis		
Positive	12.8	(54)
Negative	7.8	(713)
HSV-2[a]		
Positive	10.1	(314)
Negative	6.9	(445)
Chlamydia		
Positive	9.0	(437)
Negative	6.6	(323)

[a] HSV-2 = Herpes Simplex Type-2

infertility services. To obtain a minimal estimate of period prevalence, we used the life-history calendars. We counted as prevalent cases those women who reported a history of infecundity and whose life-history calendars had an interval of at least 24 months of unprotected sexual activity that extended into the year prior to interview. By this definition, 2.2 per cent of currently married women 25–44 years of age were infecund in 1984.

Discussion

In this study, 8.1 per cent of Costa Rican women 25 to 59 years of age had a history of difficulty in becoming pregnant at some point in their lives. This figure compares with 12.5 per cent of women with such a history in March-banks's analysis of a population-based study of US women 20–54 years of age (Marchbanks 1989). Only 5.4 per cent of Costa Rican women had consulted a physician for an infecundity problem, and 3.2 per cent of all women reported having a physician's confirmation and diagnosis. The difference in responses to these three questions suggests that clinic-based information on infecundity would underestimate the extent of infecundity in Costa Rica.

In 1984 approximately 2.2 per cent of married Costa Rican women 25–44 years of age were currently infecund, representing a potential demand for infertility services by 5100 women. However, this is an underestimate of the need for infertility services, because the survey did not include women 15–24 years of age. More importantly, since 70 per cent of women in union currently use contraceptives (Rosero-Bixby and Oberle, 1989) a large but unknown number of contraceptors may be infecund but will not discover this unless they stop using contraception and attempt to become pregnant.

Since this population-based study was not specifically designed to characterize infecundity, the sample size may have been inadequate to detect differences in infecundity in various demographic subgroups. By comparing women's life-history calendars with their responses to the questions on infecundity, we can obtain some idea of the consistency of the direct questions on infecundity. Overall, 93 per cent of women with a history of infecundity reported on the calendar a sexually active, infecund interval in which they used no contraception. Only five women with a history of infecundity did not have segments of unprotected sexual intercourse on their life-history calendars, but four of these five women had possible explanations for the lack of calendar evidence of infecundity. Three had used a rhythm method for several years and may in fact have used the rhythm method as a contraceptive initially and then later used a menstrual calendar while trying to conceive. An additional woman had been sterilized in 1981 and may have regretted this decision.

In summary, in this secondary analysis of a population-based control series, women with two or more lifetime sex partners were more likely to report a history of infecundity than completely monogamous women. A higher proportion of women with serological evidence of infection with one of three sexually transmitted diseases reported a history of infecundity. Had we had information on the clinical classification of infecundity, we would expect an even stronger association between the serological evidence of past infection and tubal infertility. The results of serological and sexual histories from this small, descriptive study are consistent with the hypothesis that sexually transmitted diseases may be associated with infecundity in Costa Rica. However, an analytical, case-control study would be necessary to explore this relationship adequately.

References

Irwin, K. L., Rosero-Bixby, L., Oberle, M. W., Lee, N. C., Whatley, A. S., Fortney, J. A., Bonhomme, M. G. (1988), 'Oral Contraceptives and Cervical Cancer Risk in Costa Rica: Detection Bias or Causal Association?' *Journal of the American Medical Association* 259: 59–64.

Larsen, S. A., Oberle, M. W., Sanchez-Braverman, J. M., Rosero-Bixby, L., Vetter, K. M. (1991), 'A Population-Based Serosurveillance of Syphilis in Costa Rica', *Sexually Transmitted Diseases* 18: 124–8.

Marchbanks, P. A., Peterson, H. B., Rubin, G. L., Wingo, P. A., and the Cancer and Steroid Hormone Study Group (1989), 'Research on Infertility: Definition Makes a Difference', *American Journal of Epidemiology* 130: 259–67.

Oberle, M. W., Rosero-Bixby, L., Lee, F. K., Sanchez-Braverman, M., Nahmias, A. J., Guinan, M. E. (1989), '*Herpes simplex* Virus Type 2 Antibodies: High Prevalence in Monogamous Women in Costa Rica', *American Journal of Tropical Medicine and Hygiene* 41: 224–9.

Ramirez, J. A., Rosero-Bixby, L., Oberle, M. W. (1987), 'Susceptibilidad al Tétanos y Rubeola en las Mujeres de Costa Rica, 1984–85', *Revista Costarricense de Ciencias Médicas* 8: 251–9.

Rosero-Bixby, L., and Oberle, M. W. (1987), 'Tabaquismo en la Mujer Costarricense, 1984–85', *Revista de Ciencias Sociales (San José)* 35: 95–102.

—— —— (1989), 'Fertility Change in Costa Rica, 1960–84: Analysis of Retrospective Lifetime Reproductive Histories', *Journal of Biosocial Science* 21: 419–32.

—— —— Lee, N. C. (1987), 'Reproductive History and Breast Cancer in a Population of High Fertility: Costa Rica', *International Journal of Cancer* 40: 747–54.

Vaessen, M. (1984), *Childlessness and Infecundity*, World Fertility Survey, Comparative Studies no. 31, International Statistical Institute, Voorburg, the Netherlands.

Vetter, K. M., Barnes, R. C., Oberle, M. W., Rosero-Bixby, L., and Schachter, J. (1990), 'Seroepidemiology of Chlamydia in Costa Rica', *Genitourinary Medicine* 66: 182–8.

9 The Effects of Exercise and Nutrition on the Menstrual Cycle

DAVID C. CUMMING

Introduction

Strenuous physical activity, particularly endurance training, is associated with delayed menarche, inadequate luteal phase, anovulatory cycles, and oligo-menorrhoea. Sub-clinical changes occur in a majority of exercising women with as little as one month of strenuous physical activity (Prior, 1982a, 1982b; Bullen et al., 1985). However, the prevalence and long-term significance of exercise-associated reproductive dysfunction are still debated. Suppression of the hypothalamic–pituitary–gonadal (HPG) axis may also occur in male runners and other athletes.

Nutritional status also influences reproduction and it appears that nutrition has a significant role in the development of exercise-associated reproductive dysfunction. The interrelationship of the various factors involved in both exercise-associated and nutritional amenorrhoea continues to be explored and is becoming clearer. The purpose of the present paper is to examine the effects of exercise on reproductive function in women and to discuss the mechanisms through which reproductive dysfunction can be influenced by changes in physical activity and nutritional status.

Delay in Menarche

Competitive athletes and ballet dancers have a delay in pubertal development and menarche when compared with non-exercising control groups or the population mean (see Fig. 9.1) (Malina et al., 1973, 1978, 1979; Warren, 1980; Frisch et al., 1980; Frisch et al., 1981; Wakat et al., 1978). The mean age of menarche was significantly later in 66 college track-and-field athletes compared with sedentary controls (in whom menarche occurred at the same age as the published norms) (Malina et al., 1973). Competition at various levels and in different sports also influences the time of menarche (Malina et al., 1978, 1979). The delay in ballet dancers far exceeds even that reported in Olympic athletes (Warren, 1980).

A range of explanations unrelated to the physical activity was initially

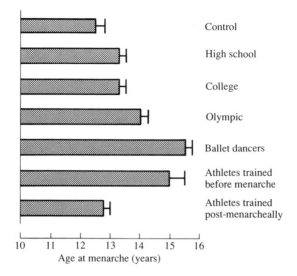

Age at menarche in control (normally sedentary) women, high school athletes, college athletes, athletes at the Montreal Olympic games, 1976, ballet dancers and two groups of swimmers and runners, divided according to whether they had begun training before menarche or post-menarcheally.

Source: The figure is a composite of several studies cited in the text.

Fig. 9.1   Exercise and age at menarche

offered for this delay in menarche. The pre-pubertal individual has a marked advantage in strength/weight ratio over her post-pubertal counterpart, which is an advantage in some sports such as gymnastics. Better neuromuscular co-ordination and a physical build with increased height, longer legs, and narrower hips are favoured by delayed puberty and may result in better athletic perform-ance (Espenschade, 1940; McNeill and Livson, 1963). Young women who mature early may socialize away from sports or physical activity within a given chronological age-group (Malina *et al.*, 1978).

Evidence, however, suggests that the physical activity itself is important in delaying the onset of menses (Frisch *et al.*, 1981). Frisch reported that the post-menarcheally trained athlete has a time of menarche similar to the general population, while her counterpart who was training pre-menarcheally has a significant delay, which is proportional to the time spent in training. The remarkable delay in menarche in ballet dancers is probably the result of their pattern of training rather than any specific effect of ballet. The age of menarche is similar in pre-menarcheally trained athletes and ballet dancers for whom long hours of practice are normal from a very young age. Warren, in a longitudinal study of teenage ballet dancers in a professional school, followed the students over 3 to 5 years (Warren, 1980). There was a clear training effect, since advancement of pubertal stages and/or resumption of menses occurred during times of inactivity. The rapid development which occurred at these times was termed 'catch-up puberty', analogous to the changes which occur during refeeding after chronic malnutrition.

Luteal Phase Inadequacy and Anovulatory Cycles

A shorter than normal luteal phase and reduced mid-luteal progesterone levels were reported in a single subject case-study of a 30-year-old woman runner during intensive training (Shangold *et al.*, 1979). Daily blood sampling in four élite teenage swimmers revealed an abbreviated luteal phase of the menstrual cycle compared with a non-exercising group of similar age (Bonen *et al.*, 1981). Progesterone levels in the swimmers failed to rise despite an LH surge, suggesting that the follicle failed to luteinize.

Two-thirds of 48 basal body temperature graphs from 14 runners in a marathon clinic were abnormal (Prior, 1982*b*). The abnormalities were equally divided between an abbreviated thermal shift (temperature rise less than 10 days) and monophasic graphs, suggesting, respectively, inadequate luteal phase and anovulation. Training runs, but not weekly mileage, were significantly longer in the two abnormal groups. Individual runners had, on separate occasions, different types of abnormal cycles.

Endometrial biopsy specimens were suggestive of inadequate luteal phase in two women runners seeking pregnancy (Prior *et al.*, 1982). Biopsy dating returned to normal when the exercise load was reduced. Salivary progesterone levels measured daily were significantly lower in 15 runner cycles compared with 19 non-exercise control cycles (Ellison and Lager, 1985). The mean weekly training load in runners was 20 km, suggesting that effects can be seen in recreational runners as well as competitive distance runners.

The unobtrusive, sub-clinical nature of these changes has been emphasized. The normal menstrual function of previously sedentary women was disrupted by 2 months of training beginning at 4 miles per day and reaching 10 miles per day by the fifth week (Bullen *et al.*, 1985). Food intake was controlled either to maintain weight or to lose weight at the rate of 0.45 kg per week. Menstrual function became abnormal in 9 of 12 subjects in the weight maintenance groups and in 15 of 16 subjects in the weight-loss group, judged on the basis of either clinical disorders (abnormal bleeding or delayed menses) or hormonal disturbances (reduced progesterone or absent LH surge). All of the runners decreased their physical activity and returned to normal menstrual function by 12 weeks after the study. While this finding is reassuring, it is unfortunate that the study could not demonstrate whether the menstrual cycle changes, once induced by a critical level of physical activity, were constant or whether they returned to a more normal pattern as the organism became adjusted to the stress of that particular level of activity.

Secondary Amenorrhoea and Oligomenorrhoea

The first significant study of secondary amenorrhoea in women runners by Feicht and colleagues was published as a letter to the editor of the *Lancet* (Feicht *et al.*, 1978). A questionnaire was sent to 400 members of collegiate track-and-field and cross-country teams, and 128 replies were received from women not taking birth-control pills. Women runners who had experienced three periods or less in the previous year were defined as having secondary amenorrhoea. The frequency of amenorrhoea thus defined, varied from 6 to 43 per cent depending upon weekly mileage (Fig. 9.2). It is a reasonable assumption that the frequency of amenorrhoea was lower in the non-responders than in those women who took the time to reply to the questionnaire, so that the actual prevalence of exercise-associated reproductive problems is likely to be significantly lower.

Speroff and Redwine (1979) found 46 of 872 (5.3 per cent) respondents to be amenorrhoeic. Only 18.6 per cent of respondents were running more than 20 miles per week and there did not appear to be an increase with increasing mileage. Dale *et al.* (1979) found the frequency of oligomenorrhoea in 'runners', 'joggers', and non-exercising controls to be respectively 34, 23, and 4 per cent. Similarly, Shangold and Levine (1982) found 16 and 2 per cent of women during marathon training to be oligomenorrhoeic and amenorrhoeic respectively, with Lutter and Cushman (1982) finding 19.3 per cent irregular and 3.4 per cent amenorrhoeic in a similar group.

The point prevalence of amenorrhoea in non-athletic women of similar age has been estimated at approximately 2 per cent (Drew, 1961; Sher, 1942; Petterson and Fries, 1973). These studies were based on carefully chosen samples from representative populations. No similar estimates are available for the frequency of oligomenorrhoea. The estimates of point prevalence of

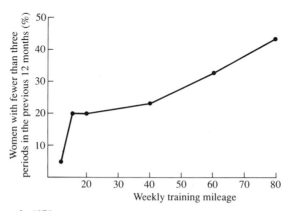

Source: Feicht *et al.*, 1978.

Fig. 9.2   The effect of weekly training mileage on the prevalence of oligomenorrhoea, defined as less than three periods in the previous year

amenorrhoea in the studies of women runners have generally relied on responses to questionnaire surveys, which may give a somewhat biased view, since it may be assumed that runners with problems may respond to the survey with greater frequency than normally menstruating runners. Based on these cross-sectional studies, some have suggested that there is not, in fact, a significant increase in exercise-associated amenorrhoea (Shangold and Levine, 1982).

Factors in Exercise-Associated Reproductive Dysfunction

The question of why menstrual irregularity should occur in runners has received considerably more attention in recent years. Amenorrhoeic runners may have significant advantages in speed compared with their normally menstruating peers (Dale *et al.*, 1979; Schwartz *et al.*, 1981), but it is not essential to develop oligomenorrhoea to be involved in exercise at the highest levels (Deuster *et al.*, 1986). There were no significant differences in cardiopulmonary function between small groups of amenorrhoeic and normally menstruating runners (Cumming and Belcastro, 1982).

Prior (1982*a*) suggested that the reproductive changes may be a hypothalamic adaptation, a change analogous to the physical conditioning that results from training. Physical conditioning clearly has benefit in the more efficient functioning of the organism. The question of whether reproductive function changes have immediate or long-term benefit(s) other than reduced fertility has been given scant attention. The !Kung San women of Southern Africa may represent the adaptation in a 'hunter-gatherer' situation. The amenorrhoea which develops is considered teleologically necessary to space the family in a manner which sustains the mothers' ability to walk 20–30 km per day, a feat which is possible carrying one child, but not with more than one child.

An alternative interpretation is that menstrual irregularity represents a stress response, perhaps making necessary metabolic facilities available to other systems. It is generally assumed that the reproductive changes are hypothalamic in origin and, from mostly anecdotal evidence, are reversible when the organism has learned to cope with the stresses which face it or when those stresses are reduced (Rebar and Cumming, 1981). Progress is being made in elucidating pathophysiological mechanisms potentially involved in exercise-associated menstrual irregularity. The various pathophysiological factors of exercise-induced changes in reproductive function will be discussed in detail, and are summarized below:

The physical stress of training and/or competing
The emotional stress of training and/or competing
Abnormalities of nutrition and energy drain
Predisposition
Altered lean–fat ratio

Loss of weight
Acute hormonal changes with exertion
Chronic hormonal effects of training

The Physical Stress of Training and/or Competition

Acute exercise is physically stressful, producing alterations in cardiac, pulmonary, and metabolic function at several sites including hepatic, pancreatic, and muscle metabolism. Minor injuries were much more common in the first group of women recruits to the US Military Academy than in their male counterparts and, over the same periods, the prevalence of amenorrhoea was extremely high (Anderson, 1979). Cross-sectional studies to determine whether increasing mileage and intensity of training increased the frequency of oligomenorrhoea have produced conflicting data and varied interpretations. Initial studies by Feicht and colleagues (1978) showed a clear increase in frequency of amenorrhoea as mileage increased. Dale *et al.* (1979) found that the frequency of oligomenorrhoea was greater in 'runners' (training volume over 30 miles per week) than in 'joggers' (5–30 miles per week). Lutter and Cushman (1982) investigated 350 women runners and found that mileage and frequency of running was greater in oligomenorrhoeic runners. In contrast, several studies found no effect of increased weekly training volume (Wakat *et al.*, 1978; Speroff and Redwine, 1979; Shangold and Levine, 1982; Schwartz *et al.*, 1981; Baker *et al.*, 1982). The question of intensity of exercise (e.g. speed of running) has received scant attention.

Prospective training studies have also tended to support the contention that most women who have regular menses when they initiate training continue to do so with increased training volume (Shangold and Levine, 1982). A series of studies from Tucson found that none of the 18 normally menstruating runners who added 50 miles per week to their training volume became amenorrhoeic, although there were clear effects on the reproductive system (Boyden *et al.*, 1982, 1983, 1984). Similarly, women in Prior's (1982*b*) study retained cycles although there were some very clear effects of training. In contrast, five of 13 regularly menstruating swimmers became oligomenorrhoeic when weekly training volume was increased from 60 to 100 km per week (Russell *et al.*, 1984*a*, 1984*b*). Training intensity and/or mileage in the genesis of the reproductive dysfunction seems to be a 'commonsense' finding but the evidence is far from conclusive.

The Emotional Stress of Training and Competing

Early authors suggested that trying to fit exercise and/or competition into a busy schedule was bound to cause psychological stress. When women runners were asked to evaluate subjectively the degree of stress associated with training, amenorrhoeic runners reported significantly more stress than their normally menstruating peers (Schwartz *et al.*, 1981). Time of menarche was normal in young musicians seeking a professional career but was delayed in ballet dancers by approximately 3 years (Warren, 1980). Assuming that the goal-oriented life-style provided a similar degree of stress for each group, the author suggested that the delay in menarche among ballet dancers was 'not entirely related to stress'.

Our early study of psychological profiles found no differences among non-exercising controls and amenorrhoeic and normally menstruating runners in any of the objective scales used to measure depression, hypochondriasis, psychasthenia, or obsessive-compulsive tendencies (Schwartz *et al.* 1981). However, in a similar study obsessive-compulsive and psychoticism scales were significantly higher in amenorrhoeic than in normally menstruating runners (Galle *et al.*, 1983). While there was no significant difference between the groups on the depression scale, a discriminant analysis suggested that this factor made the strongest independent contribution to reproductive dysfunction after the height/weight ratio, with weight change being the third contributor. None of the scores in any of the runners was indicative of a clinical problem.

Exercise has been used as a form of therapy in treating stress. Psychological advantages of physical activity include better stress management, reduction of depression, improved self-esteem, an improved feeling of well-being, and a heightened sense of personal control. However, more recently concern over psychological dependence on running was voiced by Morgan (1979), who termed the need to continue running against medical advice as 'negative addiction'. As with many aspects of exercise, the question of psychological benefits versus problems suggests that physical activity may be a two-edged sword. It seems likely that the benefit is real but that an equally real set of psychological problems may occur under certain circumstances. There is, however, scant evidence that the menstrual irregularity associated with physical activity has as its primary origin either psychological or psychiatric problems. Even when differences in psychological well-being have been shown between normally menstruating and amenorrhoeic runners, these differences have statistical, rather than clinical, relevance.

Body Composition, Nutrition, Reproduction, and Physical Activity

Although the role of nutrition and body composition in determining the onset and maintenance of normal reproductive function has been explored extensively in animals (Kirkwood *et al.*, 1987), ethical constraints have limited reports on humans to indirect, observational data. Over the last century, the mean menarcheal age has declined as more young women enter puberty at an early age (Tanner, 1962, 1981; Brown, 1966). The change has been accompanied by an increase in stature clearly apparent in school-age children (Tanner, 1962). Menarche has roughly corresponded with physical size rather than chrono-logical age, and, thus, women are achieving menarche at approximately the same physical size as their mothers but at an earlier age (Frisch, 1972). The trend towards earlier menarche may now have halted (Tanner, 1981; Damon, 1974). In geographical locations where the pattern of nutrition has not changed over many years (e.g. some Inuit, Lapp, and East Indian populations), the age of menarche has not changed over at least a generation (Bojilen and Bentzoin, 1968). Famine and starvation from warfare have provided short-term nutritional stresses. In these situations, the reproductive consequences (amenorrhoea and/or infertility) were first seen in women whose nutrition was likely to have been marginal prior to the event (Stein and Susser, 1975).

These observations have provided circumstantial evidence that nutrition and/or body composition may have an effect on the timing of menarche. In 37 582 women of varied ethnic backgrounds in a single geographical area, the reported age of menarche correlated with economic level and its attendant variables (e.g., level of nutrition) rather than race: women from lower socio-economic groups had later menarche (Weir *et al.*, 1971). Diets inferior in protein, carbohydrate, and fat throughout childhood, compared with the diets of European girls, probably cause the delay of over one year in the mean menarcheal age of rural and urban Bantu girls in South Africa (Baanders-Van Halewin and de Ward, 1968). Dietary differences could also be responsible for the difference in menarcheal age between the urban and the rural Bantu girls. Urban–rural differences in menarcheal age have been reported in other countries where the diet has been of borderline adequacy (Wolanski, 1968; Kantero and Widholm, 1971).

In Western countries, the most likely cause of dietary inadequacy in the peripubertal period is self-induced. Dieting, self-induced weight loss, and low body weight are clearly associated with delayed menarche (Kennedy, 1969). Where dietary inadequacy was observed in the USA, there was an effect on the age of physical and reproductive maturity (Dreizen *et al.*, 1967). The mean age of menarche was 12.4 years where the diet was adequate and 14.5 years where there was protein–calorie malnutrition. This was accompanied by delayed skeletal maturation and smaller stature. When puberty is delayed despite adequate nutrition, increased stature and a linear physique is usually found (McNeill and Livson, 1963).

Based on these observations linking poor nutrition with delayed age of menarche, it was suggested that, even in circumstances where nutrition is not in question, the age at which menarche occurs is more closely related to body weight than to chronological age, and, initially, body weight was suggested as a trigger for the onset of menarche (Frisch and Revelle, 1971). However, maturation involves a relative decrease in body water throughout puberty (Fries-Hansen, 1956), suggesting a relative gain in body fat. Calculations of total body water and lean and fat body mass were made for each of three pubertal milestones (growth spurt, peak height velocity, and menarche) using a formula based on height and weight (Frisch *et al.*, 1973). There was a relative increase in body fat compared with lean mass between the initiation of the adolescent growth spurt and menarche (Frisch *et al.*, 1973). The increase in body fat roughly corresponded to the energy requirements of pregnancy and three months of breastfeeding, a finding which was considered to have teleological significance (Frisch, 1984). It was also found that late maturers gain fat more slowly than early maturers, focusing attention on percentage of body fat as a trigger controlling the timing of menarche. The data upon which the theory was based are cross-sectional and were derived rather than observed. Some studies have supported the theory (Wishik, 1977), but detailed criticisms of the minimal body fat hypothesis have been published. The variability of subjects in Frisch's own study can be seen from her scattergrams (Frisch and Revelle, 1971). Others have disputed the repeatability of the original data (Billewicz *et al.*, 1976; Johnston *et al.*, 1975), the accuracy of the methodology (Reeves, 1979; Cumming and Rebar, 1984), and the statistical validity of the conclusions (Johnston *et al.*, 1975; Trussell, 1978).

Frisch (1985) has suggested four mechanisms through which fat may modify the functioning of the hypothalamic–pituitary–gonadal axis. First, fat tissue may influence the conversion of androgens to oestrogens (Siiteri and MacDonald, 1973). Since adrenarche takes place some time before menarche (Ducharme *et al.*, 1976), it may be assumed that androgenic precursors will be available. There are other tissues which convert androgens to oestrogens, but adipose tissue perhaps represents the most significant extragonadal source of oestrogen, at least in post-menopausal women (Siiteri and MacDonald, 1973). The increase in oestrone, the main oestrogen derived from peripheral androgen precursors, begins some three to six years prior to menarche, and the rise is progressive and linear throughout puberty (Saez and Morera, 1973; Bidlingmaier *et al.*, 1973; Gupta, 1975), suggesting that precursor availability may be a more significant drive than the late increase in body fat. The second factor suggested was that increasing fat can modify the direction of oestrogen metabolism to more or less potent forms (Fishman *et al.*, 1975). These were at non-physiological extremes of obesity and anorexia nervosa. Third, obese women have diminished SHBG (serum hormone binding globulin) levels (Plymate *et al.*, 1981); again, this is a non-physiological extreme. SHBG levels are lower in pubertal children and adults than in pre-pubertal children (Forest and Bertrand, 1972; Moll and Rosenfeld, 1979). The transition is gradual, beginning at about the age of 9–10 years, and the decrease in SHBG is related to increasing testosterone levels, suggesting that this factor and not body fat is responsible for the decreased SHBG levels (Bartsch *et al.*, 1980). Finally, it was observed that fat tissues are capable of storing steroid hormones (Kaku, 1969). How this may affect circulating levels of oestrogen and their interaction with the pituitary is unclear.

Puberty is underway long before the onset of menses, and it is clear from Warren's (1980) data that it is not just menarche which is delayed but, specifically, early maturation of the gonadotrophin-releasing hormone (GnRH)–pituitary axis. The initiation of puberty, as opposed to menarche, is not critically dependent upon the attainment of a specific body composition, though it may be inhibited by malnutrition or perhaps a relative excess of energy output over intake. Menarche occurs when there is sufficient variability in oestrogen levels to permit endometrial build-up and breakdown. This is ultimately dependent upon the acquisition of pulsatile release of GnRH (Boyar *et al.*, 1972), release of a biologically more active gonadotrophin (Lucky *et al.*, 1980), reduction of negative feedback (Winter and Faiman, 1973*b*; Winter *et al.*, 1978; Kelch *et al.*, 1973), acquisition of positive feedback mechanisms (Winter *et al.*, 1978; Reiter *et al.*, 1974; Winter and Faiman, 1973*b*), increasing sex steroid levels (Ducharme *et al.*, 1976; Saez and Morera, 1973; Bidlingmaier *et al.*, 1973; Gupta, 1975; Jenner *et al.*, 1972; Lee *et al.*, 1977), and cyclic variation of sex steroids and gonadotrophins (Winter and Faiman, 1973*b*; Hansen *et al.*, 1975).

The initiation of all these physiological developments precedes both the peak height velocity and menarche by some considerable time, and the linear increments in circulating sex steroids do not appear to be significantly modified during later puberty when peripheral fat deposition would be expected to exert an influence. The progressively rising sex steroid levels may be responsible for some of the physical changes which may occur, for example, the growth spurt and the deposition of fatty tissue responsible for the usual female shape (in the breasts and over the abdomen and buttocks) (Winter *et al.*, 1978). If one accepts that there is a temporal association, then the data can be interpreted in two ways in addition to the Frisch hypothesis. There may be a predetermined growth pattern which arranges that the completion of reproductive maturity should occur at the time when physical growth is completed. Alternatively, the rising levels of sex steroids could influence the body composition, rather than body composition influencing the timing of menarche. If the attainment of a minimal percentage of body fat is a necessary prerequisite for menarche, reaching the threshold will not *per se* be sufficient to trigger menarche. The maturation of the HPG (hypothalamic–pituitary–gonadal) axis remains essential and is independent (Crawford and Osler, 1975).

The possibility may also be entertained that it is not body composition but the lack of a dietary component which is important in the development of amenorrhoea or delay in puberty. Although malnutrition is associated with reduced gonadotrophin levels both pre-pubertally (Chakravarty *et al.*, 1982; Kulin *et al.*, 1984) and after maturation (Vigersky *et al.*, 1977; Beumont *et al.*, 1976), short-term fasting in obese women did not change serum gonadotrophin levels despite increases in renal luteinizing hormone (LH) and follicle-stimulating hormone (FSH) excretion (Beitins *et al.*, 1980). Short-term fasting in human males and animals has suggested reductions in pituitary release of gonadotrophins (Klibanski *et al.*, 1981; Dubey *et al.*, 1986). Attempts to define specific nutrients associated with reduced gonadotrophin levels have met with mixed and somewhat inconclusive results (Steiner, 1987).

Despite the theoretical arguments, low body weight, dieting, weight loss, and reduced body fat have been associated with both primary and secondary amenorrhoea (Fries *et al.*, 1974; Kennedy, 1969). Studies of the percentage of body fat in amenorrhoeic and normally menstruating runners have generally supported the association of low body fat with amenorrhoea. Data calculated from skinfold thickness at three sites indicated that amenorrhoeic runners had lower percentages of body fat than normally menstruating runners, who, in turn, were leaner than untrained women (Schwartz *et al.*, 1981). Using a nomogram based on height and weight, ballet dancers with secondary amenor-rhoea were significantly leaner than those with regular cycles (Frisch *et al.*, 1980). Amenorrhoeic athletes were lighter, had less body fat, and had lost more weight following the onset of running than their normally menstruating counterparts (Dale *et al.*, 1979; Schwartz *et al.*, 1981; Speroff and Redwine, 1979). However, other studies have failed to find any connection between reduced body fat and amenorrhoea (Shangold and Levine, 1982; Deuster *et al.*, 1986; Baker *et al.*, 1981).

Published studies of body composition in amenorrhoeic runners have used several different methods of calculation, whose use is based on assumptions that it is possible to measure accurately the skinfold thickness, that the chosen sites are representative of overall body fat, and that the formula chosen to calculate body fat is accurate over the range of subjects to be examined. There is a large, method-specific variation in estimates of body fat which is reflected in groups of amenorrhoeic and normally menstruating runners and normally menstruating controls (Cumming and Rebar, 1984). Differing conclusions can be drawn from the same population depending on the means of calculation. Only one study has utilized the hydrostatic method, the 'gold standard' of methods of calculating percentage body fat, to determine the percentage of body fat in runners with menstrual dysfunction or normal cycles. The findings supported the theory that menstrual irregularity in exercise was associated with a lower percentage of body fat (Carlberg *et al.*, 1983). However, low body fat is not invariably associated with reduced percentage of body fat.

Injuries preventing exercise in amenorrhoeic young ballet dancers precipitated menarche or were followed by resumption of menses in the absence of any weight change (Warren, 1980). Warren postulated that the significant energy drain of exercise may delay menarche or result in amenorrhoea without altering body composition. There is anecdotal evidence that a relatively small change in weight around the critical level may regulate menstruation, since a swimmer and runners can control menses through a change in weight over 1–2 kg (Frisch *et al.*, 1981; Schwartz *et al.*, 1981). It seems unlikely that such a small alteration in the lean–fat ratio alone can influence menstrual function. Other endocrine changes accompany the decrease in weight and fasting, and these may influence the central regulation of menstrual function. Altered diets were observed in runners beginning training pre-menarcheally (Frisch *et al.*, 1981). Schwartz and colleagues (1981) reported significant reductions in the protein content of the diets of amenorrhoeic runners compared with the diets of normally menstruating runners. Others have suggested that a reduction in fat intake may be important (Deuster *et al.*, 1986).

It is clear that the role of various factors in relation to diet, critical body weight or body composition, and loss of weight remain to be clarified. The relative imprecision of dietary evaluation, the dispute over body-fat evaluation methodology, and the conceptual barrier erected by the body-fat theory must all be dealt with before progress can finally resolve the complex interrelationships between reproduction, nutrition, and body composition.

Predisposition to Menstrual Irregularity

Women with reproductive dysfunction induced by exercise tend to be younger than those reporting regular menstrual cycles (Dale *et al.*, 1979; Lutter and Cushman, 1982; Schwartz *et al.*, 1981; Baker *et al.*, 1981). Exercise at a young age may influence both the timing of menarche and subsequent menstrual function while continuing to exercise (Frisch *et al.*, 1981). Women with regular cycles before beginning exercise have less tendency to develop irregularity (Schwartz *et al.*, 1981; Shangold and Levine, 1982; Lutter and Cushman, 1982). Athletes who have had a previous pregnancy seem less likely to experience disruption of the menstrual cycle (Schwartz *et al.*, 1981; Shangold and Levine, 1982; Lutter and Cushman, 1982; Baker *et al.*, 1981). The consistency of these findings suggests a predisposition to menstrual irregularity in some women. It is unclear how this might be investigated further.

The Effect of Exercise and Training on the Hormonal Control of the Hypothalamic–Pituitary–Gonadal Axis

Changes in the endocrine functioning of the HPG axis associated with chronic training and with acute exercise have been explored in some detail (Schwartz *et al.*, 1981; Cumming and Rebar, 1985). Acute exercise is physically stressful, producing changes in cardiac, pulmonary, and metabolic function. It is difficult to view short-term, acute-exercise-induced alterations in reproductive hormone levels as involved in the physiological adjustments to improve muscle or cardio-pulmonary function.

Comparisons of hormonal function between amenorrhoeic and normally menstruating runners have generally supported the suggestion that the mechanism of change is hypothalamic, with reduced or normal levels of LH and FSH. Levels of plasma oestradiol, SHBG, and LH in 6 amenorrhoeic runners were lower than levels in 14 control runners and 12 non-runners with normal cycles (Baker *et al.*, 1981). Levels of DHEA (dihydro-epiandrosterone), DHEAS (dihydro-epiandrosterone sulphate), androstenedione, cortisol, FSH, and prolactin were measured, and no differences were found among the groups. Schwartz *et al.* (1981) observed LH, but not FSH, levels to be higher in 12 amenorrhoeic runners than in normally menstruating runners in the early follicular phase of the cycle. Although the basal steroid levels did not differ among the groups, the ratio of oestrone to oestradiol was significantly increased in both amenorrhoeic and normally menstruating runners compared with non-running controls. In comparison with women with hypothalamic amenorrhoea, amenorrhoeic runners had significantly higher levels of LH and DHEAS and significantly lower levels of thyroid-stimulating hormone (TSH). These findings suggest that exercise-associated amenorrhoea may be a distinct entity or that the pathophysiological process leading to amenorrhoea may be heterogeneous.

Warren (1980) observed an apparent dichotomy in pubertal development which emerged when aspects of sexual maturation other than age at menarche were examined. Tanner's staging of pubic hair was appropriate for age but breast development was delayed, suggesting that the initiation of all the ovarian events of puberty are delayed, not just menarche. The pattern of delay is different from that which occurs in idiopathic delay of puberty where adrenarche and thelarche are both delayed (Copeland *et al.*, 1977). Adrenal androgen levels have been reported to be reduced in women with hypothalamic amenorrhoea not associated with exercise and in women with premature ovarian failure compared with age-matched controls (Cumming *et al.*, 1979). In contrast, DHEAS levels were normal in women with exercise-associated reproductive dysfunction (Schwartz *et al.*, 1981). The subtle differences between exercise-associated and other forms of primary and secondary amenorrhoea indicate the complexity of hypothalamic–pituitary–ovarian interaction.

The cross-sectional, single sample studies have some very obvious flaws. Reproductive hormone release is pulsatile in the short term and cyclic in the longer term. Single sample studies are inferior to those which permit an evaluation of the dynamic nature of the HPG axis. Few dynamic studies of the HPG axis in amenorrhoeic athletes have been performed. Long-term, prospective studies of the effect of physical activity are superior to cross-sectional studies, and several such studies have been carried out.

The first prospective investigations did not substantiate the previous finding that increasing mileage resulted in an increasing frequency of amenorrhoea, but they reported that a majority of cycles in such women may be anovulatory or have an inadequate luteal phase (Prior, 1982*b*). Cycles were shorter, with reduced mid-luteal gonadotrophin levels and statistically insignificant reductions in gonadotrophin response to GnRH. A similar series of investigations from Boyden and colleagues followed the effects of increasing training volume on a group of normally menstruating runners as they prepared for a marathon (Boyden *et al.*, 1982, 1983, 1984). The subjects were tested on days 8–11 in the late follicular phase at baseline (mean 15 miles per week) and when weekly mileage had reached 30 and 50 miles higher than baseline. The various reports showed that:

1. Total body weight did not change, but the subjects became leaner. As might be anticipated, lean weight increased by a mean of 2.7 kg, while fat mass decreased by 1.8 kg.

2. Basal prolactin levels decreased, but serum LH and FSH levels were unchanged by the increasing exercise load.
3. Serum oestradiol levels decreased, but testosterone and oestrone levels did not significantly decrease.
4. Gonadotrophin responses to GnRH decreased with increasing training volume.
5. Prolactin responses to thyrotrophin-releasing hormone (TRH) increased with increasing training volume.
6. There was a subjective decrease in menstrual volume or duration of flow.

These studies can be criticized because of the choice of days 8–11 of the cycle to perform dynamic studies. At this time the oestradiol levels should be increasing, and, since there was some variability in the cycles as mileage increased, the changes which were observed resulted from this rather than hypothalamic–pituitary suppression. The evidence from Prior's studies (1982a, 1982b) suggests that ovulation was occurring later in the cycle. The basal and dynamic hormonal changes which were reported by Boyden *et al.* (1983, 1984a, 1984b) could then have been the result of performing the studies at physiologically distinct times of the cycle.

A cross-sectional investigation from Finland was performed on 12 endurance-trained runners matched with 11 control women and 12 joggers matched with 7 control women in the late luteal phase of the cycle (Ronkainen, 1985). This investigation found that basal oestradiol and progesterone levels, as well as serum gonadotrophin responses to GnRH and prolactin responses to TRH and the dopamine receptor antagonist, metoclopramide, were significantly lower during the hard training season in the 12 endurance-trained women runners than in the 11 controls.

A longitudinal study from Finland compared high and low training seasons (Ronkainen *et al.*, 1985). Single samples were obtained from runners and controls on five occasions at specific times of the menstrual cycle. The study found some effects of hard training on the HPG axis but also found that there was a significant seasonal variation in the groups between the spring and fall periods, suggesting that the photoperiod may also influence the axis. Such a change could be significant in Oulu, Finland, where there is large variation in the daylight hours between winter and summer, but is less likely to be an influence in areas where there is less seasonal variation in the length of daylight.

The initiation of the normal menstrual cycle is dependent upon pulsatile release of GnRH, usually demonstrable as an LH pulse at 90–120 minute intervals in late luteal and early follicular phases (Yen *et al.*, 1972; Marshall *et al.*, 1984). Chronically altered frequency and amplitude of LH pulsatile release has been observed in the early follicular phase of the cycle in normally menstruating women runners (Fig. 9.3) (Cumming *et al.*, 1985a). Acute exercise further reduced the frequency of LH pulses (Cumming *et al.*, 1985b). LH pulse patterns are also disrupted in resting amenorrhoeic runners (Veldhuis

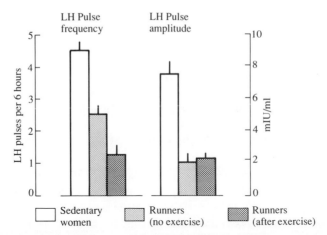

The pulse frequency is progressively reduced across the groups while the pulse amplitude is lower in runners in both situations but not further reduced by acute exercise.

Source: Composite figure from studies cited in the text.

Fig. 9.3   LH pulse frequency and amplitude in normally sedentary women, runners at rest, and runners following 60 minutes of running at 60% of maximal aerobic capacity

et al., 1985). These three studies provided clear evidence for the first time that the mechanism for exercise-associated reproductive dysfunction involved hypothalamic inhibition. Several neurotransmitters have been postulated to be involved including catechol oestrogens, dopamine, and an endogenous opiate, most popularly β-endorphin.

Neurotransmitter Involvement in Exercise-Associated Menstrual Dysfunction

Neurotransmitter control of the menstrual cycle is complex and involves catecholamines, catecholoestrogens, endogenous opiates (EO), and probably other neuromodulators. Evidence strongly suggests that dopamine and EO exert an inhibitory influence physiologically during the menstrual cycle and inappropriately in women with hypothalamic amenorrhoea. Administration of pharmacological doses of the enkephalin analogue DAMME results in a pulse pattern remarkably similar to that which we observed in normally menstruating women in the early follicular phase of the menstrual cycle (Grossman *et al.*, 1981). Peripheral β-endorphin/β-LPH (lipo-protein hormone) levels are chronically elevated at times of intensive training when reproductive dysfunction is more common (Fig. 9.4) (Russell *et al.*, 1984*b*).

Various forms of acute exercise release endogenous opiates from the pituitary (Cumming and Wheeler, 1987). The wide range of possible EO effects has encouraged research into their role in exercise performance, psychological and

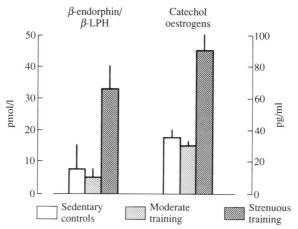

Source: Russell *et al.*, 1984*b*.

Fig. 9.4   The peripheral levels of B-endorphin/B-LPH and catechol oestrogens in sedentary women, swimmers during moderate training (60km/week), and swimmers during strenuous training (100km/week)

behavioural effects (including mood, appetite changes, exercise 'addiction', and pain perception), and a variety of hormonal changes including exercise-associated reproductive dysfunction. In perhaps the most controversial investigation, Carr and colleagues (1981) suggested that the plasma β-endorphin/β-LPH response to acute exercise increased in women with training. The conclusion was criticized because the relative load was kept constant, and power output increased as fitness increased (Farrel, 1981). Since, collectively, several investigations have suggested that the opiate response varies with workload (Cumming and Wheeler, 1987), it may be that the increased opiate response to exercise was not due to any increase in the endogenous capacity to secrete β-endorphin.

Most studies have shown that plasma opiate levels respond to physical activity, but what is the physiological significance of the increase? The presence of β-endorphin in cerebrospinal fluid at higher concentrations than in the peripheral blood and the poor penetration of β-endorphin through the blood–brain barrier implies a separately regulated central nervous system (CNS) manufacture (Nakao *et al.*, 1980; Rapoport *et al.*, 1980). Evaluation of the possible effects of any exercise-induced change must take into account the probability that peripheral levels do not enter into the CNS and the possibility that CNS changes may be quite different.

For peripheral levels of β-endorphin to affect hypothalamic function, it would be necessary for the peripheral levels to enter through the blood–brain barrier. Pharmacological doses of β-endorphin (1000 times physiological) and DAMME reduce circulating LH levels in the follicular phase of the cycle (Reid *et al.*, 1981; Stubbs *et al.*, 1978). Because of the low transfer into the CNS (Wiler *et al.*, 1979), it may be assumed that the mild increases in β-endorphin levels associated with exercise would not influence hypothalamic function. It is, however, also possible that the retrograde portal blood flow may carry endogenous opiates to the hypothalamus. A more likely explanation is that the increase in peripheral opiate levels is accompanied by an increase in hypo-thalamic β-endorphin.

It might be assumed that administration of opiate antagonists to amenorrhoeic runners would clarify the question. Unfortunately, evidence has been conflict-ing. Some studies have indicated that there is no alteration in gonadotrophin levels with an infusion of naloxone, while others have reported an increase in pulsatile LH release (Cumming and Rebar, 1983; Dixon *et al.*, 1984; McArthur *et al.*, 1980). The popular view that high peripheral EO levels, induced by the increased stress of more intensive training, relate to a central inhibitory effect remains to be proven.

Peripheral dopamine levels also increase with exercise (Van Loon, 1983), and dopamine also inhibits GnRH–pituitary action, presumably at the hypo-thalamic level. Interacting with endogenous opiates, they appear to exert an inhibitory tone on LH levels at times in the menstrual cycle and inappropriately in hypothalamic amenorrhoea. Other than the paper from Ronkainen (1985), which suggested a decreased serum prolactin response to metoclopramide in hard training runners compared with controls, little investigation has been carried out.

Catechol oestrogen levels have been shown to be elevated with β-endorphin in swimmers when their training load is increased from 60 to 100 km per week (Russell *et al.*, 1984*b*). Catechol oestrogens also appear to inhibit GnRH-gonadotrophin release (Merriam *et al.*, 1983) and have, therefore, been impli-cated in exercise-associated reproductive dysfunction. There is no direct evidence linking the peripheral increase in catechol oestrogens with central activity.

It is tempting to believe that the neurotransmitters are involved in the hypothalamic–pituitary alterations of exercise, but their involvement at present is purely conjecture. It is also likely that the common concept of a single neurotransmitter (e.g. an endogenous opiate) being responsible for menstrual dysfunction in exercise is simplistic.

Pathophysiology of Exercise-Associated Reproductive Dysfunction: A Synthesis

The evidence from LH pulse studies and from longitudinal studies of dynamic HPG axis function suggests that strenuous physical activity in women is associated with an inhibition of normal GnRH-gonadotrophin release, with secondary reductions in circulating sex steroids. In some situations, where there is an accompanying factor such as excessive thinness, nutritional inad-equacy, or hypothalamic immaturity, the sub-clinical changes become overt, with reduced frequency of menses, delayed onset of pubertal maturation, or amenorrhoea. The reversibility of this menstrual dysfunction with decreasing activity was assumed several years ago (Rebar and Cumming, 1981), and no evidence has refuted that assumption.

Anxiety over long-term sequelae of exercise-associated hypogonadism has tended to increase. Osteoporosis may well be a significant complication, but, equally important, anorexic tendencies may be part of the effect of exercise, and anorexia nervosa may be confused with exercise-associated hypogonadism. Some benefits have been suggested, such as reductions in the prevalence of hormone-dependent tumours and diabetes mellitus. Physical activity also provides a useful tool to explore hypothalamic–pituitary regulation of the ovaries, since it has become clear that exercise does form a reversible stress which alters HPG function in a substantial number of athletes. There is little doubt that exercise will continue to play an important role in the lives of pre-pubertal and reproductive age individuals. We should continue to explore the beneficial and harmful consequences of physical activity and, perhaps more importantly, be able to separate problems which are truly caused by exercise from those which occur because of an underlying problem and surface when exercise is part of the life-style.

References

Anderson, J. L. (1979), 'Women's Sports and Fitness Programs at the U.S. Military Academy', *Physical and Sports Medicine* 7(4): 72–8.

Baanders-Van Halewin, E. A., de Ward, F. (1968), 'Menstrual Cycles shortly after Menarche in European and Bantu Girls', *Human Biology* 40: 314–22.

Baker, E. R., Mathur, R. S., Kirk, R. F., and Williamson, H. O. (1981), 'Female Runners and Secondary Amenorrhea: Correlation with Age, Parity, Mileage and Plasma Hormonal and Sex-Hormone-Binding Globulin', *Fertility and Sterility* 36: 183–7.

————————— Landgrebe, S. C., Moody, L. O., and Williamson, H. O. (1982), 'Plasma Gonadotropins, Prolactin, and Steroid Hormone Concentrations Immediately After a Long Distance Run', *Fertility and Sterility* 38: 38–41.

Bartsch, W., Horst, H.-J., Derwahl, K. M. (1980), 'Interrelationships Between Sex-Hormone Binding Globulin and 17-β Estradiol, Testosterone, 5-α Dihydrotestosterone, Thyroxine and Triiodothyronine in Prepubertal and Pubertal Girls', *Journal of Clinical Endocrinology and Metabolism* 50: 1053–6.

Beitins, I. Z., Shah, A., O'Loughlin, K., Johnson, L., Ostrea, T. R., Van Wart, S., and McArthur, J. W. (1980), 'The Effects of Fasting on Serum and Urinary Gonadotropins in Obese Postmenopausal Women', *Journal of Clinical Endocrinology and Metabolism* 51: 26–34.

Beumont, P. J., George, G. C., Pimstone, B. L., and Vinik, A. I. (1976), 'Body Weight and the Pituitary Response to Hypothalamic Releasing Hormones in Patients with Anorexia Nervosa', *Journal of Clinical Endocrinology and Metabolism* 43: 487–96.

Bidlingmaier, F., Wagner-Barnack, M., Butenandt, O., and Knorr, D. (1973), 'Plasma

Estrogens in Childhood and Puberty Under Physiologic and Pathologic Conditions', *Pediatric Research* 7: 901–7.

Billewicz, W. S., Fellowes, H. M., and Hytten, C. (1976), 'Comments on the Critical Metabolic Mass and the Age of Menarche', *Annals of Human Biology* 3: 51–9.

Bojilen, K., and Bentzoin, M. (1968), 'Influence of Climate and Nutrition on Age at Menarche: A Historical Review and Modern Hypothesis', *Human Biology* 40: 69–85.

Bonen, A., Belcastro, A. M., Ling, W. Y., and Simpson, A. A. (1981), 'Profiles of Selected Hormones During the Menstrual Cycles of Teenage Athletes', *Journal of Applied Physiology* 50: 545–51.

Boyar, R., Finkelstein, J., Roffwarg, G., Kapen, S., Weitzman, E., and Hellman, L. (1972), 'Synchronization of Augmented Luteinizing Hormone Secretion with Sleep during Puberty', *New England Journal of Medicine* 287: 582–6.

Boyden, T. W., Pamenter, R. W., Gross, D., Stanforth, P., Rotkis, T. C., and Wilmore, J. H. (1982), 'Prolactin Responses, Menstrual Cycles, and Body Composition of Women Runners', *Journal of Clinical Endocrinology and Metabolism* 54: 711–14.

—— —— Stanforth, P., Rotkis, T. C., and Wilmore, J. H. (1983), 'Sex Steroid and Endurance Running in Women Runners', *Fertility and Sterility* 39: 629–632.

—— —— —— —— —— (1984), 'Impaired Gonadotropin Responses to Gonadotropin Stimulating Hormone in Endurance-Trained Women', *Fertility and Sterility* 41: 359–63.

Brown, P. E. (1966), 'The Age of Menarche', *British Journal of Social and Preventive Medicine* 20: 9–14.

Bullen, B. A., Skrinar, G. S., Beitins, I. Z., von Mering, G., Turnbull, B. A., and McArthur, J. W. (1985), 'Induction of Menstrual Disorders by Strenuous Exercise in Untrained Women', *New England Journal of Medicine* 312: 1349–53.

Carlberg, K. A., Buckman, M. T., Peake, G. T., and Riedesel, M. L. (1983), 'Body Composition of Oligo/Amenorrheic Athletes', *Medical Science and Sports Exercise* 15: 215–17.

Carr, D. B., Bullen, B. A., Skrinar, G. S., Arnold, M. A., Rosenblatt, M., Beitins, I. Z., Martin, J. B., and McArthur, J. W. (1981), 'Physical Conditioning Facilitates the Exercise-Induced Secretion of Beta-Endorphin and Beta-Lipotropin in Women', *New England Journal of Medicine* 305: 560–3.

Chakravarty, I., Sreedhar, R., Ghosh, K. K., Card, D., and Bulusu, S. (1982), 'Circulating Gonadotropin Profile in Severe Cases of Protein Calorie Malnutrition', *Fertility and Sterility* 37: 650–4.

Copeland, P. C., Paunier, L., and Sizonenko, P. C. (1977), 'The Secretion of Adrenal Androgens and Growth Patterns of Patients with Hypogonadotropic Hypogonadism', *Journal of Pediatrics* 91: 985–90.

Crawford, J. D., and Osler, D. C. (1975), 'Body Composition at Menarche: The Frisch–Revelle Hypothesis Revisited', *Pediatrics* 56: 449–58.

Cumming, D. C., and Belcastro, A. N. (1982), 'The Reproductive Effects of Exercise', *Current Problems in Obstetrics and Gynecology* 5(8): 1–42.

—— and Rebar, R. W. (1983), 'Effects of Exertion on Reproductive Function', *American Journal of Industrial Medicine* 5: 113–25.

—— —— (1984), 'Lack of Consistency in the Indirect Methods of Estimating Body Fat', *Fertility and Sterility* 41: 739–42.

—— —— (1985), 'Hormonal Changes with Acute Exercise and with Training in Women', *Seminars in Reproductive Endocrinology* 3: 55–64.

—— and Wheeler, G. D. (1987), 'Endorphins and Exercise', *Seminars in Reproductive Endocrinology* 5: 171–179.

—— Rebar, R. W., Hopper, B. R., and Yen, S. S. (1982), 'Evidence for an Influence of the Ovary on Circulating Dehydroepiandrosterone Sulfate Levels', *Journal of Clinical Endocrinology and Metabolism* 54: 1069–71.

—— Vickovic, M. M., Wall, S. R., and Fluker, M. R. (1985a), 'Defects in Pulsatile LH Release in Normally Menstruating Runners', *Journal of Clinical Endocrinology and Metabolism* 60: 810–12.

—— —— —— (1985b), 'The Effect of Acute Exercise on Pulsatile Release of Luteinizing Hormone in Women Runners', *American Journal of Obstetrics and Gynecology* 153: 482–5.

Dale, E., Gerlach, D. H., and Wilhite, A. L. (1979), 'Menstrual Dysfunction in Distance Runners', *Obstetrics and Gynecology* 54: 47–53.

Damon, A. (1974), 'Larger Body Size and Earlier Menarche: The End May be in Sight', *Social Biology* 21: 8–11.

Deuster, P. A., Kyle, S. B., Moser, P. B., Vigersky, R. A., Singh, A., and Schoemaker, E. B. (1986), 'Nutritional Intakes and Status of Highly Trained Amenorrheic and Eumenorrheic Women Runners', *Fertility and Sterility* 46: 636–43.

Dixon, G., Eurman, P., Stein, B., Schwartz, B., and Rebar, R. W. (1984), 'Hypothalamic Function in Amenorrheic Runners', *Fertility and Sterility* 42: 377–83.

Dreizen, S., Spirakis, C. N., and Stone, R. E. (1967), 'A Comparison of Skeletal Growth and Maturation in Undernourished and Well Nourished Girls Before and After Menarche', *Journal of Pediatrics* 70: 256–63.

Drew, F. L. (1961), 'The Epidemiology of Secondary Amenorrhea', *Journal of Chronic Diseases* 14: 396–401.

Dubey, A. K., Cameron, J. L., Steiner, R. A., and Plant, T. M. (1986), 'Inhibition of Gonadotropin Secretion in Castrated Male Rhesus Monkeys (Macaca mulatta) Induced by Dietary Restriction: Analogy with the Prepubertal Hiatus of Gonadotropin Release', *Endocrinology* 118: 518–25.

Ducharme, J. R., Forest, M. G., de Peretti, E., Sempe, M., Collu, R., and Bertrand, J. (1976), 'Plasma Adrenal and Gonadal Sex Steroids in Human Pubertal Development', *Journal of Clinical Endocrinology* 42: 468–76.

Ellison, P. T., and Lager, C. (1985), 'Exercise-Induced Menstrual Disorders', *New England Journal of Medicine* 313: 825–6.

Espenschade, A. (1940), 'Motor Performance in Adolescence', *Monographs in Social Research and Child Development* 5: 1–126.

Farrel, P. A. (1981), 'Exercise and the Endogenous Opioids', *New England Journal of Medicine* 305: 1591–2.

Feicht, C. B., Johnson, T. S., Martin, B. J., Sparkes, K. E., and Wagner, W. W., Jr. (1978), 'Secondary Amenorrhoea in Athletes', *Lancet* 2: 1145–6.

Fishman, J., Boyar, R. M., and Hellman, L. (1975), 'Influence of Body Weight on Estradiol Metabolism in Young Women', *Journal of Clinical Endocrinology and Metabolism* 41: 489–91.

Forest, M. G., and Bertrand, J. (1972), 'Studies of the Binding of Dihydrotestosterone (17-β-Hydroxy-5α Androstane-3-One) in Human Plasma in Different Physiological Conditions and the Effect of Medroxyprogesterone (17-Hydroxy 6-αmethyl-4-Pregnene-3, 20 Dione, 17-Acetate)', *Steroids* 19: 197–214.

Fries, H., Nillius, S. J., and Petterson, F. (1974), 'Epidemiology of Secondary Amenorrhea', *American Journal of Obstetrics and Gynecology* 118: 473–9.

Fries-Hansen, B. J. (1956), 'Changes in Body Water Compartments During Growth', *Acta Paediatrica* 101 (supplement): 1–67.

Frisch, R. E. (1972), 'Weight at Menarche: Similarity for Well Nourished and Undernourished Girls at Differing Ages, and Evidence for Historical Constancy', *Pediatrics* 50: 445–50.

—— (1984), 'Body Fat, Puberty and Fertility', *Biological Review* 59: 161–88.

—— (1985), 'Body Fat, Menarche and Reproductive Ability', *Seminars on Reproductive Endocrinology* 3: 45–54.

—— and Revelle, R. (1971), 'Height and Weight at Menarche and Hypothesis of Critical Body Weights and Adolescent Events', *Science* 169: 397–9.

—— —— and Cook, S. (1973), 'Components of Weight at Menarche and the Initiation of the Adolescent Growth Spurt in Girls: Estimated Total Body Water, Lean Body Weight and Fat', *Human Biology* 45: 469–83.

—— Wishak, G., and Vincent, L. (1980), 'Delayed Menarche and Amenorrhea in Ballet Dancers', *New England Journal of Medicine* 303: 17–19.

—— Gotz-Wellbergen, A., McArthur, J. W., Albright, T., Witschi, J., Bullen, B., Birnholz, J., Reed, R. B., and Hermann, H. (1981), 'Delayed Menarche and Amenorrhea of College Athletes in Relation to Age of Onset of Training', *Journal of the American Medical Association* 246: 1559–63.

Galle, P. C., Freeman, E. W., Galle, M. G., Huggins, G. R., and Sondheimer, S. J. (1983), 'Physiologic and Psychologic Profiles in a Survey of Women Runners', *Fertility and Sterility* 39: 633–9.

Glasser, W. (1976), *Positive Addition*, Harper and Row, New York.

Grossman, A., Moult, P. J. A., Gaillard, R. C., Delitala, G., Toff, W. D., Rees, L. H., and Besser, G. M. (1981), 'The Opioid Control of LH and FSH Release: Effects of a Metenkephalin Analogue and Naloxone', *Clinical Endocrinology* 14: 41–7.

Gupta, D. (1975), 'Changes in Gonadal and Adrenal Steroid Patterns During Puberty', *Clinical Endocrinology and Metabolism* 4: 27–56.

Hansen, J. W., Hoffman, H. J., and Ross, G. T. (1975), 'Monthly Gonadotropin Cycles in Premenarcheal Girls', *Science* 190: 161–3.

Jenner, M. R., Kelch, R. P., Kaplan, S. L., and Grumbach, M. M. (1972), 'Hormonal Changes in Puberty, IV: Plasma Estradiol, LH and FSH in Prepubertal Children, Pubertal Females, and Precocious Puberty, Premature Thelarche, Hypogonadism and in a Child with Feminizing Ovarian Tumor', *Journal of Clinical Endocrinology and Metabolism* 34: 521–30.

Johnston, F. E., Roche, A. F., Schell, L. M., Norman, H., and Wettenhall, B. (1975), 'Critical Weight at Menarche: Critique of a Hypothesis', *American Journal of the Diseases of Childhood* 129: 19–23.

Kaku, M. (1969), 'Disturbance of Sexual Function and Adipose Tissue in Obese Females', *Sanfujinka No. Jissai, Practice of Gynaecology and Obstetrics* 18: 212–18.

Kantero, R.-L., and Widholm, O. (1971), 'The Age of Menarche in Finnish Girls in 1969', *Acta Obstetrica Gynaecologica Scandanavica* 14 (supplement): 7–18.

Kelch, R. P., Kaplan, S. L., and Grumbach, M. M. (1973), 'Suppression of Urinary and Plasma FSH by Exogenous Estrogens in Prepubertal Children', *Journal of Clinical Investigation* 52: 1122–8.

Kennedy, G. C. (1969), 'Interactions Between Feeding Behavior and Hormones During Growth', *Annals of the New York Academy of Science* 157: 1049–61.

Kirkwood, R. F., Cumming, D. C., and Aherne, F. X. (1987), 'Nutrition and Puberty in the Female', *Proceedings of the Society of Nutrition* 46: 177–92.

Klibanski, A., Beitins, I. Z., Badger, T., Little, R., and McArthur, J. W. (1981), 'Reproductive Function During Fasting in Men', *Journal of Clinical Endocrinology and Metabolism* 53: 258–63.

Kulin, H. E., Bwibo, N., Mutie, D., and Santner, S. J. (1984), 'Gonadotropin Excretion During Puberty in Malnourished Children', *Journal of Pediatrics* 105: 325–8.

Lee, P., Xenakis, T., Winer, J., and Matsenbaugh, S. (1976), 'Puberty in Girls: Correlation of Serum Levels of Gonadotropins, Prolactin, Androgens, Estrogens and Progestins with Physical Changes', *Journal of Clinical Endocrinology and Metabolism* 43: 775–84.

Lucky, A. W., Rich, B. H., Rosenfeld, R. L., Fang, V. S., and Roche-Bender, N. (1980), 'LH Bioactivity Increases more than Immunoreactivity during Puberty', *Journal of Pediatrics* 97: 205–13.

Lutter, J. M., and Cushman, S. (1982), 'Menstrual Patterns in Female Runners', *Physical and Sports Medicine* 10(9): 60–72.

McArthur, J. W., Bullen, B. H., Beitins, I. Z., Pagano, M., Badger, T. M., and Klibanski, A. (1980), 'Hypothalamic Amenorrhea in Runners of Normal Body Composition', *Endocrine Research Communications* 7: 13–25.

McNeill, D., and Livson, N. (1963), 'Maturation Rate and Body Build in Women', *Child Development* 34: 25–32.

Malina, R. M., Harper, A. B., Avent, H. H., and Campbell, D. E. (1973), 'Age at Menarche in Athletes and Non-athletes', *Medicine and Science in Sports* 5: 11–13.

—— Spirduso, W. W., Tate, C., and Baylor, A. M. (1978), 'Age at Menarche and Selected Menstrual Characteristics in Athletes at Different Competitive Levels and in Different Sports', *Medicine and Science in Sports* 10: 218–22.

—— Bouchard, C., Shoup, R. F., Demirjian, A., and Larviere, G. (1979), 'Age at Menarche, Family Size and Birth Order in Athletes at the Olympic Games, 1976', *Medicine and Science in Sports* 11: 354–8.

Marshall, J. C., Kelch, R. P., Sauder, S. E., Barkan, A., Reame, N. E., and Khoury, S. (1984), 'Pulsatile Gonadotropin-Releasing Hormone (GnRH): Studies of Puberty and the Menstrual Cycle', in F. Labrie and L. Proulx (eds.), *Endocrinology: Proceedings of the 7th International Congress of Endocrinology, Quebec City, 1–7 July 1984*, Amsterdam and New York, Excerpta Medica: 25–32.

Merriam, G. R., Pfeiffer, D. G., Loriaux, D. L., and Lipsett, M. B. (1983), 'Catechol Estrogens and the Control of Gonadotropin and Prolactin Secretion in Man', *Journal of Steroid Biochemistry* 29: 619–25.

Moll, G. W., Jr., and Rosenfeld, R. L. (1979), 'Testosterone Binding and Free Plasma Androgens Under Physiological Conditions: Characterization by Flow Dialysis Technique', *Journal of Clinical Endocrinology and Metabolism* 49: 730–6.

Morgan, W. P. (1979), 'Negative Addiction in Runners', *Physical and Sports Medicine* 7(2): 56–70.

Nakao, K., Nakai, Y., Oki, S., Matsubara, S., Konishi, T., Nishitani, H., and Imura, H. (1980), 'Immunoreactive β-endorphin in Human Cerebrospinal Fluid', *Journal of Clinical Endocrinology and Metabolism* 50: 230–3.

Petterson, F., and Fries, H. (1973), 'Epidemiology of Secondary Amenorrhea', *American Journal of Obstetrics and Gynecology* 117: 80–6.

Plymate, S. R., Fariss, B. L., Bassett, M. L., and Matej, L. (1981), 'Obesity and its Role in Polycystic Ovarian Syndrome', *Journal of Clinical Endocrinology and Metabolism* 52(6): 1246–8.

Prior, J. C. (1982a), 'Endocrine "Conditioning" with Endurance Training', *Canadian Journal of Applied Sports Science* 7: 148–57.

—— (1982b), 'Menstrual Cycle Changes with Training: Anovulation and Short Luteal Phase', *Canadian Journal of Applied Sports Science* 7: 173–7.

—— Ho Yuen, B., Clement, P., Bowie, L., and Thomas, J. (1982), 'Reversible Luteal Phase Changes Associated with Marathon Training', *Lancet* 1: 269–70.

Rapoport, S. I., Klee, W. A., Pettigrew, K. D., and Ohno, K. (1980), 'Entry of Opioid Peptides into the Central Nervous System', *Science* 207: 84–6.

Rebar, R. W., and Cumming, D. C. (1981), 'Reproductive Function in Women Athletes', *Journal of the American Medical Association* 246: 1590.

Reeves, J. (1979), 'Estimating Fatness', *Science* 204: 881.

Reid, R. L., Hoff, J. D., Yen, S. S. C., and Li, C. H. (1981), 'Effects of Exogenous b.h*-Endorphin on Pituitary Hormone Secretion and Disappearance Rate in Normal Human Subjects', *Journal of Clinical Endocrinology and Metabolism* 52: 1179–84.

Reiter, E. O., Kulin, H. E., and Hamwood, S. M. (1974), 'The Absence of Positive Feedback Between Estrogen and Luteinizing Hormone in Sexually Immature Girls', *Pediatric Research* 8: 740–5.

Ronkainen, H. (1985), 'Depressed Follicle Stimulating Hormone, Luteinizing Hormone, and Prolactin Responses to the Luteinizing Hormone Releasing Hormone, Thyrotropin-Releasing Hormone, and Metoclopramide Test in Endurance Runners in the Hard-Training Season', *Fertility and Sterility* 44: 755–9.

—— Pakarinen, A., Kirkinen, P., and Kauppila, A. (1985), 'Physical Exercise-Induced Changes and Season-Associated Differences in the Pituitary–Ovarian Function of Runners and Joggers', *Journal of Clinical Endocrinology Metabolism* 60: 416–22.

Russell, J. B., Mitchell, D., Musey, P. I., and Collins, D. C. (1984a), 'The Relationship of Exercise to Anovulatory Cycles in Female Athletes: Hormonal and Physical Characteristics', *Obstetrics and Gynecology* 63: 452–6.

—— —— —— —— (1984b), 'The Role of β-Endorphins and Catechol Estrogens on the Hypothalamic–Pituitary Axis in Female Athletes', *Fertility and Sterility* 42: 690–5.

Saez, J. M., and Morea, A. M. (1973), 'Plasma Oestrogens Before Puberty in Humans', *Acta Paediatrica Scandanavica* 62: 84.

Schwartz, B., Cumming, D. C., Riordan, E., Selye, M., Yen, S. S., and Rebar, R. W. (1981), 'Exercise-Associated Amenorrhea: A Distinct Entity?' *American Journal of Obstetrics and Gynecology* 141: 662–70.

Shangold, M. M., and Levine, H. S. (1982), 'The Effect of Marathon Training on Menstrual Function', *American Journal of Obstetrics and Gynecology* 143: 862–9.

—— Freeman, R., Thysen, B., and Gatz, M. (1979), 'The Relationship Between Long-Distance Running, Plasma Progesterone and Luteal Phase Length', *Fertility and Sterility* 31: 130–3.

Sher, N. (1942), 'Causes of Delayed Menstruation and its Treatment', *British Medical Journal* 1: 347–9.

Siiteri, P. K., and MacDonald, P. C. (1973), 'Role of Extraglandular Estrogen in Human Endocrinology', in S. R. Geiger, E. B. Astwood, and R. O. Greep (eds.), *Handbook of Physiology*, Section 7, Endocrinology: 615–29, American Physiological Society, Washington, DC.

Speroff, L., and Redwine, D. B. (1979), 'Exercise and Menstrual Dysfunction', *Physical and Sports Medicine* 8 (5): 42–52.

Stein, Z., and Susser, M. (1975), 'Fertility, Fecundity, Famine: Food Rations in the Dutch Famine 1944/5 have a Causal Relationship to Fertility and Probably to Fecundity', *Human Biology* 47: 131–54.

Steiner, R. A. (1987), 'Nutritional and Metabolic Factors in the Regulation of Reproductive Hormone Secretion in the Primate', *Proceedings of the Nutrition Society* 46: 159–75.

Stubbs, W. A., Delitala, G., Jones, A., Jeffcoate, W. J., Edwards, C. R., Ratter, S. J., Besser, G. M., Bloom, S. R., Alberti, K. G. (1978), 'Hormonal and Metabolic Responses to an Enkephalin Analogue in Normal Man', *Lancet* 2: 1225–7.

Tanner, J. M. (1962), *Growth in Adolescence*, 2nd edn., Blackwell Scientific, Philadelphia, Pa.

—— (1981), 'Menarcheal Age', *Science* 214: 614.

Trussell, J. (1978), 'Menarche and Fatness: A Re-examination of the Critical Body Composition Hypothesis', *Science* 200: 1506–13.

Van Loon, G. R. (1983), 'Plasma Dopamine: Regulation and Significance', *Federal Proceedings* 42: 3012–18.

Veldhuis, J. D., Evans, W. S., Demers, L. M., Thorner, M. O., Wakat, D., and Rogol, A. D. (1985), 'Altered Neuroendocrine Regulation of Gonadotropin Secretion in Women Distance Runners', *Journal of Clinical Endocrinology and Metabolism* 61: 557–63.

Vigersky, R. A., Andersen, A. E., Thompson, R. H., and Loriaux, D. L. (1977), 'Hypothalamic Dysfunction in Secondary Amenorrhea Associated with Simple Weight Loss', *New England Journal of Medicine* 297: 1141–5.

Wakat, D. K., Sweeney, K. A., and Rogol, A. D. (1978), 'Reproductive System Function in Women Cross Country Runners', *Medicine and Science in Sports* 14: 263–9.

Warren, M. P. (1980), 'The Effects of Exercise on Pubertal Progression and Reproductive Function in Girls', *Journal of Clinical Endocrinology and Metabolism* 51: 1150–57.

Weir, J., Dunn, J. E., Jr., and Jones, E. G. (1971), 'Race and Age at Menarche', *American Journal of Obstetrics and Gynecology* 111: 594–6.

Willer, J. C., Boureau, F., Dauthier, C., and Bonora, M. (1979), 'Study of Naloxone in Normal Awake Man: Effects on Heart Rate and Respiration', *Neuropharmacology* 18: 469–72.

Winter, J. S. D., and Faiman, C. (1973a), 'Pituitary–Gonadal Relations in Female Children and Adolescents', *Pediatric Research* 7: 948–53.

—— —— (1973b), 'The Development of Cyclic Pituitary–Gonadal Function in Adolescent Females', *Journal of Clinical Endocrinology and Metabolism* 37: 714–18.

—— —— and Reyes, F. I. (1978), 'Normal and Abnormal Pubertal Development', *Clinical Obstetrics and Gynecology* 21: 67–86.

Wishik, S. M. (1977), 'The Implications of Undernutrition During Pubescence and Adolescence on Fertility', in K. S. Moghissi and T. N. Evans (eds.), *Nutritional*

Impacts on Women Throughout Life with Emphasis on Reproduction: 23–9, Harper and Row, Hagerstown, Md.

Wolanski, N. (1968), 'Environmental Modification of Human Form and Function', *Annals of the New York Academy of Science* 134: 826–40.

Yen, S. S. C., Tsai, C. C., Naftolin, F., Vandenberg, G., and Ajabor, L. (1972), 'Pulsatile Patterns of Gonadotropin Release in Subjects with and without Ovarian Function', *Journal of Clinical Endocrinology and Metabolism* 34: 671–5.

10 Fertility Following Contraceptive Use

GEORGE R. HUGGINS

The issue of fertility following contraceptive use is of the utmost importance to any patient or couple seeking advice as to the best method of contraception. Few things are as disheartening to a couple and their physician as the discovery of an infertility problem after having postponed childbearing. The late discovery of an unsuspected infertility problem often occurs in patients who have utilized long-term steroidal contraception, an intra-uterine device (IUD), or a combination of these two methods. Contraception usage today is heavily concentrated on oral contraceptives and intra-uterine devices. In addition to the preventive contraceptive methods, approximately one million elective abortions are performed each year in the United States (Centers for Disease Control, 1987).

Oral contraceptives, IUDs, and therapeutic abortions have been implicated in a number of possible complications which involve not only immediate morbidity and mortality, but also subsequent effects on fertility. Of equal concern is the question of possible chromosomal damage and resulting foetal malformations following the use of a contraceptive method, although these issues will not be considered here.

Abortion

Future Fertility

There have been conflicting reports in the literature regarding the effect of therapeutic abortion on future fertility. Special attention has been given to the incompetent cervical os, increased prematurity rates, and pelvic adhesions which may produce infertility. Studies using a number of different methodologies have reached different conclusions, ranging from 'no significant increase in relative risk' in Japan (Hayashi and Momose, 1966) to 'a markedly increased risk of infertility' in Greece (Trichopoulos *et al.*, 1976: 649). Studies from Japan (Glenc, 1974) for example, have reported secondary infertility rates varying from 1 per cent to 7.6 per cent. This general range is within the normal experience for patients with full-term pregnancies.

The association between induced abortion and ectopic pregnancy is confounded by the rapidly increasing incidence of sexually transmitted diseases, including PID, and the changing availability of abortions. For patients whose abortions have not been complicated by infections or retained products, there appears to be little evidence of increased risk of subsequent ectopic pregnancy.

Hogue *et al.* (1982) conducted a comprehensive review of world experience prior to 1982 and summarized a number of specific outcomes, including low birth-weight, prematurity, and spontaneous abortions in subsequent pregnancies. Tables 10.1, 10.2, and 10.3 summarize nine cohort studies that compared the outcomes of second pregnancies after vacuum aspiration terminations, with the outcomes of first pregnancies among comparable women who elected to carry their first pregnancy to term.

TABLE 10.1. *Selected results of nine studies describing the impact of first-trimester induced abortion of a woman's first pregnancy on the rate of low birth-weight[a] in the second pregnancy*

Study	Study period	Relative risk (abortion cohort and primary comparison group)	95% confidence interval
Abortion cohort studies			
Hogue, 1975	1968–72	1.2	(0.5–2.6)
Lean et al., 1977	1974–7	1.4	(0.74–2.6)
Meirik and Bergstrom, 1983	1970–8	0.95	(0.5–1.8)
Logrillo et al., 1980	1970–7	1.4	(1.0–1.9)
Chung et al., 1989	1970–8	0.90	(0.48–1.7)
Pregnancy cohort studies			
Daling and Emanuel, 1977	1972–6	0.88	(0.45–1.7)
WHO, 1979	1976–8	1.2	(0.58–2.6)
WHO, 1979	1976–8	1.3	(0.64–2.5)
Lerner and Varma, 1981	1976–80	0.99	(0.82–1.2)
Obel, 1979	1967–73	0.80	(0.39–1.6)

[a] <2500 or 2501 g depending on study.

These studies show remarkably consistent results. For all three pregnancy outcomes, the relative risks range close to 1. The 95 per cent confidence intervals include or touch 1 for all estimates. With this large number of diverse populations showing similar results, the current evidence supports the conclusion that vacuum aspiration abortion has no effect on low birth-weight, premature delivery, or mid-trimester spontaneous abortion in the subsequent pregnancy.

Studies of pregnancy outcomes after multiple abortions yield conflicting results and the data on subsequent pregnancies in patients who undergo second trimester abortions is still too sparse to draw definitive conclusions. Further large-scale studies are needed before these risks can be better defined.

TABLE 10.2. *Selected results of six studies describing the impact of first-trimester induced abortion of a woman's first pregnancy on the rate of premature delivery in the second pregnancy*

Study	Study period	Relative risk (abortion cohort and primary comparison group)	95% confidence interval
Abortion cohort studies			
Meirik and Bergstrom, 1983	1970–8	0.97	(0.57–1.6)
Logrillo *et al.*, 1980	1970–7	0.75	(0.28–2.0)
Chung *et al.*, 1989	1970–8	0.57	(0.32–1.0)
Pregnancy cohort studies			
Daling and Emanuel, 1977	1972–6	0.96	(0.56–1.6)
WHO, 1979	1976–8	1.9	(0.93–4.1)
WHO, 1979	1976–8	1.0	(0.47–2.2)
Lerner and Varma, 1981	1976–80	1.1	(0.50–2.3)

TABLE 10.3. *Selected results of five studies describing the impact of first-trimester induced abortion of a woman's first pregnancy on the rate of mid-trimester spontaneous abortion of the second pregnancy*

Study	Study period	Relative risk (abortion cohort and primary comparison group)	95% confidence interval
Abortion cohort studies			
Logrillo *et al.*, 1980	1970–7	n.a.	n.a.
Chung *et al.*, 1989	1970–8	0.72	(0.36–1.5)
Pregnancy cohort studies			
Harlap *et al.*, 1979	1974–6	1.4	(0.76–2.7)
WHO, 1979	1976–8	0.71	(0.16–3.1)
WHO, 1979	1976–8	0.90	(0.19–4.3)
Lerner and Varma, 1981	1976–80	0.79	(0.14–4.5)

Asherman's Syndrome

Asherman's syndrome (the presence of intra-uterine synechiae or adhesions which produce clinical symptoms such as menstrual abnormalities, infertility, and habitual abortion) has in the past been relatively rare and, when described, has been high correlated with pre-existing intra-uterine infections associated with dilation and curettage. The incidence seems to have been under-reported, as was confirmed in a comprehensive report by Klein and Garcia (1973).

March and Israel (1976) reported on ten amenorrhoeic patients who had undergone early, elective, first-trimester termination of pregnancy without immediate post-operative complications. All patients had had normal menses prior to pregnancy. These patients developed post-abortal amenorrhoea ranging in duration from 15 to 18 months.

Fertility rates following treatment for this condition are discouraging. Wood and Pena (1964) reported that menses returned in only five out of nine cases with only two having successful full-term pregnancies. Bergman (1961) reported a conception rate of only 30 per cent; half of these pregnancies were carried to term. Klein and Garcia (1973), using a similar method of therapy (i.e. insertion of a Foley catheter and exogenous administration of oestrogens), restored normal menses in six out of seven patients treated. Only three of these patients conceived and successfully carried a pregnancy to term.

Oral Contraceptives

The return of spontaneous menses in patients who have discontinued oral contraceptives (OCs) is usually prompt, occurring within 6 to 10 weeks in the vast majority of patients. Rice-Wray et al. (1967) reported that approximately 70 per cent of patients ovulated during their first spontaneous cycle and 98 per cent by the third cycle. This return of menses does not appear to be either dose- or time-related.

Vessey et al. (1976) reported a delayed return of fertility in oral contraceptive users as compared with diaphragm users or IUD users. The delay was more marked in nulliparous women than in multiparous women. However, as the authors stated, the number of patients studied was too small to permit a final evaluation of the potential risk. Further analysis of the fertility patterns among these patients two years later (Vessey et al., 1978) confirmed a temporary impairment of fertility after discontinuing oral contraceptives. This effect was smaller among multiparous women and had become negligible in nulligravidas by 42 months. Linn et al. (1982) analysed pregnancy rates in 3214 women after the cessation of contraception: the conception rate for prior pill users was lower than for users of all other forms of contraception. These differences disappeared by 12 months. They concluded that while there might be some temporary delay in the return of fertility in former pill users there was no evidence of long-term impairment.

As early as 1966 Shearman reported the syndrome of prolonged secondary amenorrhoea in patients who had taken oral contraceptives. The cause of what has been referred to as 'post-pill amenorrhoea' has, as yet, to be firmly established. In the ensuing years a number of observations have been made concerning this syndrome: (1) it does not appear to be related to any particular type of hormone; (2) it is not time-related, having been reported in patients who had taken oral contraceptives for as short a period as 3 months; and (3) it does not appear to be dose-related, since it has been reported in patients taking various doses of both combined and sequential oral contraceptive preparations.

The incidence of this syndrome depends in part what particular time-period the investigator uses before the patient is diagnosed as having post-pill amenorrhoea. Larsson-Cohn (1969) and Petterson *et al.* (1973) reported amenorrhoea in 0.7 to 0.8 per cent of their patients who had discontinued oral contraceptives for at least 6 months. In the latter study, which examined the epidemiology of secondary amenorrhoea in a large group of women in Sweden, the prevalence of amenorrhoea lasting 6 months or more in the general population was 1.8 per cent. The authors concluded that the incidence of secondary amenorrhoea is very low, and they were unable to arrive at a statistical correlation between the use of oral contraceptives and subsequent amenorrhoea.

The majority of patients with post-pill amenorrhoea respond to Clomid administration with evidence of apparent ovulation and the return of menses. The most responsive patients are those with adequate endogenous oestrogen production. However, a relatively large percentage of patients who resume regular menstruation after clomiphene therapy do not achieve a pregnancy. Shearman (1975) studied 61 amenorrhoeic patients treated with clomiphene citrate. This treatment resulted in a pregnancy rate of 43.6 per cent. Unfortunately, 14 patients who achieved a pregnancy subsequently developed persistent amenorrhoea.

Certain patients with secondary amenorrhoea will also develop galactorrhoea and have high levels of serum prolactin (PRL). Shearman *et al.* (1978) carried out a study on the pathogenesis of PRL-secreting pituitary adenomas. 42 women with amenorrhoea/prolactinaemia had histologically verified pituitary adenomas. The authors hypothesized that the oestrogen content of OCs presented a greater oestrogenic stimulus than either the normal menstrual cycle or pregnancy. This relative hyperoestrogenic state might stimulate the growth of occult pituitary tumours. 74 per cent became symptomatic in the immediate post-partum period, during OC use, or shortly after discontinuation of OCs. Shearman believed that these data suggested that oestrogens may facilitate the expression of a pre-existing lesion.

This suggested association between the use of OCs and pituitary adenomas was noted by other small studies before 1980. Because of the paucity of data on this important issue, the Pituitary Adenoma Study Group (1983) was established. This group undertook a large, multi-centre, case-control investigation to further analyse the relationship between OCs and PRL-secreting pituitary adenomas. Three case-groups, consisting of 212 women with adenomas, 119 hyperprolactinaemic patients with amenorrhoea and/or galactorrhoea with normal or equivocal tomograms, and 205 normo-prolactinaemic women with amenorrhoea and/or galactorrhoea, were matched to neighbourhood control subjects. No association was found between OC use and the development of pituitary adenomas within any of the three study groups. The relative risks were 1.33, 1.35, and 0.67, respectively. Further study was recommended to establish whether OCs may promote the growth of a pre-existing lesion.

Shy *et al.* (1983) conducted a case-control study of 72 women with pituitary prolactinaemia matched to 303 neighbourhood controls selected by random-digit dialling. A major confounding variable was menstrual pattern. When those patients who were using OCs only for contraception were compared to never-users, there was no increased risk of pituitary adenoma (relative risk, 1.3). When patients who were using OCs for menstrual irregularity were compared to never-users, there was a significantly increased risk of pituitary adenoma (relative risk, 7.7; confidence interval, 3.7 to 17.0). The data suggest that those patients taking OCs to correct a menstrual disturbance may have had a pre-existing, undiagnosed prolactinoma.

On the basis of currently available data, there appears to be no increased risk of development of a pituitary adenoma in normal patients taking OCs. The question of whether women with menstrual irregularity taking OCs represent a high-risk group for these lesions remains unresolved.

Intra-uterine Devices

A significant percentage of infertile patients have lesions that are potentially correctable with surgery. Usually the presence of tubo-ovarian, peri-tubal, and other associated pelvic adhesions can be related to one or more episodes of pelvic inflammatory disease (PID).

The use of the Grafenberg intra-uterine device (IUD) and its modifications in the early 1900s was condemned and its use discontinued primarily because of an unacceptably high incidence of acute pelvic inflammatory disease associated with mortality. Following the introduction of modern intra-uterine devices in the early 1960s, the question of whether the IUDs cause an increased incidence of clinical or sub-clinical pelvic inflammatory disease resurfaced.

The Dalkon Shield was withdrawn from use in 1974 in part because of reports of serious pelvic infections with the subsequent death of some pregnant patients who continued to wear the device. One possible explanation for this outcome may be the multi-filament tail appended to the device, which acts as a wick, drawing fluid and viable bacteria into the intra-uterine cavity. Tatum *et al.* (1975) have demonstrated this wick-like effect and have cultured both aerobic and anaerobic bacteria from the intra-uterine portion of the string. In addition, they reported that more than 35 per cent of the devices studied showed breaks in the sheath of the tail within the intra-uterine cavity. Speculation persists, however, as to whether the multi-filament tail is the sole cause of the development of pelvic inflammatory disease.

Mishell *et al.* (1966) have shown that the insertion of an intra-uterine device contaminates each patient's intra-uterine cavity with bacteria. Over a short period of time, however, the uterus is apparently able to cleanse and sterilize its environment through multiple biological mechanisms.

Taylor *et al.* (1975) described a syndrome of unilateral tubo-ovarian abscess in 16 patients wearing IUDs. In none of these patients was gonococcus cultured. Unilateral tubo-ovarian abscess has, as a general rule, been a rare clinical condition except when it follows the development of other unilateral pelvic disease or pelvic surgery. The observations by Taylor *et al.* (1975) were confirmed in several other institutions in which the occurrence of unilateral pelvic abscess was also associated with a high incidence of IUD usage. This relationship was not confirmed by a more recent study, however, (Burkman *et al.*, 1981; Lee *et al.*, 1983).

Faulkner and Ory (1976) studied a group of febrile and afebrile patients seen in an emergency room with a diagnosis of pelvic inflammatory disease. These patients were then matched with control patients seen in the same area, who had complaints other than abdominal pain or discomfort and who had no pathological gynaecological diagnosis. The results revealed a significantly higher proportion of IUD users among the febrile cases of pelvic inflammatory disease than among controls (38 per cent versus 11 per cent, respectively). Faulkner and Ory concluded that an IUD user is approximately four times more likely to develop pelvic inflammatory disease than a non-user.

The WHO Study (1979) of PID associated with fertility regulatory agents included 12 centres in both developed and developing countries. Among parous women from developed countries, the increased relative risk of a first episode of PID associated with IUD use was 4.1, while among women from developing countries it was 2.3. The risk of developing subsequent episodes of PID was two to three times higher than the risk of the first episode, but it did not differ significantly between IUD users and non-users.

One problem inherent to studies such as these is the possible over-reporting of diagnoses of pelvic inflammatory disease in a clinic population. Jacobson and Westrom (1960) compared the results of laparoscopic and clinical diagnoses of pelvic inflammatory disease in Sweden. They found that among patients suspected of having pelvic inflammatory disease, visual confirmation could be made in only 65 per cent of the cases. This experience has been shared in our own institution by physicians at all stages of training and expertise. Unfortunately, clinical acumen in the diagnosis of pelvic inflammatory disease is not totally satisfactory.

Although there are studies which fail to show an association between IUD use and PID, most clinical and epidemiological studies over the past 20 years have shown that IUD users face a greater risk of developing acute PID than non-users. Some of the earlier studies may have overestimated this risk because they included barrier contraceptive users and oral contraceptive users among the control population. These contraceptive methods protect against PID and so may bias the estimated increase in relative risk for IUD users.

Acute salpingitis predisposes women to the development of infertility primarily from occlusion of the fallopian tubes by post-inflammatory adhesion formation. The degree of infertility is directly related to both the severity and number of episodes. The incidence of infertility following one episode of mild salpingitis is 6.1 per cent, after moderate salpingitis, 13 per cent, and after a single episode of severe salpingitis 30 per cent (Westrom, 1980).

Tietze and Lewitt (1970) were unable, however, to demonstrate impaired fertility among women who discontinued the intra-uterine device because of a desire for pregnancy: over 30 per cent conceived within one month, approximately 60 per cent within three months, and almost 90 per cent within one year. Tatum and Connell (1986) reported a cumulative pregnancy rate of 84.6 per cent in one year among 553 women who had Copper-Ts removed in order to establish another pregnancy. The figures reported in these studies are within the same range for all women attempting to achieve a pregnancy. These authors concluded that short-term use (one to three years) of an intra-uterine device does not impair future fertility.

While there were few data prior to 1984 that showed a direct association between use of an intra-uterine device and infertility, more recent studies have found just such a connection. Daling *et al.* (1985) investigated the relationship between IUD use and subsequent infertility among US nulligravid women. The cases consisted of 159 nulligravid women with tubal infertility, who were matched for age and race with 159 women who conceived their first child at the time the infertile women were trying to become pregnant. The analysis adjusted for cigarette smoking, number of sexual partners, and income. A higher percentage of cases (35 per cent) than controls (14 per cent) reported ever having used an IUD. The relative risk was 2.6 (Table 10.4).

The highest risk among ever-users was seen with the Dalkon Shield (relative risk, 6.8). This excess risk, compared to the Copper IUD, Lippes Loop, and Saf-T-Coil users, was also present among patients who had only used one type of device. The smallest increase in risk was found among users of Copper IUDs. The relative risk was 1.9, with a 95 per cent confidence interval of 0.9 to 4.0, for women who had ever used a Copper IUD. The relative risk was 1.3, with a 95 per cent confidence interval of 0.6 to 3.0, for women who had only used a Copper IUD. The authors concluded that the use of the Dalkon Shield intra-uterine device significantly increased the risk of infertility. The increased relative risk of infertility among copper-containing IUD users was not significant.

Cramer *et al.* (1985) conducted a large, multi-centre case-control study including as cases 283 nulliparous women with primary tubal infertility and 69 women with secondary tubal infertility. The controls were 3833 women admitted for delivery at the seven collaborating hospitals. Potential confounding factors including region, year of menarche, religion, education, and number of sexual partners were controlled for in the analysis.

The use of any kind of IUD before a live birth was associated with a statistically significant increase in the risk of primary tubal infertility

TABLE 10.4. *IUD use in women with primary tubal infertility and in controls, according to type of IUD*

	Cases		Controls		Relative risk	95% confidence interval
	%	No.[a]	%	No.[a]		
Ever used						
Any IUD	35.2	56	13.8	22	2.6	1.3–5.2
Dalkon Shield	14.5	23	2.5	4	6.8	1.8–25.2
Copper IUD	17.6	28	10.1	16	1.9	0.9–4.0
Lippes Loop/Saf-T-Coil IUD	9.4	15	2.5	4	3.2	0.9–12.0
Only used						
Dalkon Shield	8.6	12	0.7	1	11.3	1.4–95.0
Copper IUD	12.1	17	8.6	11	1.3	0.6–3.0
Lippes Loop/Saf-T-Coil IUD	7.1	10	0.7	1	4.4	0.5–41.8

[a] One control did not know the type of IUD used; one case did not know the first type of IUD used but later used a Copper IUD.

Source: Daling *et al.*, 1985.

(Table 10.5). When number of sexual partners was also considered, there was no increase in the risk of primary tubal infertility among IUD users who reported having only one sexual partner (Table 10.6).

Summary

The incidence of post-operative infection following first-trimester therapeutic abortion in the United States is low. However, increasing numbers of women are undergoing repeated pregnancy terminations, and their risk for subsequent pelvic infections may be multiplied with each succeeding abortion. The incidence of prematurity due to cervical incompetence or surgical infertility following first-trimester pregnancy terminations is not increased significantly. Asherman's syndrome may occur following non-septic therapeutic abortion. The pregnancy rate following treatment of this syndrome is low.

TABLE 10.5. *Relation of IUD use to the risk of primary tubal infertility*

Type of device	Relative risk	95% confidence interval	Value of P
Dalkon Shield only	4.3	1.7–6.1	0.0002
Lippes Loop or Saf-T-Coil only	4.2	1.7–5.2	0.0002
Copper device only	1.6	1.1–2.4	0.01
Other or combination	2.4	1.1–3.0	0.03
Non-copper IUD	3.2	1.7–3.4	<0.0001

Source: Cramer *et al.*, 1985.

TABLE 10.6. *Relation of number of sexual partners and IUD use to the risk of primary tubal infertility*

IUD use	Relative risk	95% confidence interval	Value of P
No IUD use			
1 partner	1.0	—	—
>1 partner	1.8	1.1–2.1	0.01
Copper IUD			
1 partner	1.0	0.5–2.7	ns
>1 partner	3.0	1.7–4.5	<0.0001
Other IUD			
1 partner	0.9	0.2–3.2	ns
>1 partner	5.4	2.7–6.5	<0.0001

Source: Cramer *et al.*, 1985.

The return of menses and the achievement of a pregnancy may be slightly delayed after oral contraceptives are discontinued, but the fertility rate is within the normal range by one year. The incidence of post-pill amenorrhoea of more than 6 months' duration is probably less than 1 per cent. The occurrence of the syndrome does not seem to be related to length of use or type of pill. Both patients who had normal menses and those who had menstrual abnormalities before they began using oral contraceptives may develop this syndrome. Patients with normal oestrogen and gonadotrophin levels usually respond with return of menses and ovulation when treated with clomiphene. However, their pregnancy rate is much lower than that of patients with spontaneous return of menses.

The criteria for defining pelvic inflammatory disease or for categorizing its severity are diverse. The incidence of pelvic inflammatory disease is higher among IUD users than among patients taking oral contraceptives or using a barrier method. At present, the effect of IUD use on future development of pelvic adhesions with resultant infertility is difficult to appraise, but recent studies suggest an increased risk of tubal infertility.

All present medical methods of contraception entail some risk to the patient. The risk of impaired future fertility with the use of any method appears to be low. Careful identification of patients who may be at high risk, such as those with a history of oligomenorrhoea or pelvic inflammatory disease, may allow the physician to suggest a method which imposes the least risk to future fertility.

References

Bergman, P. (1961), 'Traumatic Intrauterine Lesions', *Acta Obstetrica Gynecologica Scandanavica* (supplement 4) 40: 1.

Burkman, R. T., and The Women's Health Study (1981), 'Association Between Intrauterine Device and Pelvic Inflammatory Disease', *Obstetrics and Gynecology* 57: 269–76.

Centers for Disease Control (1987), 'Surveillance Summaries', *Morbidity and Mortality Weekly Report*: 36: 1SS–53SS.

Chung, C. S., Steinhoff, P. G., Mi, M. P., and Smith, R. G. (1989), 'Long-Term Effects of Induced Abortions', paper presented at the 105th Annual Meeting of the American Public Health Association, Washington, DC.

Cramer, D. W., Schieff, I., Schoenbaum, S. C., Gibson, M., Belisle, S., Albrecht, B., Stillman, R. J., Berger, M. J., Wilson, E., Stadel, B. V., and Seibel, M. (1985), 'Tubal Infertility and the Intrauterine Device', *New England Journal of Medicine* 312 (15): 941–7.

Daling J. R., and Emanuel, I. (1977), 'Induced Abortion and Subsequent Outcome of Pregnancy in a Series of American Women', *New England Journal of Medicine* 297: 1241–5.

—— Weiss, N. S., Metch, B. J., Chow, W. H., Soderstrom, R. M., Moore, D. E., Spadoni, L. R., and Stadel, B. V. (1985), 'Primary Tubal Infertility in Relation to the Use of an Intrauterine Device', *New England Journal of Medicine* 312 (15): 937–41.

Faulkner, W. L., and Ory, H. W. (1976), 'Intrauterine Devices and Acute Pelvic Inflammatory Disease', *Journal of the American Medical Association* 235: 1851–3.

Glenc, F. (1974), 'Course of Pregnancy Following Abortion', *Polski Tygodnik Lekarski* 29: 991–2.

Harlap, S., Shiono, P. H., Ramcharan, S., Berendes, H., and Pellegrin, F. (1979), 'A Prospective Study of Spontaneous Fetal Losses After Induced Abortion', *New England Journal of Medicine* 301: 677–81.

Hayashi, M., and Momose, K. (1966), 'Statistical Observation on Artificial Abortion and Secondary Sterility', in Y. Loya (ed.) *Harmful Effects of Induced Abortion*: 35–43, Family Planning Association of Japan, Tokyo.

Hogue, C. J. R. (1975), 'Low Birthweight Subsequent to Induced Abortion: A Historical Prospective Study of 948 Women in Skopje, Yugoslavia', *American Journal of Obstetrics and Gynecology* 123: 675–81.

—— Jr. Cates, W., and Tietze, C. (1982), 'The Effects of Induced Abortion on Subsequent Reproduction', *Epidemiologic Reviews*, 4: 66–94.

Jacobson, L., and Westrom, L. (1960), 'Objectivized Diagnosis of Acute Pelvic Inflammatory Disease', *American Journal of Obstetrics and Gynecology* 105: 1088.

Klein, S. M., and Garcia, C. R. (1973), 'Asherman's Syndrome: A Critique and Current Review', *Fertility and Sterility* 24: 722–35.

Larsson-Cohn, U. (1969), 'The Length of the First Three Menstrual Cycles After Combined Oral Contraceptive Treatment', *Acta Obstetrica Gynecologica Scandanavica* 48: 416–22.

Lean, T. H., Hogue, C. J. R., and Wood, J. (1977), 'Low Birthweight After Induced Abortion in Singapore', abstract of a paper presented at the annual meeting of the American Public Health Association, Washington, DC; published in the programme supplement: p. 102.

Lee, N. C., Rubin, G. L., Ory, H. W., and Burkman, R. T. (1983), 'Type of Intrauterine Device and the Risk of Pelvic Inflammatory Disease', *Obstetrics and Gynecology* 62: 1–6.

Lerner, R. C., and Varma, A. O. (1981), 'Prospective Study of the Outcome of Pregnancy Subsequent to Previous Induced Abortion', Downstate Medical Center, State University of New York, New York.

Linn, S., Schoenbaum, S. C., Monson, R. R., Rosner, B. B., and Ryan, K. J. (1982), 'Delay in Conception for Former "Pill" Users', *Journal of the American Medical Association* 247: 629–32.

Logrillo, V. M., Quickenton, P., Therriault, G. D., and Ellrott, M. A. (1980), *Effect of Induced Abortion on Subsequent Reproductive Function*, New York State Health Department, Albany.

March, C. M., and Israel, R. (1976), 'Intrauterine Adhesions Secondary to Elective Abortion', *Obstetrics and Gynecology* 48: 422–4.

Meirik, O., and Bergstrom, R. (1983), 'Outcome of Delivery Subsequent to Vacuum Aspiration Abortion in Nulliparous Women', *Acta Obstetrica Gynecologica Scandanavica* 62: 499–509.

Mishell, D. R., Bell, J. H., Good, R. G., and Moyer, D. L. (1966), 'The Intrauterine Device: A Bacteriologic Study of the Endometrial Cavity', *American Journal of Obstetrics and Gynecology* 96: 119–26.

Obel, E. (1979), 'Pregnancy Complications following Legally Induced Abortion', *Acta Obstetrica Gynecologica Scandanavica* 58: 485.

Petterson, F., Fries, H., and Nillinus, J. S. (1973), 'Epidemiology of Secondary Amenorrhea', *American Journal of Obstetrics and Gynecology* 117: 80–6.

Pituitary Adenoma Study Group (1983), 'Pituitary Adenomas and Oral Contraceptives: A Multicenter Case-Control Study', *Fertility and Sterility* 39: 753–60.

Rice-Wray, E., Correu, S., Gordoviski, J., Esquiver, J., and Goldzieher, J. W. (1967), 'Return of Ovulation after Discontinuance of Oral Contraception', *Fertility and Sterility* 18: 212.

Shearman, R. P. (1966), 'Amenorrhea after Treatment with Oral Contraceptives', *Lancet* 2: 1110–11.

—— (1975), 'Secondary Amenorrhea after Oral Contraceptives Treatment and Followup', *Contraception* 11: 123.

Shearman, B. M., Harris, C. E., Schlechte, J., Duello, T. M., Halmi, N. S., VanGilder, G., Chapler, F. K., and Granner, K. D. (1978), 'Pathogenesis of Prolactin-Secreting Pituitary Adenomas', *Lancet* 2: 1019–1021.

Shy, K. K., McTierman, A. M., Daling, J. R., and Weiss, N. S. (1983), 'Oral Contraceptive Use and the Occurrence of Pituitary Prolactinoma', *Journal of the American Medical Association* 249: 2204–7.

Tatum, H. J., and Connell, E. B. (1986), 'A Decade of Intrauterine Contraception, 1976 to 1986', *Fertility and Sterility* 46: 173–92.

—— Schmidt, F. H., and Phillips, D. (1975), 'Morphological Studies of Dalkon Shield Tails Removed from Patients', *Contraception* 11: 465–77.

Taylor, E. S., McMillan, J. H., Greer, B. E., Droegemueller, W., and Thompson, H. E. (1975), 'The Intrauterine Device and Tubo-Ovarian Abscess', *American Journal of Obstetrics and Gynecology* 123: 338–48.

Tietze, C., and Lewitt, S. (1970), 'Evaluation of Intrauterine Devices: Ninth Progress Report of the Cooperative Statistical Program', *Studies in Family Planning* 55: 1–40.

Trichopoulos, D., Handanos, N., Danezis, J., Kalandidi, A., and Kalapothaki, V. (1976), 'Induced Abortion and Secondary Infertility', *British Journal of Obstetrics and Gynaecology* 83: 645–50.

Vessey, M. P., Doll, R., Peto, R., Johnson, B., and Wiggins, P. (1976), 'A Longterm Follow-Up Study of Women Using Different Methods of Contraception: An Interim Report', *Journal of Biosocial Science* 8: 373–427.

—— Wright, N. H., McPherson, K., and Wiggins, P. (1978), 'Fertility after Stopping Different Methods of Contraception', *British Medical Journal* 1: 265–7.

Westrom, L. (1980), 'Incidence, Prevalence and Trends of Pelvic Inflammatory Disease and Its Consequences in Industrialized Countries', *American Journal of Obstetrics and Gynecology* 138: 880–92.

WHO (1979), (World Health Organization Task Force on the Sequelae of Abortion), 'Gestation, Birthweight, and Spontaneous Abortion in Pregnancy After Induced Abortion', *Lancet*, 1: 142–5.

Wood, J., and Pena, G. (1964), 'Treatment of Traumatic Uterine Synechiae', *International Journal of Fertility* 9: 405–10.

11 Toxic Substances, Conception, and Pregnancy Outcome

MICHAEL J. ROSENBERG

The last decade has witnessed a growing interest in the effects of physical, chemical, and biological agents to which people are exposed in the environment, particularly in the workplace. This attention has come about for several reasons. In the United States today some 109 million men and women between the ages of 15 and 44 work with more than 70 000 chemical, biological, and physical agents. Only a small fraction of these have been evaluated for their reproductive toxicity, but dramatic examples of reproductive problems leave little doubt that these agents can exert powerful adverse effects.

The magnitude of reproductive problems attributable to these agents cannot be gauged with data presently available. Yet the relationship between occupation and reproduction has become a prominent concern for two reasons. First, the number of women in the work-force has been increasing in both relative and absolute terms. In the United States, for example, women now comprise half the work-force, up from 31 per cent in 1970 (Wessel, 1989). Similar increases are occurring throughout the industrialized world. Second, there are a decreasing number of children in each family, and first pregnancies are being delayed until later in the reproductive years. These trends are placing greater urgency on assuring that each pregnancy occurs when planned and produces a healthy child.

Assessing Reproductive Impairments

Although many endpoints have been used in the clinical study of reproductive impairments, they fall into three groups: difficulty in becoming pregnant, increased rates of pregnancy loss, and birth or developmental defects, as detailed below:

Infecundability
1. Sexual dysfunction: libido, potency
2. Sperm abnormalities: number, motility, morphology
3. Amenorrhoea
4. Anovulatory menstrual cycles
5. Infertility
6. Time to conceive

Foetal loss
  1. Early (≤20 weeks)
  2. Late (21+ weeks)
Birth or developmental disorders
  1. Intra-partum death
  2. Low birth-weight (<2500 g)
  3. Birth defects: major, minor
  4. Chromosomal abnormalities
  5. Death in first week of life
  6. Death in first month of life
  7. Death in first year of life
  8. Childhood morbidity
  9. Childhood malignancy
(Taken from Rosenberg, 1986.)

Indices of difficulty in becoming pregnant include both infertility and time required for conception. Use of either measure as an endpoint is complicated by factors such as frequency of intercourse, intermittency of contraceptive use, and the fact that these impairments may be due to social or medical problems that are unrelated to environmental exposures.

Pregnancy loss is the most common and most studied adverse outcome. Retro-spective studies have traditionally relied on pregnancy loss because approxim-ately 15 per cent of recognized pregnancies end spontaneously, making detection of increases above the background rate easier than with other, less frequent outcomes. This tool has recently been improved by the development of a highly sensitive urine immuno-radiometric assay for β-hCG, which allows the use of daily urine samples to detect pregnancy as soon as implantation occurs (Wilcox *et al.*, 1988). An important advantage of this method is its ability to detect pregnancies so briefly viable that a woman might never have recognized she was pregnant. This effectively increases the frequency of foetal loss that can be detected, which decreases sample size requirements (Table 11.1). The possibility of following relatively small groups of women with virtually complete ascertain-ment of pregnancy and foetal loss introduces a powerful new tool for prospective studies of agents of concern.

Birth or developmental defects are infrequent occurrences: considered to-gether, defects occur at a rate of approximately 3 per cent. But since no one agent causes increases in all defects, individual defects must be studied. The most frequent of these occur at a rate of approximately 1 per cent, and most are much less common. Their rarity makes birth defects a difficult endpoint because of the very large sample sizes required (Table 11.1). Developmental defects are similarly rare, difficult to define objectively, and seldom used.

Reproductive studies may also be complicated by methodological difficulties (US Congress, 1985). First, as noted, many outcomes require large numbers of subjects to detect group differences reliably. Sample size requirements are often further increased by the presence of common, extraneous, potentially

TABLE 11.1. *Sample size required to detect doubling in adverse reproductive outcomes*

Outcome	Background rate (%)	Sample size[a]
Fecundability		
Infertility	10	436 couple-years
Pregnancy loss		
After implantation	31	218 pregnancies
≤20 weeks' gestation	15	322 pregnancies
21+ weeks' gestation	2	1856 pregnancies
Birth/developmental defects		
Birth weight <2500 g	7	586 live births
Major birth defects (all)	3	1262 live births
Neural tube defect	1	3638 live births
Infant death (≤1 year)	2	1856 live births

[a] Divided evenly between exposed and unexposed groups, one-sided α.
Source: Rosenberg, 1986.

confounding factors such as smoking and alcohol consumption. Second, the infrequency of outcomes and the often preliminary nature of such studies favour a case-control design, necessitating retrospective determination of exposure. Accurate assessment of exposures may be difficult when participants are aware of the hypothesis being investigated, as is often the case with preliminary investigations. Third, the adverse effects of other common exposures, such as sexually transmitted diseases, contraception, smoking, and alcohol, may overshadow those agents under investigation. Such factors need to be evaluated for their confounding effects and controlled as necessary. Collectively, these difficulties may produce conflicting results even when a real hazard exists, particularly when the effect is subtle.

Logistical problems may exacerbate these difficulties or present pitfalls of their own in carrying out reproductive studies. They include the need to find populations exposed to the agent under investigation which are large enough to fulfil sample size requirements and are stable enough to allow reasonable follow-up. A problem with occupational setting is that the large plants sometimes necessary for sufficient sample size are often those where exposures are well controlled. Higher exposures are more common at smaller plants, which less often monitor exposures or provide non-mandated protective equipment.

Animal Toxicology and Biological Markers

Because of the considerable expense and difficulty of studying reproductive hazards in humans, human studies have been supplemented by animal studies. Animals offer the advantage of short reproductive cycles, and their use also allows for control of important exposure factors, including time, route, and dose of administration; number of doses; and other factors such as maternal age or nutritional deficiencies (Kurzel and Centulo, 1985). In addition, certain studies are not possible among humans because of ethical considerations or patient needs. Although toxicology testing on animals has proved to be an important means of identifying toxicity among humans, variations between test animals and humans raises uncertainty about the degree to which animal results can be extrapolated to people. Despite a study that compared the effects of 175 substances in 14 animal species and in humans and that produced a predicted positive value of 75–100 per cent and a predicted negative value of 64–91 per cent (Jelovsek *et al.*, 1989), animal studies continue to be under-appreciated.

More recent efforts have sought to identify markers for exposure, effect, and susceptibility to reproductive hazards among animals and humans. Such markers might identify an incipient disease or disability and help clarify dose-response relationships. Furthermore, they may be more accessible than currently available means. Although some markers seem particularly promising—for example, the examination of sperm morphology to identify genetic alterations—most are in the early stages of development, and we need considerably greater experience to be able to gauge their utility and limitations. The subject of such markers has recently been reviewed by the National Academy of Sciences (1989).

Studies in Humans

Despite the limitations discussed, a number of associations have been reasonably well established as impairing reproduction (Table 11.2) (Kurzel and Centulo, 1985; Rosenberg, 1986; Rosenberg *et al.*, 1987). Among men, these include exposure to solvents (ethylene glycol ethers), polychlorinated biphenyls, heavy metals (notably lead and arsenic), pesticides (kepone), nitrous oxide, alcohol, chemotherapeutic agents, and ionizing radiation. Relationships are less well studied among women, but established relationships have been shown with exposure to anaesthetic gases, ethylene oxide, viral agents, mercury, lead, and organic solvents. Questions have recently been raised about women in the semiconductor manufacturing industry (Pastides *et al.*, 1988), and women doing heavy labour (Goulet and Theriault, 1987). But studies that lack confirmation from others must be interpreted with extreme caution because of common weaknesses of reproductive studies including inadequate sample size and poor response rates; potential for selection bias, often unquantified; inadequate characterization of and control for potential confounding factors; and poor characterization of exposure (Rosenberg *et al.*, 1987).

In addition, a number of studies involving large numbers of exposures are liable to produce significant indications of risk. For example, a study of work during pregnancy, which involved 22 761 single live births, found a significant

TABLE 11.2. *Occupational agents with reproductive toxicity in man or animal*

Agent	Uses or potential exposures	Reproductive effects			
		Humans		Animals (but no human evidence)	
		Males	Females	Males	Females
Anaesthetic gases (including halothane)	Hospital operating room; dental clinics; veterinary surgeries	Impaired fertility	Impaired fertility; spontaneous abortion		
Arsenic	Manufacture of copper, lead, or alloys; glass, insecticides or fungicides		Menstrual disorders; spontaneous abortion		
Benzo[a]pyrene	Reagent for determination of cadmium			Testicular damage; impaired fertility	Oestrus cycle disorders
Benzene	Manufacture of chemicals, dyes, or other organic compounds; artificial leather, varnishes, lacquers; solvents		Spontaneous abortion; impaired fertility; menstrual disorders	Testicular damage	
Beryllium	Aerospace fabrications		Maternal death		
Boron	Weatherproofing; preservative; cosmetics		Impaired fertility		
Cadmium	Plating; photo-electric cells; dentistry	Testicular damage		Testicular atrophy	Fetotoxic; ovarian atrophy infertility
Carbon monoxide	Persons exposed to automobile fumes		Low birth-weight		
Chloroform	Solvent for oils, fats, resins, rubber		Impaired fertility		Fetotoxic
Chloroprene	Rubber manufacturers	Decreased libido; impotence			Fetotoxic
Dichloromethane	Degreasers and cleaners				Fetotoxic; low birth-weight
Epichlorophydrin	Solvent for resins, gums, paints, varnishes, and lacquers			Reduced fertility	Testicular damage
Ethylene dibromide	Fruit fumigators; gasoline fumes				Testicular atrophy
Ethylene dichloride	Solvent for rubber, fats, oil; extract for tobacco				Fetotoxic

TABLE 11.2. (*cont.*)

Ethylene oxide	Fumigant; sterilizing agents for surgical instruments; fungicide		Menstrual disorders; low birth-weight		Spontaneous abortion
Formaldehyde	Resins, leather, rubber, metals or wood; workers in pathology laboratories		Menstrual disorders; spontaneous abortion; low birth-weight		
Hormones (androgens, oestrogens, progestogens, synthetic hormones)	Pharmaceutical workers or researchers		Ectopic pregnancy; spontaneous abortions		
Lead	Automobile or aircraft exhaust fumes	Decreased libido		Spontaneous impotence; testicular damage or infertility	Abortion
Manganese	Manufacture of steel, glass, ink, dry-cell batteries, ceramics, paint, rubber, welding rods, wood preservatives	Decreased libido		Impotence	
Mercury		Decreased libido; impotence	Low birth-weight		Fetotoxic and embryo-toxic
Pesticides (including carbaryl, dibromochloro-propane, kepone, malathion, 2, 4, 5-T)	Insecticides	Testicular damage or infertility			
Polybrominated biphenyls (PBBs)	Fire retardant in plastics, wood preservatives, electrical insulations			Impaired fertility	Fetotoxic
Polychlorinated biphenyls (PCBs)	Insulating materials in transformers and capacitators; hydraulic fluid		Menstrual disorders		
Selenium	Photography; electronic components, instruments; rubber manufacture				Fetotoxic

TABLE 11.2. (*cont.*)

Agent	Uses or potential exposures	Reproductive effects			
		Humans		Animals (but no human evidence)	
		Males	Females	Males	Females
Styrene	Manufacture of plastics, synthetic rubber, resins, insulators		Menstrual disorders		
Toluene	Manufacture of benzoic acid, benzaldehyde, explosives, dye	Decreased libido; impotence	Menstrual disorders; low birth-weight		
Vinyl chloride	Manufacture of vinyl chloride, polyvinyl chloride, and related products	Decreased libido; impotence	Low birth-weight		
Xylene	Solvent				Fetotoxic

Source: Rosenberg, 1986.

association of pre-term births and infants of low birth-weight with work involving heavy lifting, shift work, long hours, or great fatigue (McDonald *et al.*, 1988). When gestational age was considered, the association with specific occupations, long working hours, and fatigue largely disappeared (Armstrong *et al.*, 1989). However, the associations with heavy lifting and shift work persisted. Another prospective study of 3901 working women found no association between adverse pregnancy outcomes and occupational categories (Ahlborg *et al.*, 1989). Finally, a third retrospective study of prematurity among 3437 French women found a significant association with strenuous working conditions (Mamelle *et al.*, 1984). Working conditions were measured by a constructed score, which varied between one and five. Prematurity was found to increase in a nearly linear fashion from a score of zero (prematurity rate 2.3 per cent) to scores of four and five (prematurity rate 11.1 per cent). The diversity of outcomes, study design, data collection, analysis, and presentation for these studies underscores the complex nature of these relationships and the need for caution and multiple studies to determine likely causation.

Visual display units (VDU) have become common in the last decade and have triggered concern about the possibility of adverse reproductive outcomes among users. Although measurements of radiation at various frequencies indicated a lack of measurable radiation (National Research Council, 1983) concern was fuelled by several reports of higher-than-expected frequencies of birth defects and spontaneous abortions among women using VDUs (Foster, 1986). While such clusters are expected on a statistical basis, the small number of subjects in cluster reports makes evaluation impossible, particularly in the emotionally charged atmosphere in which such preliminary investigations are often conducted. One such investigation in which the author was involved recorded a higher-than-expected number of spontaneous abortions among VDU users without apparent cause. Following the institution of a programme to monitor all pregnancies, the frequency of spontaneous abortions was found to be substantially lower than chance would permit. This finding is similar to that of another situation, this time involving women drinking solvent-contaminated drinking water. An initial study indicated a significant excess of adverse reproductive outcomes (Swan *et al.*, 1989), but follow-up study which investigated a second contaminated area revealed a deficit of such outcomes, leading to the conclusion that the solvent was not likely to have caused the excess number of adverse outcomes observed in the first study (Wrensch *et al.*, 1990).

Larger studies of exposure to VDUs have presented conflicting results, but are generally reassuring about the absence of VDU hazards. A retrospective study of 817 pregnancies among Michigan clerical workers using self-reported work histories found no adverse effects from VDU exposure (Butler and Brix, 1986). A later case-control study using interview information about VDU and other exposures found a slightly elevated odds ratio of approximately 1.2 in three different exposure groups, without suggestion of a dose-response relationship (McDonald *et al.*, 1986). Recall bias may have contributed to these findings. A 1989 matched case-control study of 334 pregnancies which ended in miscarriages and 664 control pregnancies revealed no effect of VDU use (Bryant and Love, 1989). Careful exposure questions among separate prenatal and postnatal control groups in this study also suggested the presence of recall bias, which might partially explain a modestly increased risk. Finally, one of the largest studies, a case-control study of miscarriage among 1583 members of a Health Maintenance Organization, found a significant elevation in the level of spontaneous abortion among women who reported working with VDUs at least 20 hours a week during the first trimester (Goldhaber *et al.*, 1988). This study found no confounding for age, smoking, alcohol, and other factors but was unable to control for other possible contributory factors such as stress. In addition, the study's reliance on self-reported exposure histories after miscarriage and the modest elevation in the odds ratio found raises the similar possibility of recall bias. Since exposure during pregnancy is a critical aspect, this issue will be unlikely to be resolved until a prospective study or a well-validated exposure history is available.

Conclusions

Collectively, studies of possible hazards to reproduction are made difficult by a host of methodological and logistical problems, the most important of which are adequate sample size and the need for unbiased exposure histories. Aside from the obvious need for caution in interpreting such studies, these difficulties point to the need for meticulously designed, conducted, and analysed studies. These limitations also emphasize the need to judge causality by broader standards that involve more than a single study, including strength of association, specificity, consistency, dose-response, relationship, temporal relationship, and biological plausibility (Schlesselman, 1987).

References

Ahlborg, G., Hogstedt, C., Bodin, L., and Barany, S. (1989), 'Pregnancy Outcome Among Working Women', *Scandinavian Journal of Work and Environmental Health* 15: 227–33.

Armstrong, B. G., Nolin, A. D., and McDonald, A. D. (1989), 'Work in Pregnancy and Birth Weight for Gestational Age', *British Journal of Industrial Medicine* 46: 196–9.

Bryant, H. E., and Love, E. J. (1989), 'Video Display Terminal Use and Spontaneous Abortion Risk', *International Journal of Epidemiology* 18: 132–8.

Butler, W. J., and Brix, K. A. (1986), 'Video Display Terminal Work and Pregnancy Outcome in Michigan Clerical Workers', paper presented at the International Conference on Work with Display Units, Stockholm, Sweden.

Foster, K. R. (1986), 'The VDT Debate', *American Scientist* 74: 163–8.

Goldhaber, M. K., Polen, M., and Hiatt, R. A. (1988), 'The Risk of Miscarriage and Birth Defects Among Women Who Use Video Display Terminals During Pregnancy', *American Journal of Industrial Medicine* 13: 695–706.

Goulet, L., and Theriault, G. (1987), 'Association between Spontaneous Abortion and Ergonomic Factors: A Literature Review of the Epidemiologic Evidence', *Scandinavian Journal of Work and Environmental Health* 13: 399–403.

Jelovsek, F. R., Mattison, D. R., and Chenn, J. J. (1989), 'Prediction of Risk for Human Developmental Toxicity: How Important are Animal Studies for Hazard Identification?', *Obstetrics and Gynecology* 74: 624–36.

Kurzel, R. B., and Centulo, C. L. (1985), 'Chemical Teratogenesis and Reproductive Failure', *Obstetrics and Gynecology Survey* 40: 397–425.

McDonald, A. D., Cherry, N. M., Delorme, C., and McDonald, J. C. (1986), 'Visual Display Units and Pregnancy: Evidence of the Montreal Survey', *Journal of Occupational Medicine* 28: 1226–31.

—— McDonald, J. C., Armstrong, B., and Cherry, N. M. (1988), 'Prematurity and Work in Pregnancy', *British Journal of Industrial Medicine* 45: 56–62.

Mamelle, N., Laumon, B., Lazar, P. (1984), 'Prematurity and Occupational Activity During Pregnancy', *American Journal of Epidemiology* 119: 309–22.

National Academy of Sciences (1989), *Biological Markers in Reproductive Toxicology*, National Academy Press, Washington, DC.

National Research Council (1983), *Video Displays, Work, and Vision*, National Academy Press, Washington, DC.

Pastides, H., Calabrese, E. J., Hosmer, D. W., and Harris, D. R. (1988), 'Spontaneous Abortions and General Illness Symptoms Among Semiconductor Manufacturers', *Journal of Occupational Medicine* 30: 543–51.

Rosenberg, M. J. (1986), 'Reproduction in the Working Environment', in B. P. Sachs, and D. Acker, (eds.), *Clinical Obstetrics: A Public Health Perspective*, PSG Publishers, Littleton, Mass: 205–32.

—— Feldblum, P. J., and Marshall, E. G. (1987), 'Occupational Influences on Reproduction: A Review of Recent Literature', *Journal of Occupational Medicine* 29: 584–91.

Schlesselman, J. J. (1987), 'Proof of Cause and Effect in Epidemiologic Studies: Criteria for Judgement', *Preventive Medicine* 16: 195–210.

Swan, S. H., Shaw, G., Harris, J. A., Epstein, D. M., and Neutra, R. R. (1989), 'Adverse Pregnancy Outcomes in Relation to Water Contamination, Santa Clara County, California, 1980–1981', *American Journal of Epidemiology* 129: 885–93.

US Congress (1985), Office of Technology Assessment, *Reproductive Hazards in the Workplace*, US Government Printing Office, Washington, DC.: OTA–BA–266.

Wessel, D. (1989), 'Census Bureau Study Finds Shifts in Fertility Patterns', *Wall Street Journal*, p. 1, col. 3.

Wilcox, A. J., Weinberg, C. R., O'Connor, J. F., Baird, D. D., Schlatterer, J. P., Canfield, R. E., Armstrong, E. G., and Nisula, B. C. (1988), 'Incidence of Early Fetal Loss of Pregnancy', *New England Journal of Medicine* 319: 189–94.

Wrensch, M., Swan, S., Lipscomb, J., Epstein, D., Fenster, L., Claxton, K., Murphy, P. J., Shusterman, D., and Neutra, R. R. (1990), 'Pregnancy Outcomes in Women Potentially Exposed to Solvent-Contaminated Drinking Water in San Jose, California', *American Journal of Epidemiology* 131: 283–300.

Part IV

Fecundability

12 Models of Fecundability*

MEREDITH L. GOLDEN

SARA R. MILLMAN

Introduction

Models of fecundability, reviewed in this paper, contribute to a basic understanding of reproductive processes and provide tools to analyse such processes quantitatively. They have applications in such diverse areas as the treatment of fertility impairments, the study of contraceptive effectiveness, and the evaluation of family-planning programmes. Our aim here is to provide a succinct overview of these models for those working in related fields and to identify directions for the further development of such models.

We start by defining our terms, giving both a general sense of what is meant by fecundability and a set of more precise specifications of the several distinct phenomena it encompasses, which are sometimes confused with one another in the literature. Our most extensive section reviews the various efforts that have been made over the last several decades to model fecundability, tracing the gradual development of demographic thinking on this topic and distinguishing those models that treat fecundability as an input into the production of such outcomes as patterns of birth spacing and cumulative fertility and those that take fecundability itself as an outcome and focus on its components or determinants. In our concluding section, we attempt to identify issues that require further work and to provide a few suggestions as to the kinds of effort that are likely to contribute most substantially to further progress.

What is Fecundability?

Most demographers working on fecundability would agree at least on the broad outline of its definition as the probability of conception, per month or per menstrual cycle, for a woman exposed to some risk of conception. When this broad outline is filled in, however, we see a number of different concepts of

* Preparation of this paper was partially supported by the Ford Foundation Endowment Grant to the Population Studies and Training Center at Brown University and by a pre-doctoral NICHD-NRSA (National Institutes of Child Health and Development, National Research Science Award) traineeship through the Carolina Population Center. Helpful comments by Roger Avery, Robert S. Chen, Jane A. Menken, and Robert G. Potter, Jr. are gratefully acknowledged.

fecundability emerging. In general, the dimensions of variation relate to exactly what should be counted as a conception and how the boundaries should be drawn to delimit exposure to risk of conception.

In describing the distinctions between the various versions of fecundability, we can do no better than to start with the definitions provided by Bongaarts (1975: 646) over a decade ago:

Fecundability is defined as the probability of a conception in a menstrual cycle, a conception being the fertilization of an ovum by a sperm . . . Fecundability is measured in women who ovulate regularly, i.e., pregnant, sterile or postpartum anovulatory women are excluded. The term natural fecundability is used in noncontracepting populations.

Since the foregoing definition has led to various interpretations, we make the following definitions:

(1) Total fecundability (TF) is the probability that any conception occurs during a cycle; this includes non-implanted fertilized ova and conceptions aborted spontaneously before the end of the cycle.

(2) Recognizable fecundability (RF) is the probability of a conception which is recognizable at the end of the conception cycle by the nonoccurrence of the menstruation. A fraction a_1 of all conceptions fails to implant or aborts before the beginning of the next cycle:

$$RF = (1 - a_1)\ TF$$

(3) Effective fecundability (EF) is the probability of a conception which will end in a live birth. A fraction a_2 of the recognizable conceptions aborts spontaneously after the first cycle of gestation; therefore,

$$EF = (1 - a_2)\ RF$$
$$= (1 - a_2)\ (1 - a_1)\ TF$$

Bongaarts further distinguishes between gross and net fecundability. Gross fecundability is that which occurs for women actually engaging regularly in intercourse. Net fecundability is the conception probability in a population in which some interruptions in exposure to intercourse occur, as a function, for example, of illness or separation.

Of these many variations on the fecundability theme, Bongaarts claims that what is most often meant by the generic label 'fecundability' is more precisely natural net recognizable fecundability: the probability of a conception lasting at least long enough to delay the next menstruation, among non-contracepting women, of whom not all are necessarily regularly exposed to intercourse. While this generalization still holds, the generic label continues to be applied to enough distinct versions of fecundability to create considerable confusion. Our first plea would be for researchers in this area to adopt and consistently apply the precise terminology suggested by Bongaarts. In our discussion of specific modelling, below, we attempt to translate the diverse presentations of the various authors into these standard terms.

A Review of Existing Fecundability Models

The models of fecundability developed by demographers fall into two major categories that have evolved along separate lines. Models in the first category treat fecundability as an input that contributes significantly to the level of some empirically observed reproductive outcome, such as the number of live births, the proportion of women conceiving, or the waiting time to conception. In some cases, these models are simple mathematical relationships. Models in the second category treat fecundability as an output and attempt to quantify the behavioural and physiological processes underlying it. These models characterize the relationship between fecundability and one or more of its determinants, e.g. coital frequency, length of the fertile period, and the probability of implantation.

Gini introduced the concept of fecundability in 1924 and attempted to estimate it as an input, calculating the proportion of women in a population conceiving within a month. Beginning in the 1960s renewed interest in fecundability led to the development of input models along different branches, each designated by an observable reproductive endpoint. The first set relates to the number of live births; the second concerns the waiting time to conception, i.e. the number of months or cycles at risk prior to conception; the third measures the length of birth intervals; the fourth focuses on the proportion of women conceiving over a designated period of time.

Attempts to model fecundability as an output began in the early 1950s when Glass and Grebenik (1954) introduced a simple probabilistic process model based on coital frequency. In the late 1960s, other researchers addressed issues of coital frequency and timing, patterns of coition related to ovulation, and other physiological and behavioural components of reproduction.

Reproductive processes are very complex. To make the subject more manageable, early models utilized simplifying assumptions such as homogeneity among women. Recent models incorporate more detailed information about reproductive variability within the population and over time. In particular, they have taken advantage of new techniques that measure the physiological components of fecundability directly, new mathematical approaches that deal with population heterogeneity, and expanded population databases that include detailed reproductive histories.

Here we briefly review a representative set of models from each category in order to trace the general evolution of such models and their contributions and limitations. For a more comprehensive review of the literature up to 1975 see Menken (1975a, 1975b). In addition, Potter and Millman (1985) present a critique of nine models of fecundability based on coital frequency. Finally, Wood and Weinstein (1986) provide an up-to-date summary of some key background papers.

Models with Fecundability as an Input Variable

Live Births

'Live birth' models are those in which fecundability is used in conjunction with other independent variables to predict the number of live births within a specified time-period. In addition, estimates of fecundability can be derived from distributions of these births. This class includes models by Brass (1958), James (1963), Ridley *et al.* (1966), Barrett (1969), Bongaarts (1977), Bhattacharya and Nath (1983, 1984), and Bhattacharya and Singh (1984).

Brass (1958) suggests that the distribution of births in human populations follows a truncated negative binomial distribution related to a Pearson Type III distribution of the expectation of bearing children among women. His basic model is:

$$\Pr(r) = (ET)$$

where r refers to the number of births; E is the expected rate of childbearing of each woman; and T represents the period of exposure to risk of conception.

Brass never specifically relates 'the expectation of bearing children' to fecundability nor does he calculate a range of values for this variable. However, he does set up a model associating the expectation of bearing children with the total number of live births. He introduces the notion that women are heterogeneous with respect to their reproductive performance. Thus, the distribution of fertility in the population tends to be skewed and can therefore be fitted to a Pearson Type III (incomplete gamma) distribution (Keyfitz, 1968). Brass provides an equation for the mean of the Type III distribution of ET, the expected number of births to a woman in the reproductive years if she were exposed to risk over the whole period:

$$ET = \frac{kb}{(1 - b)}$$

where k and b are two parameters of the distribution for which no direct interpretation was provided.

James (1963) extends Brass's model of the mean of the distribution of ET in the population to estimate mean fecundability:

$$E = \frac{kb}{300\,(1 - b)}$$

where 300 represents the number of ovulatory cycles for which a woman is at risk of conception during her reproductive life-span. Accepting Brass's basic assumptions, James applies the extended model to the observed distribution of births among the Hutterites. He assumes that for all women the post-partum period of sterility is 3.6 months and determines that b is about 0.914 and k is approximately 2.01. These inputs yield an EF (effective fecundability) estimate of 0.07. A change in post-partum sterility to 6.1 months increases fecundability only marginally to 0.08. James then considers the effect of spontaneous abortions on fecundability and concludes that, if 20 per cent of recognized pregnancies had resulted in foetal loss, the mean *RF* (recognizable fecundability) estimate for the Hutterites may have been just over 0.10. The relatively low level of fecundability may have resulted from lower levels of coital frequency among the Hutterites, the assumption of a short, 25-day menstrual cycle, the inclusion of observations from the entire reproductive span rather than the first birth interval, and the consideration of pregnancies resulting in foetal loss.

Stochastic models have also been used to relate fecundability and other inputs to the number of live births per individual within a period of time and the distribution of intervals between them. Barrett (1969) simulates the reproductive history of a cohort of 1000 women from the beginning of marriage until the end of childbearing using Monte Carlo techniques. He tests the sensitivity of his model to changes in a number of important variables such as probability of sterility, probability of foetal loss, age at menopause, and length of post-partum sterility based on pregnancy outcome. Initially, *RF* is assigned the value of 0.20 per lunar month. A comparison of the simulation results with data from the Census of Ireland (1911) is made to check whether fecundability is over- or underestimated (Barrett, 1969). In additional simulations, Barrett introduces heterogeneity of fecundability into the model. The fecundability of each woman is based on a random number selected from a uniform distribution of *RF* between 0 and 0.21.

Bongaarts (1977) presents a deterministic model that describes the sequence of transitions through reproductive states that every woman is assumed to make from her own birth to the birth of her children. These include fecundable, pregnant, post-partum, and other non-susceptible states. The probabilities of transitions between reproductive states exactly determine the incidence of reproductive events. These probabilities may change with age and time. Bongaarts also describes his model in terms of seven intermediate fertility variables leading to age-specific birth-rates. These inputs include natural fecundability, contraceptive effectiveness, abortions, post-partum amenorrhoea, natural sterility by age, marital disruption and remarriage, and age at first marriage.

Bongaarts develops a model of the distribution of intervals from marriage to first birth and fits it to the observed distribution in eighteenth-century Canada (Henripin, 1954). Heterogeneity is considered with respect to fecundability, but not with respect to other reproductive determinants. The population is comprised of three subgroups whose *RF* levels are 50 per cent, 100 per cent, and 150 per cent of the mean *RF* for all ages, 0.31, based on earlier work (Bongaarts, 1975).

Bhattacharya and Nath (1983) specifically address the issue of heterogeneity in models that describe the number of births to a woman over long observational periods. While fecundability seems to follow a gamma-distribution over the short term, models that incorporate this assumption do not always give an adequate fit for long reproductive intervals. Bhattacharya and Nath suggest that the distribution of fecundability in a population may, in fact, not be unimodal. Therefore, subgroups of the population may have mean fecundabilities based on different distributions.

Bhattacharya and Nath test their hypothesis by assuming that fecundability in the population is a mixture of two distinct distributions. They use a model of the number of births to a woman within a specific time-period based on one developed by Singh *et al.* (1973). They extend it to incorporate variations in the length of non-susceptible periods following foetal loss. The new model is then calibrated with data from a 1978 sample survey of rural development and population growth in India. It includes only births occurring to women between the ages of 20 and 35. Through maximum likelihood estimation (MLE) techniques, the authors estimate that about 85 per cent of the population have high *RF* with a mean of 0.70 and the rest have low *RF* with a mean of 0.25.

In a subsequent paper, Bhattacharya and Nath (1984) develop another live-birth model that takes into account the effect of parity on several determinants of fertility, including foetal loss, non-susceptible periods, and fecundability. Estimates of these fertility parameters are determined by applying MLE techniques both to simulated data and to observed data from the 1978 Indian sample survey (Bhattacharya and Nath, 1984). The null hypothesis, that women of all parities share the same fecundability (estimated as 0.50), does not provide a good fit. An adequate fit is obtained, however, when the population is divided into two parity-dependent subgroups. The first includes fecund women at zero parity who share an estimated *RF* of 0.31. The second consists of fecund women at higher parity levels whose *RF* is 0.60. Possible explanations for the lower fecundability for zero-parity women include the young age at marriage in Indian Society and the Indian custom of women returning home to their parents for long periods of time.

In addition to parity, other demographic characteristics such as age and marital duration can also affect fertility determinants. Bhattacharya and Singh (1984) explore how the different age-groups in the population vary in terms of sterility, foetal loss, and fecundability. They use models of the number of live births to couples within a set time-period based on models developed by Singh *et al.* (1973) and Sheps and Menken (1973). Inputs for the models include the number of coitions within a time-interval, the distribution of the number of conceptions, the probability of foetal loss, and the length of non-susceptible periods following a pregnancy.

The findings of Bhattacharya and Singh (1984) indicate that fecundability levels change with a woman's age: increasing after menarche, reaching a maximum in the early 20s, staying on a plateau until 30, and then declining. Depending on the specified level of foetal loss, their 'effective' fecundability levels vary from 0.84 (20–5-year-olds with a 0.20 probability of foetal loss) to 0.20 (40–5-year-olds with a 0 to 0.20 probability of foetal loss). Their definition of 'effective' fecundability, however, does not correspond to Bongaarts's

(1975): it appears not to be limited to conceptions resulting in live births. Bhattacharya and Singh conclude that age may contribute to changes in biological, behavioural, and environmental factors that affect coital frequency, pregnancy wastage, duration of post-partum periods, incidence of ovulatory cycles, and secondary sterility.

Waiting Time to Conception

Another group of models relate to the waiting time to conception, that is the length of the period that begins when a woman is first exposed to the risk of conception and ends when conception occurs. These events are difficult to pinpoint in time. Marriage or cessation of contraception typically denotes the beginning of the period at risk. The endpoint is usually designated as the month when a recognized conception occurs or 9 months prior to a live birth. Potter and Parker (1964), Sheps (1964), Majumdar and Sheps (1970), Barrett (1971), Suchindran (1972), Bongaarts (1975), Suchindran and Lachenburch (1975), and Menken (1975a) have contributed to the development of this class of models.

In a homogeneous population, fecundability is the same for all women. Assuming that fecundability is also constant over time, the waiting time to conception is geometrically distributed, and its mean is the reciprocal of fecundability. Given heterogeneity with respect to fecundability, however, it is necessary to make explicit assumptions about the underlying distribution of fecundability across women in the population.

Potter and Parker (1964) develop a model to predict the 'time required to conceive', which they define as the months exposed to the risk of conception plus the month of conception. They assume that the frequency of different fecundability values is distributed within the population according to unimodal Type I (Beta Type) geometric curve, as suggested by Henry (1961). The proportion of couples, f(p), with a fecundability level of p is denoted as

$$f(p) = \frac{p^{a-1}(1-p)^{b-1}}{B(a, b)}$$

where $0 < p \leq 1$ and $B(a, b)$ is the beta-coefficient with $a, b > 0$.

The authors calculate the mean and variance of the time to conception for women included in the Princeton Fertility Study (Potter and Parker, 1964). Only women who began their exposure to conception after a deliberate cessation of contraception are included in the application. The fitted model yields different *RF* levels for women in terms of the number of months at risk of conception. These range from 0.26 at the start of exposure (0 months) to 0.05 after 48 months. Initially, the sample of women have widely varying fecundabilities as indicated by a large standard deviation, 0.13. As time goes on, the more fecund women drop out of the population leaving a fairly homogeneous group of less fecund women still at risk (with a standard deviation of 0.03).

Sheps (1964) examines characteristics of rates of conception in a heterogeneous population. She assumes that fecundability has a continuous frequency distribution, but relaxes the assumption by Potter and Parker (1964) of a specific shape. Given a homogeneous population, the fecundability p is the probability of waiting zero months to conceive and the corresponding mean waiting time is $(1 - p)/p$ months. In a heterogeneous population, however, the mean number of months to conception assumes a (compound) geometric distribution and is denoted as

$$M = E\left(\frac{1}{p}\right) - 1 = \frac{(1 - p')}{p'}$$

where $E(1/p)$ is the reciprocal of the harmonic mean and p' is the harmonic mean of fecundability. Utilizing harmonic means, Sheps shows that the mean waiting time in a heterogeneous population is longer than indicated by the arithmetic mean of the distribution. Also, the variance in waiting times for heterogeneous populations is greater than that of a homogeneous population with the same mean. MLE estimates are derived for this model with data from the analysis by Potter and Parker of the Princeton Fertility Study. The estimated harmonic mean of RF is 0.187 for women who began their exposure period after cessation of contraception and 0.096 for women who never started contraception.

Majumdar and Sheps (1970) suggest an alternative to the use by Potter and Parker of the 'method of moments', which they claim generates unreliable estimates of the parameters of the Pearson Type I geometric distribution of fecundability. Maximum likelihood estimation (MLE) techniques are applied to data from the Princeton Fertility Study and the Hutterites. Although MLE estimates fit the data better than the method of moments estimates, the fit is still poor. Majumdar and Sheps attribute this either to model deficiencies (e.g. the unrealistic assumption that fecundability remains constant over time) or to sampling problems (e.g. over-representation of women with short waiting times). Their MLE approach generates both arithmetic and harmonic means of fecundability for three sets of data. The first set of data consists of women in the Princeton Fertility Study whose exposure period begins with the cessation of contraception. The estimated arithmetic mean RF is 0.373 ± 0.015, and the estimated harmonic mean RF is 0.118 ± 0.027. The second set of Princeton data, women who conceived prior to using contraception, have corresponding values of 0.246 ± 0.017 and 0.043 ± 0.027. Finally, the Hutterites have an arithmetic mean EF of 0.270 ± 0.019 and a harmonic mean EF of 0.207 ± 0.015.

Bongaarts (1975) develops a method for estimating mean fecundability from the distribution of first birth intervals, that is, the time intervals from marriage or cessation of contraception to the first birth. He presents two models of the distribution of the 'exposure interval', based on probability distribution functions of the waiting times in both fecundable and non-susceptible states. According to Bongaarts, non-susceptible states result from any recognized pregnancies that terminate without a live birth and their associated periods of post-partum amenorrhoea. The models assume that non-susceptible periods are geometrically distributed. Bongaarts uses Leridon's (1973) estimate that

16.2 per cent of recognized pregnancies during the first birth interval result in a late spontaneous abortion.

The first model assumes that the population of women is homogeneous: for any particular state, all women share the same monthly transition probability. The second extends the first model to permit heterogeneity with respect to fecundability: subgroups of the population have different levels of fecundability. The probability distribution function of fecundability is assumed to be a modified beta-distribution which is completely determined given the mean and variance of fecundability. For a heterogeneous population, the exposure interval distribution is modelled as

$$e(z) = \sum_{n=1}^{m} F(f_n)\, e(z\,|\,f_n)$$

where $F(f_n)$ is the probability distribution function of fecundability of the nth subpopulation and $e(z\,|\,f_n)$ is the probability distribution function of the exposure interval in the nth subpopulation.

Bongaarts applies the model to data on 5 historical populations (from the seventeenth to nineteenth centuries) from Crulai, Tourouvre au Perche (France), Geneva, Tunis, and Quebec (Canada). Bongaarts uses an iterative approach whereby a computer checks 26 values of the fecundability mean and variance to determine the best fit of the model and the empirical data. The results for mean *RF* range from 0.18 to 0.31. Bongaarts uses the simple relationship, $RF = (1 - a_1)TF$, to determine the mean *TF*. Assuming that the proportion of all conceptions failing to implant or aborting before the next cycle (a_1) is 0.35 (James, 1978), he calculates that *TF* varies from 0.28 to 0.48.

Suchindran and Lachenbruch (1975) address the problem of truncated data in estimating fecundability. In most data-sets, not all of the women at risk of conception have conceived by the end of the observation period. Ignoring this situation, models often assume that the waiting times are known for the entire population at risk. Suchindran and Lachenbruch develop an algorithm for calculating both the moment and MLE estimates from truncated samples. Women are considered heterogeneous with respect to reproductive processes. Fecundability in the population is described by a beta-distribution, and the distribution of times to conception for truncated data is characterized by a truncated Type I geometric distribution.

Suchindran and Lachenbruch apply their model to an arbitrarily truncated version of the data on the American Hutterites and two subgroups from the Princeton Fertility Study used by Majumdar and Sheps (1970). For the Hutterite data truncated at six months, the mean *EF* estimates generated by the moment and MLE procedures are 0.307 and 0.279, respectively. For those women in the Princeton Fertility Study who stopped contraception prior to their exposure period, the MLE estimate of *RF* for a 24-month truncation is 0.336. As in the other studies, those women who do not contracept prior to the start of their exposure period have a lower *RF* estimate. Also truncated at 24 months, their MLE estimate of *RF* is 0.236. Suchindran and Lachenbruch compare their estimates with those derived by Majumdar and Sheps (1970) for complete samples of the same data-sets. The estimates of fecundability for both complete and truncated samples are similar, though the truncated samples indicate higher variation.

Menken (1975*a*) suggests use of the Sheps and Menken MLE procedure for models based on waiting time to conception. This procedure is especially designed to deal with short observation periods. It is particularly appropriate for developing countries where records or recall of reproductive events may be poor. Menken applies the Sheps and Menken MLE procedure to data from an intensive prospective study of birth interval dynamics in Bangladesh from 1969 to 1971 (Chen *et al.*, 1974). She goes on to compare the Sheps and Menken MLE estimates of a beta-distribution from censored data to the fecundability estimates obtained by three other methods: (1) the Pearl Index for models based on the proportion of women conceiving; (2) the MLE when the duration of post-partum amenorrhoea is considered a constant; and (3) the D'Souza convolution model (1973) applied to closed birth intervals. In addition, Menken examines the effect of temporary spousal separations on fecundability.

Estimates of *RF* calculated by the Sheps and Menken MLE procedure are similar to those generated by the Pearl Index. They both generated arithmetic and harmonic means of *RF* of about 0.07, indicating a relatively low level for Bangladesh. The application of the Pearl Index to data that exclude censored observations, however, results in a 100 per cent overestimate of fecundability. By contrast, the MLE estimate based on a constant duration of post-partum amenorrhoea underestimates fecundability. Finally, D'Souza's procedure (1973), when applied to closed intervals only, produces invalid estimates. The exclusion of censored observations from the Bangladesh data causes substantial selection bias. Including only women with live births effectively selects women with shorter intervals, shorter post-partum periods, and higher fecundability than is representative of the population as a whole. However, when the D'Souza procedure is applied to data without substantial selection bias it produces valid estimates of fecundability in Bangladesh.

Two other findings by Menken are particularly noteworthy. First, adjustment for the non-susceptible periods due to temporary spousal separation leads to a 20 per cent higher level of fecundability in the total population and a 7 per cent higher level in women under 30. Second, examination of conception rates by calendar month indicates seasonality of fecundability. Menken suggests that spousal separation should be accounted for more accurately in future work. In a related paper, she explores the effects of seasonal migration on fecundability estimates (Menken, 1979).

Birth Intervals

Birth-interval models are similar to models based on waiting time to conception, the key difference being that their endpoint is a live birth rather than conception. Fecundability estimates based on birth intervals must take into account periods of non-susceptibility such as length of pregnancy and post-partum amenorrhoea for both live births and foetal losses. D'Souza (1973) provides one of the best examples of this class of models.

D'Souza develops a model in which the interval between live births is considered the sum of a 'standardized mean time to conception' of a live birth and a 'standardized dead time' (periods of non-exposure). Given a non-contracepting population with low foetal loss, the standardized mean time to conception is $1/\alpha$ and the standardized fecundability is its reciprocal. D'Souza applies the model to historical data from Bavarian villages (late nineteenth century) and the American Hutterites (mid-twentieth century), including only women who have completed families of four or more children. He divides these populations into subgroups by age before using MLE techniques to estimate standardized fecundability. Standardized fecundability seems analogous to Bongaarts's definition of *EF*.

The model generates values of standardized fecundability for one of the Bavarian populations which range from 0.036 for women over 41 years old to 0.278 for women under 25 years old. By contrast, the Hutterites have a slightly higher value for the oldest age-group, 0.068, and a much lower value, 0.163, for the youngest. D'Souza claims that his results for the Hutterites are compatible with those of Sheps (1965), who estimates their harmonic mean fecundability to be 0.185, excluding women with foetal losses. According to Menken (1975*a*), the success of D'Souza's model depends upon the availability of accurate records of reproductive events. This type of data cannot easily be obtained from large, single-round surveys or from couples with poor recall of such information.

Proportion of Women Conceiving

Fecundability is sometimes estimated from the proportion of women conceiving within a specified time-period, usually at monthly intervals. Models by Gini (1924), Sheps (1964), Bongaarts (1975), and Goldman *et al.* (1985) are representative of this class.

In a homogeneous population, the proportion of women who conceive in the first month of exposure to the risk of conception is equivalent to fecundability p. The proportion who conceive in the second month of exposure is p times those women still at risk, $p(1 - p)$. Thus, fecundability remains constant, though the expected proportion of the population conceiving each month declines geometrically (Sheps, 1964). In a heterogeneous population, the proportion of women who conceive in the first month of exposure is equivalent to the arithmetic mean fecundability of the population. Assuming that the fecundability of an individual woman remains constant over time, the proportions that conceive in the second and following months of exposure are smaller than would be expected in a homogeneous population. This discrepancy is due to the fact that generally the more fecund women in a heterogeneous population conceive before the less fecund women, so that those women remaining at risk each succeeding month have a lower mean level of fecundability.

Sheps (1964) asserts that it is possible to characterize the distribution of fecundability in a population from the proportion of women conceiving in each of the first three months of exposure. Accordingly, Sheps uses the Princeton Fertility Study data as presented by Potter and Parker (1964) to calculate MLE estimates of fecundability. For women whose exposure period begins after the cessation of contraception, fecundability estimates for the first three months are 0.397, 0.160, and 0.098, respectively. For women whose exposure period preceded any contraception, the mean fecundability estimates are smaller: 0.282, 0.124, and 0.116.

Bongaarts (1975) develops a short procedure to estimate the mean *EF*. He uses the ratio of births in the first year of marriage, excluding those prior to the ninth month, to all first births. Fecundability estimates derived from five historical populations by fitting a model of waiting times are compared with those generated by this alternative approach. The results are nearly identical.

Goldman *et al.* (1985) estimate mean fecundability for eight countries in Latin America and Asia included in the World Fertility Survey. They consider the proportion of zero-parity women with live-birth conceptions in the first 12 or 48 months following marriage. The authors use Bongaarts's (1975) short procedure to estimate *RF*. They assume that fecundability is heterogeneous in the population and follows a beta-distribution. Adjustments are made for foetal wastage. In addition, women are divided into two groups based on whether their marriage took place 0–1 year or 2–4 years prior to the study. The estimated *RF* for the first group ranges from 0.23 to 0.35 and for the second group from 0.17 to 0.26.

Models with Fecundability as an Output Variable

Coital Frequency, Timing, and Patterns

Numerous models consider fecundability as an output dependent upon variations in coital frequency, coital timing relative to ovulation, and coital patterns over the inter-menstrual period. This class of models includes important contributions by Glass and Grebenik (1954), Lachenbruch (1967), Glasser and Lachenbruch (1968), Barrett and Marshall (1969), Barrett (1971), Trussell (1977), Schwartz *et al.* (1980), and Potter and Millman (1986).

Glass and Grebenik (1954) developed a probabilistic model that calculates *TF* in terms of the number of coitions within the inter-menstrual period. They arbitrarily fix the length of the inter-menstrual period at 24 days and the length of the fertile period at 4 days. They consider sperm viable and motile only on the day of coitus, but indicate how to relax this restriction. If coition occurs within the fertile period, it is assumed that conception will take place. Their model states the chance of n coitions not resulting in conception as:

$$p' = \frac{\binom{20}{n}}{\binom{24}{n}} = \frac{20!}{24!} \frac{(24-n)!}{(20-n)!}$$

Therefore, the probability of conception is simply $(1 - P')$. Using four hypothetical values of coital frequency (5, 10, 15, and 20), Glass and Grebenik calculate the probability of conception for two broad patterns of coitus: (1) coitus occurring any time in the inter-menstrual period (lower limit) and (2) coitus not occurring more than once in any 24-hour period (upper limit). The values of *TF* range from a lower limit of 0.598 at five coitions to an upper limit of 0.999 with 20 coitions per inter-menstrual period.

Lachenbruch (1967) estimates the probability of conception in terms of when and how often coitus occurs in a 4-day fertile period: 2 days prior to ovulation, the day of ovulation, and 1 day post-ovulation. Coitus on other days of the menstrual cycle is considered to be inconsequential. The day of ovulation is determined by its distribution based on Farris's (1956) data, but weighted for ovulations later in the cycle. Lachenbruch develops two models assuming different 'shapes' of the fertile period. Model *A* has a broad fertile period, that is to say, the probabilities of conception are fairly similar over the 4 days: 0.10, 0.20, 0.30, and 0.20 for days $D - 2$ to $D + 1$, respectively. Model *B* has a peaked fertile period, so that the probabilities of conception vary widely over the different days of this period: 0.05, 0.30, 0.50, and 0.05. Since coital frequencies change over the inter-menstrual cycle (Udry and Morris, 1968), Lachenbruch considers 8 different hypothetical distributions or patterns of coitions. Frequencies of intercourse between five and 12 times a cycle (Kinsey *et al.*, 1953) are considered.

Using micro-simulation techniques to estimate *TF*, Lachenbruch incorporates probabilities of three events: timing of intercourse near ovulation, timing of ovulation in the cycle, and occurrence of conception given the prior two events. His general model for the probability of conception is

$$P = \sum_{j=10}^{20} q_j \left(P^*_{j-2}\, r_{j-2,j} + P^*_{j-1} r_{j-1,j} + P_j r_{j,j} + P^*_{jr1+1} r_{j+1,j} \right)$$

where q_j is the probability of ovulation of day i; $r_{i,j}$ is the probability that conception occurs given intercourse on day i and ovulation on day j; and P^*_j is the probability that intercourse occurs on day j assuming no replacement in sampling, that is, intercourse occurs not more than once on any one day.

Lachenbruch determines estimates of *TF* for different frequencies (five to 12) and patterns (each of the eight distributions) of intercourse per cycle under the two models (*A* and *B*) describing the shape of the fertile period. Based on a sample size of 1000 simulated couples, his fecundability estimates range from 0.14 to 0.42 for a broad fertile period and 0.046 to 0.45 for a peaked fertile period. These results indicate that fecundability estimates vary greatly depending on the different frequencies and patterns of intercourse in the cycle. Lachenbruch points out that his models do not fully reflect the complexities of reproduction. Inputs such as the length of the menstrual cycle and the time of ovulation may be considerably more variable in human populations than in the model. He suggests that more data are needed on the occurrence of anovulatory cycles, the effect of frequency of coitus on sperm counts, and the range of monthly coital patterns.

Barrett and Marshall (1969) examine the risk of conception on different days of the menstrual cycle. In their model, they make two key assumptions. The first is that the probability of conception as a consequence of coitus on a particular day is independent of the probability of conception on any other day. Thus, the probability of conception after two acts of intercourse, on day *i* and day *j*, for example, leads to a combined probability of conception:

$$P_{ij} = P_i + P_j - P_iP_j$$

where P_i is the probability of conception during a cycle with intercourse on day *i* only. The second assumption is that all combinations of days of coitus are equally likely for a set number of coitions. Their model of the probability of conception for a given cycle is

$$1 - P = \pi\beta_ix_i$$

where $\beta_i = 1 - \alpha_i$ and $x_i = 1$ if coitus occurred on day *i* of the cycle and 0 otherwise. This can also be written as

$$\log_e (1 - P) = \sum \gamma_ix_i$$

where $\gamma_i = \log_e\beta_i$.

Data from 241 British married couples with at least one child prior to the observation period are used to compare the number of coitions on specific days relative to ovulation with the corresponding number of conceptive or non-conceptive cycles. The authors determine that the probability of conception is significantly different from zero only on the five days prior to ovulation, but also consider the day following ovulation as part of the fertile period. Their model generates levels of recognizable, not total, fecundability, since foetal losses in the first month are not detected. Foetal losses in the second and later months are counted as conceptions here, where in other models early losses are often missed. Assuming that coitus occurs only once in the fertile period, the probabilities of conception during the fertile period are 0.13, 0.20, 0.17, 0.30, 0.14, and 0.07 for each of the days −5 to +1, respectively. Barrett and Marshall also use the same coefficients (γ_i) derived by MLE for the 6 days to calculate fecundability levels for different patterns of coitus:

$$1 - P = \exp(-0.14x_{-4.5} - 0.22x_{-3.5} - 0.19x_{-2.5} - 0.35x_{-1.5} - 0.15x_{-0.5} \\ - 0.07x_{-0.5})$$

where the midpoint of the first post-ovulatory day is represented by $i = 0.5$. *RF* estimates range from 0.68 for daily coitus to 0.14 for weekly coitus. The authors also explore whether or not the probabilities of conception on the six different days surrounding ovulation are independent. Given one to six coitions during this period with any combination of days equally likely, the observed and expected probabilities are closely matched, indicating independence.

Barrett (1971) extends Barrett and Marshall's model to determine the effect of a woman's age on the relationship between fecundability and coital frequency. Two groups of women from the same British data-set are considered. Group 1 consists of women aged 30 and under; group 2 includes women older than 30. Assuming an 8-day fertile period with coitus occurring only once, Barrett uses quantal regression to calculate the daily probabilities of conception for each age-group. For the younger women, the risk of conception for days -7 to $+1$, respectively, are 0.056, 0.00, 0.086, 0.305, 0.125, 0.317, 0.111, and 0.082. The corresponding values for older women are 0.038, 0.049, 0.146, 0.022, 0.113, 0.200, 0.084, and 0.095.

Given the probabilities of conception for each day of the fertile period, Barrett estimates for each age-group the levels of *RF* for different patterns of coitus. The group of younger women has a 0.16 probability of conception with coitus once a week and a 0.71 probability with coitus once a day. For the older group, the corresponding values are 0.10 and 0.55. Overall, the fecundability levels for older women are about 30 per cent lower. Barrett also looks at the effects of coital frequency and pattern using two different sets of daily conception probabilities (relative to ovulation) developed by Lachenbruch. *RF* estimates are within the range already calculated, 0.11 to 0.68, based on weekly versus daily coitus, respectively.

Trussell (1977) addresses the causes of variability in fecundability across populations by examining the effects of timing and frequency of intercourse. He attempts to improve upon studies by Barrett (1971), Glasser and Lachenbruch (1968), and Lachenbruch (1967). The conditional probabilities of conception are considered for both a 4-day and a 6-day fertile period. Mean levels of *RF* are determined from a micro-simulation of the reproductive histories of 5000 women. They are stated in terms of the average number of coitions per cycle and contraceptive effectiveness. Given no contraception and a longer fertile period (a smoothed version of the Barrett and Marshall 1969 data), mean fecundability ranges from 0.11 for 2.74 coitions per cycle to 0.415 for a coital frequency of 10.74. For a shorter fertile period (Lachenbruch, 1967), the corresponding range is from 0.098 to 0.367.

Schwartz *et al.* (1980) recommend a model based on the conditional independence of coitus on different days given that the ovum was fertilizable and viable. They assert that the risks of conception from different acts of coitus are not statistically independent. Models that incorrectly assume independence yield higher levels of *RF* than feasible considering Leridon's (1977) estimated rates of early spontaneous abortion. The authors improve upon past efforts by incorporating three key probabilities into their extended model. The first is the probability P_o that ovulation produces a fertilizable ovum; the second is the probability P_f that fertilization takes place; the third is the probability P_v that the fertilized egg is maintained until recognized, i.e. for at least six weeks. Their model of recognizable fecundability *P* combines these probabilities as follows,

$$P = P_o\, P_f\, P_v.$$

The authors assume that only P_f is affected by coital pattern and, therefore, $P_o P_v = k$. They recognize that the value of *k* depends on a woman's age and estimate that the average value for all women is 0.52. All cycles are considered to be statistically independent. They also consider the probability of conception after two coitions, one on day *i* and one on day *j*, written as

$$P_{ij} = P_i + P_j - P_iP_j/k.$$

Schwartz *et al.* (1980) fit their model to the Barrett and Marshall (1969) data. This yields estimates of the daily conditional probabilities of fertilization P_{fi} for each day of the fertile period. For a 7-day fertile period, from day −6 to +1, the P_{fi} values are 0.08, 0.27, 0.38, 0.38, 0.65, 0.27, and 0.13. The corresponding daily probabilities of conception P_i are 0.04, 0.14, 0.20, 0.20, 0.34, 0.14, and 0.07. These values are quite similar to Barrett and Marshall's estimates for a 6-day fertile period. However, the new model gives a range for *RF* from 0.16 for coitus once a week to 0.49 for coitus every day, whereas Barrett and Marshall's corresponding estimates are 0.14 and 0.68. Thus, fecundability as estimated by Schwartz *et al.* does not increase as greatly with frequency of coitus as suggested by Barrett and Marshall, whose model considered coital days statistically independent in terms of fertilization probabilities.

Estimates of the effects of coital frequency, timing, and patterns on fecundability depend to a great extent on what assumptions are made about the physiological parameters of reproduction. Model inputs are often arbitrarily assigned values based either on small sample populations or limited knowledge of biological systems. Focusing on the relationship between the length of coital intervals and fecundability, Potter and Millman (1986) examine the effects of particular input values on fecundability predictions. They present seven different models with various assumptions regarding the timing of ovulation in the cycle and the length of fertilization and impregnation periods. The fertilization period refers to the time within a favourable cycle that a viable spermatozoa may penetrate a viable ovum. The impregnation period is the interval co-extensive with or included within the fertilization period during which insemination may result in a recognized pregnancy. Ovulation is considered to occur either 'early' or 'late' in the cycle. The fertilization period is allowed to range from a minimum of 48 hours to a maximum of 66 hours. Included within the fertilization period is the impregnation period which may range from 24 to the full 66 hours. Within both of these periods, there are optimum times when the respective probability of each of these events occurring is 1.0.

Potter and Millman consider the redundancy of two coitions within the same fertile period. One model assumes that if two coitions occur more than 6 hours prior to ovulation, then the one closest to the time of ovulation always causes fertilization. Other models assign more probability to the likelihood that the earlier coitus is responsible for fertilization. It is assumed that several factors remain constant across populations and time, even though variability no doubt exists. These include times for sperm capacitation (6 hours), ovum viability (24 hours), sperm viability (48 hours), and penetration by capacitated sperm (1–2 hours).

The seven models are used to calculate fecundability levels for three different lengths of inter-coital intervals: 66, 48, and 24 hours. Although Potter and Millman refer to 'recognized pregnancies' in their paper, recognition occurs at the time of implantation, much earlier than usually detected. Since conceptions that abort in the post-implantation period are included in their estimates of fecundability, their definition seems closely related to Bongaarts's 'total fecundability' (1975). The first set of fecundabilities assumes that only the coition nearest to ovulation can cause fertilization. The 66-hour inter-coital period, permitting only one coition in the fertilization period, produces a fecundability of 0.364 for all the models. The 48-hour inter-coital period yields a range of fecundabilities from 0.357 to 0.500. Finally, a 24-hour inter-coital period has estimates ranging from 0.250 to 0.714.

The inclusion of the possibility that early coitions contribute to fertilization leads to lower fecundability levels in general. The extent of the decline depends on the attributes of the different models. For an inter-coital interval of 24 hours, the diminished levels of fecundability run from 0.125 to 0.571. Potter and Millman conclude that the marginal gains in fecundability with higher rates of coitus may be less at high coital levels than at low coital levels due to the redundancy of coitions within the same fertile period. Although there is no decisive evidence of the effect of ageing gametes on fecundability, the authors point to new insights regarding possible changes in fecundability based on inter-coital intervals. They recommend additional data collection, rather than further modelling, to resolve unsettled issues in this area.

Comprehensive Physiological and Behavioural Components

Wood and Weinstein (1986) present a new theoretical model of the physio-logical and behavioural components of age-specific fecundability. Their model stems from previous work relating frequency of intercourse with fecundability (Barrett and Marshall, 1969; Glasser and Lachenbruch, 1968; Lachenbruch, 1967; Potter, 1961; Tietze, 1960; and Glass and Grebenik, 1954). Age-related changes in physiological functions and reproductive behaviour, however, were not incorporated into these early models. Bongaarts (1976, 1977) and Bongaarts and Potter (1983) have considered how age affects fecundability with an empirical approach based on waiting times. Wood and Weinstein extend these prior efforts to predict fecundability as a function of its own determinants. They provide estimates for the various components of fecundability and also test the sensitivity of fecundability to changes in these values.

Many of the determinants of fecundability change with age, across populations, and by marital duration. Wood and Weinstein recognize the importance of these variations. However, given the problems of modelling such complexities they focus primarily on the issue of age dependency and otherwise assume homogeneity within the population. They also consider the determinants of fecundability to be independent. Finally, the study population is restricted to non-contracepting, currently married, sexually active women who are fecund (neither pregnant nor lactating).

Wood and Weinstein present the following model:

$$\text{Pr}_j\,(c) = \sum_{n=0}^{\infty} \text{Pr}_j\,(c\,|\,N = n)\,\text{Pr}_j\,(N = n)$$

where c is the event that conception occurs to a woman of j years and N is the number of times intercourse occurs during a cycle. The probability that a conception occurs during one ovulatory cycle for a woman aged j years, $\text{Pr}_j(c)$, is thus a function of the two primary components of fecundability: the susceptibility component, $\text{Pr}_j(c\,|\,N = n)$, and the exposure component, $\text{Pr}_j(N = n)$. The susceptibility component refers to how fecund a woman is, or, more specifically, the probability of a conception given N number of coitions during one cycle. It can be written, in turn, as the combination of three other probabilities.

$$\text{Pr}_j\,(c\,|\,N = n) = \sum_{i=1}^{n} \text{Pr}_j\,(c\,|\,I = i)\,\text{Pr}_j\,(I = i\,|\,N = n,o)\,\text{Pr}_j\,(o)$$

where $\text{Pr}_j(c\,|\,I = i)$ is the probability of conception given the number of coitions in the fertile period; $\text{Pr}_j(I = i\,|\,N = n,o)$ is the probability that coitus occurs in the fertile period given the number of coitions in one cycle; and $\text{Pr}_j(o)$ is the probability that the cycle is ovulatory. The exposure component, $\text{Pr}_j (N = n)$, indicates the probability of N number of coitions actually occurring in a cycle. Other factors taken into account include: the chance that a conception results from a single intercourse in the fertile period; the probability that a conceptus dies prior to birth; the expected cycle length for women at age j; the expected length of the fertile period for women at age j; and the number of fertile periods either partially or totally encompassed by a 30-day month.

Wood and Weinstein use a variety of sources to estimate values for the components of fecundability and to develop a reference population. The probability that a woman at age *j* is post-menarcheal and pre-menopausal is based on US data collected by Treloar (1974). Treloar *et al.* (1967) provide data on mean cycle length by age. Their estimates of the probability that a cycle is ovulatory are based on over 30 000 cycles from a sample of US women (Vollman, 1977). The authors also consider models of the viability of the ovum and sperm (Royston, 1982). Finally, age-specific estimates for the length of fertile periods and the probability that coitus during the fertile period leads to conception are from clinical studies that detect ovulation and early pregnancy.

The authors conclude that an appropriate estimate of the average probability of conception from coitus on any one day of the fertile period is 0.60. The range of embryonic and foetal loss by age is based on nine geographically dispersed study populations. An estimated average level of loss across all age-groups is 0.30. The total non-susceptibility period for a foetal loss derived from a fetal life-table study (French and Bierman, 1962) is the sum of gestational length and post-partum amenorrhoea, respectively 3.7 and 0.30 weeks on average, or roughly a total of 4 weeks. Age-specific coital frequencies for 'standard marital exposure' are from the Swedish schedule used by Coale and McNeil (1972). The mean age of marriage is fixed at 23 years of age, following a typical European pattern. In addition, a 'maximal exposure' scenario is considered that assumes daily acts of intercourse during the fertile period.

From the composite reference characteristics of the determinants of fecundability, Wood and Weinstein determine estimates of *TF* and *EF* by age under both maximum and marital exposure regimes. The variation of fecundability due to marital duration is also examined for the case of standard marital exposure. Under maximum exposure, mean *EF* is 0.32 and mean *TF* is 0.66. Under standard marital exposure, mean *EF* is 0.27 (mean *TF* is not calculated). Estimates of fecundability are compared to those observed by other researchers (Bongaarts and Potter, 1983; Bendel and Hua, 1978; and Leridon, 1977).

Finally, Wood and Weinstein conduct a series of sensitivity tests to determine the degree to which age-specific *EF* estimates vary given a reasonable range of values for specific determinants. The components examined include: age at first marriage, level of intra-uterine mortality, late menarche and early menopause, long ovarian cycles, frequent anovulatory cycles, length of the fertile period, and probability that one coition leads to conception. They conclude that *EF* varies under both exposure scenarios with changes in foetal loss and frequency of anovulatory cycles. For marital exposure, the length of the fertile period and the probability that one coition leads to conception also affect fecundability. From the model, it is clear that not only variations in coital behaviour, but also variations in ovarian function and in foetal loss affect fecundability over a woman's reproductive life-span.

Summary

The models reviewed in this paper generate widely divergent estimates of fecundability ranging from 0.00 to 0.999. Table 12.1 summarizes these estimates according to model classification and type of fecundability. More detailed tables are presented in a related paper by the authors (Golden and Millman, 1988). In general, sources of variation in fecundability may be associated with differences in research methodologies and population characteristics. The former category includes modelling strategies, sampling techniques, and issues of data quality. The latter refers to those characteristics—physiological, behavioural, demographic, and environmental—that affect the actual level of fecundability in a population. Examples of possible sources of variation in estimates of fecundability are listed below:

Research Methodologies: Differences in Modelling

- Type or definition of fecundability: total, recognizable, or effective
- Model classification: number of live births, waiting time to conception, birth intervals, proportion of women conceiving, coital characteristics, comprehensive components
- Estimation techniques: method of moments vs. MLE procedures
- Treatment and basic unit of time: discrete vs. continuous time; menstrual cycle, calendar month, lunar month, or fixed number of days
- Period of observation: first sexual union to first pregnancy or birth (within or regardless of marriage), x number of years of marriage, women between two given ages (e.g. 20 to 35 years old), or the entire reproductive life-span (from menarche to menopause assuming exposure to the risk of conception)
- Modelling fecundability as heterogeneous vs. homogeneous within a population

TABLE 12.1. *Summary of fecundability estimates by type and model classification*

Model Classification	Type of Fecundability		
	Total	Recognizable	Effective
Number of live births	—	0.00–0.84	0.07–0.76
Waiting time to conception	0.28–0.48	0.043–0.336	0.207–0.307
Birth intervals	—	—	0.036–0.278
Proportion of women conceiving	—	0.039–0.397	0.181–0.315
Coital frequency, timing, and patterns	0.050–0.999	0.00–1.00	—
Comprehensive physiological and behavioural components	0.66	—	0.27–0.32
All models	0.050–0.999	0.00–1.00	0.036–0.76

- Underlying distribution of fecundability fitted to a data-set: Pearson Type I geometric (beta-) distribution, Pearson Type III (incomplete gamma-) distribution, and non-symmetric triangular distribution
- Treatment of fecundability and its determinants over time: secular trends and age effects

Research Methodologies: Differences in Data Collection

- Completeness and reliability of data from sample population: data-collection method (retrospective vs. prospective, large- vs. small-scale, single vs. multiple round survey), truncated data-set (e.g. censoring of women whose conception times are longer than the observational period), selection bias (e.g. over-representation of women with high fecundability), misclassification bias (e.g. differences in detection and reporting of ovulation, early spontaneous abortions, and pregnancy), and recall bias (e.g. poor memory of coital frequency, contraceptive use, and conceptions not ending in live births)
- Representativeness of sample or study population with respect to the larger population (e.g. quality of sampling techniques)

Population Characteristics: Differences in Underlying Determinants Affecting Actual Levels of Fecundability

- Physiological parameters of reproduction: ages at menarche and menopause, incidence of anovulatory cycles, length of inter-menstrual and fertile periods, shape of fertile periods, viability of gametes, blood incompatibilities, intra-uterine environment, and length of gestation and post-partum amenorrhoea by pregnancy outcome
- Behavioural attributes: marital duration, spousal separation due to illness or seasonal migration, family-planning practices including breastfeeding, attitudes toward induced abortions, and coital frequency and patterns
- Demographic profile: age structure, racial and ethnic composition, parity, educational attainment, and access to quality prenatal care
- Environmental exposures: reproductive toxins, physical factors such as high altitude effects, and seasonal climatic changes such as temperature

A detailed account of how each of these sources of variation may affect fecundability estimates is beyond the scope of this paper. Indeed, the effects of many of these factors, while potentially substantial, are currently unknown. Research on fecundability seems to have ignored the more difficult questions regarding reproductive processes. Most of the existing models only describe their methodological procedures and assumptions briefly. The choice of input variables and their values vary greatly, often without any meaningful explanation of their selection.

Wood and Weinstein (1986) offer a new, more comprehensive approach to modelling fecundability. They consider how changes in each of several key determinants of fecundability affect its estimate. The selection of values for these variables is based on ranges either observed in populations or determined from biomedical knowledge of reproductive processes. Not all the sources of variation in fecundability are addressed by Wood and Weinstein, but their approach provides a prototype for more extensive research.

If estimates of fecundability are to provide useful measures of the reproductive health of an individual or population, it is essential, at the very least, for researchers to state explicitly both their methodological approaches and their assumptions regarding fecundability and its determinants. Demographers and medical researchers might also consider standardizing with respect to certain key determinants of fecundability, for example, age, parity, marital duration, and contraceptive use. Controlling for differences in these factors will make it possible to compare fecundability estimates across populations more rigorously.

Conclusions

Over the last several decades two strands of fecundability modelling have developed. The first has estimated fecundability levels from the outcomes of fecundability, such as the proportion of women conceiving in a single month of exposure, the distribution of waiting time to conception, parities attained within some specified duration, and birth intervals. The second strand takes fecundability itself as an outcome of such determinants as the frequency and timing of intercourse and the probability that a menstrual cycle is ovulatory. Within each of these lines of research, development over time has been in the direction of ever greater complexity. Simplifying assumptions such as that of homogeneity among women over time have been relaxed. As a result, recent models come closer to reflecting reality than those produced by earlier efforts. Achievement of a still more accurate understanding of fecundability will probably require further increases in complexity. For instance, more work is needed to describe the interdependence among determinants of fecundability. Such advances in modelling will need to be supported by the accumulation of more extensive and more detailed empirical evidence on each of the components of fecundability and on their interrelationships.

Among the aspects of fecundability requiring further attention, we identify several as particularly important. These include: variation in the detection of conception; criteria for identifying those at risk of conception and their periods of exposure; applications to populations in which at least some members use contraception; treatment of couples rather than women as the reproductive unit; and the effects of age, seasonality, and toxic exposures on fecundability.

Theory often defines the occurrence of any conception at all as the event of interest, that is, researchers often wish to estimate total fecundability. However, those conceptions leading to early foetal wastage may never be observed. A focus on effective fecundability, or the probability of a conception leading to a live birth, is one response to this problem: such conceptions are unlikely to go unnoticed! Recognizable fecundability, or the probability of a conception lasting long enough to lead to some delay in the next menstruation, represents a compromise position. In practice, however, the proportion of conceptions that survive long enough to cause a menstrual delay is less than one and undoubtedly varies widely across populations and over groups within populations. One might also expect that for those whose lives do not make it important to keep track of the passage of time, pregnancies may not be detected or acknowledged until considerably later. In these groups or populations, 'recognizable fecundability' will be underestimated, especially if the incidence of early spontaneous abortions is high. Therefore, cross-national or educational-group comparisons of fecundability may be seriously distorted by variations in the detection and reporting of conceptions.

Difficulties in defining who should be included in fecundability studies relate to problems in specifying coital exposure and sterility. Attempts to limit the study population to those at risk of conception often lead to an exclusive focus on married women, which may be problematic in situations where:
1. population estimates are desired;
2. much exposure takes place outside formal unions; and
3. union status may be affected by reproductive performance.

A further limitation is to exclude those who, although married, are temporarily not at risk of conception due to separation or illness; alternatively, current modelling can capture such situations as a reduction in the frequency of intercourse. Whatever her exposure to intercourse, a woman is at risk of conception only in an ovulatory menstrual cycle. Thus, the principle is generally accepted that women who are sterile or post-partum anovulatory, as well as those who are pregnant, should be excluded from fecundability calculations. These points, although not controversial, may be problematic in their implementation. Neither sterility nor post-partum anovulation is directly observed. Procedures to identify women in either of these states differ from study to study and may be subject to considerable error.

Most fecundability estimates incorporate a further restriction to those intervals in which no contraceptive use occurs. Where it is the underlying physiological ability to reproduce that is of interest, contraception only obscures the picture. However, if past reproductive performance is a cause of current contraceptive use, fecundability of non-users of contraception cannot be assumed to correspond to that which would be experienced by users if they were not contracepting. Furthermore, exclusion of contraceptors does not guarantee that estimates obtained will reflect only the underlying physiological reproductive capacity even for non-contraceptors. The timing and frequency of intercourse affect fecundability, and varying patterns may be deliberately adopted by those wishing to minimize or maximize the probability of conception.

'Natural fecundability' may be affected by volition, although it is generally interpreted as non-volitional.

As modelling efforts become increasingly complicated, it is important for those carrying out the work to keep in mind that would-be consumers of their insights may not be mathematically inclined nor familiar with their technical jargon. Clearly defined and reasonably standard terminology would reduce confusion, as would provision of verbal translations of mathematical formulae. Since the complexity of modelling is sure to increase, high priority needs to be placed on consistency of definition and clarity of presentation.

References

Barrett, J. C. (1969), 'A Monte Carlo Simulation of Human Reproduction', *Genus* 25: 1–22.

—— (1971), 'Fecundability and Coital Frequency', *Population Studies* 25: 309–13.

—— and Marshall, J. (1969), 'The Risk of Conception on Different Days of the Menstrual Cycle', *Population Studies* 23: 455–61.

Bendel, J.-P., and Hua, C.-I. (1978), 'An Estimate of the Natural Fecundability Ratio Curve', *Social Biology* 25: 210–27..

Bhattacharya, B. N., and Nath, D. C. (1983), 'A Probability Model for Number of Births and its Application in Estimation of Fecundability for a Heterogeneous Population', *Janasamkhya* 1(2): 163–71.

—— —— (1984), 'An Extension of a Parity-Dependent Model for Number of Births and Estimation of Fecundability', *Mathematical Biosciences*, 71(2): 201–16.

—— and Singh, K. K. (1984), 'A Modification of a Model for Number of Births and Estimation of Age Specific Fecundability and Sterility', *Janasamkhya* 2(1): 1–18.

Bongaarts, J. (1975), 'A Method for the Estimation of Fecundability', *Demography* 12: 645–60.

—— (1976), 'Intermediate Fertility Variables and Marital Fertility Rates', *Population Studies* 30: 227–41.

—— (1977), 'A Dynamic Model of the Reproductive Process', *Population Studies* 30(3): 59–73.

—— and Potter, R. G. (1983), *Fertility, Biology and Behavior: An Analysis of the Proximate Determinants*, Academic Press, New York.

Brass, W. (1958), 'The Distribution of Births in Human Populations', *Population Studies* 12: 51–72.

Chen, L. C., Ahmed, S., Gesche, M., and Mosley, W. H. (1974), 'A Prospective Study of Birth Interval Dynamics in Rural Bangladesh', *Population Studies* 28: 277–97.

Coale, A. J., and McNeil, D. R. (1972), 'The Distribution by Age at First Marriage in a Female Cohort', *Journal of the American Statistical Association* 67: 743–9.

D'Souza, S. (1973), 'Interlive Birth Intervals of Non-Contraceptive Populations: A Data Analytic Study', *Social Action* 23: 404–25.

Farris, E. J. (1956), *Human Ovulation and Fertility* (Lippincott, Philadelphia).

French, F. E., and Bierman, J. M. (1962), 'Probabilities of Fetal Mortality', *Public Health Report* 77: 835–47.

Gini, C. (1924), 'Premières recherches sur la fécondabilité de la femme', *Proceedings of the International Mathematical Congress, Toronto*, ii: 889–92.

Glass, D. V., and Grebenik, E. (1954), 'The Trend and Pattern of Fertility in Great Britain: A Report on the Family Census of 1946', *Papers of the Royal Commission on Population*, vi HMSO, London.

Glasser, J. H., and Lachenbruch, P. A. (1968), 'Observations on the Relationship between Frequency and Timing of Intercourse and the Probability of Conception', *Population Studies* 21: 23–31.

Golden, M. L., and Millman, S. R. (1988), *Comparison of Models and Estimates of Fecundability*, working paper no. 88 (forthcoming), Population Studies and Training Center, Brown University, Providence, RI.

Goldman, N., Westoff, C. F., and Paul, L. E. (1985), 'Estimation of Fecundability from Survey Data', *Studies of Family Planning* 16: 252–61.

—— —— —— (1987), 'Variations in the Natural Fertility: The Effect of Lactation and other Determinants' *Population Studies* 41: 127–46.

Henripin, J. (1954), *La population Canadienne au début du XVII siècle*, Institut national d'études démographiques cahier no. 22, Presses Universitaires de France, Paris.

Henry, L. (1961), 'La fécondité naturelle: Observation–théorie–résultats', *Population* 16(4): 663.

James, W. H. (1963), 'Estimates of Fecundability', *Population Studies* 17: 57–65.

—— (1978), 'Length of the Human Fertile Period', *Population Studies* 32: 187–94.

Keyfitz, N. (1968), *Introduction to the Mathematics of Population*, Addison-Wesley, Reading, Mass.

Kinsey, A. C., Pomeroy, W., Martin, C., and Gebhard, P. (1953), *Sexual Behavior in the Human Female*, Saunders, Philadelphia.

Lachenbruch, P. A. (1967), 'Frequency and Timing of Intercourse: Its Relation to the Probability of Conception', *Population Studies* 21: 23–31.

Leridon, H. (1973), *Aspects biométriques de la fécondité humaine*, Institut national d'études démographiques cahier no. 65, Presses Universitaires de France, Paris.

—— (1977), *Human Fertility: The Basic Components*, University of Chicago Press, Chicago.

Majumdar, H., and Sheps, M. C. (1970), 'Estimators of a Type I Geometric Distribution from Observations on Conception Times', *Demography* 7: 349–60.

Menken, J. A. (1975a), 'Estimating Fecundability', Ph.D. dissertation, Princeton University, Princeton, NJ.

—— (1975b), 'Biometric Models of Fertility', *Social Forces* 54: 52–65.

—— (1979), 'Seasonal Migration and Seasonal Variation in Fecundability: Effects on Birth Rates and Birth Intervals', *Demography* 16: 103–20.

Potter, R. G., Jr. (1961), 'Length of the Fertile Period', *Milbank Memorial Fund Quarterly* 39: 132–62.

—— and Parker, M. P. (1964), 'Predicting the Time Required to Conceive', *Population Studies* 18: 99–116.

—— and Millman, S. R. (1985), 'Fecundability and the Frequency of Marital Intercourse: A Critique of Nine Models', *Population Studies* 39: 461–70.

—— —— (1986), 'Fecundability and the Frequency of Marital Intercourse: New Models Incorporating the Ageing of Gametes', *Population Studies* 40: 159–70.

Ridley, J. C., Sheps, M. C., Lingner, J. W., and Menken, J. A. (1966), 'On the Apparent Subfecundity of Non-Family Planners, *Social Biology* 16(1): 24–8.

Royston, J. P. (1982), 'Basal Body Temperature, Ovulation and the Risk of Conception, with Special Reference to the Lifetimes of Sperm and Egg', *Biometrics* 38: 397–406.

Schwartz, D., MacDonald, P. D. M., and Heuchel, V. (1980), 'Fecundability, Coital Frequency, and the Viability of Ova', *Population Studies* 34: 397–400.

Sheps, M. C. (1964), 'On the Time Required for Conception', *Population Studies* 18: 85–97.

—— (1965), 'An Analysis of Reproductive Patterns in an American Isolate', *Population Studies* 19: 65–80.

—— and Menken, J. A. (1973), *Mathematical Models of Conception and Birth*, University of Chicago Press, Chicago.

Singh, S. N., Bhattacharya, B. N., and Joshi, P. D. (1973), *Journal of Indian Social and Agricultural Statistics* 25: 91.

Suchindran, C. M. (1972), *Estimators of Parameters in Biological Models of Human Fertility*, Institute of Statistics Mimeo Series no. 849, University of North Carolina at Chapel Hill, Chapel Hill, NC.

—— and Lachenbruch, P. A. (1975), 'Estimates of Fecundability from a Truncated Distribution of Conception Times', *Demography* 12: 291–301.

Tietze, C. (1960), 'Probability of Pregnancy Resulting from a Single Unprotected Coitus', *Fertility and Sterility* 11: 485–8.

Treloar, A. E. (1974), 'Menarche, Menopause and Intervening Fecundability', *Human Biology* 46: 89–107.

—— Boynton, R., Behn, B., and Brown, B. (1967), 'Variation of the Human Menstrual Cycle through Reproductive Life', *International Journal of Fertility* 12: 77–126.

Trussell, J. (1977), 'Natural Fertility: Measurement and Use in Fertility Models', in H. Leridon and J. Menken (eds.), *Natural Fertility*: 50–5, Ordina Editions, Liège, Belgium.

Udry, J. R., and Morris, N. M. (1968), 'Distribution of Coitus in the Menstrual Cycle', *Nature* 220: 593.

Vollman, R. (1977), *The Menstrual Cycle*, Saunders, Philadelphia.

Wood, J. W., and Weinstein, M. (1986), *A Model of Age-Specific Fecundability*, research report no. 86–101, Michigan Population Studies Center, University of Michigan, Ann Arbor, Mi.

13 Age Patterns of Fecundability*

MAXINE WEINSTEIN

JAMES WOOD

CHANG MING-CHENG

Fecundability is defined as the probability that a couple will conceive during a month of exposure to unprotected intercourse, given that both partners are biologically able to conceive (Gini, 1924). Fecundability is of demographic importance because it determines a substantial portion of every birth interval, the so-called fecund waiting time to next conception. In a homogeneous population (that is, a group of couples all with the same fecundability), the relationship is simple: the mean waiting time is the inverse of fecundability. Thus, if fecundability is 0.25, couples can expect to experience an average of four months of regular intercourse before conceiving. As we shall see below, the heterogeneous case is more complicated—and more interesting—but the basic point still holds: fecundability determines the distribution of waiting times to conception.

Fecundability is of special interest because, with lactational anovulation, it is one of the principal points of intersection between the biological and the behavioural determinants of fertility. On the biological side, the female partner must be experiencing regular ovarian cycles and her cycles must produce viable eggs (at least occasionally) for conception to occur, while in the male, sperm must be motile and of sufficient quantity. In addition, since pregnancies cannot be detected until about the time of implantation, the apparent value of fecundability will be influenced by the level of pre-implantation intra-uterine loss, which reflects both maternal and paternal factors. The primary behavioural determinants of fecundability are, obviously, the overall frequency of intercourse and the way in which it is distributed across the cycle.

It is now well established that apparent fecundability varies in a systematic fashion with the age of the female partner, rising rapidly to a peak during the early 20s and then declining slowly to zero at about the time of menopause (Bendel and Hua, 1978). However, there is a remarkable lack of agreement about the cause of these changes, in particular whether they are attributable primarily to changes in coital frequency or to changes in the female's physiological ability to begin and maintain a pregnancy (cf. Bendel and Hua, 1978;

* We gratefully acknowledge the programming assistance of Paul Friday and the comments and suggestions of Patricia Johnson and Jane Menken. This research was supported by NIHCD grant R01-HD-20989.

James, 1979). Researchers affiliated with CECOS (Centres d'Étude et de Conservation des Ovules et du Sperme Humain) in France have claimed that, in women undergoing artificial insemination with donor sperm, the probability of conception declines markedly with age even when coital frequency is held constant (Schwartz and Mayaux, 1982); those familiar with the controversy sparked by this claim (Bongaarts, 1982; Menken *et al.*, 1986) will appreciate how difficult it is to interpret the available empirical evidence on this point.

In this paper, we attempt to partition the decline in fecundability with advancing age into its physiological and behavioural components in order to determine which components are more important in causing the decline. Later in the paper, we focus on one particular aspect of the behavioural component, namely couple-to-couple variation in coital rates, to ascertain how it contributes to the decline and to heterogeneous fecundability in general. In view of the well-known difficulties in measuring fecundability directly (Goldman *et al.*, 1985), we address these questions using a mathematical model of fecundability.

For simplicity, we treat fecundability as if it were a function of the female, but not the male, partner's physiology, although both male and female characteristics will be allowed to affect the behavioural component. This is not to deny that age-related changes in male physiology may be important, but merely to reduce the analysis to manageable proportions. We will also distinguish apparent from total fecundability (or what might be called 'measurable' versus 'real' fecundability) and deal with both in our analyses.[1] Because early embryonic loss affects the former but not the latter, the age pattern of the two need not be the same.

Background

Several features of female reproductive physiology relevant to fecundability are known to vary with age. Most obviously, the probability that a woman is both post-menarcheal and pre-menopausal is highly age-dependent: in US women this probability rises sharply from near zero at age 10 to almost one by age 18 and then declines again after age 37, approaching zero by age 56 (Treloar, 1974). The length of ovarian cycles is also likely to change with age, being longer and more variable at peri-menarcheal and peri-menopausal ages (Lenten *et al.*, 1984a). Cycle length can affect fecundability by determining how many, if any, ovulations and fertile periods occur within a fixed period of exposure. And, of course, cycles vary in quality as well as length. There is a higher probability of a cycle being anovulatory at early ages and, to a lesser

---

[1]   To define these terms more exactly, total fecundability is the probability of a conception during a month of exposure to unprotected intercourse, regardless of the outcome of the pregnancy, while apparent fecundability is the conditional probability of conception during a month of exposure, given that the conceptus survives long enough to be detected by standard clinical techniques.

degree, late ages as well; in addition, cycles during the first few years following menarche tend to be characterized by short or otherwise insufficient luteal-phase increases in progesterone (Lenten *et al.*, 1984*b*). Since luteal sufficiency is a primary consideration in the ability to maintain a pregnancy during its earliest stages, this aspect of ovarian function should influence the level of pre-implantation embryonic loss and, thus apparent (though not total) fecundability.

The level of early embryonic loss is known to increase after maternal age 25, a pattern which appears to have been quite stable over at least the past two generations (Wilcox *et al.*, 1981). This effect of maternal age, which persists even when paternal age and parity are controlled (Selvin and Garfinkel, 1976), partly reflects an increasing risk of chromosomal aberrations caused by meiotic non-disjunction (Jacobs, 1982), although characteristics of the uterus may also be important after age 40 (Stein, 1985). Chromosomal aberrations are known to be particularly common among abortuses of low gestational age (Jacobs, 1982). Some studies have suggested that the probability of intra-uterine loss is also elevated in teenage pregnancies, most likely because of luteal insufficiency (Harlap *et al.*, 1980). On functional grounds, one would expect such losses to be concentrated early in gestation as well.

We have estimated the age pattern of foetal loss from nine studies (as detailed in Wood and Weinstein, 1988) to derive the curve in Fig. 13.1. Since these studies undoubtedly underestimate the overall frequency of foetal loss, we have adjusted the curve upward to yield a probability of early embryonic death in women aged 20–4 equal to 0.3, in conformity with recent studies (Edmonds *et al.*, 1982; Miller *et al.*, 1980; Wilcox *et al.*, 1985; Whittaker *et al.*, 1983) of sub-clinical loss based on assays of human chorionic gonadotrophin (see Chapter 18, below).[2] We assume that the age pattern of sub-clinical loss parallels the curve in Fig. 13.1 (though at a higher level), a reasonable assumption given what we know about the aetiology of early losses.

There are at least three important dimensions of variation in coital behaviour within marriage—wife's age, husband's age, and marital duration—and coital rates have been found to decline with all three (Fig. 13.2 and 13.3). Unfortunately, the three are highly correlated with each other, and it has proved difficult to determine which is most important (Udry and Morris, 1978; Udry, 1980; Jasso, 1985). We shall avoid this issue for the moment and, at least initially, treat these three effects as if they were independent.

When the necessary data are available, they reveal substantial couple-to-couple heterogeneity in coital rates, net of age and duration effects (James, 1981). Heterogeneity in coital behaviour is important insofar as it induces heterogeneity in fecundability. As mentioned earlier, in the case of random

---

[2] Here we adjust Wilcox's preliminary estimate of 0.20–0.25 for the probability of sub-clinical loss upwards slightly to correct for the fact that the assay system with which he works still misses pregnancies that terminate during the first week of gestation, despite being the most sensitive and specific assay currently available.

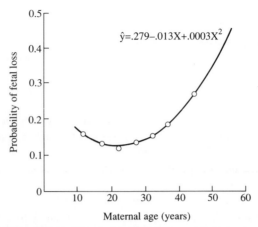

Open circles represent pooled data from nine populations, each adjusted to yield an overall loss across all ages of 150 per 1000 conceptions. The solid curve is a quadratic equation fit to these data by OLS (r^2 = 0.998).

Source: Wood and Weinstein, 1988.

Fig. 13.1   The age pattern of embryonic and foetal loss in women from populations in which induced abortion is not a competing risk

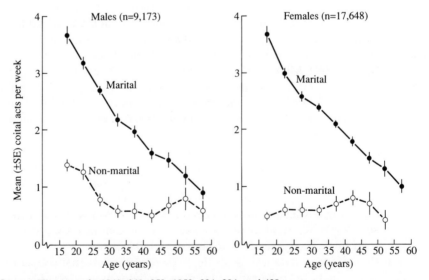

Source: Kinsay *et al*., 1948: 248, 252; 1953: 334, 394, and 439.

Fig. 13.2   Age pattern of marital and non-marital coital frequency, US males and females, 1938–47

homogeneous fecundability, there is a simple inverse relationship between fecundability and the expected waiting time to conception. When couple-to-couple variation (or month-to-month variation in the same couple) is purely

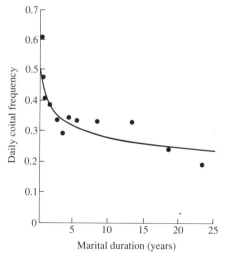

Solid curve represents a linear regression fit by OLS to a log-log plot of these data ($r^2 = 0.838$).

Source: James, 1983, reporting data originally collected by J. R. Udry.

Fig. 13.3 The relationship between daily coital frequency and the duration of marriage in 1430 currently married US women

random, this relationship is not altered, save that now the expected waiting time to conception is the inverse of the mean fecundability rather than some constant value of fecundability (Sheps, 1964). When, however, there exist systematic and persistent differences in fecundability among couples, the entire distribution of waiting times is altered (Fig. 13.4). The distribution becomes more right-skewed, and the mean waiting time to conception may be increased substantially (Sheps, 1964).[3]

The potential importance of heterogeneity in coital rates for the decline in apparent fecundability with age is now obvious. If heterogeneity increases with age—as would occur, for example, if the number of couples who abstain from intercourse increases with age or marital duration—then the mean waiting time to conception may be lengthened accordingly. Any analysis which failed to take this change in heterogeneity into account would yield an apparent, but artefactual, decline in fecundability with age.

Whenever the proper analytical tools have been used to look for it, considerable heterogeneity in fecundability has been detected.[4] As a rule, mean waiting times appear to be between 20 and 90 per cent longer than expected under homogeneous fecundability (Leridon, 1977: 34). To date, however, no one knows how much of this heterogeneity is attributable to variation in coital rates

[3] More precisely, the mean waiting time in the heterogeneous case is equal to the inverse of the harmonic mean fecundability (Sheps, 1964). With heterogeneity, the harmonic mean must be smaller than the arithmetic mean, so the expected waiting time is correspondingly increased.

[4] The one apparent exception to this generalization involves data from Bangladesh analysed by Menken (1975).

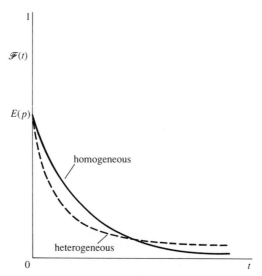

p in the homogeneous case equals $E(p)$ in the heterogeneous case.

Fig. 13.4 An idealized representation of the distribution of conception waits under homogeneous fecundability (solid curve) and heterogeneous fecundability (broken curve)

or whether it increases with age or marital duration. We will explore these issues below.

A Mathematical Model of Fecundability

We give a highly condensed presentation of our model here since the full details appear elsewhere (Wood and Weinstein, 1988). In general, the model accurately embodies our current understanding of ovarian function and coital behaviour. However, we make four simplifying assumptions which may need to be modified in future work: (1) the conditional risk of intercourse (in the sense of Glasser and Lachenbruch, 1968) is constant, so that acts of intercourse are independent in occurrence; (2) the probability of intercourse is unaffected by cycle day, so the suggestion of Hedricks *et al.* (1987) that coital rates increase at mid-cycle is not considered; (3) multiple inseminations on a single day are equivalent to a single insemination on that day;[5] and (4) the probability of conception from a single insemination does not vary across the fertile period (cf. Chapter 12, above).

[5] Although this assumption is unlikely to be strictly true, it appears that the probability of conception does not increase proportionately with the number of inseminations when all occur on the same day; presumably this reflects exhaustion of sperm reserves in the male (Alfred Spira, personal communication).

Let c be the event that conception occurs in one ovarian cycle of exposure to unprotected intercourse. Then

$$\Pr(c) = \sum_{n=0}^{\infty} \Pr(c \mid N = n) \Pr(N = n) \tag{1}$$

where N is the number of acts of unprotected intercourse per cycle. This equation partitions the probability of conception into two independent components, which might be called the 'behavioural' component, $\Pr(N = n)$, and the 'physiological' component, $\Pr(c \mid N = n)$. The physiological component can be further partitioned as

$$\Pr(c \mid N = n) = \sum_{i=1}^{n} \Pr(c \mid I = i) \Pr(I = i \mid a, N = n, o) \Pr(o) \tag{2}$$

where o is the event that a cycle is ovulatory and I is the number of times that intercourse occurs during one fertile period. If acts of intercourse are independent, then

$$\Pr(I = i \mid a, N = n, o) = \binom{n}{i} (F/C)^n (C/F - 1)^{n-i}, i = 0, \ldots, n \tag{3}$$

where F is the length of the fertile period and C is total cycle length (both in days).

The probability of conception can now be found as follows. Let $P_r(i)$ be the conditional probability that exactly r days with at least one act of intercourse occur in the fertile period, given that $I = i$. Then

$$p_r(i) = \binom{F}{r}\binom{i-1}{r-1} \Big/ \binom{F+i-1}{i}, r = 1, \ldots, F. \tag{4}$$

If a is the probability that conception occurs from a single day of intercourse during the fertile period, then

$$\Pr(c \mid I = i) = \sum_{r=1}^{F} [p_r(i)a \sum_{k=1}^{r}(1 - a)^{k-1}], i > 0 \tag{5}$$

and

$$\Pr(c \mid I = 0) = 0.$$

The probability of conception per cycle can be converted into total fecundability (the probability of conception per month) as shown by Wood and Weinstein (1988); apparent fecundability (P_a) is then related to total fecundability (p) as

$$P_a = p (1 - s)/(1 + pgs) \tag{6}$$

where s is the probability of sub-clinical intra-uterine death per conception and g is the duration of the non-susceptible period associated with each sub-clinical death. Assuming that no time is added to the birth interval by sub-clinical loss, which would seem to be one of the defining characteristics of such loss, then $g = 0$ and equation (6) reduces to

$$P_a = p(1 - s). \tag{7}$$

Small values of g, in the order of a week to ten days, have very little impact on the value of p_a.

In the applications to follow, we permit age-related variation in several major physiological determinants of fecundability, including the probability of being both post-menarcheal and pre-menopausal, the probability that a cycle is ovulatory given that the woman is post-menarcheal and pre-menopausal, the expected length of the cycle, and the probability of sub-clinical embryonic loss. All are allowed to vary according to the patterns that have been observed in normal, healthy Western women.[6]

For the first part of the results section, in which we use the model to estimate the relative contributions of behaviour and biology to the decline in fecundability with age, we assume that there is no systematic heterogeneity among couples in coital rates, although there can be purely random variation both among couples and from cycle to cycle for any particular couple. Under this model, the number of acts of intercourse per cycle follows a Poisson distribution, such that

$$\Pr(N = n) = [\exp(-mC) \cdot (mC)^n]/n!, n = 0, 1, 2, \ldots . \tag{8}$$

where m is the mean daily probability of intercourse. In what follows, m will be treated as a function of wife's age, husband's age, and marital duration, either jointly or separately. An alternative specification of the model, which we call 'maximal exposure', assumes that intercourse occurs every single day of the cycle. Under this specification, coital frequency is held constant at its maximum level while physiology is allowed to vary. Thus the maximal exposure model can be thought of as a model of pure fecundity.

Results

The Contributions of Physiology and Coital Behaviour

To assess the relative contributions of female physiology and coital behaviour to the age-related decline in fecundability, we examine how fecundability

[6] For the age pattern of variation in cycle length and in onset of menarche and menopause, we use the data of Treloar *et al.* (1967) and Treloar (1974). Estimates of the probability that a cycle at each age is ovulatory are taken from Vollman (1977). As detailed above, the probability of sub-clinical embryonic loss is set at 0.3 for women aged 20–5 and then allowed to vary at other ages according to the curve in Fig. 13.1. We assume that the length of the fertile period and the conditional probability of conception given a day of intercourse within the fertile period are 4 and 0.6, respectively, following the analysis of Royston (1982). We do not allow these figures to vary with age, for the simple if unsatisfying reason that no one has yet attempted to document such variation.

changes with age (1) when exposure is held constant while physiology varies and (2) when physiology is held constant while exposure varies.

Constant exposure. In controlling coital frequency we consider two cases. First, we assume that intercourse occurs at least once a day throughout the cycle (i.e. maximal exposure); we then set coital frequency at its expected value for a wife aged 25.

The results for the maximal exposure case are shown in Fig. 13.5 (top panel). In the absence of intra-uterine mortality, fecundability under maximal exposure is determined by the effects of cycle length, the probability that a woman is post-menarcheal and pre-menopausal, the probability that a cycle is ovulatory, and the joint effects of the length of the fertile period and the probability that intercourse during the fertile period will result in conception. Because most of these factors change with age, total fecundability varies over the reproductive span even when coital frequency is held constant. Before age 25 and after age 40 total fecundability changes rapidly; between these ages it is remarkably stable. Indeed, total fecundability appears to rise slightly to a peak during the late 30s. At this peak, however, total fecundability is still less than one owing to less-than-certain conception following each insemination and a non-zero probability that a particular month of exposure contains no fertile periods.

Because apparent fecundability is affected by sub-clinical foetal loss, its age pattern under maximal exposure is markedly different from that of total fecundability (Fig. 13.5, top panel). Since the risk of intra-uterine mortality increases after age 25, apparent fecundability begins to decline some 15 years earlier than total fecundability. Over the entire reproductive span, apparent fecundability averages about 54 per cent of total fecundability; between ages 20 and 40, it averages 67 per cent of total fecundability.

Maximal exposure is, of course, an unlikely scenario. We therefore investigate a second case in which we hold the daily probability of intercourse constant over all ages at its expected value for a wife aged 25 (Fig. 13.5, bottom panel).[7] Although the overall shape of the curves is similar to those produced by the maximal exposure model, fecundability is substantially lower, as would be expected. Instead of rising to a peak of 0.96, total fecundability reaches only 0.62. Apparent fecundability reaches a maximum value of 0.42, whereas under the assumption of daily intercourse it attained 0.68.

The important point here is that fecundability varies considerably with age even when coitus is held constant. Apparent fecundability declines after age 25, and this decline is clearly attributable to intra-uterine mortality, not to other aspects of ovarian function. When we remove the effects of intra-uterine mortality, the decline does not begin until about age 40.

Constant physiology. We next investigate the effects of varying coital frequency while holding female physiology constant at the level estimated for wife's age 25. We allow coital frequency to vary by age of wife, age of husband,

---

[7] This expected probability of intercourse is interpolated from the data of Kinsey *et al.* 1953: 394.

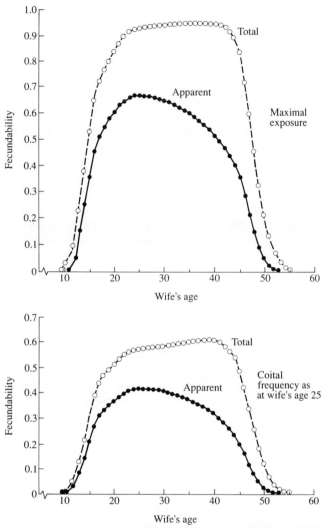

Top panel: maximal exposure or daily intercourse; bottom panel: coital frequency held constant at the level observed in married US women aged 25.

Fig. 13.5   Model predictions of age-specific total and apparent fecundability when coital frequency is held constant and female reproductive physiology is allowed to vary

and duration of marriage as shown in Fig. 13.2 and 13.3. Since we do not have access to data on US couples from which to estimate the joint influence of these three variables, we examine their separate effects here.

The Kinsey data suggest an approximately linear decline in coital frequency with both husband's and wife's ages, while the data for coital frequency relative to marital duration show a sharp decline over the first few years of marriage followed by a slower decline at higher durations. Not surprisingly, the predicted fecundabilities under these coital patterns follow similar curves when physiology is held constant (Fig. 13.6). The effects of wife's and husband's ages are virtually identical: apparent fecundability declines almost linearly with increasing age, from a maximum of just under 0.5 at age 16 to a minimum of about 0.2

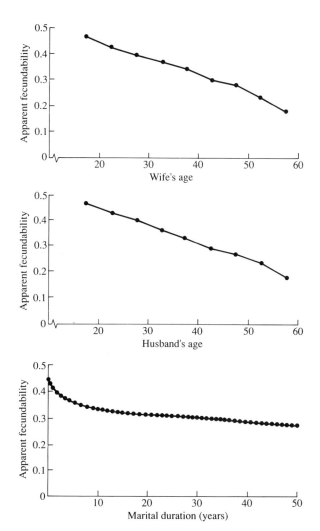

Coital frequency varies by wife's age (top panel), husband's age (middle panel), and duration of marriage (bottom panel).

Fig. 13.6   Model predictions of age-specific apparent fecundability when female reproductive physiology is held constant at wife's age 25 and coital frequency is allowed to vary

at age 56. Duration of marriage (Fig. 13.6, bottom panel) induces a far smaller decline in apparent fecundability, from about 0.45 to slightly less than 0.3. As might be predicted, most of this decline occurs within the first five years of marriage.

In Fig. 13.7*A*, we compare the effects of physiology and coital behaviour directly. While declining coital frequency is clearly of some importance in explaining the drop in fecundability between ages 25 and 35, physiological factors become increasingly important at higher ages. Another way to show the same thing is to calculate the fraction of the decline in apparent fecundability after age 25 attributable to physiological changes in the female (Fig. 13.7*B*). This fraction increases almost linearly between ages 30 and 45, and reaches almost 50 per cent by age 35. Before age 35 most of the decline must be due to changes in coital behaviour, but after that age the decline is primarily biological. And, as we have already noted, it principally reflects the increasing risk of early embryonic loss.

The Effect of Heterogeneity in Coital Behaviour

We turn now to a consideration of couple-to-couple variation in coital rates as a possible source of heterogeneity in apparent fecundability. In order to invest-igate the effects of such variation, we consider three distinct cases. The first case is that of constant intercourse, in which each cycle of exposure contains exactly the mean number of acts of intercourse per cycle. That is,

$$\Pr(N = n) = \begin{cases} 1, \text{if } n = \text{mean no. acts/cycle} \\ 0, \text{otherwise.} \end{cases} \tag{9}$$

The second case is that of Poisson variation in the number of acts of intercourse per cycle, which was described in equation (8). This case can be thought of as purely random variation in coitus, either among couples or from month to month for any single couple. Finally, we consider the case of systematic heterogeneity or 'greater than Poisson variation' in coital rates. For this case, we either use an empirical distribution of coital rates where appropriate or, following the suggestion of James (1981), assume that coitus follows a negative binomial distribution:

$$\Pr(N = n) = \binom{k+n-1}{k-1} (M/K)^n (1 + M/K)^{-(K+n)}, n = 0,1,2, \ldots \tag{10}$$

where M and K are parameters to be estimated by the method of moments. This distribution can arise if our population of couples consists of several subgroups, within which Poisson variation holds, but among which mean coital rates differ (Johnson and Kotz, 1969: 124–5).[8] As James (1981) has pointed out, and as we shall show below, equation (10) gives a good fit to real data on coital rates.

---

[8] More precisely, the negative binomial model assumes that the Poisson parameter mC in equation (8) varies among subgroups as a gamma random variable.

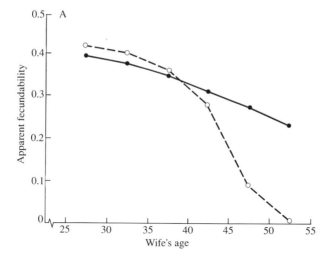

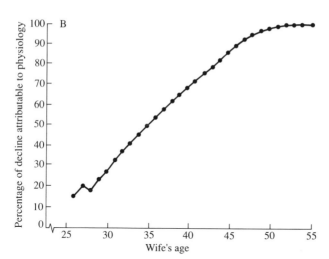

In *A* reproductive physiology is held constant at wife's age 25 while coitus varies by wife's age (solid line), and coitus is held constant at wife's age 25 while reproductive physiology varies by wife's age (broken line). While in *B* the fraction of the age-related decline in apparent fecundability after age 25 is attributable to changes in female reproductive physiology.

Fig. 13.7   A comparison of two sets of model predictions of age-specific apparent fecundability and the fraction of age-related decline in apparent fecundability attributable to changes in female reproductive physiology

As we would expect on theoretical grounds (Sheps, 1964), constant intercourse and Poisson variation yield virtually identical results—identical, in fact, to the second decimal place.[9] It is only the introduction of systematic heterogeneity that makes a difference.

To examine this effect, we first make use of empirical data on variation in coital frequency. These data were collected in Taiwan at the beginning of 1986 in an island-wide survey of 4312 ever-married women between ages 20 and 50. Included in the questionnaire was a series of self-administered questions,[10] one of which asked that the respondent report the number of times she and her husband had had sexual intercourse during the last month. Fewer than 2 per cent of the respondents refused to answer this question. In the analyses to follow, we use a subset of 4090 women currently married for the first time, for whom age could be determined to the nearest year. Table 13.1 gives the mean and variance of reported monthly coital frequencies for these women by five-year age-groups.

We use the Taiwan data to compare three levels of variation in coital behaviour: (1) one in which the number of acts of intercourse is constant each month and equal to the observed mean for each age; (2) one in which the number of acts varies as a Poisson random variable with parameter equal to the observed mean; and (3) one in which we use the observed distributions of coital frequency by five-year age-groups and marital duration category at each age. Since the observed variances in number of acts are consistently greater than the observed means, the third situation represents one of systematic heterogeneity among couples.

To compare these three levels of variability, we move from estimates of

TABLE 13.1. *Reported coital frequency in the last month, women aged 20–49 in current first marriages, Taiwan, 1986*

Age	Mean	Variance	N
20–24	5.08	11.29	435
25–29	4.52	8.47	898
30–34	4.05	6.60	1000
35–39	3.57	5.76	766
40–44	2.76	3.03	537
45–49	2.23	3.24	454

[9] In these applications, we assumed that the frequency of intercourse was determined primarily by marital duration, following the pattern in Fig. 13.3. At each age, the expected distribution of marital durations was found using Rodriguez and Trussell's (1980) reparameterization of the Coale–McNeil marriage model, with a mean age at first marriage equal to 23 and a variance of 43.

[10] We have no direct way of estimating the reliability of the responses, although about 37 per cent of the respondents were illiterate and were asked the questions by the interviewer. Controlling for age, the reported distributions of coital frequencies for these women were quite similar to those for women who completed the forms for themselves.

fecundability itself to the implied estimates of waiting times to conception. For the first two levels, the waiting time is simply the reciprocal of expected fecundability. For the third, heterogeneous level, it is the weighted average of the reciprocal of fecundability for each coital frequency and marital duration and age category.

The expected waiting times to a reported conception—that is, the waiting times associated with apparent fecundability—are shown in Table 13.2 for all three levels of variation.[11] A comparison of the homogeneous and heterogeneous cases, which should be most dissimilar, reveals differences in expected waiting times that do not exceed two months. In the Taiwan case, then, the observed heterogeneity in coital behaviour induces, at most, about a 15 per cent increase in the expected waiting time to conception, only a fraction of the increase reported in most empirical studies of conception waits.

TABLE 13.2. *Expected waiting times to conception by age under three assumptions about variability in coital rates*

Wife's age	Expected waiting time (months)		
	Constant	Poisson	Heterogeneous
20–24	4.28	4.39	4.58
25–29	4.61	4.51	4.66
30–34	4.79	4.96	5.08
35–39	5.57	5.84	5.95
40–44	8.47	9.48	9.72
45–49	32.34	32.37	34.21

These results suggest an interesting question: How much variation in coital rates is needed in order to generate the amount of heterogeneity that has actually been observed in waiting times to conception, assuming that there is no other source of variation? We examine two cases in order to explore this question.

First, we take the Taiwan example and increase the variance in coital rates while maintaining the observed mean. But of course we need the entire $\Pr(N = n)$ distribution for our model, not just the mean and variance. Here we resort to the negative binomial model given by equation (10), a model which provides a good fit to the Taiwan data (Fig. 13.8) and which is fully specified by two parameters, the mean and variance. In the second example, we use data on US couples collected as part of the 1974 Family Planning Evaluation Project and reported by Udry *et al.* (1982). Here, too, we apply the negative binomial model on the assumption that it should provide a good fit to these data. Unfortunately, we do not have the full set of data on US couples to test the fit of

[11] The differences between the constant and Poisson times are attributable to rounding: for the constant application, integral values of coital frequency must be used.

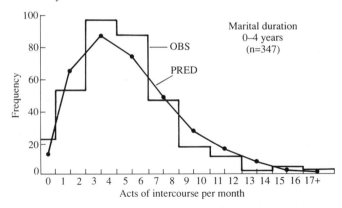

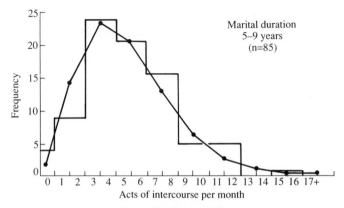

The top panel shows women with marital duration 0–4 years; goodness of fit test: log-likelihood ratio test statistic = 22.7, d.f. = 6, $P < 0.01$. The bottom panel shows women with marital duration 5–9 years; goodness of fit test: log-likelihood ratio test statistic = 5.9, d.f. = 4, $0.5 < p < 0.1$.

Fig. 13.8   Fit of the negative binomial distribution to coital data reported by Taiwanese women aged 20–4

the model, but the model does well when applied to other data on US couples (James, 1981). For both the Taiwan and US cases, we confine our attention to wives aged 20–4, and in the Taiwan case we use only marital durations 0–4 and 5–9 years.

The results of these applications are shown in Table 13.3. For Taiwan, with a mean monthly coital rate at age 20–4 of 5.1, doubling the variance in coital frequency increases the expected waiting time to conception by a little more than one-fourth, from about 4.5 to 5.7 months. In the United States, with a higher mean coital rate of 11.6, a 50 per cent increase in the variance raises the waiting time by just under one-quarter. In other words, quite massive increases in couple-to-couple variation in coital rates generate levels of heterogeneity in the associated waiting times that are still small compared with the observed

TABLE 13.3. *Expected waiting times to conception under varying assumptions about heterogeneity in coital frequency, women aged 20–4*

Population	Ratio of simulated to observed variance	Waiting time (months)
Taiwan 1986	1.0	4.47
	1.5	4.86
	2.0	5.68
United States 1974	0.5	2.59
	1.0	2.84
	1.5	3.52

levels of heterogeneity. From this point of view, variation in coital behaviour appears unlikely to be an important source of heterogeneous fecundability within populations. It is unlikely to contribute much to the age-related decline in fecundability.

Discussion

According to our analyses, variation in coital behaviour has surprisingly little impact on the age pattern of fecundability, especially after age 35. This conclusion is, of course, heavily model-dependent. If our model is incorrect, the conclusion is suspect. However, we believe the model is a good one that captures the major features of the physiological and behavioural determinants of fecundability. There is no indication that our conclusion is an artefact of any simplifying assumptions.

We conclude, then, that the decline in fecundability after age 25 is determined, at least in part, by declining female fecundity; after age 35, declining fecundity plays the dominant role. Between ages 25 and 40, moreover, the decline in fecundity is caused virtually exclusively by an increasing risk of early embryonic loss, not by an inability to conceive.

We further conclude that heterogeneity in coital rates is unlikely to be an important cause of heterogeneous fecundability. It should be stressed that fecundability appears to be markedly heterogeneous in most empirical studies. In the light of our analyses, we suggest that this heterogeneity also has a physiological source. Sensitivity tests of our model indicate that differences among women in the level of intra-uterine mortality and in the incidence of anovulatory cycles, as well as in total cycle length, are potentially important sources of this heterogeneity (Wood and Weinstein, 1988).

Lest anyone accuse us of suggesting that sex is unimportant, we stress that our results pertain strictly to patterns of variation within particular populations. Differences in average rates of intercourse on the order of those observed between human populations—Taiwan and the United States, for example—may have a substantial demographic impact. Such inter-population differences have not been addressed in this paper.

References

Bendel, J.-P., and Hua, C. (1978), 'An Estimate of the Natural Fecundability Ratio Curve', *Social Biology* 25: 210–27.

Bongaarts, J. (1982), 'Infertility after Age 30: A False Alarm', *Family Planning Perspectives* 14: 75–8.

Edmonds, D. K., Lindsay K. S., Miller, J. F., Williamson, E., and Wood, P. J. (1982), 'Early Embryonic Mortality in Women', *Fertility and Sterility* 38: 447–53.

Gini, C. (1924), 'Premières recherches sur la fécondabilité de la femme', *Proceedings of the International Mathematical Congress* ii: 880–92.

Glasser, J. H., and Lachenbruch, P. A. (1968), 'Observations on the Relationship Between Frequency and Timing of Intercourse and the Probability of Conception', *Population Studies* 22: 399–407.

Goldman, N., Westoff, C. F., and Paul, L. E. (1985), 'Estimation of Fecundability from Survey Data', *Studies of Family Planning* 16: 252–9.

Harlap, S., Shiona, P. H., and Ramcharan, S. (1980), 'A Life Table of Spontaneous Abortions and the Effects of Age, Parity, and other Variables', in I. H. Porter and E. B. Hook (eds.), *Human Embryonic and Fetal Death*, Academic Press New York: 145–58.

Hedricks, C., Piccinino, L. J., Udry, J. R., and Chimbira, T. H. K. (1987), 'Peak Coital Rate Coincides with Onset of Luteinizing Hormone Surge', *Fertility and Sterility* 48: 234–8.

Jacobs, P. A. (1982), 'Pregnancy Losses and Birth Defects', in C. R. Austin and R. V. Short (eds.), *Embryonic and Fetal Development*, Cambridge University Press, Cambridge: 289–98.

James, W. H. (1979), 'The Causes of the Decline in Fecundability with Age', *Social Biology* 26: 330–4.

—— (1981), 'Distributions of Coital Rates and of Fecundability', *Social Biology* 28: 334–41.

—— (1983), 'Decline in Coital Rates with Spouses' Ages and Duration of Marriage', *Journal of Biosocial Science* 15: 83–7.

Jasso, G. (1985), 'Marital Coital Frequency and the Passage of Time: Estimating the Separate Effects of Spouses' Ages and Marital Duration, Birth and Marriage Cohorts, and Period Influences', *American Sociological Review* 50: 224–41.

Johnson, N. L., and Kotz, S. (1969), *Distributions in Statistics*, i. *Discrete Distributions*, Wiley, New York.

Kinsey, A. C., Pomeroy, W. B., and Martin, C. E. (1948), *Sexual Behavior in the Human Male*, Saunders, Philadelphia, Pa.

—— —— —— and Gebhard, P. H. (1953), *Sexual Behavior in the Human Female*, Saunders, Philadelphia, Pa.

Lenten, E. A., Landgren, B.-M., Sexton, L., and Harper, R. (1984a), 'Normal Variation in the Length of the Follicular Phase of the Menstrual Cycle: Effect of Chronological Age', *British Journal of Obstetrics Gynaecology* 91: 681–5.

—— Landgren, B.-M., and Sexton, L. (1984*b*), 'Normal Variation in the Length of the Luteal Phase of the Menstrual Cycle: Identification of the Short Luteal Phase', *British Journal of Obstetrics Gynaecology* 91: 685–9.

Leridon, H. (1977), *Human Fertility: The Basic Components*, University of Chicago Press, Chicago.

Menken, J. (1975), 'Estimating Fecundability', Ph.D. dissertation, Princeton University, Princeton, NJ.

—— Trussell, J., and Larsen, U. (1986), 'Age and Infertility', *Science* 233: 1389–94.

Miller, J. F., Williamson, E., Glue, J., Gordon, Y. B., Grudzinskas, J. G., and Sykes, A. (1980), 'Fetal Loss After Implantation: A Prospective Study', *Lancet* 2: 554–6.

Rodriguez, G., and Trussell, J. (1980), 'Maximum Likelihood Estimation of the Parameters of Coale's Model Nuptiality Schedule from Survey Data', *World Fertility Survey (WFS) Technical Bulletin*, no. 7, World Fertility Survey, London.

Royston, J. P. (1982), 'Basal Body Temperature, Ovulation and the Risk of Conception, with Special Reference to the Lifetimes of Sperm and Egg', *Biometrics* 38: 397–406.

Schwartz, D., and Mayaux, M. J. (1982), 'Female Fecundity as a Function of Age', *New England Journal of Medicine* 307: 404–8.

Selvin, S., and Garfinkel, J. (1976), 'Paternal Age, Maternal Age, and Birth Order and Risk of a Fetal Loss', *Human Biology* 48: 223–30.

Sheps, M. C. (1964), 'On the Time Required for Conception', *Population Studies* 18: 85–97.

Stein, Z. A. (1985), 'A Woman's Age: Childbearing and Child Rearing', *American Journal of Epidemiology* 121: 327–342.

Treloar, A. E. (1974), 'Menarche, Menopause and Intervening Fecundability', *Human Biology* 46: 89–107.

—— Boynton, R. E., Behn, B. G., and Brown, B. W. (1967), 'Variation of the Human Menstrual Cycle through Reproductive Life', *International Journal of Fertility* 12: 77–126.

Udry, J. R. (1980), 'Changes in the Frequency of Marital Intercourse from Panel Data', *Archives of Sexual Behaviour* 9: 319–25.

—— Morris, N. M. (1978), 'Relative Contributions of Male and Female Age to the Frequency of Marital Intercourse', *Social Biology* 25: 128–34.

—— Deven, F. R., and Coleman, S. J. (1982), 'A Cross-National Comparison of the Relative Influence of Male and Female Age on the Frequency of Marital Intercourse', *Journal of Biosocial Science* 14: 1–6.

Vollman, R. F. (1977), *The Menstrual Cycle*, W. B. Saunders, Philadelphia, Pa.

Whittaker, P. G., Taylor, A., and Lind, T. (1983), 'Unsuspected Pregnancy Loss in Healthy Women', *Lancet* 1: 1126–7.

Wilcox, A. J., Treloar, A. E., and Sandler, D. P. (1981), 'Spontaneous Abortion over Time: Comparing Occurrence in Two Cohorts of Women a Generation Apart', *American Journal of Epidemiology* 114: 548–53.

—— Weinberg, C. R., Wehmann, R. E., Armstrong, E. G., Canfield, R. E., and Nisula, B. C. (1985), 'Measuring Early Pregnancy Loss: Laboratory and Field Methods', *Fertility and Sterility* 44: 366–74.

Wood, J. W., and Weinstein, M. (1988), 'A Model of Age-specific Fecundability', *Population Studies* 42: 85–113.

Part V

Infertility and Assisted Conception

14 Artificial Insemination with Frozen Donor Semen: A Model to Appreciate Human Fecundity

CECOS FÉDÉRATION

JAQUES LANSAC

Since Georges David founded the first sperm-bank in Paris in 1973, a network of twenty sperm-banks called CECOS (Centre for the Study and Preservation of Eggs and Sperm) has been established in France to serve the entire country.

Structure, Functions, and Policy of CECOS

The CECOS centres are located in university hospitals, but they do not fall under hospital jurisdiction. Rather, they are managed by an administrative board that includes representatives from each hospital's administration, social workers, and various related medical disciplines, such as gynaecology, genetics, endocrinology, bacteriology, and epidemiology.

CECOS has three functions: (1) the preservation of a husband's semen for artificial insemination (AIH) or *in vitro* fertilization (IVF); (2) the preservation of semen for artificial insemination by a donor (AID); and (3) the cryopreservation of embryos and oocytes. The research programme focuses on the problems of cryopreservation, donor recruitment, donor semen, requests for artificial insemination, data collection, and the use of these findings to improve the efficacy of our procedures.

Semen Preservation: The 'Nouvelle Politique' of CECOS

CECOS policy states that semen donation is an anonymous gift for which no payment is received, as is the case of organ donation. Only married men under the age of 55, who have one or more normal children and whose spouse consents, are accepted as donors. These requirements offer several advantages:

1. They provide an additional guarantee of donor fertility and lower the risk of hereditary disease.

2. The men respond honestly when their personal and family medical histories are collected. This information is collected during their initial visit, when they also undergo a physical examination.
3. As a population, these men have a low risk of carrying the AIDS virus. Since 1985, none of the more than 3000 semen donors have had a positive HIV serology. An additional 3250 women were inseminated with frozen sperm before 1985; of those studied, none has had a positive HIV serology.

CECOS centres collect only a limited number of ejaculates—usually five or six—from a single donor over about a month's time. This policy limits the number of children born to the same donor to five, thus reducing the risk of consanguinity (David and Price, 1980; David, 1984).

Donor Selection

Donor selection is necessary to eliminate: (1) infertile and subfertile donors; (2) donors carrying an infectious disease who might present a risk to the recipient; and (3) donors carrying a hereditary disease who might present a risk to any child that is conceived. Fatherhood may be regarded as a guarantee of the donor's fertility. The ultimate criterion, however, is semen analysis, especially post-thaw mobility.

Bacteriological analysis is used to minimize the risk of transmitting an infectious disease. This includes a semen culture to check for the presence of pathogenic bacteria, particularly *Escheria coli* and *Neisseria gonorrhoeae*, *Chlamydia trachomatis*, and viruses such as herpes and hepatitis. Since August 1985, the law has also mandated a serology for HIV.

The possibility of transmitting hereditary diseases can be eliminated by genetically screening donors, both with karyotypes and family and personal histories. Obviously, there has to be some threshold set: if every carrier of a recessive gene was rejected and if all heterozygotes could be detected, there would be no qualified donors left.

Therefore, the CECOS system classifies prospective donors into three categories: (1) rejected; (2) accepted without restriction; and (3) accepted with a specific risk factor. The family or personal histories of donors in the last group have disclosed some disorder of genetic origin, such as allergy. Before using semen from this kind of donor, the family and personal histories of the recipient are checked to ensure that they do not reveal the same disorder.

Indications for AID

Only couples are accepted; unmarried women and homosexual couples are refused. The main reason for using AID is the infertility of the husband. In 60 per cent of all cases the husband suffers from irreversible azoospermy, and his sterility is clear. When the semen is not azoospermic but only of poor quality, it is more difficult to draw a definite conclusion about the husband's sterility. In such cases, the duration of infertility, the woman's age, and the failure of artificial insemination by the husband and of *in vitro* fertilization attempts are also considered. The couple's evaluation also includes an interview with a psychiatrist working with the centre. The purpose of this interview is not to pass judgement on the motivation for the couple's request, but rather to reveal cases of psychological pathology. Fewer than 5 per cent of all requests for AID are refused. The reasons for these refusals are unproven male sterility, female infertility, and psychological disorders.

The Insemination Procedure

Gynaecologists working for CECOS, for the hospital, or in private practice carry out the inseminations. It is essential to determine the optimal day for conception. The simplest way to do this is to examine the basal body temperature curve, along with cervical dilatation, the abundance of cervical mucus, and spinnbarkheit.

When it is time to perform the insemination, the straw containing the frozen sample is removed from the liquid nitrogen and allowed to thaw for a few minutes at 37.5 °C. After cutting off one end of the straw, it is placed in an insemination device with which the semen can be slowly injected directly into the cervix. Only one sample per cycle is used during the first two months of AID.

Collection and Analysis of Data on AID

CECOS has centralized all information on donors, requesting couples, inseminations, the occurrence and evolution of conceptions, and the condition of children at birth. The patients have been classified in one of four categories, as described by Schwartz and Mayaux (1980):

1. Lost to follow-up. Women for whom no data has been received since the last insemination cycle, so final results are not known.
2. Success. Women who conceived, based on 21 days of hyperthermia, an elevation of the hCG rate, or clinical or echographical signs of pregnancy.
3. Drop-out. Women who have withdrawn from the AID programme.
4. Open case. Women whose next treatment cycle has not yet taken place. If more than one year has elapsed since the last treatment cycle, the patient is classified in the drop-out category.

The following rates have been calculated:

1. The rates of successes, open cases, and drop-outs per cycle.
2. Mean success and drop-out rates for all cycles.
3. Cumulative success rates calculated by the life-table method. The effective success rate takes drop-outs into account, while the theoretical success rate ignores them.

Fig. 14.1 displays the results of the French CECOS Fédération in 1986. There were 1938 pregnancies among the 2872 women treated with AID. It is clear that the success rate decreases each month, as the most fertile women become pregnant in the first cycles. The women who are not pregnant after two years of AID have a very low success rate.

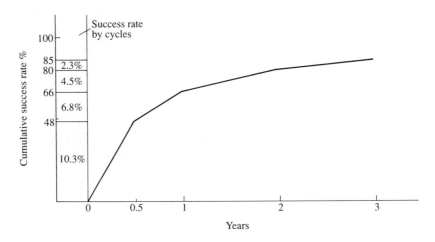

There were 1938 pregnancies.

Source: French CECOS Fédération, 1986.

Fig. 14.1   Cumulative success rate (conceptions/cycle) for 2872 women undergoing AID

AID: A Model to Appreciate Human Fecundity

France has a population of 55 million. Since 1980 requests for AID have been stable, running at about 3000 annually in the CECOS system. Each year 2000 pregnancies are conceived with frozen donor semen and 800 new donors are selected. The CECOS system for the collection and analysis of data has allowed us to determine the best day for conception, the importance of various cervical factors, female fecundity both as a function of women's age and as a function of semen characteristics, and the value of *in vitro* fertilization as a way to speed conception.

The 'Best' Day for Conception

It is critical to know which cycle day is 'best' for conception. The CECOS French Fédération AID protocol recommends a simple intra-cervical insemination using one dose of frozen semen and no accompanying therapy during the first two menstrual cycles. Among 821 cycles recorded for 529 women, the pregnancy rate per cycle was 12 per cent (Schwartz *et al.*, 1979). Cycle days

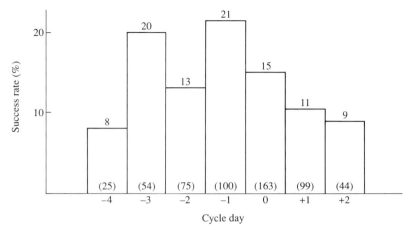

Numbers of inseminations are shown in parentheses.

Source: Schwartz *et al*., 1979.

Fig. 14.2   AID success rate according to cycle day among 821 cycles with a single insemination

were numbered with respect to the last day of hypothermia. The highest success rates were obtained on days −1 (21 per cent) and −3 (20 per cent), although day zero had the highest frequency of insemination (Fig. 14.2).

These results may not be considered significant as the numbers are low. They are worth mentioning, however, in comparison with the results published by Barrett and Marshall (1969), who used a different approach. They studied the results of natural insemination in a series of 241 couples, for whom they obtained a total of 1898 temperature curves together with the dates of intercourse. In most cycles several acts of intercourse occurred during the fertile period, but the authors were able to estimate the probability of fertilization for each cycle day by using a mathematical model that did not specify which act of intercourse was responsible for conception. Barrett and Marshall's results are reproduced in Fig. 14.3 together with the present results. The similarities are striking.

Value of the Cervical Factors

Three factors—dilatation of the cervix, abundance of cervical mucus, and spinnbarkheit—were studied in the same series of 821 AID cycles described above. Conception rates were 14 per cent when the cervix was dilated (vs. 8 per cent, $p < 0.05$); 15 per cent when there was abundant mucus (vs. 6 per cent), and 18 per cent when spinnbarkheit was 10 cm (vs. 9 per cent) (Table 14.1) (Schwartz *et al*., 1979). In our study, the relatively high success rate on day −3 appeared to be particularly marked for cases with little cervical mucus (24 per

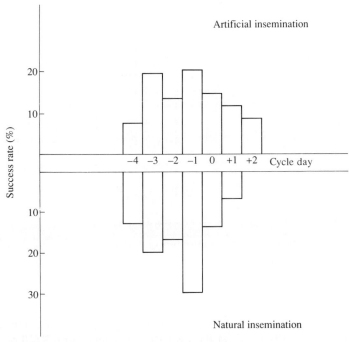

Sources: Barrett and Marshall, 1969; Schwartz *et al.*, 1979.

Fig. 14.3   Success rate according to cycle day, with artificial and natural insemination

TABLE 14.1. *AID success rate by cervical score (%),*
among 821 cycles with a single insemination

	No		Yes		*p<*
Cervix dilated	8	(227)	14	(508)	0.05
Abundant cervical mucus	6	(243)	15	(533)	0.001
Spinnbarkheit >10	9	(470)	18	(258)	0.001

Note: Numbers of inseminations (or cycles) are shown in parentheses
Source: Schwartz *et al.*, 1979.

cent vs. 15 per cent with abundant mucus). This result presents some difficulties in interpretation.

Female Fecundity as a Function of Semen Characteristics

There are three possible approaches to studying female fecundity as a function of semen characteristics. We can either look at the success rate as a function of the husband's semen, or at the success rate as a function of the characteristics of the frozen semen used for AID, or at the success rate as a function of previous AID cycles.

Success rate as a function of husband's semen. The success rate for AID varies with the properties of the husband's semen in an unexpected way (see Table 14.2). The success rate is significantly higher (10 per cent, $p < 0.02$) for women whose husbands are azoospermic than for women whose husbands are severely oligospermic but retain the ability, although extremely reduced, to fertilize their wives (Emperaire *et al.*, 1981). The success rate for this latter group is 7.2 per cent per cycle.

TABLE 14.2. *AID success rate according to quality of husband's semen*

Husband's semen	Conception rate per cycle (%) (Number of inseminations or cycles)
Azoospermia	10.1
(N = 95)	(N = 626)
Severe oligospermia	7.2
(N = 45)	(N = 348)
	$p < 0.07$

Source: Emperaire *et al.*, 1981.

Hyperfertile women married to oligospermic men may become pregnant after exposure to their husbands' semen, with the likelihood of pregnancy increasing with the duration of exposure. Thus, they may never need to apply for AID. The loss of these hyperfertile women skews the fertility of the remaining group of women with oligospermic husbands who do undergo AID. This, of course, does not hold true for women married to azoospermic men: the fertility of these women exactly reflects that of the general population. Thus, a difference in the mean fertility of the two groups of women probably accounts for the difference in their success rates.

Success rate as a function of frozen semen characteristics. This study examined 1438 ejaculates from 342 donors and 15 364 insemination cycles (David *et al.*, 1980; Mayaux *et al.*, 1985). The sperm count (m), volume (v), pre-freeze mobility, and post-thaw mobility were evaluated for each ejaculate; the morphology of the first ejaculate of each donor was also evaluated.

The success rate increased steadily with the sperm count, pre-freeze mobility, and post-thaw mobility (Table 14.3). Success rates were stable for volumes up to 5.5 ml and for proportions of abnormal forms up to 40 per cent. After that, success rates decreased. Of all the abnormal sperm forms considered, only the microcephalics and those with irregular heads were found to be linked to the success rate. This is not surprising, since it is likely that these anomalies affect the mobility of the spermatozoa. They are associated with ultra-structural changes of the flagella seen in electron microscopy.

TABLE 14.3. *Mean success rates for AID according to characteristics of donor semen*

Sperm count		Pre-freeze mobility		Post-thaw mobility	
$n10^6$ml	% success rate by cycles	$m0$ %	% success rate by cycles	$m1$ %	% success rate by cycles
<100	8.1	<70	6.5	<45	7.1
100–50	9.6	70–5	9.0	45–50	8.1
150–200	10.8	80–5	11.9	55–60	12.4
>200	11.3	>85	16.4	>60	18.1

Note: The sample includes 1438 ejaculates used in 15 364 cycles.
n = Sperm count; m = percentage of motile sperm.

Source: Mayaux *et al.*, 1985.

Because most of the characteristics studied were correlated, a multiple stepwise regression was carried out to determine the relative importance of each variable. The most predictive variable was post-thaw mobility, followed by percentage of microcephalics. The other variables contribute no further information, especially at a given post-thaw mobility. The pre-freeze mobility and, consequently, the loss in mobility have no influence on the success rate.

It is difficult to know to what extent these results reflect the conditions of natural reproduction. However, AID with frozen semen provides the best means of separating male and female factors, since a single donor inseminates several women. At the same time, AID offers a unique opportunity to test the fecundity of a specific sample with known characteristics, an aspect not to be neglected when considering the intra-individual variability of different ejaculates from the same man. In conclusion, we propose that mobility can be regarded as the most useful predictor of male fertility.

Success rate as a function of previous AID cycles.   (David and Price, 1980; David *et al.*, 1980; David, 1984). During the first six cycles, the mean success rate is 10.3 per cent, depending partly on chance and partly on factors already discussed. Later, the success rate decreases; after 24 cycles, it is 2.3 per cent per cycle (Table 14.1). The success rate was considerably lower for women inseminated for a first pregnancy than for women seeking a second or third pregnancy (Table 14.4) (CECOS Fédération and LeLannou, 1987). This suggests that the former group includes some hypofertile women.

Female Fecundity as a Function of Age

A decrease in female fecundity beyond a certain age is generally acknowledged, but supporting data on natural reproduction are scarce. The study group included 2193 women who received AID in 11 CECOS centres between 1973 and 1980 and who had azoospermic husbands (CECOS Fédération *et al.*, 1982). They were divided into four age-groups: 25 and younger (371 women),

TABLE 14.4. *AID success rates for first and succeeding pregnancies*

	Number of cycles	Number of pregnancies	Success rate by cycles (%)
First pregnancy			
1980	5255	511	9.8
1986	17 987	1296	7.2
Second and third pregnancies			
1980	509	82	16.3
1986	5731	642	11.2

Note: The authors of the studies were Georges David in 1980 and the CECOS Fédération in 1986.

Source: CECOS Fédération and LeLannou, 1987.

26–30 (1079 women), 31–5 (599 women), and 36 and older (144 women). The curve of the cumulative success rate was similar for the two youngest age groups. However, this curve showed a significant decrease in the cumulative success rate for women in the 31–5 age-group (53.6 per cent after twelve cycles vs. 73 per cent for the younger women). Similar decreases with age were observed for the mean conception rate per cycle (6.5 per cent vs. 11 per cent for the younger group) (Table 14.5).

Any attempt to study female fecundity as a function of age must face two major problems. First, the effect of a woman's age must be separated from associated variables such as coital pattern and husband's age. Second, the age of the woman may itself introduce a kind of selection bias. For AID, this is especially true for husbands who have reduced fertility but are not sterile (as has been discussed above). This is why only women with azoospermic husbands undergoing AID were studied. The characteristics of the donors and the number of inseminations per cycle were similar for all age-groups.

Is *in vitro* Fertilization a Faster Way to Become Pregnant?

AID frequently fails: after one year of treatment, 44 per cent of women are still not pregnant. The success rate decreases slowly over time, declining to just 2.3

TABLE 14.5. *AID success rates by age of woman among 2193 nulliparous women with azoospermic husbands*

Age (N)	<25 (371)	26–30 (1079)	31–5 (599)	>35 (144)
Mean success rate per cycle (%)	11.0	10.5	9.1	6.5
Cumulative success rate after 12 cycles (%)	73.0	74.1	61.5	53.6

Source: CECOS Fédération *et al.*, 1982.

per cent during the third year of treatment. Success rates are highest for women who are less than 35 years old, are married to azoospermic husbands, and have no fertility problems.

Usually, after six to 12 unsuccessful AID treatment cycles, an evaluation is carried out to discover the reason for the failure. This includes an examination of the cervical mucus and the pattern of ovulation, as well as a celioscopy to look for endometriosis, peritoneal adhesions, or LUF (luteinized unruptured follicle) syndrome. When the hysterography or the celioscopy shows tubal lesions or if the woman is more than 35 years old and dysovulating, we recommend *in vitro* fertilization with donor semen (IVF-D).

Table 14.6 lists the results of IVF-D in four groups of women; the CECOS Fédération group has the largest series in France (de Mouzon *et al.*, 1987). The pregnancy rate by puncture is 15.6 per cent, while the success rate by replacement is 24.7 per cent. Only 4.4 straws are needed to obtain a pregnancy, as compared to 24 for AID. With the same ejaculate, the pregnancy rate is 33.3 per cent after puncture with the IVF-D technique vs. 9.2 per cent per AID treatment cycle.

TABLE 14.6. *Results of* in vitro *fertilization using donor semen*

Author	Number of punctures	Number of oocytes	Pregnancy rate by puncture	Pregnancy rate by replacement
Mahadevan and Trounson 1984 (frozen semen)	29	61	10.3	13.6
Mahadevan and Trounson 1984 (fresh semen)	76	138	8.0	12.2
COHEN et al., 1985	55	211	31.0	31.5
CECOS 1986	632	2065	15.6	24.7

It is not surprising that IVF-D has better results than IVF with oligoastheno-spermic semen, because the donor is fertile. However, the pregnancy rate for IVF-D is also better than that for IVF with tubal pathology (15.6 per cent vs. 11.1 per cent obtained by FIVNAT (IVF with husband's sperm) in 1986) (de Mouzon *et al.*, 1987). The frozen semen technique does not reduce the success rate as Cohen *et al.* (1985) found. The pregnancy rate by AID cycle was 8.1 per cent in 1986 in the CECOS Fédération. During the same year, the pregnancy rate by puncture in IVF-D was 15.6 per cent. Possible explanations for the difference include the use of better semen (post-thaw mobility 60) and better synchronization in IVF. Mattei (1987) studied AID and IVF-D pregnancy rates using the same ejaculates (Table 14.7). Not only are the results better in IVF-D (33.3 per cent vs. 9.2 per cent for AID), the technique also requires less semen to produce a pregnancy (4 straws vs. 24.4 for AID).

When a woman suffers from tubal infertility and her husband's fertility is also impaired, IVF-D is the only solution. If the woman's tubes are normal,

TABLE 14.7. *Pregnancy rates after IVF-D and AID using the same ejaculates*

	Number of punctures	Number of semen samples	Number of pregnancies	Pregnancy rate by puncture	Number of semen samples per pregnancy
IVF-D	105	155	35	33.3	4.4
AID	108	244	10	9.2	24.4

Source: Mattei and CECOS Fédération, 1987.

however, is AID or IVF-D the better technique? AID is simpler, less expensive, and easy to do each month. IVF-D is more complicated, expensive, and, practically speaking, is limited to three or four punctures per year. In our CECOS practice, the cumulative pregnancy rate after one year of AID was 63.2 per cent vs. 39.7 per cent after three IVF punctures. During the second year of treatment, the results were the same. In the third year, IVF-D seems to be the best technique, with a 14.3 per cent success rate vs. 8.4 per cent with AID (Table 14.8). Cryopreservation of the embryo may increase the success rate in IVF. Therefore, except for tubal lesions and women more than 37 years old, it seems easier to practise AID. After 12 cycles without pregnancy, there is an indication for IVF-D, especially if the woman is 35 years old or more, has dysovulation, or has a gynaecological infertility factor.

Conclusion

It is difficult to know to what extent the results of the CECOS studies approximate to those of natural reproduction. However, AID with frozen donor semen now appears to provide the best means of minimizing the influence of associated variables and other sources of bias. The most fertile women become pregnant during the first cycles, if they are actively trying to conceive. The best days for conception are $J-3$ and $J-1$. Pregnancy rates are highest when the cervix is dilated, there is abundant cervical mucus, and spinnbarkheit 10. A woman is more hypofertile if she unsuccessfully tries to become pregnant during many cycles, is over 35 years old, or has a husband with good semen. The most useful predictor of male fertility is spermatozoa

TABLE 14.8. *Life-table cumulative pregnancy success rates (%) for AID and IVF-D by treatment years*

	First year	Second year	Third year
AID			
(12 cycles/year)	63.22	23.99	8.37
IVF-D			
(3 IVF/year)	39.74	23.8	14.31

mobility. IVF offers an alternative technique, either to obtain pregnancy more quickly or to maximize the chances of success in hypofertile couples.

References

Barrett, J. C., and Marshall, J. (1969), 'The Risk of Conception on Different Days of the Menstrual Cycle', *Population Studies* 23: 455–60.

CECOS Fédération, and LeLannou, D. (1987), 'Bilan d'activité des CECOS', *Contraception, Fertilité, Sexualité* 15: 693–5.

CECOS Fédération, Schwartz, D., and Mayaux, M. J. (1982), 'Female Fecundity as a Function of Age: Results of Artificial Insemination in 2193 Nulliparous Women with Azoospermic Husbands', *New England Journal of Medicine* 306: 404–6.

Cohen, J., Edwards, R. G., and Fehilly, C. B. (1985), 'In Vitro Fertilization Using Cryopreserved Donor Semen in Cases where both Partners are Infertile', *Fertility and Sterility* 43(4): 570–4.

David, G. (1984), 'Artificial Insemination by Donor (AID)' in E. Steinberger and G. Fropese (eds.), *Reproductive Medicine*: 319–26, Serono Symposia no. 29, Raven Press.

—— and Price, W. S. (1980), *Human Artificial Insemination and Semen Preservation*, Plenum Press, New York and London.

—— Czyglik, F., Mayaux, M. J., and Schwartz, D. (1980), 'The Success of AID and Semen Characteristics: Study on 1489 Cycles and 192 Ejaculates', *International Journal of Andrology* 3: 613–19.

Emperaire, J. C., Gauzere-Soumireau, E., Ussel, L., and Audebert, A. (1981), 'Insemination par donneur et fertilité féminine', *Journal de Gynaecologie, Obstetrique et Biologie de la Reproduction* 10: 717–27.

Mahadevan, M. M., and Trounson, A. O. (1984), 'The Influence of Seminal Characteristics on the Success Rate of Human *in Vitro* Fertilization', *Fertility and Sterility* 43: 400–5.

Mattei, A., and Fédération Francaise des CECOS (1987), 'La Fecondation *in vitro* avec sperme de donneur (FIV. D): Bilan de l'activité des CECOS durant l'année 1986', *Contraception, Fertilité, Sexualité* 15 (7–8): 706–8.

Mayaux, M. J., Schwartz, D., and Czyglik, F. (1985), 'Conception Rate According to Semen Characteristics in a Series of 15,364 Insemination Cycles', *Andrologia* 17(1): 9–15.

Mouzon de, J., Belaich-Allart, J., Dubuisson, J. B., Montagut, J., Testart, J., Bachelot, A., and Piette, C. (1987), 'Dossier FIVNAT: Analyse des resultats 1986. Generalites, indications, stimulations, rand de la tentative, age de la femme', *Contraception, Fertilité, Sexualité* 15 (7–8): 740–6.

Schwartz, D., and Mayaux, M. J. (1980), 'Mode of Evaluation of Results in Artificial Insemination and Semen Preservation', in G. David, and W. S. Price (eds.), *Human Artificial Insemination and Sperm Preservation*, Plenum Press, New York: 197–210.

—— —— (1982), 'Female Fecundity as a Function of Age', *New England Journal of Medicine* 306: 404–6.

—— —— Martin-Boyce, A., Czyglik, F., and David, G. (1979), 'Donor Insemination: Conception Rate According to Cycle Day in a Series of 821 Cycles with a Single Insemination', *Fertility and Sterility* 31: 226–9.

15 Hormonal Regulation in *in Vitro* Fertilization

GARY D. HODGEN

During the late 1960s Bob Edwards and his colleagues fixed on the idea that *in vitro* fertilization and embryo transfer in humans would provide enormous therapeutic and scientific opportunities. While this was not altogether a new idea, he, along with the clinician Patrick Steptoe, was the first to persevere in the face of both peer and public ridicule as well as seemingly insurmountable technical problems. We should recall that, early on, public tolerance for such endeavours was slight indeed. The situation changed dramatically in the summer of 1978 with the birth of Louise Brown in Oldham, England. At last Edwards and Steptoe had succeeded in one case with *in vitro* fertilization and embryo transfer. While we were all amazed (some were sceptical; others were dubious) at this great achievement, it had arrived not unlike so many other medical advances: that is, through many years of preliminary animal and human studies, ultimately brought to clinical application through heroic effort and rigorous scientific study. But these events are best recorded by Edwards himself. Even so, it must be noted that the practical utility of *in vitro* fertilization and embryo transfer on a broad scale required radical revisions of the initial procedures in order to achieve anything approaching a reliable treatment. Much of this presentation is taken from earlier summaries (Hodgen, 1986; Veeck, 1986).

In less than seven years, more than 1000 children worldwide were born to couples treated by *in vitro* fertilization and embryo transfer. Although exact statistics are difficult to compile, surely several hundred more ongoing pregnancies have derived from extra-corporeal fertilization. The utility of this procedure continues to increase. Accordingly, *in vitro* fertilization and embryo transfer is no longer an experimental technique; rather, it is a recognized medical procedure. Indeed, some states in the USA require health insurance carriers to offer coverage specifically designed for *in vitro* fertilization and embryo transfer treatment. Although US federal guidelines for this treatment have lagged since the 1979 DHEW (Department of Health, Education, and Welfare) Ethics Advisory Board Report, many states, as well as local institutional review boards, have adopted regulatory standards and oversight committees for both clinical service and research involving *in vitro* fertilization and embryo transfer. Moreover, professional societies and organizations concerned with reproductive health have made specific recommendations on the ethical and legal issues surrounding *in vitro* fertilization and embryo transfer and some of its caveat procedures. There continues to be a moral debate which gains balance and perspective from the collective input of widely divergent opinions. At the epicentre of this controversy are research objectives that require access to human embryonic tissue: the desire for new discoveries about the treatment and prevention of disease comes into conflict with primordial feelings of intrusion upon the very essence of being human. The choices are difficult at best.

Indications for *in Vitro* Fertilization

In vitro fertilization was first applied to patients with uncorrectable tubal disease; however, now the indications extend to a variety of disorders as listed below:

1. Generally healthy husband and wife
2. Accessible ovaries
3. A normally functioning uterus
4. Normal or correctable menstrual function
5. Wife under age 40
6. An uncorrected problem
   - *a*. Tubal
   - *b*. Inadequate sperm for normal reproduction but not azoospermia
   - *c*. Endometriosis
   - *d*. Undiagnosed by available methods
   - *e*. Diethylstilbestrol exposure
   - *f*. Cervical hostility
   - *g*. Immunological
   - *h*. Anovulation
   - *i*. Other

(Jones 1985).

Much of this presentation is taken from the work of Howard Jones, Jr. and his colleagues, who pioneered this work in the USA.

Tubal Disease

Some 615 of the first 825 treatment cycles (75 per cent) at the Eastern Virginia Medical School (EVMS), Norfolk were for tubal disease. Essentially all patients had failed conventional therapy, and many had had multiple laparotomies. All eggs were harvested by laparoscopy. It is of significance that the tubal disease group had the lowest pregnancy rate by cycle (18.4 per cent) excluding the male factor and by transfer (22.3 per cent) among the five major diagnostic groups in the EVMS series. Furthermore, the transfer rate of 82 per cent was the lowest of the major diagnostic categories—excluding couples with a male problem (Table 15.1).

These low rates probably reflect the extent of pelvic disease. Some 122 cycles (20 per cent) were aspirated from patients who had only one remaining ovary, and partial availability of ovaries was common. Seventy-two cycles were aspirated among patients with a secondary diagnosis which by itself could have been responsible for the infertility. However, neither a single remaining ovary, nor a secondary diagnosis, nor a combination of the two seemed to influence the pregnancy rate.

Male Infertility

Absolute criteria for a semen examination which characterizes infertility remain undescribed. Nevertheless, most patients in this category have repeated sperm counts with less than 20 million sperm. Good motility seems to be an essential requirement, as penetration of the zona seems impossible without it.

Screening of two to three samples prior to admission into the programme is helpful. Continuing pregnancies have occurred from specimens which yield 1.5 million actively motile sperm after swim-up. There has also been a good correlation between pregnancy and a positive hamster penetration test. Although fertilization, in our experience, can occur with as few as 12 500 sperm from a euspermic man, present evidence suggests that this number may be far too few for an oligospermic specimen.

Presently, there are not completely reliable criteria which can discriminate oligoasthenospermic specimens with fertilizing capability from those without. Nevertheless, *in vitro* fertilization offers the only opportunity for pregnancy for some oligoasthenospermic men. Among the first 65 couples treated as EVMS whose primary problem seemed to rest with the male, 41 (63 per cent) also had a contribution factor in the female as well. As with tubal ligation, this secondary factor did not seem to influence the end result.

Couples with a male factor experienced a very low rate of transfer (49 per cent) compared to other diagnostic categories (Table 15.2). However, if the procedure reached the transfer stage, the pregnancy rate was quite comparable to that in other groups.

Among the male group, the total number of eggs harvested was quite comparable to other groups. However, the number of eggs transferred in the group was the lowest of any category, suggesting that even when fertilization occurred it did so with a lesser efficiency than in other groups (Tables 15.1 and 15.2).

Endometriosis

All patients in this category have had prior endocrinological and/or surgical therapy without achieving a pregnancy. Among 55 cycles aspirated at EVMS

TABLE 15.1. *IVF results by category of infertility, Norfolk, January 1981–September 1984 (Series 1–16)*

Category of infertility	No. of cycles	No. of transfers	% with transfer	No. of pregnancies	Pregnancies/ cycle (%)	Pregnancies/ transfer (%)
Tubal	615	504	82	113	18.4	22.3
Male	65	32	49	11	16.9	34.3
Endometriosis	55	48	87	14	25.5	29.2
Undiagnosed	37	32	86	11	29.7	34.3
DES	33	30	91	8	24.2	26.6
Cervical	9	8	89	1	11.1	12.5
Immunological	7	6	86	2	28.6	33.3
Anovulation	4	4	100	1	25.0	25.0

Source: Jones (1985).

TABLE 15.2. *IVF results for couples with male factor infertility, Norfolk, January 1981–September 1984 (Series 1–16)*

Category of infertility	No. of cycles	No. of transfers	No. of Pregnancies	Pregnancies/ cycle (%)	Pregnancies/ transfer (%)
All	65	32	11	16.9	34.3
Single diagnosis	24	10	3	12.5	30.0
With secondary diagnosis	41	22	8	19.5	36.4

Source: Jones (1985).

with a primary diagnosis of endometriosis, 38 had endometriosis as the sole diagnosis while 17 also had secondary problems. However, the transfer rate and pregnancy rate by cycle or by transfer was not influenced by the secondary factor (Table 15.3). There were only minor differences in the number of eggs collected and transferred between the two endometriosis categories and between endometriosis patients and patients in other categories.

A classification problem complicates the evaluation of the usefulness of *in vitro* fertilization for patients with endometriosis. In a review of the EVMS material through June 1984, Chillik and his associates (1985) noted that there were three different groups of patients. The first comprised patients who had a history of therapy for endometriosis, but at the time of harvest laparoscopy during the *in vitro* programme were found not to have any active disease. These patients had turned to the EVMS programme because they had not become pregnant following the original therapy for the endometriosis. There were 15 such cycles with 12 transfers and five pregnancies (33 per cent by cycle; 42 per cent by transfer). A second group of 14 patients, who had previously been treated for endometriosis, were found at the time of laparoscopy in the *in vitro* programme to still have considerable residual active disease. In this group there was but one pregnancy (which ended in a first trimester abortion) among 14 cycles which resulted in 11 transfers (7 per cent by cycle; 9 per cent by

TABLE 15.3. *IVF results of women with endometriosis, Norfolk, January 1981–September 1984 (Series 1–16)*

Category of infertility	No. of cycles	No. of transfers	No. of Pregnancies	Pregnancies/ cycle (%)	Pregnancies/ transfer (%)
All	55	48	14	25.5	29.2
Single diagnosis	38	34	10	26.3	29.4
With secondary diagnosis	17	14	4	23.5	28.6

Source: Jones (1985).

transfer). A third group of 10 patients, originally classified as having undiagnosed infertility on the basis of a previous work-up, had minimal endometriosis at the time of harvest laparoscopy in the *in vitro* programme. All of these patients were transferred and there were 6 pregnancies (60 per cent by cycle; 60 per cent by transfer). Thus, a detailed categorization of patients is essential to understand the indications for *in vitro* fertilization among patients with endometriosis.

In view of the success with *in vitro* fertilization among patients with minimal endometriosis and the success of *in vitro* fertilization in patients above the age of 35 (see below), it is possible that *in vitro* fertilization should be considered as the primary therapy for patients above the age of 35 with minimal endometriosis. However, the situation among patients over age 35 with active disease is less clear.

Undiagnosed

By definition, these patients have been investigated by contemporary diagnostic techniques, and no identifiable cause for their infertility has been found. All patients must have had examinations of the semen, post-coital tests, hysterosalpingograms, timed endometrial biopsies with basal temperature charts, and laparoscopic examinations without revealing any abnormality. All patients (husband and wife) must have a negative examination for anti-sperm antibodies in the serum.

While the number of patients is small, the results for the undiagnosed group at EVMS were higher than for any other diagnostic category (29.7 per cent by cycle; 34.3 per cent by transfer cycle). This good result probably reflects the fact that this group had a larger number of eggs transferred per cycle than any other diagnostic group (Table 15.1).

Diethylstilbestrol (DES)

Exposure to DES is a problem confined almost exclusively to the United States. Anomalous involvement after exposure to DES *in utero* occurs at various points along the mullerian ducts. Many of these patients will have had ectopic pregnancies and salpingectomies, some bilateral, due to deformities of the fallopian tubes. Many will have some degree of deformity in the endometrial cavity. Some will have deformities of the cervix.

Overall, the results at EVMS (24.2 per cent by cycle; 26.6 per cent by transfer) were comparable to the other groups. Because of the deformity of the uterine cavity, a high miscarriage rate was anticipated. However, of eight pregnancies, only one terminated prior to viability. The number of eggs transferred in this group was comparable to that of other groups. Muasher and his associates (1984) have reported these cases in detail.

Cervical Factors

Some patients immobilize the sperm of the husband and donor sperm, and there is no satisfactory explanation. In this group, by definition, there are no anti-sperm antibodies in the serum of these women or their husbands. This is a puzzling group as intra-uterine insemination with washed sperm does not often achieve a pregnancy. Nevertheless, by *in vitro* fertilization one such patient at EVMS became pregnant.

Immunological

As used here, the term 'immunological infertility' is meant to imply that the female partner has anti-sperm antibodies in the serum. In one patient at EVMS, the follicular fluid was tested and found to contain anti-sperm antibodies in a concentration comparable to the peripheral serum. This patient nevertheless became pregnant and has delivered. One other patient became pregnant, but aborted.

Anovulation

Anovulatory patients refractory to standard methods of ovulation induction can be treated successfully by *in vitro* fertilization.

Indications for Variations in the Basic Procedure

The Use of Donor Sperm

Donor sperm have been used for many years to inseminate the female partner when a couple's infertility is due to the inadequate sperm of the male partner. The same can be done in a programme of *in vitro* fertilization. However, there must also be some abnormality in the female that demands such fertilization. Several programmes have used this technique successfully. Since, however, it requires that both partners have a particular combination of fertility problems, its use will be limited.

The Use of Donor Eggs

There are several circumstances which make it impossible to harvest eggs from the female partner. These include patients with congenital absence of the ovaries (streak gonads), patients with premature menopause (perhaps even a normal menopause), or bilateral oophorectomy for whatever reason. Patients with blocked pelves obstructing laparoscopic harvest not amenable to surgical correction may be candidates for ultrasonic guided egg harvest, but even some of these may need and benefit from a donor egg.

If a patient is without oocytes, she will require suitable substitution therapy with oestrogen and progesterone to mimic normal ovarian function. This has been achieved in both monkeys and women. If the recipient has normal ovarian function, synchronization of donor and recipient is required. This has been done in monkeys and women in the programme at EVMS.

The Problem of Ovarian Inaccessibility

Some patients have pelvic disease so extensive that the ovaries are either partially or totally inaccessible to laparoscopic egg harvest. When these are relatively minor avascular adhesions, they can be released by laparoscopic techniques either at the time of a preliminary screen or at the time of egg harvest. Other patients may be suitable candidates for ultrasonic guided transvesical or transvaginal egg harvest. However, until these techniques produce pregnancy rates equal to those available with laparoscopic harvest, there remains a place for a preliminary laparotomy with a goal of making available the ovaries for laparoscopic harvest.

In properly selected patients, the results of such a procedure are acceptable. Such a procedure involves ovarian liberation, the removal of the tubes, if any, and suspension of the ovaries by severing the utero-ovarian ligaments and suturing them to the round ligaments so that the ovary rests on the uterus more or less at the site of the excised tube. Finally, it is usually necessary to suspend the uterus. In the event adhesions re-form to obstruct a subsequent laparoscopic approach, the ovaries should be ideally situated for a transvesical ultrasound guided approach.

As of September 1984 in the programme at EVMS, 54 patients had such a preliminary laparotomy. At the time of writing, 37 of these patients had come to subsequent laparotomy; 14 (38.8 per cent) became pregnant. However, a total of 55 laparoscopies were carried out among these 37 patients. As one patient became pregnant twice, the pregnancy rate per laparoscopy was 15/55 (27 per cent).

Effect of Age

It has been recognized for years that natural fertility decreases with age, substantially so beginning at about the age of 35. Therefore, it has been customary practice not to offer surgical therapy for infertility to patients above the age of 35. Many *in vitro* fertilization programmes, including the one at EVMS, began with the same rule with respect to age. However, this rule was gradually violated, and in the EVMS programme the pregnancy rate for patients in the age bracket 36–9 has been better than that for any other age-group. Indeed, pregnancies have occurred at age 40 and above. For example, our oldest mother was 42 years of age at delivery. Of significance is the finding that in the small series of patients aged 40 and over, the abortion rate was no greater than for the younger age-group (Table 15.4). However, Edwards and Steptoe have found that among patients above age 40 the expectancy of pregnancy is diminished and associated with a high abortion rate. Thus, it seems that there is uncertainty about the application of *in vitro* fertilization to patients at or about the age of 40 years. With this caveat in regard to age, some self-evident criteria and indications based on the EVMS experience are stated on p. 244.

TABLE 15.4. *IVF results by women's age,*
Norfolk, January 1981–September 1984
(Series 1–16)

Age	Pregnancies/ transfer cycle (%)	Abortions/ pregnancies (%)
<26	0/3 (0)	—
26–30	35/153 (23)	8/35 (23)
31–5	80/352 (23)	26/80 (32)
36–9	40/132 (30)	12/40 (30)
>40	6/27 (22)	2/6 (33)
Total	161/667 (24)	50/161 (31)

Source: Jones (1985).

Procedures of *in Vitro* Fertilization

The initial success with *in vitro* fertilization began with the collection of one egg from the single dominant follicle of the natural ovarian/menstrual cycle (Fig. 15.1), but it soon became evident that raising pregnancy rates to practically useful levels would usually require aspiration of several pre-ovulatory eggs from each patient. This change has had more to do with improving the outcome of *in vitro* fertilization than any other primary revision in procedures. This change resulted in the transfer of multiple embryos, which, in turn, enhanced changes for achieving viable pregnancies (Table 15.5).

Methods of Ovarian Stimulation

The large number of stimulation protocols tested for *in vitro* fertilization patients precludes a practical description of each one. Accordingly, I have

TABLE 15.5. *Multiple pregnancy rates rise along with the pregnancy rate as the number of embryos transferred increases*

No. of embryos transferred	Pregnancy rate/ transfer cycle (%)	Multiple pregnancy rate (%)
1	14	1
2	22	4
3	29	9
4	31	15
5	33	21
6	35	28

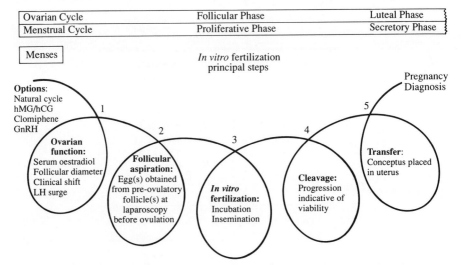

Fig. 15.1   The five principal steps of *in vitro* fertilization and embryo transfer procedure

drawn heavily from a recent summary by Georgeanna Jones and colleagues (1984) in grouping comparisons of various procedures, several of which have been used successfully worldwide by different *in vitro* fertilization and embryo transfer teams.

Three basic methods have been used for stimulation of multiple oocyte retrieval: (1) clomiphene citrate with or without human chorionic gonadotrophin (hCG); (2) clomiphene citrate plus human menopausal gonadotrophin (hMG) plus hCG; and (3) hMG plus hCG. At the present time, most *in vitro* fertilization programmes have abandoned the use of clomiphene citrate alone, because the number of oocytes obtained, the pregnancy rates, and the cycle cancellation rates were not as satisfactory as with other methods of stimulation. More recently, the majority of the Australian teams, as well as those in Europe and the United States, have used clomiphene citrate plus hMG plus hCG. Here at EVMS, hMG plus hCG stimulation has been used almost from the beginning of the programme.

Clomiphene citrate plus hCG.   Monitoring for clomiphene citrate plus hCG-stimulated cycles was reported early on by Trounson and Wood (1981). These investigators relied on ultrasound as their major method of monitoring, although urinary oestrogen and LH (luteinizing hormone) assays were also obtained. Thus, 50 to 150 mg clomiphene citrate was administered daily beginning at about days 3 to 5 of the cycle, and hCG was administered when the ultrasound indicated the largest follicular diameter was 20 mm or more. If the LH surge was detected, the cycle was usually cancelled. Oestrogen assays in serum were estimated to be 400 pg/ml times the number of the follicles visualized on ultrasound; thus, if three follicles were visualized, the serum oestrogen should be approximately 1200 pg/ml.

Clomiphene citrate plus hMG plus hCG.   Clomiphene citrate is given at 50 to 150 mg per day beginning at about day 5 of the cycle. Two ampoules of hMG, 75 IU each of FSH (follicle-stimulating hormone) and LH, are given on days 6, 8, and 10 of the cycle. Follicular ultrasound and serum oestrogens are the major methods used for monitoring; typically, hCG is given when two 15 mm follicles are seen. The Women's Hospital group in Melbourne, Australia has individualized cases by using serum oestradiol and biological parameters to determine when to give hCG. It is important to realize that each *in vitro* fertilization team may favour minor variations in these generic protocols.

hMG plus hCG.   Here at EVMS, hMG (75 IU each of FSH and LH) was given at the rate of two ampoules of Pergonal daily beginning on cycle day 3 in patients having a cycle of 28 days ±3 days. The hMG was administered as needed im (intramuscularly) at 16.00 hours after the oestradiol values were reported at 15.00 hours. hMG was discontinued or decreased as determined by monitoring. This protocol produced good responses in many patients, but did not optimize the results in several subgroups. Accordingly, in recent months we have intensified evaluations of FSH-rich stimulation protocols.

'Pure' FSH plus hMG plus hCG.   Preliminary findings indicate that many patients treated with greater amounts of FSH relative to LH, especially early in the stimulation protocol, became pregnant in the EVMS *in vitro* fertilization programme. Current results favour the pure FSH plus hMG plus hCG over all other regimens tested. Whether pure FSH (Metrodin), alone or in combination with hMG and/or hCG (by a protocol yet to be evaluated), will ultimately prove superior to previous regimens for certain patients is being tested.

Rationale for the Treatment Regimen

The period from day 3 to day 5 was chosen for beginning most regimens because the dominant follicle is typically not selected before about day 6. Thus, this period is usually right to accommodate two or three additional follicles from the maturing cohort of follicles developing concurrently. Two ampoules of hMG per day were given because, in prior experience with ovulation induction, this amount stimulated patients with minimal hypothalamic pituitary function within an 8- to 10-day period. Importantly, by starting with the highest amount of hMG estimated to be necessary and then reducing the dose, if indicated, the stimulation is more manageable than starting with a low dosage and later increasing it.

Cycles are monitored by all parameters available for the estimation of follicle growth and development, which should, theoretically, parallel maturation of the oocyte. These include serum oestradiol levels; the biological response of the individual to the oestradiol, measured by peripheral end-organ responses such as maturation of the vaginal cells and changes in cervical mucus; and the number of follicles and their anatomic growth as measured by daily ultrasound.

Follicular ultrasound measurement.   The diameter of the hMG-stimulated follicles was found by ultrasound to be smaller than anticipated, based on the size of the dominant follicle in the natural cycle. The average diameter of the largest follicles when hMG was discontinued was 13.7 mm ± 1.4 SD and 15.1 mm ± 1.5 SD when hCG was given, as compared to 15 mm and 21 mm in the natural cycle. The clarity of the follicular borders is also somewhat obscured by the oedema which occurs in the hMG/hCG-stimulated ovary. Although the ultrasound is invaluable in determining the side in which the largest follicles occur, their location, and their number, it has not been used at EVMS as a primary monitoring method. Here, it may influence the discontinuation of the hMG by ± 1 day. However, other *in vitro* fertilization teams rely quite adequately on ultrasound as their principal tool for patient monitoring.

Monitoring Patient Response.   The ideal time for discontinuing the hMG depends very much on individual patient response. Three patient response categories were identified and arbitrarily regarded as low, intermediate, and high. These categories related the serum oestradiol values to the peripheral oestrogen effect. It was determined that hMG should be discontinued in the majority of patients (comprising the intermediate group) when the oestradiol E_2 was 300 pg/ml or above, if the peripheral biological oestrogen response (vaginal and cervical) had occurred. In the high responder group, hMG should be discontinued when 600 pg/ml or above of serum oestradiol is reached, without regard for biological response (Fig. 15.2). In the low responder group, hMG should be discontinued if there is a biological response up to 3 days ahead, even if serum oestradiol values are below 300 pg/ml (Fig. 15.3).

The aetiology of the characteristic high, intermediate, or low patient response to hMG resides in the complex physiology of the hypothalamic–pituitary–ovarian axis. It is not due to a higher total hMG dosage given to the high responders, because the high responders require less dosage over a shorter period of time to induce a comparable effect on both the biological E_2 response and oestradiol and progesterone synthesis. Note that the degree of steroidogenesis in the luteal phase reflects responses in the follicular phase (Fig. 15.4).

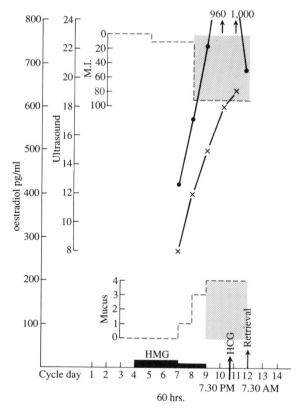

The symbols are the same as in Fig. 2. The patient does not show an oestrogen shift in the peripheral response until the serum oestradiol is above 600 pg/ml. Mucus = cervical mucus score; hMG = Human menopausal gonadotrophin; hCG = Human chorionic gonadotrophin; Ultrasound = measurement of follicular diameter.

Source: Jones *et al.*, 1984.

Fig. 15.2   A woman with a high response to hMG stimulation

Importantly, recent findings (Fig. 15.5) suggest that co-administration of a GnRH antagonist with gonadotrophin, to achieve a state approaching reversible 'medical hypophysectomy', may markedly reduce the individual variability of response to FSH or FSH:LH mixtures.

Unimportance of the FSH:LH Ratio

I must begin by assuring you that this remains an unsettled issue. However, the present trend of interpretations of recent data (Fig. 15.6) indicates that the amount of FSH is much more significant than the amount of LH. Thus, the ratio of FSH to LH *per se* may be a futile consideration. Adequate ovarian response clearly requires more FSH in some patients than others. What is less

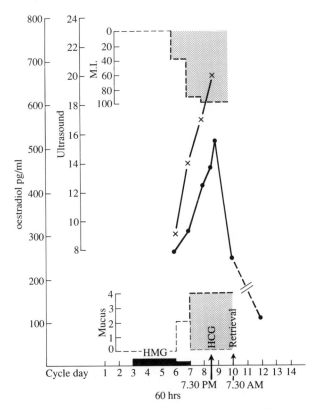

The symbols are the same as in Fig. 15.2. The patient has had an oestrogen shift in the peripheral response for 48 hours but the serum oestradiol has not reached 300 pg/ml.

Source: Jones *et al.*, 1984.

Fig. 15.3   A woman with a low response to hMG stimulation

obvious is how much LH is required to support optimal folliculogenesis for *in vitro* fertilization therapy, or whether LH is needed at all. Ongoing studies may show that extra amounts of FSH will directly compensate for an overt LH deficiency.

One myth that deserves to be laid to rest is that a major variable in patient response is the FSH:LH ratio in commercial preparations of hMG. There may be as much as a 25 per cent variation (usually about 10 per cent) in FSH:LH biopotency among particular batches of hMG preparations. However, the enormous variation in the sensitivity of individual patients to exogenous gonadotrophins is so overwhelming as to extinguish the minor impacts of differences in the medications themselves. Besides, patient monitoring is structured to accommodate the need for increasing or decreasing the stimulation regimen based on individualized responses. Thus, while some variation in the bioavailability of FSH and/or LH is surely inherent to all commercial hMG

Norfolk series 2–6, tubal

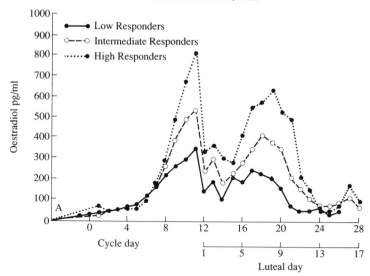

Norfolk series 2–6, tubal

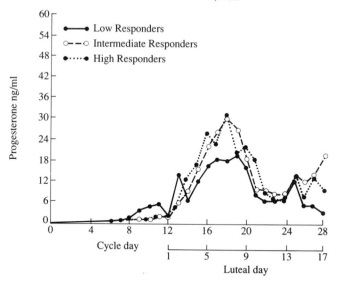

Both the luteal oestradiol (*A*) and progesterone (*B*) reflect the patterns of the steroidogenesis in the follicular phase of the cycle indicating that the responses are dependent upon the initial response to the hMG stimulus, perhaps favouring a receptor theory.

Source: Jones *et al.*, 1984.

Fig. 15.4   The patterns of steroidogenesis in the follicular phase after hMG stimulation

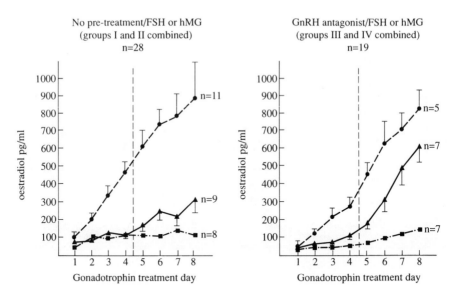

No pre-treatment/FSH or hMG
(groups I and II combined)
n=28

GnRH antagonist/FSH or hMG
(groups III and IV combined)
n=19

Gonadotrophin treatment day

Gonadotrophin treatment day

The panels represent the composite of groups I and II versus groups III and IV, i.e. those that did not receive and those that did receive pre-treatment and concurrent treatment with the GnRH antagonist. Among responders, AUC computations for days 1 to 4 and days 5 to 8 (comparing fast and slow responders), analysis of variance, and Kramer's modification of Duncan's multiple range test showed a significant difference ($p < 0.05$) between responses during treatment with the GnRH antagonist. n = the number of subjects for AUC analysis, whereas the number of subjects for daily mean oestradiol values may be greater. Coefficients of variation among responders for total AUC in groups I to IV were 63.1, 70.5, 43.1, and 28.3, respectively. Without GnRH antagonists (groups I and II) or gonadotrophin treatment with GnRH antagonist (groups III and IV) the AUC coefficients of variation were 69.0 and 47.0, respectively. ●, fast responder; ▲, slow responder; ■, non-responder.

Source: Kenigsberg *et al.*, 1984*b*.

Fig. 15.5   Comparison of women who received pre-treatment with GnRH antagonist with those who did not

preparations, its contribution to overall results with *in vitro* fertilization is obscured by much larger factors. Moreover, radio-immunoassay of FSH and LH levels in hMG medications is erroneous, misleading, and irrelevant to patient response, which depends strictly on the biologically active molecular forms of FSH and LH present there. Although certain patients do respond similarly in subsequent cycles, others depart radically, despite repeating the exact protocol in the same woman (Table 15.6).

Oocyte Maturation in Culture

With hMG stimulation, the cohort of follicles is seldom completely synchron-ized. One may, therefore, obtain a number of immature oocytes associated with the pre-ovulatory oocytes. Although the fertilization rate of immature

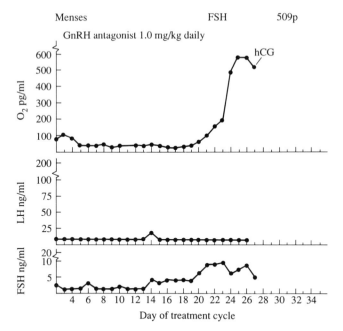

Plasma oestradiol exceeded 300 pg/ml, qualifying the subject as a responder; but since the level of 300 pg/ml was not reached on or before gonadotrophin treatment day 5, this monkey was classified as a slow responder. The shaded area corresponds to gonadotrophin treatment days 1 to 8.

Source: Kenigsberg *et al.*, 1984*b*.

Fig. 15.6   Representative serum hormone values in a typical group III subject

oocytes is not high (Table 15.7), varying the duration of time in culture before fertilization can improve the success rate. Those oocytes judged to be more mature (germinal vesicle breakdown), may require only 12 hours in culture for polar body extrusion. More immature oocytes (with germinal vesicles) may need up to 32 hours for polar body extrusion. Fertilization should not be attempted before polar body extrusion. Ability to mature such oocytes allows an increased number of concepti to be transferred. As previously reported, pregnancies resulting from only immature oocytes matured *in vitro* have occurred but may be few in number.

The Surrogate LH Surge

hCG is usually required after hMG is discontinued. In choosing the time for aspiration, ovulation will begin within approximately 36 to 40 hours of hCG administration. In the EVMS programme, oocyte aspiration is done at 07.50 hours; therefore, hCG is usually administered between 19.00 and 21.00 hours, 34–6 hours before the aspiration schedule. If ultrasound and other parameters indicate that follicle maturation is progressing normally, hCG is administered

TABLE 15.6. *Hormonal parameters in IVF/ET patients relating oocyte yield to plasma steroid levels*

No.	Cycle no.	Pre-hCG E_2	Number of mature follicles	Luteal Phase	
				E_2 PCG/ML	Progesterone NG/ML
1	(1)	1660	3	1100	21
	(2)	840	2	650	17
2	(1)	2390	5	1580	17
	(2)	3700	2	780	21
3	(1)	1310	3	400	12
	(2)	940	2	620	16.5
4	(1)	1280	2	435	1.2
	(2)	980	1	470	6
5	(1)	1810	6	1310	20
	(2)	3020	3	870	50
6	(1)	150	3	420	12
	(2)	1590	2	680	12.5
7	(1)	1420	5	630	14
	(2)	1000	3	530	
8	(1)	770	3	265	12
	(2)	520	6	520	15.5
9	(1)	800	2	680	5.5
	(2)	133	4	1040	30
10	(1)	3320	5	1010	31
	(2)	1260	?	35	38

Source: Cohen, J., personal communication (1985).

50 hours after the last hMG injection. If the ultrasound shows a rapidly increasing follicular size or the serum E_2 reaches a plateau, hCG may be given between 30 and 32 hours after the last hMG injection. Timing of the hMG to hCG interval has been varied throughout several series. A study of the results when the interval was shortened without specific indications suggested that, although the numbers of fertilizable eggs retrieved is about the same whether the interval is long or short, as are fertilization, cleavage, and transfer rates, the pregnancy rate per cycle and per transfer is higher after a 50- or 60-hour interval. Therefore, the hMG to hCG interval should be shortened only by specific indications as stated above.

hCG, which substitutes for the LH surge in the natural cycle, initiates the resumption of oocyte meiosis, the nuclear change which signals oocyte maturation. This requires approximately 28 hours from the beginning of the LH surge and 36 hours from the administration of hCG. From this study, it seems that an interval of 50 to 60 hours between discontinuing hMG stimulation and the administration of hCG may represent the time necessary for cytoplasmic

TABLE 15.7. *Results of attempts to mature and fertilize human oocytes* in vitro *as compared to attempts to fertilize pre-ovulatory oocytes during the same period*

	Immature		Pre-ovulatory	
	No.	%	No.	%
Total number oocytes	74		216	
Failed maturation	10	13.5		
Inseminated before completion of maturation	2	2.7		
Failed fertilization after maturation	5	6.8	27	12.5
Fertilized with more than 2 pronuclei	6	8.1	19	8.8
Failed cleavage after apparently normal fertilization	7	9.5	6	2.8
Total number of concepti undergoing fertilization and transfer	44	59.5	165	76.4
Transferred with cleavage	35	79.5	165	100
Transferred at pronuclear or post-pronuclear stage before cleavage	9	20.5	0	0

Note: Procedures were attempted from 1 September 1982 to 31 July 1983.
Source: Veeck *et al.*, 1983.

oocyte maturation to be completed within the 36 hours after hCG administration. Recent work by Moor and associates in Cambridge (1983) would seem to substantiate this theory. The oocytes obtained after a shortened hMG/hCG interval did not seem to show a difference in nuclear maturation but only in the ability to induce a normal pregnancy. It would, therefore, seem that germinal vesicle breakdown and polar body extrusions representing nuclear maturation are not influenced by the hMG-to-hCG time-interval.

In the first 31 EVMS cycles monitored, with LH serum values taken every 4 hours after the serum oestradiol level indicated an LH surge might be expected, it was found that no LH surge occurred (Fig. 15.7). LH has not been used, therefore, in monitoring patients in the subsequent series. Oocyte aspiration for *in vitro* fertilization has been performed in 207 cycles stimulated by hMG with this method, and no spontaneous ovulation has occurred before the administration of hCG.

Blockade, Delay, or Attenuation of the LH Surge

The finding that hMG stimulation is associated with failure of the LH surge in response to normal or above normal amounts of oestradiol over a 48-hour period in women with normal feedback mechanisms is consistent with the findings of other investigators. Fowler and co-workers (1978) stated that the LH surge 'seldom occurs after hMG stimulation of normally menstruating women'. These are the only investigators who have had a large experience with hMG stimulation in normally ovulating women. When normally ovulating

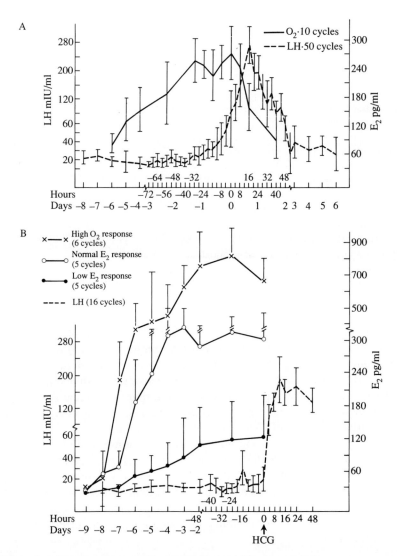

Relation of serum LH peak to serum oestradiol surge in the normal cycle.

Relation of serum LH to oestradiol in 16 hMG stimulated cycles followed by hCG ovulation induction.

A, Serum LH (dashed line) and 17–oestradiol (solid line) in spontaneous cycles (control group) normalized to the time of initial LH rise (over 60 mIU/ml). Time 0 = time of initial LH rise. *B*, serum LH (dashed line) and 17–oestradiol (solid line) in hMG/hCG-stimulated cycles, normalized to the time of hCG administration (day 0). The three different oestradiol responses are represented. All cycles resulted in aspiration of pre-ovulatory oocytes.

Source: Ferraretti *et al.*, 1983.

Fig. 15.7   A comparison of serum hormone levels in spontaneous and hMG/hCG-stimulated cycles

women are stimulated with various types of hMG stimulation in various phases of the cycle, if a single follicle is stimulated or if stimulation over 2000 pg/ml of oestradiol is accomplished, an LH surge may occur; otherwise, spontaneous LH surges are unlikely to occur.

With hMG induction of ovulation in anovulatory women, although hCG administration is usually necessary, it has long been recognized that ovulation can occasionally occur without administration of hCG, particularly in those patients with polycystic ovarian disease in whom inappropriate LH surges occur spontaneously. Schoemaker and co-workers (1978) demonstrated the inhibition of LH secretion in anovulatory patients receiving 'pure' pituitary FSH. The assumption, therefore, is that LH suppression is mediated by the FSH content of the hMG administered and is not a direct LH inhibition by LH. The inhibition of the LH surge in hMG-stimulated cycles is apparently not an absolute one, but is related to the amount of oestradiol that is stimulated, balanced by the number of follicles that are stimulated.

In the hMG-treated cycles, those follicles from which a pre-ovulatory oocyte is retrieved show a decreased size, both by ultrasound and by amount of follicular fluid aspirated. Channing and associates (1983) analysed follicular fluid from these pre-ovulatory follicles and found decreased levels of steroids (oestradiol, progesterone, and androstenedione) in relation to those found in the natural cycle, and increased levels of inhibin-like activity. This was from three to ten times the amount found in the dominant follicle of the natural cycle. Although porcine follicular fluid 'inhibin' preferentially blocks pituitary FSH release, it may also inhibit LH if given in sufficient amounts.

It may, therefore, be postulated that the suppressive effect of hMG on the LH surge is related to the increased amount of an inhibin-like protein produced by the hMG-stimulated follicles. We have advanced this theory after determining that administration of pure FSH blocks the FSH and LH surge release in monkeys with normal cycles presenting ovarian hyperstimulation. We have further pinpointed the origin of this suppression at the ovarian level. In contrast, oophorectomized, hMG-stimulated monkeys showed normal FSH and LH responses to a GnRH or oestradiol stimulation. Blockade of pituitary LH secretion during hMG-induced hyperstimulation is highly transient after ovariectomy. The proof of this hypothesis awaits purification and identification of the follicular factor(s).

Endometrial Development in a Pharmacological Milieu

The greatest inefficiency in the programme for *in vitro* fertilization is found in the step beyond transfer. Why does implantation fail to occur in 75 per cent of cycles? The two obvious possibilities are that: (1) the endometrium is defective and unable to receive an implantation signal or (2) the oocyte is defective and unable to signal the endometrium.

It was initially assumed that there was no problem with the endometrium in the hMG-stimulation cycle as the majority of women show progesterone serum values in excess of those found in the natural cycle. Nevertheless, in cycles in which oestradiol is also significantly above that seen in the natural cycle, it is possible that there could be a physiological imbalance in the stimulation of the endometrium. Endometrial biopsies were, therefore, performed on 22 patients who for one reason or another did not receive a conceptus transfer. These biopsies were dated according to the Noyes criteria by three separate pathologists who had no knowledge of the history of the patients. The day of follicular aspiration was arbitrarily designated as cycle day 14 to correspond with the presumed ovulation date in the natural cycle. One biopsy was taken on day 14, one on day 15, and the other twenty biopsies were taken on day 16, the day on which transfer would have occurred. Biopsies obtained on days 14 and 15 were reported as proliferative endometrium, as was one biopsy taken on day 16. Five of the biopsies taken on day 16 were 'in phase' by histologic dating, in contrast to eleven which were dated one, two, or three days in advance of normal.

The biopsy dates were then compared to the serum progesterone values, and a good correlation between the dating and the serum progesterone was found (Table 15.8). Serum progesterone values of patients at the time of transfer might, therefore, be used as an estimate of whether the endometrium into which the conceptus was transferred was advanced or in phase at the time of transfer. Those cycles in which pregnancy occurred were associated with high progesterone values, similar to values seen in the cycles with the advanced endometrial patterns.

It must be recalled that after *in vitro* fertilization, typically a four-cell conceptus is transferred on the 16th cycle day. In contrast, in the natural cycle a blastocyst arrives in the uterus on the 17th or 18th cycle day. Therefore, during *in vitro* fertilization with hMG stimulation, a conceptus is being transferred

TABLE 15.8. *Serum progesterone levels at the time of the endometrial biopsy*

No. of cycles	Day of endometrial biopsy			Progesterone ng/ml (mean)
	14[a]	15	16	
2	Proliferative			1.3
3		Proliferative		2.2
1			Proliferative	1.3
4			Secretory 16	5.2
5			Secretory 17	8.3
3			Secretory 17–18	16.2
2			Secretory 18	14.7
1			Secretory 19–20	20.8

[a] Follicular aspiration day.

Source: Garcia *et al.*, 1984.

into a uterine endometrium which may be one-to-three days advanced (Fig. 15.1) in relation to conceptus development.

A study of the luteal progesterone values indicates that progesterone values on the day of aspiration, day 14, and through day 17 are similar in the pregnant, non-pregnant, and advanced endometrial biopsy groups of patients. However, by day 19, one day after conceptus transfer, there is a statistically significant increase in progesterone values in those patients who become pregnant (Fig. 15.8).

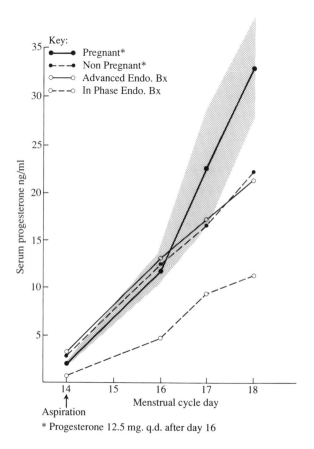

* Progesterone 12.5 mg. q.d. after day 16

The shadowed area represents the P levels, ±SE, of the pregnant group after hMG/hCG-stimulated cycles during early luteal phase. Notice how P levels of the non-pregnant and 'advanced' endometrial biopsy groups were within the same range of the pregnant group on the 14th and 16th menstrual cycle day. By day 17, P levels were lower in the non-pregnant and advanced endometrial biopsy groups, but were still within the 1 SE. All day-18 P levels are significantly lower than the pregnancy levels.

Source: Garcia *et al.*, 1984.

Fig. 15.8   A comparison of serum progesterone values in pregnant and non-pregnant women after hMG/hCG-stimulated cycles

The finding that serum progesterone values are significantly elevated in the fertile cycles by even one day after transfer needs further study. If this can be substantiated it is hard to escape the conclusion that the embryo, even at this early state, is signalling to reinforce the function of the corpus luteum and to prevent luteolysis.

Pregnancy Rates

The ultimate success of *in vitro* fertilization and embryo transfer therapy can be judged only by the take-home-rate of normal healthy babies. In order to evaluate the efficacy of these pregnancy statistics, it is necessary to compare the pregnancy rates of the *in vitro* fertilization programme with the expectancy of pregnancy and abortion in any one normal cycle of pregnancy exposure. When studies in the literature are evaluated, it can be seen that *in vitro* results are approaching those of normal reproduction (Fig. 15.9). However, because of the ability to transfer more than one conceptus, it is theoretically possible that when optimum conditions are known and achieved, the normal pregnancy rate of 25 per cent may be exceeded by *in vitro* fertilization.

Although the pregnancy rate for *in vitro* fertilization is beginning to approach the normal expectancy for any given exposure cycle, there are still many unknowns, and both technical and theoretical problems remain to be solved. Chief among these are determining the best method to stimulate multiple follicle maturation for oocyte retrieval and improving the monitoring to ensure

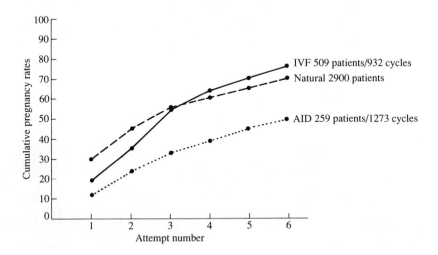

Source: Jones, 1985

Fig. 15.9   A comparison of cumulative pregnancy rates of *in vivo*, *in vitro*, and AID fertilization

retrieval of the most mature oocyte. However, in addition to improving upon current methods of stimulation and monitoring, it is important to make an effort to improve the culture media with the goal of improved oocyte cyto-plasmic maturation.

The state of the art for *in vitro* fertilization today is aiming towards the induction of a more predictable stimulation pattern. Recognition of the high, intermediate, or low response patterns of an individual patient to hMG stimulation, and perhaps also to clomiphene citrate, may be crucial. Patient individualization should result in increased pregnancy rates and fewer mis-carriages, which now comprise up to 30 per cent of all confirmed pregnancies. Also, the problems associated with the failure of implantation after transfer seem to be with the normalcy and stage of maturation of the oocyte itself, more than with the endometrium.

Unique Research Opportunities

It may be enlightening to point out that until the era of successful *in vitro* fertilization in patients, perhaps less than ten people had ever seen a living human pre-implantation embryo. Except for the few early observations of Hertig and colleagues (1959), scarcely any investigative forays have permitted direct study of the early human conceptus. Indeed, it was the clinical utility of *in vitro* fertilization and embryo transfer for infertility treatment which simul-taneously provided the professional impetus and the ethical justification for crossing this threshold.

With the advent of *in vitro* fertilization has come access, for the first time, to the substrates requisite for renewal of human life. From this setting, research opportunities emerge at two levels: (1) clinical investigations aimed at improv-ing and extending the therapeutic success of *in vitro* fertilization or its direct caveats to benefit infertile couples; and (2) basic research concerned with the fundamental processes operating during activation of development, differen-tiation of the embryo, maternal immune tolerance, and response to the genomic signals which orchestrate timely gene expression and repression. Among the former group are improvements in ovarian stimulation protocols, cryopreservation of embryos, oocyte maturation *in vitro* (Fig. 15.10), and egg or embryo donation. Current clinical indications for the latter are as follows (see also Fig. 15.11):

1. Inaccessible ovaries
2. Genetic disease
3. Contra-indications for IVF
4. Ovarian dysgenesis
5. Premature menopause
6. Surgical castration
7. Failed IVF

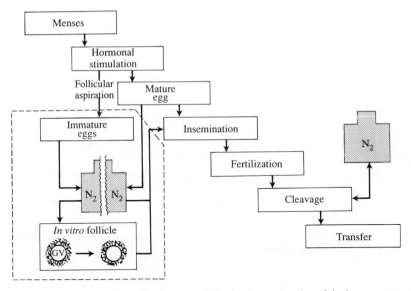

A high scientific priority is the technology permitting *in vitro* maturation of the immature oocyte

N_2 = liquid nitrogen; GV = germinal vesicle

Fig. 15.10   The process of *in vitro* fertilization

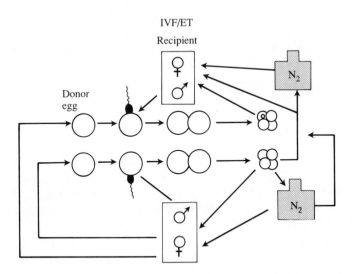

N_2 = liquid nitrogen

Fig. 15.11   A series of possible methods of egg or embryo donation

However, the latter research opportunities have potential significance at and beyond the brink of our current scientific anticipation. Indeed, this newly acquired access to human gametes and pre-implantation embryos provides the basis for direct study of the human germinal line: the origins of both teratogenic and genetic defects (lethal and non-lethal), the process of oncogenesis, and even ageing itself. Whereas development of somatic cell gene therapy is virtually upon us, it is not unreasonable to predict the manipulation of human germinal material for disease diagnosis and prevention by the onset of the twenty-first century, less than a decade away. Through the confluence of molecular biology and reproductive medicine, these opportunities surely rival the most monumental achievements in the medical sciences, including the contributions of Pasteur early in the last century and of Watson and Crick in this one.

A few examples will make my point. Cancer biologists are making a persuasive case that 20 to 30 oncogenes may spawn the aggressive behaviour of virulent tumour cells. Often these malignant tissues are able to preferentially sequester a vast blood supply, avoid immune rejection by the host, and elaborate unique gene products such as chorionic gonadotrophin and alpha foetoprotein that reflect re-activation of embryonic genes, long dormant after completion of intra-uterine life. The parallels between oncogenesis and embryogenesis and foetal development are known to be extensive, including angiogenic expressions of the implanting blastocyst, the immune privilege of gestation, the co-presence of unique trophoblastic hormones (hCG) with alpha foetal hepatic proteins (AFP), and, finally, persistence of an accelerated mitogenic status. It is imperative to learn whether viral vectors are passed between generations along the human germinal line itself.

We have only begun to appreciate how these new investigative endeavours radiate outward from current *in vitro* fertilization and embryo transfer therapy. While the treatment of human infertility remains at the epicentre of these activities, past and current achievements may pale beside the nascent realities previously trapped within the inaccessible human embryo. That profound ethical, social, and legal concerns are raised by human embryo research is obvious. This, too, is a unique and special challenge to mankind, because the preservation and protection of what is human can be described and regarded in so many ways.

References

Channing, C. P., Liu, C. Q., Evans, V., Gabliano, P., Jones, G. S., Veeck, L. L., and Jones, H. W. (1983), 'Decline of Follicular Oocyte Maturation Inhibitor Coincident with Maturation Achievement of Fertilizability of Oocytes Recovered at Midcycle of Gonadotrophin-Treated Women', *Proceedings of the National Academy of Science*, 80: 4184.

Chillik, C. R., Acosta, A. A., Garcia, J. E., Perera, S., van Dem, J. H., Rosenwaks, Z., and Jones, H. W. (1985), 'The Role of *in Vitro* Fertilization in Infertile Patients with Endometriosis', *Fertility and Sterility* 44: 56.

Ferraretti, A. P., Garcia, J. E., Acosta, A. A., and Jones, G. S. (1983), 'Serum LH During Ovulation Induction for *in Vitro* Fertilization in Normally Menstruating Women', *Fertility and Sterility* 40: 742.

Fowler, R. E., Edwards, R. G., Walters, D. R., Chan, S. T. H., and Steptoe, P. C. (1978), 'Steriodogenesis in Preovulatory Follicies of Patients Given Human Menopausal Gonadotrophin', *Journal of Endocrinology* 77: 161.

Garcia, J. E., Acosta, A. A., Hsiu, J. G., and Jones, H. W., Jr. (1984), 'Advanced Endometrial Maturation after Ovulation Induction with Human Menopausal Gonadotropin/Human Chorionic Gonadotropin for *in Vitro* Fertilization', *Fertility and Sterility* 41: 31.

Hertig, A. T., Rock, J., Adams, E. G., and Menkin, M. C. (1959), 'Thirty-Four Fertilized Human Ova, Good, Bad, and Indifferent, Recovered from 210 Women of Known Fertility', *Pediatrics* 23: 202–11.

Hodgen, G. D. (1986), 'Hormonal Regulation in *in Vitro* Fertilization' *Vitamins and Hormones* 43: 251–82.

Jones, G. S. (1984), 'Update on *in Vitro* Fertilization', *Endocrine Reviews* 5: 62.

—— Garcia, J. E., and Rosenwaks, Z. (1984), 'The Role of Pituitary Gonadotrophins in Follicular Stimulation and Oocyte Maturation in the Human', *Journal of Clinical Endocrinology and Metabolism* 59: 178.

Jones, H. W., Jr. (1985), 'Indications for *in Vitro* Fertilization', in H. W. Jones, Jr., G. S. Jones, G. D. Hodgen, and Z. Rosenwaks (eds.), In Vitro *Fertilization, Norfolk* ii, Williams and Wilkins, Baltimore, Md., 1–7.

Kenigsberg, D., Littman, B. A., Williams, R. F., and Hodgen, G. D. (1984), 'Medical Hyphophysectomy, II: Variability of Ovarian Response to Gonadotrophin Therapy', *Fertility and Sterility* 42: 116.

Moor, R. M., Crosby, I. M., and Osborn, J. B. (1983), 'Growth and Maturation of Mamalian Oocytes', in P. G. Crosignal, and B. L. Rubin (eds.), In Vitro *Fertilization and Embryo Transfer*, Serono Clinical Coloquia on Reproduction and Academic Press, London, 39.

Muasher, S., Garcia, J. E., and Jones, H. W. (1984), 'Experience with Diethystilbestrol-Exposed Infertile Women in a Program of in Vitro Fertilization', *Fertility and Sterility* 42: 20.

Schoemaker, J., Wentz, A. C., Jones, G. E., Dudin, N. H., and Sapp, R. C. (1978), 'Stimulation of Follicular Growth with "Pure" FSH in Patients with Anovulation and Elevated LH Levels', *Obstetrics and Gynecology* 51: 270.

Trounson, A., and Wood, C. (1981), 'Extracorporeal Fertilization and Embryo Transfer', *Clinical Obstetrics and Gynecology* 8: 681.

Veeck, L. L. (1986), *Atlas of Human Oocyte and Early Conceptus*, Williams and Wilks, Baltimore, Md.

—— Wortham, J. W., Witmyer, J., Sandow, B. A., Acosta, A. A., Garcia, J. E., Jones, G. S., and Jones, H. W., Jr. (1983), 'Maturation and Fertilization of Morphologically Immature Oocytes in a Program of *in Vitro* Fertilization', *Fertility and Sterility* 39: 594.

16 Conception Probability and Pregnancy Outcome in Relation to Age, Cycle Regularity, and Timing of Intercourse

ALFRED SPIRA

BEATRICE DUCOT

MARIE-LUCE GUIHARD-MOSCATO

NADINE JOB-SPIRA

MARIE-JEANNE MAYAUX

JAQUELINE MÉNÉTRIER

JEANINE WATTIAUX

Fertility regulation and infertility work-ups must take into account various factors which may be related to the components of fecundability. This paper presents the results of four different epidemiological studies and reviews the current state of knowledge about the probability of conception and pregnancy outcome in relation to age (both male and female), cycle regularity, and the timing of intercourse. Spontaneous abortions, congenital malformations, the sex ratio, and twinning are all considered.

Materials and Methods

Results from four studies will be presented. Those studies are described below.

Cohort Study (GEFCO)

This prospective study recruited couples who were trying to conceive by placing articles and advertisements in newspapers from 1979 to 1982. Initially, general information about the man, the woman, and the couple was collected, in part through questionnaires filled out by the couples themselves. The women then filled out and sent in a temperature curve chart for each menstrual cycle, recording on it acts of intercourse and other relevant events. The couples also supplied information on the progress and outcome of any pregnancies, including the results of the midwife's or paediatrician's examination at birth.

There were 2361 couples who agreed to participate in the study. When the data were analysed, 1246 of the couples (53 per cent) had established a pregnancy, with a known outcome in 1200 cases (97 per cent). Of the pregnancies with known outcomes, 148 ended in spontaneous abortions and 1052 in live births. There were 33 infants born with malformations (A. Spira *et al.*, 1985).

The analysis of all events during the menstrual cycle was based on the data recorded on the temperature charts. The same person analysed all the temperature curves, without knowledge of the outcome of any pregnancies. One important parameter of the analysis was the duration of the hypothermic phase, beginning on the first day of the menses and ending on day 0, the last low point before the nadir. The analysis considered all acts of intercourse up to day 21 of the cycle, selecting as the 'time of insemination' the one that occurred nearest to the nadir during the fertile period (day -7 to day $+3$) or, in the case of *ex aequo*, the one occurring before the nadir. When a woman reported that her menstrual cycles commonly varied in length by four days or more around the average, her cycles were classified as 'irregular'. The probability of conception was calculated as the conception rate during the first cycle.

Artificial Insemination Study (AID)

This study is based on a programme of artificial insemination with donor semen (AID) established in 1973. The women studied had husbands suffering from azoospermia or severe oligospermia and hence judged to be permanently sterile. All the women had at least one insemination during the fertile period, using frozen semen from donors who were married and aged 45 or younger. The data available for analysis were collected from 1973 to 1980 and concerned 1112 women, 13 280 cycles, and 342 donors (David *et al.*, 1980).

During the first two cycles of the programme, one insemination per cycle was performed on the day considered most appropriate, that is, the last day of hypothermia according to the temperature curves. Thereafter, there were no limitations on inseminations. Hence, the analysis of the time of insemination is restricted to those first two cycles. The probability of conception has been defined as the success rate per cycle.

Retrospective Study (RETRO)

This study is based on data collected from June 1980 to June 1982 in questionnaires completed anonymously by couples themselves. Questionnaires were systematically distributed to women during their first consultation for pregnancy at 13 maternity clinics and hospitals in Paris. Questionnaires were also sent to all women residing in a department in the Paris region who had registered a pregnancy (which is mandatory in France). The couples completed the questionnaires during the twentieth week of pregnancy, on average. Of the 5108 questionnaires collected, 54 per cent came from the maternity clinics and hospitals and 46 per cent from women who had registered their pregnancies.

The following information was collected: age, gravidity, parity, coital pattern, last contraceptive method used and the date it was discontinued, the initial date of intercourse without protection in the planning of the pregnancy, and the date of the last menstrual period. To simplify matters, the date of conception was defined as that of the last menstrual period. The average fertility of the various groups was evaluated by their fecundability, i.e. the proportion of women conceiving during their first cycle.

Generally, initial exposure to the risk of conception was adopted as a starting date. Depending on the couple, this could be either when they stopped using contraception or when they began having intercourse without protection. (Some couples, independently or on the advice of a physician, observed a waiting period after they stopped using contraception; during that time they employed techniques such as abstinence, withdrawal, and condoms.) These delays were termed 'cessation of precautions'.

Of the total sample of 5108, 1710 women were excluded from the analysis for various reasons. The study was concerned only with the fertility of couples who were planning a pregnancy, so the 675 cases of unwanted pregnancy were dropped. Another 505 couples did not know when the woman was first exposed to the risk of conception, either because they did not use contraception or could not remember when they stopped using contraception or taking precautions. The method of contraception was unidentified in 70 more cases, while the 460 foreign women were excluded to create a homogeneous group. Thus, the analysis was restricted to 3398 native French women (N. Spira *et al.*, 1985).

In Vitro Fertilization Study (IVF)

The data presented here are extracted from an international survey of the pregnancy outcomes of *in vitro* fertilization. The first report focused on ectopic pregnancies and covered the pregnancies obtained by 21 IVF teams from the time their centres opened until 31 December 1984. The aim of the second report was to give a worldwide overview of the obstetric outcomes for IVF conducted in 1985. Of the 120 IVF units asked to participate, 80 centres agreed to collaborate, and data from 55 centres was available for analysis. The final report included all clinically detected pregnancies (i.e. pregnancies determined biochemically were excluded) in 21 IVF centres over the years 1979 to 1985 and in another 34 centres for the year 1985 only.

All centres filled out questionnaires and sent them for processing to the Unit Santé Publique–Epidémiologie–Reproduction Humaine of the Institut National de la Santé et de la Recherche Médicale, Kremlin-Bicetre, France. The following data were provided for each pregnancy: the age of the woman, her obstetric history, the indication for IVF, the condition of her fallopian tubes, the mode and timing of the stimulation used for the conception cycle, the transfer date, and details on oocyte collection and pregnancy outcomes. When a woman had more than one pregnancy during the period studied, only the first was included in the analysis. The survey found a total of 2342 pregnancies, of which 13 (0.6 per cent) were excluded for lack of data on the outcome of the pregnancy. The analysis includes the remaining 2329 pregnancies (J. Cohen *et al.*, 1986).

Results

Male Age

Table 16.1 summarizes the results for the five pregnancy outcomes studied according to male age. There was no significant relationship between male age and any of the outcomes. In all four studies, however, male age was concentrated between 20 and 40 years of age, so that it would be difficult to show any effect at older ages.

TABLE 16.1. *Conception probability and pregnancy outcome according to male age, various studies*

	Male age					
	<20	20–4	25–9	30–4	35–9	40+
Probability of conception (%)						
GEFCO	—	18	17	16	14	17
AID	—	9	8	10	8	9
RETRO	21	33	39	41	35	24
Spontaneous abortions (%)						
GEFCO	—	16	12	11	11	18
AID	—	19	20	18	12	19
Malformations (%)						
GEFCO	—	4.3	3.0	3.1	1.4	4.6
Sex ratio						
GEFCO	—	94	93	126	95	91
Twinning (%)						
GEFCO	—	1.2	1.8	0.4	1.4	4.5

Female Age

Table 16.2 looks at the relationship between female age and the five pregnancy outcomes studied.

Probability of conception. Although the levels of fecundability vary according to the different protocols, the three studies which include this information exhibit the same trend. In the GEFCO and AID studies, the probability of

TABLE 16.2. *Conception probability and pregnancy outcome according to female age*

	Female age						Signific-ance ($p \leqslant$)
	<20	20–4	25–9	30–4	35–9	40+	
Probability of conception (%)							
GEFCO	10	19	16	14	13		0.001
AID	—	11	11	9	7		0.01
RETRO	28	33	41	37	33		0.001
Spontaneous abortions (%)							
GEFCO	10	15	10	12	17		
AID	—	19	15	22	25		0.05
IVF	—		23		28	27	0.05
Malformations (%)							
GEFCO	0.0	3.7	4.1	1.0	0.0		
AID	—	0.9	2.1	2.6	2.0		
IVF	—		1.9		2.9	6.1	
Sex ratio							
GEFCO	50	94	105	103	100		
AID	—	172	102	103	123		
IVF	—		107		124	78	
Twinning (%)							
GEFCO	0.0	1.7	1.2	1.5	0.0		
AID	—	4.1	3.8	2.9	0.0		
IVF	—		2.1		1.7	1.8	

conception peaks in the 20–4 year age-group; in the RETRO study, it peaks in the 25–9 year age-group. In all three studies, there is a significant decline after these peaks.

Spontaneous abortions. Once again, the three studies considered show the same trend, with spontaneous abortions increasing significantly after age 35. This effect seems to be more important in the GEFCO group (a 38 per cent increase) than in the AID and IVF groups. Moreover, the increase is marked in the GEFCO group only after age 35, while the increase begins in the other two groups as early as age 30.

Malformations. As is well known, the rate of malformations increases with maternal age. Our data does not illustrate this trend, however, because of the small number of cases involved.

Sex ratio. No relationship between maternal age and sex ratio could be shown.

Twinning rate. Because ovulation is frequently induced in artificial insemination and *in vitro* fertilization, these studies are not suitable for studying twinning rates. The GEFCO study, which looked at 'natural reproduction', did not reveal any association between female age and the twinning rate.

Cycle Regularity

In the three studies considered, cycles are termed 'regular' when the difference between the longest and shortest cycles was four days or less. When the difference in length was greater, the cycles have been termed 'irregular'. Thus, the regularity of the cycles is a characteristic of the woman herself. Table 16.3 summarizes the results.

TABLE 16.3. *Conception probability and pregnancy outcome according to cycle regularity*

	Cycle regularity		
	Regular	Irregular	Significance ($p \leqslant$)
Probability of conception (%)			
GEFCO	18	14	0.05
AID	9	9	
RETRO	39	31	0.001
Spontaneous abortions (%)			
GEFCO	13	12	
AID	18	18	
Malformations (%)			
GEFCO	1.8	5.6	0.01
AID	2.7	1.0	
Sex ratio			
GEFCO	91	119	0.05
AID	111	115	
Twinning (%)			
GEFCO	1.1	1.5	
AID	5.7	1.7	0.01

Probability of conception.   In the 'natural reproduction' studies (GEFCO and RETRO), fecundability is slightly higher among women with regular cycles. The increase in fecundability is of the same order of magnitude in both studies (28 per cent and 25 per cent, respectively). Such an increase is not observed in the AID study.

Spontaneous abortions.   Rates showed no relation to cycle regularity.

Malformations.   The risk of malformation was significantly increased ($R = 3.1$) among women with irregular cycles in the GEFCO study. This increase remains significant after taking into account confounding factors, such as maternal age.

Sex ratio.   The observed sex ratio is higher for women with irregular cycles, but the difference is significant only in the GEFCO study.

Twinning rate.   The results are contradictory: the GEFCO study found no association between the twinning rate and cycle regularity, while the AID study found the twinning rate to be lower for women with irregular cycles.

Time of Insemination

There were too few cases to study the relationship between time of insemination and the rates of malformation and twinning. Table 16.4 presents the results for conception probability and spontaneous abortions.

Probability of conception. In the GEFCO study, the results clearly show that the probability of conception reaches a maximum on day 0, which is the estimated day of the temperature shift. The conception rate is low on days −6 and −5, rises to an intermediate level on day −4, reaches a plateau on days −3 to +1, subsides to an intermediate level once again on day +2, and then declines to a low level.

The same general pattern is shown by the AID results. The plateau is shorter, however, lasting only from day −3 to day 0, and the maximum is observed on day −1.

Spontaneous abortions. In 'natural reproduction' (the GEFCO study), the spontaneous abortion rate is twice as high for conceptions occurring after the temperature shift (days +2 and +3) as for conceptions taking place earlier. Artificial insemination yields completely different results, although the trend is not significant. In the AID study, the spontaneous abortion rate is highest when conception takes place before the temperature shift, on days −4 to −2.

Sex ratio. There appears to be no relation at all between the sex ratio and the time of insemination.

Discussion

The four studies described here offered the advantage of large samples and allowed us to test the stability of the reported relationships. All together, about

TABLE 16.4. *Conception probability and pregnancy outcome according to the time of insemination*

Time of insemination (days in relation to the shift)	Probability of conception (%)		Spontaneous abortions		Sex ratio	
	GEFCO	AID	GEFCO	AID	GEFCO	AID
−6	14	—	11	—	129	
−5	17	—		—		
−4	25	8	10	27		57
−3	33	17		21	63	145
−2	32	13	11	23	141	154
−1	34	21	13	17	79	94
0	36	15	11	15	117	132
+1	34	9	12	14	83	84
+2	26	8	24	17	88	180
+3	19	—	29	—		
Significance ($p \leqslant$)	0.01	0.05	0.05			

8000 couples (or pregnancies) have been studied, and consistent results have been observed.

Paternal Age

It has been shown that an age-related reduction in sperm production occurs during meiosis in humans, as well as in Leydig and Sertoli cells (Johnson, 1986). This decrease seems to be regular, and no threshold value seems to exist (Johnson *et al.*, 1984). Based on the work of Johnson and colleagues (1984), sperm production decreases about 1 per cent annually after age 20. Thus, a young man with a sperm count of 100 million/ml should only reach a sperm count of 40 million/ml about 60 years later, by the time he is in his 80s. The standard deviation of this decrease, however, is quite large. The study of sperm characteristics in men supposed to be normal for their age has shown no significant decrease in semen volume and sperm count with age, and a decrease only in sperm motility, which begins to decline after 45 years of age (Schwartz *et al.*, 1983). Anderson (1975) has shown that there is no clear upper age limit on fertility in males, corresponding to menopause in females, but rather a general, almost linear, decline after 42.5 years of age.

In 50 to 60 per cent of all cases of spontaneous abortion, the conceptus is cytogenetically abnormal. It is well established that a relationship does exist between maternal age and these chromosomal aberrations. It is believed that in couples with repeated pregnancy losses (as opposed to infertility), women are more frequently affected cytogenetically than men. This is because chromosomal aberrations in males more often prevent them from fathering a child than cause pregnancy wastage. More than 15 per cent of azoospermic men have a chromosome abnormality (F. L. Cohen, 1986). Gene mutations seem to be statistically related to the age of the father, after taking into account maternal age and birth order. Such disorders as achondroplasia, Apert's syndrome, Mengan's syndrome, progeria, and haemophilia *A* can be related to paternal ageing. Some have speculated that Duchenne muscular dystrophy could also result from paternal ageing. In this case, the first mutation would appear in the grandfather, be transmitted to his daughters, and then be expressed in about half of his grandsons (Hutton and Thompson, 1970).

Ruder (1985) has reported a significant paternal age effect (independent of birth order and maternal age) in the sex ratio of live births among whites in the United States: the male to female sex ratio declines as paternal age increases. According to James (1987), this effect could be related to declining male androgen levels during the ageing process.

Maternal Age

It is difficult to study the effect of female age on the probability of conception for a variety of reasons, the main one being that social factors, including methods to control fertility, may have a greater impact than any biological effect. Historical studies, however, all indicate a decline in fertility with age (Guttmacher, 1939; Eaton and Mayer, 1953; Tietze, 1957). These results have been confirmed by more recent studies, in which only 24 per cent of women under age 25 required longer than 12 months to conceive, as opposed to 34 per cent of women aged 25–9 and 45 per cent of women aged 30 and over (Hendershot, 1984).

The 'natural reproduction' studies (GEFCO and RETRO) found the same decline in fertility with maternal age as did the 'artificial reproduction' studies. AID is of particular interest, because in many couples the husband is azoospermic. In this situation, the women may be considered 'normal'—or at least as normal as a single woman chosen at random from the general population. AID results are likely to underestimate the chances of conception because of the nature of the treatment and use of cryopreserved semen, but even so they are exactly the same as the results of natural reproduction.

In vitro fertilization studies also offer a special insight into fertility, especially when limited to couples who turn to IVF because of bilateral tubal occlusion. In this case, both the woman's ovarian function and the man's spermatogenesis can be assumed to be normal, unless there is a relation between infection and gametogenesis. The study of such cases in France has found that the probability of conception declines after age 37. This decline seems to be related to a decrease in the mean number of available oocytes (even after stimulation), to a decrease in the proportion of ova fertilized, and to a decrease in the effectiveness of the implantation process (de Mouzon *et al.*, 1987).

It is also possible that the consequences of pelvic inflammatory disease (PID) reduce the chances of conception. Tubal disease seems, even if it is not the first cause of infertility, to account for 15 to 20 per cent of these cases in developed countries (Hull, 1985; A. Spira, 1986). This factor is clearly related to age, as the probability of its occurrence increases with time. Thus it would predominantly affect older women, who have had prolonged exposure to such influences.

The relationship between maternal age and the risk of spontaneous abortion has been well documented (Lazar *et al.*, 1971). The evidence suggests that an increase in the incidence of chromosomally abnormal foetuses is responsible for the higher rate of spontaneous abortions among older women (Alberman *et al.*, 1976). The proportion of aborted foetuses with chromosomal abnormalities more than doubles from 8 per cent among women under age 20 to 17 per cent among women over age 40. While there has been much discussion in the literature about the respective roles of age and gravidity in producing abnormal embryos, Wilcox and Chaden (1982) have clearly demonstrated that the apparent effect of gravidity is artefactual. It is also clear from the literature that the frequency of chromosomally normal abortions rises with age, especially after age 37 (Stein *et al.*, 1980), which suggests a decline in uterine function.

The relation between maternal age and trisomy 21 has also been well documented (Juberg, 1984). In general, the frequency of spontaneous abortions with trisomic abnormalities rises with age. Here, however, the rise begins in the teenage years and increases exponentially until age 40. Thus, the shapes of the curves for chromosomally normal and trisomic abortions are dissimilar, both in the age at which the upward climb begins and in the relative risk between the extremes of age (Stein *et al.*, 1980). From these observations Stein (1985: 334) concludes that

in women the effect of aging on the quality of the ovum and, hence, on the viability of the embryo, appears at younger ages than does the effect of aging on the function of the uterus and its capacity to support the embryo. This is contrary to expectations based on the findings of most studies with laboratory animals.

There is also a well-known relationship between increasing maternal age and the risk of a congenital defect at birth. This risk has been extensively examined both in prospective and retrospective studies (Saxen *et al.*, 1974), from which it can be concluded that the risk is greater for women over age 40. It is interesting to note that the other prognostic factors are a history of stillbirths and abortions, the birth of other children with defects, and the threat of spontaneous abortion.

At least three different hypotheses have been proposed to explain this relationship. The first proposes that the risk of exposure to teratogen rises with increasing time, i.e. with age. Since the thalidomide problem in Europe in the 1960s, many researchers have focused on the relationship between malformations and the consumption of drugs early in pregnancy. These studies have been disappointing because, first, very few drugs (corticosteroids, aspirin) have been linked to the occurrence of congenital anomalies and, second, it has been nearly impossible to distinguish between the effects of the drug itself and the disease for which the drug was prescribed. The other hypotheses are the same as those proposed for spontaneous abortions.

Numerous analyses from 1926 to 1969 have yielded confusing and contradictory results with regard to the effects of birth order, paternal age, and maternal age on the sex ratio. Most of these reports, however, do not indicate any relationship between maternal age and the sex ratio at birth, when correctly taking into account confounding variables. This is also the case in the three studies we were able to analyse.

The relationship between maternal age and the twinning rate is not significant in our set of data. This relationship is, in fact, rather complex. The rate of dizygotic twinning routinely rises with maternal age, starting with the younger age-groups and becoming even more pronounced after age 30. Reproductive failures, however, become more important after age 30, even more so after age 35. As a consequence of these two phenomena, the rate of dizygotic twinning increases until about age 35 and then plummets dramatically, as dizygotic pregnancies are transformed into monozygotic pregnancies (Lazar *et al.*, 1978).

Cycle Regularity

The most important results from our studies relate to cycle regularity. This variable is significantly related to the probability of conception, the rate of congenital abnormalities, the sex ratio, and the twinning rate.

The relationship between cycle regularity and the probability of conception is significant only in 'natural reproduction' studies. In the 'artificial reproduction' programmes, the use of ovulation induction and hormonal treatments obviously modifies cycle characteristics.

There are at least two potential reasons why fecundability is higher when cycles are regular. First, regular cycles make it easier for couples who are trying to conceive to increase the frequency of intercourse during the fertile period. Second, cycle irregularity may reflect oocyte maturation problems or a hormonal imbalance. This second hypothesis is supported by other results: both the rates of malformations and twinning were higher among women with irregular cycles. The higher risk of congenital abnormalities for women with irregular cycles could, however, also be due to a longer delay between intercourse and conception. If couples do deliberately increase the frequency of intercourse during the supposed fertile period in the cycle, the existence of regular cycles would minimize the delay between intercourse and conception. This kind of interaction could also explain why this relationship is not found in the AID group.

It is surprising that the incidence of twinning is higher among women with regular cycles. However, Hemon *et al.* (1979) has reported similar results: 24 per cent of the mothers of singletons had irregular cycles, as compared to 15 per cent of the mothers of twins. While Treloar (1967), followed by Vollman (1977) and Bean *et al.* (1979), has stressed that there are large discrepancies between objectively reported and subjectively reported characteristics of the menstrual cycle, there is no reason why such a bias should exist in prospective studies like GEFCO and AID.

The relationship between cycle regularity and pregnancy outcome, especially the occurrence of congenital malformations, does not disappear even when other important variables are taken into account.

Time of Insemination

The relation between the time of insemination and the probability of conception has been extensively studied by many authors, and a complete review has been proposed by Potter and Millman (1986). When coital frequencies are low enough to make multiple coitions during the same fertile period unlikely, there is good agreement among several published models of fecundability. It is less certain what happens to fecundability at higher coital frequencies. Obviously, the higher the coital frequency, the shorter the delay between intercourse and conception, but this deserves further study.

Our results indicate that, as expected, the conception probability remains almost constant from day −3 to day +1 in 'natural reproduction'. The results are slightly different in AID with frozen semen, but this difference can be explained by the use of frozen semen and the modifications (including hormonal treatments) introduced by the AID programme. It would be interesting to study the effect of the delay between insemination and ovulation in women artificially inseminated with their husband's semen, but no such studies have been undertaken. This type of study would not only increase our knowledge of artificial insemination, but might also lead to practical improvements to artificial insemination programmes.

The most important study of the ageing of gametes and the risk of spontaneous abortion remains that of Guerrero and Lanctot (1972), who showed that the probability of spontaneous abortions was low for days around ovulation. These results suggest that the ageing of gametes, both spermatozoa and ova, are a cause of spontaneous abortion. Our results agree in part with those of Guerrero and Lanctot. In the GEFCO study, the probability of spontaneous abortion was raised only for late conceptions (days +2 and +3), when ovum ageing may be suspected. In the AID study, by contrast, the probability of spontaneous abortions was raised for early conceptions, raising the possibility of spermatozoon ageing.

These apparently contradictory results are less surprising since a similar contradiction appeared in Guerrero's (1974) study of the relationship between the time of insemination and the sex ratio at birth. This study found that when insemination took place on day 0, artificial insemination led to a higher sex ratio, while natural reproduction resulted in a minimal sex ratio. This is another proof of the important differences that may exist between 'natural' and 'artificial' reproduction or, at least, between fresh and cryopreserved semen. In our studies, however, there was no relationship at all between the time of insemination and sex ratio. This disagrees with the results of both Guerrero (1974) and Harlap (1979) results.

Conclusion

Natural reproduction is limited by a variety of factors, the most important of which seems to be the high incidence of spontaneous abortions. Some biological and behavioural factors, such as those studied in this paper, seem to be important risk factors for spontaneous abortion. Environmental factors, however, are supposed to be more important, especially considering their relationship with early embryo losses. The results of this study indicate that their importance must be evaluated while taking into account factors such as age, cycle regularity, and timing of intercourse.

References

Alberman, E., Creasy, M., Elliott, M., and Spicer, C. (1976), 'Maternal Factors Associated with Fetal Chromosomal Anomalies in Spontaneous Abortion', *British Journal of Obstetrics and Gynaecology* 83: 621–7.

Anderson, B. A. (1975), 'Results from Ireland prior to 1911', *Population Index* 41: 561–6.

Bean, J. A., Leeper, J. D., Wallace, R. B., Cherman, B. M., and Jagger, H. (1979), 'Variations in the Reporting of Menstrual Histories', *American Journal of Epidemiology*, 109: 181–5.

Cohen, F. L. (1986), 'Paternal Contribution to Birth Defects', *Nursing Clinics of North America* 21: 49–64.

Cohen, J., Mayaux, M. J., Guihard-Moscato, M. L., and Schwartz, D. (1986), 'In Vitro Fertilization and Embryo Transfer: A Collaborative Study of 1163 Pregnancies on the Incidence and Risk Factors of Ectopic Pregnancies', *Human Reproduction* 1: 255–8.

David, G., Czyglik, F., Mayaux, M. J., Martin-Boyce, A., and Schwartz, D. (1980), 'Artificial Insemination with Frozen Sperm: Protocol, Method of Analysis and Results for 1188 Women', *British Journal of Obstetrics and Gynaecology* 87: 1022–8.

de Mouzon, J., Belaisch-Allart, J., Dubuisson, J. B., Montagut, J., Testart, J., Bachelot, A., and Piette, C. (1987), 'Dossier FIVNAT: Analyse des résultats 1986. Géneralités, Indications, Stimulations, Rang de la Tentative, Age de la Femme', *Contraception, Fertilité, Sexualité* 15: 740–5.

Eaton, J. W., and Mayer, A. J. (1953), 'The Social Biology of very High Fertility among the Hutterites: The Demography of a very Unique Population', *Human Biology* 25: 206–64.

Guerrero, R. (1974), 'Association of the Type and Time of Insemination Within the Menstrual Cycle with the Human Sex at Birth', *New England Journal of Medicine* 291: 1056–9.

—— and Lanctot, C. A. (1972), 'Aging of Fertilizing Gametes and Spontaneous Abortion', *American Journal of Obstetrics and Gynecology* 113: 263–7.

Guttmacher, A. F. (1939), 'Factors Affecting Normal Expectation of Conception', *Journal of the American Medical Association* 161: 855–60.

Harlap, S. (1979), 'Gender of Infants Conceived on Different Days of the Menstrual Cycle', *New England Journal of Medicine* 300: 1445–8.

Hemon, D., Berger, C., and Lazar, P. (1979), 'The Etiology of Human Dizygotic Twinning with Special Reference to Spontaneous Abortions', *Acta Geneticae Medicae et Gemellologiae* 28: 253–8.

Hendershot, G. E. (1984), 'Maternal Age and Overdue Conceptions', *American Journal of Public Health* 74: 35–8.

Hull, M. G. R., Glazener, C. M. A., and Kelly, N. J. (1985), 'Population Study of Causes, Treatment and Outcome of Infertility', *British Medical Journal* 291: 1693–7.

Hutton, E. M., and Thompson, M. W. (1970), 'Paternal Age and Mutation Rate in Duchenne Muscular Dystrophy', *American Journal of Human Genetics* 26a: 22 (summer).

James, W. H. (1987), 'Sex Ratio, Paternal Age and Duration of Marriage', *American Journal of Human Genetics* 40: 287.

Johnson, L. (1986), 'Spermatogenesis and Aging in the Human', *Journal of Andrology* 7: 331–54.

—— Petty, C. S., and Neaves, W. B. (1984), 'Influence of Age on Sperm Production and Testicular Weight in Men', *Journal of Reproduction and Fertility* 70: 211–18.

Juberg, R. C. (1984), 'Origin of Non-disjunction in Trisomy 21 Syndrome: All Studies Compiled, Parental Age Analysis and International Comparisons', *American Journal of Human Genetics* 16: 111–16.

Lazar, P., Hemon, D., and Berger, C. (1978), 'Twinning Rate and Reproduction Failures', in A. R. Liss (ed.), *Twin Research: Biology and Epidemiology*: Academie des Sciences, Paris: 125–32.

—— Gueguen, S., Boué, J., and Boué, A. (1971), 'Sur la distribution des ages de 715 mères ayant eu un avortement spontané précoce', *Comptes Rendus Hebdomadaires des Séances de l'Academie des Sciences Serie A* 272: 2852–5.

Potter, R. G., and Millman, S. R. (1986), 'Fecundability and the Frequency of Marital Intercourse: New Models Incorporating the Aging of Gametes', *Population Studies* 40: 159–70.

Ruder, A. (1985), 'Paternal Age and Birth Order Effect on the Human Secondary Sex Ratio', *American Journal of Human Genetics* 37: 362–72.

Saxen, L., Klemetti, A., and Haro, S. (1974), 'A Matched Pair Register for Studies of Selected Congenital Defects', *American Journal of Epidemiology* 100: 297–306.

Schwartz, D., Mayaux, M. J., Spira, A., Moscato, M. L., Jouannet, P., Czyglik, F., and David, G. (1983), 'Semen Characteristics as a Function of Age in 833 Fertile Men', *Fertility and Sterility* 3: 530–5.

Spira, A. (1986), 'Epidemiology of Human Reproduction', *Human Reproduction* 1: 111–15.

—— Spira, N., Papiernik-Berkauer, E., and Schwartz, D. (1985), 'Pattern of Menstrual Cycles and Incidence of Congenital Malformations', *Early Human Development* 11: 317–24.

Spira, N., Spira, A., and Schwartz, D. (1985), 'Fertility of Couples Following Cessation of Contraception', *Journal of Biosocial Science* 17: 281–90.

Stein, Z. A. (1985), 'A Woman's Age: Childbearing and Child Rearing', *American Journal of Epidemiology* 121: 327–42.

—— Kline, J., and Susser E. (1980), 'Maternal Age and Spontaneous Abortion', in I. H. Porter, and E. B. Hook (eds.), *Human Embryonic and Fetal Death*: 107–27, Academic Press, New York.

Tietze, C. (1957), 'Reproductive Span and Rate of Reproduction among Hutterite Women', *Fertility and Sterility* 8: 89–97.

Treloar, A. (1967), 'Variations of the Human Menstrual Cycle through Reproductive Life', *International Journal of Fertility* 12: 77–126.

Vollman, R. F. (1977), *The Menstrual Cycle*, Saunders, Philadelphia, Pa., London and Toronto.

Wilcox, A. J., and Chaden, B. C. (1982), 'Spontaneous Abortion: The Role of Heterogeneous Risk and Selective Fertility', *Early Human Development* 7: 165–78.

Part VI

Causes and Frequency of Foetal Loss

17 Biological Causes of Foetal Loss

JOE LEIGH SIMPSON

SANDRA CARSON

Some 10 to 15 per cent of recognized pregnancies are lost during the first trimester, and an additional 2 to 3 per cent are lost later in pregnancy. In addition, many conceptions are lost before they are even recognized clinically. We shall first consider the frequency of foetal wastage during various stages of gestation. Thereafter, we shall review the causes of spontaneous abortions, emphasizing factors that serve as potential confounding variables. Clinical management is reviewed elsewhere (Carson and Simpson, 1990).

Pre-clinical Losses

That foetal loss rates occur prior to clinical recognition of pregnancy can be concluded from several studies. The first study prospectively utilizing sensitive β-hCG (human chorionic gonadotropin) assays to determine frequencies of losses was that of Miller *et al.* (1980). These investigators studied 197 ovulating women aged 25–35 years. Beginning 21 days after the previous menses and continuing until menstruation or pregnancy, urinary β-hCG assay was performed on alternate days in 623 cycles. Pregnancy was defined as either a single value of 5 μg/L or as 2 values of 2 μg/L. In 152 of the 623 cycles, β-hCG was sufficiently elevated to justify the diagnosis of pregnancy. However, in only 102 of 152 (67 per cent) was pregnancy appreciated clinically. Of the 102 conceptions showing clinical evidence of pregnancy, 14 were later lost (14 per cent). The overall frequency of losses (clinical and sub-clinical) was 43 per cent.

Using a different assay, Edmonds *et al.* (1982) tested women 21 days after their last menstrual period. Of 198 ovulatory cycles, 118 were characterized by elevated β-hCG. However, only 51 of the 118 (43 per cent) women with a β-hCG value of 56 IU/L subsequently showed clinical evidence of pregnancy. Of these 51, six (12 per cent) experienced clinically recognized abortions.

Performing β-hCG serum radio-immunoassay 25 days after the previous menses, Whittaker *et al.* (1983) studied 226 cycles in 91 women. Neither women in the follicular phase nor men showed values greater than 4 mU/mL. Of the 226 cycles, 92 were characterized by β-hCG 16 mU/mL or greater; 85 of the 92 (92 per cent) had clinically recognized pregnancy, revealing a pre-clinical loss rate much lower than observed by Edmonds *et al.* (1982) and

Miller *et al.* (1980). Of the 85, 11 (13 per cent) terminated in spontaneous abortion.

A slightly different design was utilized by one of us in a National Institutes of Child Health and Development (NICHD) collaborative cohort prospective study (Mills *et al.*, 1988). The sample consisted of women identified before pregnancy. Pregnancy tests were usually performed 16 days after ovulation was confirmed by basal body temperature analysis (two days after expected menses); no participant was more than 35 (gestational) days pregnant. Foetal loss rates (pre-clinical and clinical) in 460 normal women proved to be only 16.2 per cent. One logical explanation for the lower loss rate we observed is that substantial selection occurs at or immediately after implantation, a stage too early to have been detected with our experimental design.

There are several potential explanations for the general phenomenon of pre-clinical losses. However, the one unequivocal explanation is morphological and genetic abnormalities in early embryos. Studies not likely to be repeated in the United States were conducted decades ago by Hertig and Rock (Hertig *et al.*, 1956, 1959; Hertig and Rock, 1973). These workers examined the fallopian tubes, uterine cavities, and endometria of women undergoing elective hyster-ectomy. All women were of proved fertility, and their mean age was 33.6 years. Coital times were recorded prior to hysterectomy. Over many years, eight pre-implantation embryos (less than 6 days from conception) were recovered. Four of these embryos were morphologically abnormal. The four abnormal embryos presumably would not have implanted. If implanted, they would not have survived very long thereafter. Similarly, nine of 26 implanted embryos (6–14 embryonic days) were morphologically abnormal, likewise presumably being unlikely to develop further.

Although currently not possible in the United States, cytogenetic analysis of early human pre-implantation embryos is performed in Europe. In aggregate, chromosomal abnormalities are observed in approximately 20 per cent of *in vitro* fertilized embryos (Angell *et al.*, 1983; Rudak *et al.*, 1985; Zenzes *et al.*, 1985; Michelman *et al.*, 1986). Reported abnormalities included monosomy, trisomy, haploidy, and polyploidy. The largest single study is that of Plachot *et al.* (1987). Of 69 human embryos recovered at the two- to eight-cell stages, relatively few embryos could actually be karyotyped. However, 3 of 68 analysed by Plachot and colleagues showed only a single pronucleus, presumably being haploid; 1 of the 3 was also monosomic for a C-group chromosome. Of 15 other embryos showing 3 or more pronuclei, 7 were grossly triploid, 3 triploid–diploid mosaics, 2 polyploid, and only 3 grossly diploid. However, none of the 3 grossly diploid embryos could be verified by full chromosomal analysis to be normal. The 50 remaining embryos showed three pronuclei; however, 37 could not be karyotyped. Of the 13 that could be karyotyped, only 5 were cytogenetically normal. We can thus conclude that chromosomal abnormalities are not only frequent, but plausibly could be responsible for many of the early morphological abnormalities documented by Hertig and Rock.

There are further animal studies consistent with this conclusion, such as those by Gropp (1973, 1975). Mice heterozygous for various Robertsonian translocations were mated to produce various monosomies and trisomies. By selective mating and sacrifice of pregnant females, both survivability and phenotypic characteristics of the various aberrant complements could be determined. In mice, as in man, autosomal monosomy proved inviable. Monosomes usually aborted within 4–5 days of conception (i.e. around implantation) (Fig. 17.1). Trisomies were lost later, with only a few (trisomies 12 and 19) surviving until live birth.

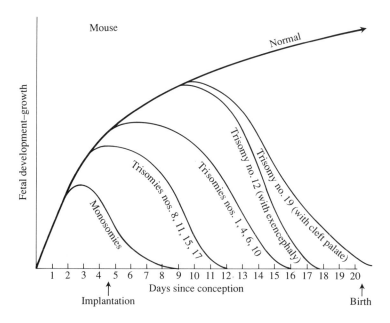

Source: Gropp, 1975.

Fig. 17.1   Relative timing for loss of murine autosomal monosomy and murine autosomal trisomy

Frequency and Timing of Clinically Recognized Losses

Clinically recognized foetal loss rates of 12–15 per cent are well documented (Simpson and Mills, 1986). However, the timing of these losses has recently been placed in doubt. Traditionally, such losses were recognized after 8 weeks' gestation on the basis of such clinical criteria as the passage of tissue (products of conception), the opening of the cervical os, uterine contractions, or bleeding. Using such criteria, Stevenson *et al*. (1959) observed that 45 per cent of losses were recognized and, hence, assumed to occur between gestational weeks 7 to 11; 30 per cent occurred between gestational weeks 12 and 15; few clinical losses were recognized before 7 weeks.

The timing of clinical losses cited above has now been shown to be erroneous. Ultrasonographical criteria make it clear that foetal demise usually occurs long before overt clinical signs are manifested. That is, foetuses aborting clinically at 10–12 weeks have usually died weeks previously. The phenomenon of a retained dead foetus in utero is termed 'missed abortion'.

One source of data that leads to the conclusion that clinically recognized losses usually represent missed abortions of perhaps 3–4 weeks were studies of obstetrical registrants routinely subjected to ultrasonography. Christiaens and Stoutenbeek (1984) identified 274 women in whom a viable pregnancy was confirmed by ultrasound at an initial obstetric visit before 10 weeks' gestation. A second ultrasound at 16 weeks revealed 3.3 per cent of these pregnancies to have been lost in the interim. Wilson *et al.* (1984) similarly studied 734 women in whom an ultrasonographically normal pregnancy was documented at their first obstetric visit (7–12 weeks). The loss rate between the initial visit and 20 weeks was 2.4 per cent. The loss rate was 4.5 per cent in women whose age was greater than 35 years, 2.5 per cent among those women aged 30–5 years, and 1.5 per cent among women under 30 years. Similar conclusions were reported by Gilmore and McNay (1985) and Cashner *et al.* (1987).

Although informative, studies of obstetrical registrants potentially suffer from methodological shortcomings regarding selection biases. Are women registering at 7–10 weeks' gestation unusually health conscious, and thus at low risk for abortion? Conversely, do such women have valid reasons to be concerned about their pregnancy, being at high risk? The prospective cohort study of Simpson *et al.* (1987) was not subject to such selection biases. In the National Institutes of Child Health and Development (NICHD) Diabetes in Early Pregnancy (DIEP) sample, subjects were recruited prior to conception; thus, biases of selection were minimized. The cohort consisted of 220 ultrasonographically-proved normal timed pregnancies of 8 weeks' gestation. The loss rate between 8 gestational weeks and delivery was 3.2 per cent, similar to data reported from studies of obstetrical registrants.

It is worth emphasizing the significance of these data to actuarially-calculated loss rates. Inasmuch as the time at which clinical recognition of abortion occurs is no longer accepted to correspond to the time of embryonic demise, certain actuarial derivations need to be altered. In particular, estimation of loss rates at a given gestational interval are invalid if their derivation utilizes data based upon the assumption that foetal demise coincides with onset of clinical symptoms. New data-sets are necessary, namely those verifying foetal demise on the basis of ultrasound criteria.

When does foetal demise occur in the 3 per cent of pregnancies lost after confirmed viability at 8 gestational weeks? One informative study is that of Tabor *et al.* (1986). Background foetal loss rates were 0.7 per cent in 30–4-year-old women confirmed by ultrasound to have viable pregnancies at 16 weeks. In the 1978 United Kingdom Amniocentesis study (Working Party on Amniocentesis, 1978), loss rates in a slightly older cohort were not dissimilar (1.1 per cent). Thus, we can conclude that perhaps two-thirds of losses occurring after the first 18 weeks of gestation are lost during gestational weeks 9–16. After 16 weeks, losses are uncommon (1 per cent) and heavily influenced by maternal risk factors such as incompetent cervix or serious systemic illnesses (e.g. lupus erythematosis).

Causes of Clinically Recognized Losses

Numerical Chromosomal Abnormalities (Aneuploidy and Polyploidy)

First Trimester. At least 50 per cent of clinically recognized pregnancy losses result from cytogenetic abnormalities. Relatively minor differences in frequencies exist among various studies, but these are readily attributable to variations in maternal age or gestational stage.

Autosomal trisomies comprise the largest single class of abnormal chromosomal complements in spontaneous abortions (Simpson and Bombard, 1987). Of all abnormal complements, 53 per cent are trisomic. Approximately 25 per cent of all abortuses are trisomic (Table 17.1). Trisomy for every chromosome except no. 1 has been reported, and trisomy for that chromosome has been observed in an eight-cell embryo (Watt *et al.*, 1987). Boué *et al.* (1976) observed that most trisomic conceptuses fail to progress beyond the stage expected for 8 gestational weeks or less. (Data cited above concerning the timing of losses are consistent with this thesis.) A few trisomies show specific anatomic features. Traditionally defined 'blighted ova' is claimed for trisomies 2, 3, 4, and 5. Group C (6–12) trisomies usually show some foetal tissue (Boué *et al.*, 1976). Cyclopia and other facial anomalies are observed in trisomy D (13–15, predominantly 13).

Trisomy has a cytological counterpart—monosomy. The latter is rarely, if ever, observed in humans. The data on humans are thus comparable to those collected by Gropp (1973, 1975), who observed that murine monosomies fail to survive implantation.

Polyploidy is the presence of more than two haploid chromosomal complements. Triploidy ($3n = 69$) and tetraploidy ($4n = 92$) occur frequently in abortuses (Table 17.1). The mean duration of survival for triploid conceptuses is about 5 weeks of embryonic life (7 weeks' gestation) (Boué *et al.*, 1976). Pathological characteristics of triploid placentas include disproportionately large gestational sac, variable cystic degeneration of placental villi, intrachorial haemorrhage, and hypotrophic trophoblasts (pseudomolar degeneration). Triploid abortuses are usually 69,XXY or 69,XXX, resulting from dispermy (Jacobs *et al.*, 1978). Tetraploid conceptuses are uncommon, rarely progressing beyond 2 to 3 weeks of embryonic life (4–5 weeks' gestation). Pathological specimens often show only chorionic vesicles (Boué *et al.*, 1976).

TABLE 17.1. *Chromosomal complements in spontaneous abortions recognized clinically in the first trimester*

Complement	Frequency	%
Normal		
46,XX or 46,XY		54.1
Triploidy		7.7
69,XXX	2.7	
69,XYX	0.2	
69,XXY	4.0	
Other	0.8	
Tetraploidy		2.6
92,XXX	1.5	
92,XXYY	0.55	
Not stated	0.55	
Monosomy X		8.6
Structural abnormalities		1.5
Sex chromosomal polysomy		0.2
47,XXX	0.5	
47,XXY	0.15	
Autosomal monosomy (G)		0.1
Autosomal trisomy		22.3
Chromosome no.		
1	0	
2	1.11	
3	0.25	
4	0.64	
5	0.04	
6	0.14	
7	0.89	
8	0.79	
9	0.72	
10	0.36	
11	0.04	
12	0.18	
13	1.07	
14	0.82	
15	1.68	
16	7.27	
17	0.18	
18	1.15	
19	0.01	
20	0.61	
21	2.11	
22	2.26	

Monosomy X is the single most common chromosomal abnormality in spontaneous abortions, accounting for 20–50 per cent of all abnormal specimens. Monosomy X occurs in 8.6 per cent of all conceptions (approximately 20 per cent of chromosomally abnormal abortions). Characteristic placental morphology includes the presence of sub-chorial thromboses and avascular or hypovascular villi (Honoré *et al.*, 1976). Embryos may consist of only an umbilical cord stump. In foetuses surviving until later in gestation, anomalies characteristic of the Turner stigmata (Simpson, 1976) may be seen: horseshoe kidney, cystic hygromas, and generalized oedema. Monosomy X occurs as a result of paternal sex chromosome loss (Chandley, 1987). This observation is consistent with, but does not explain, the inverse maternal age effect characteristic of 45,X.

Although the frequencies of various chromosomal abnormalities seem well accepted, a few caveats are in order. One difficulty is the impossibility of determining the status of abortuses that fail to grow in culture. Could failures be disproportionately represented by chromosomal abnormalities? Indeed, this is not an illogical hypothesis, given growth retardation being characteristic of 45,X and possibly autosomal trisomy (Simpson and LeBeau, 1981). Guerneri *et al.* (1987) utilized chorionic villus sampling to recover tissue from women shown by ultrasound to have a foetal demise (i.e. prior to clinical manifestation); culture success rates were higher (90 per cent) than usual (60–70 per cent), and 77 per cent of samples showed cytogenetic abnormalities. On the other hand, cytogenetically normal abortuses might preferentially have failed to grow because they were infected, although the nature of the study by Guerneri and colleagues makes this possibility unlikely. Another difficulty is determining whether the material (villi or membrane) being cultured truly reflects embryonic status. In chorionic villus sampling (CVS), we and others have observed cytogenetic abnormalities that were not confirmed upon culturing embryonic tissue. In particular, there is growing recognition that 45,X cells and certain lethal trisomies (e.g. +16) in villi need not necessarily indicate an abnormal embryo.

Second and Third Trimester. It would be of great interest to know the prevalence of chromosomal abnormalities in losses occurring in pregnancies known to have been viable at 8 weeks' gestation. As is already apparent, however, the high frequency of missed abortion in the first trimester invalidates previous attempts to correlate precisely the frequency of chromosomal abnormalities with gestational interval. Even taking into account the phenomenon of missed abortions, however, the frequency of chromosomal errors in losses recognized between 16 and 28 weeks seems to be less than that observed in losses recognized earlier (Ruzicska and Cziezel, 1971; Warburton *et al.*, 1980). In the second trimester, one also observes chromosomal abnormalities similar to those observed in liveborn infants: trisomies 13, 18, and 21; monosomy X; and sex chromosomal polysomies. Moreover, anatomical findings in such abortuses are reminiscent of those present in aneuploid liveborns.

The frequency of chromosomal abnormalities in third trimester losses (traditionally designated stillborn infants) is about 5 per cent. This frequency is far less than that observed in earlier abortuses, but still higher than in liveborns (0.6 per cent). The database supporting this contention is relatively large. One illustrative study is that of Sutherland *et al.* (1974), who found that 7.2 per cent of perinatal deaths ($n = 153$) could be attributed to a chromosomal abnormality. Kuleshov (1976) published cytogenetic data on 175 of 315 infants dying in the perinatal period. 12 (6.9 per cent) of the 175 were chromosomally abnormal: three of 22 (13.6 per cent) ante-partum deaths, three of 61 (4.9 per cent) intra-partum deaths, and six of 92 (6.5 per cent) neonatal deaths. The author further studied 607 premature infants, 2.5 per cent of which were chromosomally abnormal. Half of the abnormalities were autosomal trisomies: nos. 13 ($n = 1$), 18 ($n = 2$), 21 ($n = 2$), and 22 ($n = 1$); monosomy X, 47,XYY, 69,XXX, and a deletion were observed once each, and there were two 46,XX/46,XY mosaics.

McLeod *et al.* (1979) studied 204 perinatal deaths, among which were 55 infants with multiple congenital anomalies. Of the 55, 30 were successfully karyotyped. Three of the 30 (6 per cent) showed an abnormal chromosomal complement: two autosomal trisomy and one triploidy. Of 124 stillborn or early neonatal deaths studied by Mueller *et al.* (1983), seven showed an abnormal chromosomal complement: three autosomal trisomy, one monosomy X, one triploidy, and two autosomal structural rearrangements. Of these seven, three were observed in infants whose abnormalities were not appreciated by gross examination (autopsy). Similar observations had previously been made by Sutherland *et al.* (1976) and by others, and presumably reflect maceration. On the basis of these data, routine cytogenetic evaluation could be recommended for all stillborns. Possible exceptions might exist if one recognizes a mutant gene (e.g. Meckel syndrome) or an isolated CNS anomaly (e.g. neural tube defect) of presumed polygenic/multifactorial aetiology (see Simpson *et al.*, 1982).

Recurrent Aneuploidy.   Numerical chromosomal abnormalities (aneuploidy) may also be responsible for recurrent foetal losses, thus constituting an important confounding variable. Such reasoning is based on observations that the complements of successive abortuses in a given family are more likely to be either consistently normal or consistently abnormal. That is, abortuses in a given family show non-random distribution with respect to chromosomal complements. If the complement of the first abortus is abnormal, the likelihood is 80 per cent that the complement of the second abortus will also be abnormal (Hassold, 1980). The recurrent abnormality is usually trisomy, but it may also be monosomy or polyploidy. These data suggest that certain couples are predisposed towards chromosomally abnormal conceptions, most of which naturally result in spontaneous abortion. On the other hand, Warburton *et al.* (1987) interpret these same data as indicating that corrections for maternal age render the phenomenon of recurrent aneuploidy statistically non-significant.

The issue remains contentious and highly relevant. If a couple were truly predisposed to recurrent aneuploidy, they might logically be at increased risk for aneuploid liveborns. The autosome trisomic in a subsequent pregnancy might not confer lethality (e.g. trisomy 16), but rather be compatible with life (e.g. trisomy 21). Available data do not allow one to determine whether liveborn aneuploidy is increased following aneuploid abortions. However, several studies suggest that the risk of liveborn trisomy 21 following a trisomic abortus is about 1 per cent (Alberman, 1981). The significance of recognizing recurrent aneuploidy for epidemiological studies is obvious, for an excess of women in this category could skew outcomes sharply.

Chromosomal Translocations

Structural chromosomal abnormalities are a well-accepted explanation for repetitive abortions and a less common explanation for losses in general. The most common structural rearrangement encountered is a translocation. Individuals with balanced translocations are phenotypically normal, but abortuses or abnormal liveborns may show duplications or deficiencies as a result of normal meiotic segregation (Fig. 17.2). Uncorrected for ascertainment, about 5 per cent of individuals (women and men) experiencing at least two abortions have a balanced translocation. Females are about twice as likely as males to show a balanced translocation (Simpson *et al.*, 1981). About 60 per cent of the translocations are reciprocal, the other 40 per cent being Robertsonian.

Among reported series, there are widely differing prevalence rates. One potential explanation for such differences is differing clinical practice. If cytogenetic studies are routinely performed on all couples experiencing recurrent foetal losses, relatively fewer translocations will be detected. By contrast, investigations restricted to couples experiencing not only abortions, but also stillborn infants or anomalous liveborn infants, will yield relatively more translocations (Simpson *et al.*, 1989) (Table 17.2). There are other unanswered questions: (1) are prevalence rates influenced by numbers of previous losses? and (2) does the occurrence of both first- and second-trimester losses affect prevalence rates?

If a balanced translocation is detected, antenatal cytogenetic studies should be offered in subsequent pregnancies. Actually, the frequency of unbalanced foetuses at 16 weeks (discovered through amniocentesis) appears to be lower if a balanced translocation is ascertained through repetitive abortions than if it is ascertained through an anomalous liveborn (Boué and Gallano, 1984).

Chromosomal Inversions

Another parental chromosomal rearrangement causing foetal loss is an inversion. In this intra-chromosomal rearrangement the order of genes is reversed. Such a rearrangement is usually caused by two chromosomal breaks, followed by reversal and reinsertion of the chromosomal segment produced by the breaks. Inversions in which break points exist on opposite sides of the centromere are

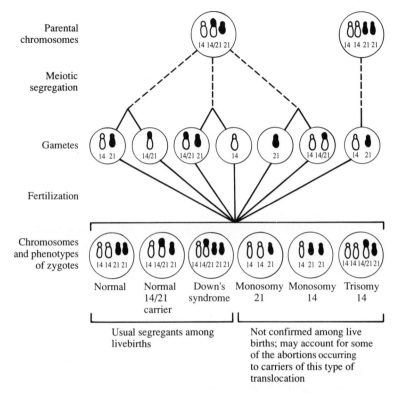

Three of the six possible gametes are incompatible with life. The likelihood that an individual with such a translocation would have a child with Down's syndrome is theoretically 33%. However, the empirical risk is considerably less.

Source: Gerbie and Simpson, 1976.

Fig. 17.2   Diagram of possible gametes and progeny of a phenotypically normal individual heterozygous for a Robertsonian translocation between chromosomes 14 and 21 (a form of D/G translocation)

TABLE 17.2. *Balanced translocations in couples experiencing repeated abortions*

Couples with or without normal liveborn		Couples with stillborn or abnormal liveborn		No subcategorization	
Female	Male	Female	Male	Female	Male
89/3712	57/3651	20/432	7/409	100/3074	65/3009
2.4%	1.0%	4.0%	1.7%	3.3%	2.1%

Source: Pooled data from Simpson *et al.* (1989) and 60 other reports.

pericentric; those in which break points are on the same side of the centromere are paracentric.

Heterozygotes for either pericentric or paracentric inversions may be normal if genes are neither lost, gained, nor altered as a result of the breaks leading to the inversion. However, individuals with inversions suffer abnormal reproductive consequences as a result of normal meiotic phenomena, namely crossing-over during meiosis I (Fig 17.3). In order for genes within inversions to pair, a

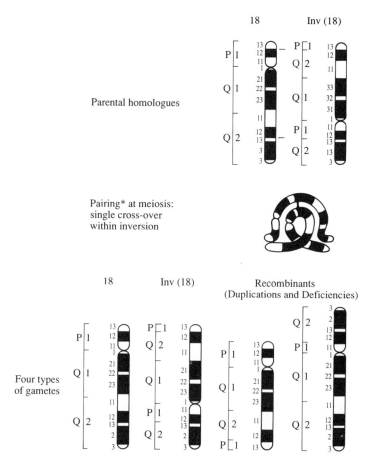

* Only two of the four strands are shown.

The inversion loop resulting from pairing during meiosis is shown. As a result, crossing over at meiosis I would be expected to produce the four types of gametes shown. Two of the four would be genetically balanced, although one would show the same inversion present in the parent. In addition, two types of gametes would be genetically unbalanced, showing complementary duplications and deficiencies. It is the chromosomal region outside the inverted segment that appears as a duplication or deletion.

Source: Martin *et al.*, 1983.

Fig. 17.3   Diagram illustrating the breakpoints leading to an inversion in chromosomes 18

loop must form during meiosis I. Crossing-over may or may not occur within an inversion loop, but it is likely to do so if the loop encompasses a large portion of the chromosome. If crossing-over occurs, certain gametes are unbalanced (Fig. 17.3).

The frequency of inversions among repeated aborters is low. However, this inversion is highly deleterious. A single crossover within a paracentric inversion results in both dicentric and acentric products. Both acentric and dicentric gametes contribute to foetal wastage. Because both outcomes are usually lethal, paracentric inversions are rarely associated with anomalous live births.

By contrast, pericentric inversions are likely to cause not only abortions but also anomalous liveborns. After crossing-over, we have noted that two of the four gametes represent the parental sequences (one normal, one inverted). The other two gametes represent recombinants, genes distal to one breakpoint deficient and genes distal to the other breakpoint duplicated (Fig. 17.3). The prevalence of pericentric inversions among couples experiencing repetitive abortions seems to be considerably lower than the prevalence of balanced translocations. Pooled data suggest that inversions exist in 0.1 per cent of females and 0.1 per cent of males experiencing repeated spontaneous abortions.

Luteal Phase (Progesterone) Deficiency (LPD)

Early pregnancy abnormalities resulting from implantation in an unsupportive endometrial environment provide a very plausible explanation for spontaneous abortion. The term luteal phase deficiency (LPD) is used to describe an endometrium manifesting inadequate progesterone effect. Such an abnormality may arise from abnormal progesterone milieu, as a result of either poor endometrial progesterone receptor function or low progesterone production. In the latter, the corpus luteum may be unable to secrete progesterone in quantities sufficient to maintain the pregnancy until placental secretion becomes self-sustaining (5 weeks post conception or 7 weeks' gestation).

Luteal phase deficiency is of unknown frequency. In fact, even its validity could be argued. The phenomenon could also merely be a secondary effect, the primary defect being an (abnormal) embryo that cannot trigger the appropriate signal for luteal function. Thus, coexistence of LPD and trisomy 16 has been reported (Wentz *et al.*, 1984). Alternatively, an abnormality in follicle-stimulating hormone (FSH) secretion could independently lead to both LPD and aneuploidy. Cytogenetic data on conceptuses that allegedly abort as a result of LPD are needed to answer this question.

Luteal phase deficiency is diagnosed on the basis of two endometrial biopsies, each showing a lag of two days or more behind that expected on the basis of timed ovulation. Treatment consists of progesterone administration or clomiphene citrate. Although these agents are believed to prevent repetitive abortion, definitive proof is actually lacking because randomized studies have not been reported.

A typical study claiming effective treatment is that of Tho *et al.* (1979). Luteal phase deficiency was diagnosed in 23 of 100 couples with repetitive abortions. Of 23 women treated with progesterone suppositories, 21 completed pregnancies. Unfortunately, there was no control group. The closest approximation was a subset of 37 couples who had no demonstrable explanation for their repetitive abortions. Of the 37, 22 were treated 'empirically' with progesterone, while 15 were not. Sixteen of the 22 treated women (73 per cent) had successful pregnancies, whereas only seven of the 15 (47 per cent) untreated women had successful pregnancies. Although the success rate following treatment was ostensibly good, it was actually only marginally better than expected on the basis of empirical recurrence risks (60–70 per cent). In fact, other studies have shown comparable or even better success rates in repeated aborters who undergo no treatment (Vlaanderen and Treffers, 1987).

Probably the most persuasive study confirming the existence of LPD is that of Daly *et al.* (1983), who ascertained the phenomenon not in aborters but rather in infertile women. Only those women with LPD showing endometria capable of being 'corrected' by progesterone retained future pregnancies; women whose endometria continued to show LPD following progesterone administration failed to carry to term.

Given the controversy in this area, treatment should be instituted only if the diagnosis is firmly documented and only after couples are apprised of claims of teratogenicity.

Thyroid Abnormalities

Decreased conception rates clearly occur with overt hypothyroidism or overt hyperthyroidism. However, data implicating sub-clinical thyroid dysfunction with foetal losses are lacking. Some studies purporting to show a relationship may be questioned on the basis of the diagnostic criteria, whereas all lack proper controls.

Diabetes Mellitus

Spontaneous abortion rates are no higher among patients with moderately well controlled diabetes mellitus than among controls. The large prospective collaborative study conducted by our group (Diabetes in Early Pregnancy Study; Mills *et al.*, 1988) was unique in that metabolic data were gathered from the fifth week of gestation. Loss rates were subjected to analysis for a host of potentially confounding variables. Overall no significant differences in loss rates existed between controls (15.6 per cent) and women with insulin-dependent diabetes mellitus. However, loss rates were significantly higher in diabetic women whose initial glycosylateal haemoglobin was <4 SD of the control mean, compared to those diabetic women who were in better control. Thus, poorly controlled diabetes mellitus is associated with increased loss rates, but not well controlled or sub-clinical diabetes mellitus.

Intra-Uterine Adhesions (Synechiae)

Intra-uterine adhesions could interfere with implantation of early embryonic development. Adhesions may follow over-zealous curretage of the uterus during the post-partum period, intra-uterine surgery (e.g. myomectomy), or endometritis. Curettage accounts for most cases, with adhesions most likely to develop when the procedure is performed 3 or 4 weeks post-partum. Affected individuals are usually suspected because of menstrual abnormalities, but 15–30 per cent show repeated abortions. If adhesions are detected in a woman experiencing repetitive losses, lysis of the adhesions under direct hyperoscopic visualization should be performed. Approximately 50 per cent of subjects conceive after surgery, but the frequency of abortions remains high.

Incomplete Mullerian Fusion

Failure of the embryologically paired mullerian ducts to fuse and canalize occurs in approximately 0.1 per cent of all females (Simpson, 1976). Uterine fusion defects (Fig. 17.4) include uterus unicornis (absence of one uterine horn), with or without a coexisting contra-lateral rudimentary hemi-uterus; uterus subseptus (persistence of a complete uterine septum); uterus bicornis bicollis (two separate uterine cavities, each of which leads to a separate cervix and separate vagina with the two vaginas separated by a septum); and completely separated hemi-uterus with not only separate cervices and separate vaginas but also separate perineal orifices. Anomalies may be diagnosed at delivery by exploration of the uterine cavity. In the non-pregnant patient, these malformations may be suspected on pelvic examination. Hystero-salpingography and hysteroscopy are of great value in determining configuration of the uterine cavity; ultrasound may be helpful.

In incomplete uterine fusion, the pregnant uterus may be unable to accommodate the growing foetus, and the placenta may implant on a poorly vascularized septum. First-trimester abortions occurring after ultrasonographic confirmation of a viable pregnancy at 8 or 9 weeks may also be plausibly attributed to uterine fusion defects. (Those occurring at 10 to 12 weeks' gestation without confirmation of prior viability are statistically more likely to represent missed abortions, foetal demise having occurred before 8 weeks' gestation.)

Uterine fusion defects are more widely accepted as a cause of second-trimester abortions, but not rigorously studied. The prevalence of abortions in patients with such defects may be as high as 20–25 per cent (Heinonen *et al.*, 1982). Loss rates may be higher with septate and bicornuate uteri than with unicornuate uteri or uteri didelphys; however, data are sparse and not gathered in prospective cohort fashion.

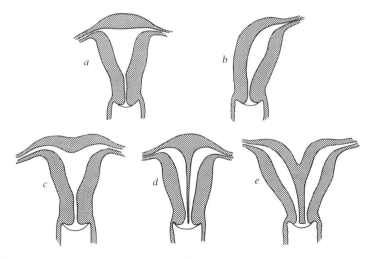

(*a*) normal uterus, fallopian tubes, and cervix; (*b*) uterus unicornis (absence of one uterine horn); (*c*) uterus arcuatus (broadening and medial depression of a portion of the uterine septum); (*d*) uterus septus (persistence of a complete uterine septum); and (*e*) uterus bicornis unicollis (two hemiuteri, each leading to same cervix).

Source: Simpson, 1976.

Fig. 17.4   Diagrammatic representation of some mullerian fusion anomalies

Women experiencing second trimester abortions and shown to have a mullerian fusion anomaly may benefit from uterine reconstruction; however, careful selection is important for optimal results.

Leiomyomas

Uterine leiomyomas are well-circumscribed, non-encapsulated benign tumours consisting of smooth muscle and varying amounts of fibrous connective tissue. The lesions are usually multiple. Although leiomyomata occur very frequently, relatively few women develop symptoms necessitating medical or surgical therapy. A contribution to pregnancy wastage is plausible but probably uncommon. Some gynaecologists erroneously conclude that the coexistence of uterine leiomyomata and reproductive losses always implies a causal relationship between the two phenomena. Actually, no solid epidemiological data exist.

The location of leiomyomata is probably more important than their size in causing abortions. Sub-mucous leiomyomas are the type most likely to cause a foetal loss, acting through several potential mechanisms: (1) thinning of the endometrium over the surface of a sub-mucous leiomyoma could predispose to implantation in a poorly decidualized site; (2) rapid growth under the hormonal milieu of pregnancy might compromise the blood supply of the leiomyoma, resulting in necrosis ('red degeneration') that in turn leads to uterine contractions and foetal expulsion; and (3) large leiomyomas may encroach upon the space required by the developing foetus, thereby leading to premature delivery through mechanisms analogous to those present in incomplete mullerian fusion. Lack of space can also lead to foetal deformations.

Myomectomy may occasionally be warranted for women experiencing repetitive second-trimester abortions. Careful patient selection is important.

Incompetent Cervix

A functionally intact cervix and lower uterine cavity is an obvious necessity for a successful intra-uterine pregnancy. Cervical incompetence is characterized by painless dilatation and effacement, usually during the mid-second or early third trimester. Cervical incompetence frequently follows antecedent traumatic events such as surgical dilatation, cervical lacerations, cervical amputations, conization, or cauterization. A history of premature cervical dilation during pregnancy suggests the diagnosis, which is not always easy to verify. Diagnosis may be confirmed in the non-pregnant state if an object of fixed diameter (e.g. no. 8 Hegar dilator) easily traverses the internal cervical os. Ultrasonography readily confirms that dilation has already occurred, but it is less helpful in identifying women destined to experience premature cervical dilatation. Various operations for correcting cervical incompetence have been proposed, with success rates approximating 80 per cent (Rock and Jones, 1977).

Infections

Infections are a well-known cause of late foetal wastage, and logically could be responsible for early foetal loss as well. Any of several mechanisms could be responsible: (1) intra-uterine foetal demise resulting from overwhelming infection; (2) micro-organisms interfering with organogenesis to such an extent that differentiation can no longer proceed; (3) fever *per se*; and (4) the teratogenic action of agents used to treat the infection. However, it remains contentious whether a given infectious agent actually caused the demise or merely arose after the foetal demise. Lack of knowledge concerning cytogenetic and endocrine status makes it almost impossible to address the above issues in a truly satisfactory fashion.

Micro-organisms associated with spontaneous abortion include *Variola*, *Vaccina*, *Salmonella typhi*, *Vibrio foetus*, *Malaria*, *Cytomegalovirus*, *Brucella Toxoplasmosis*, *Mycoplasma hominis*, *Chlamydia trachomatis*, and *Ureaplasma urealyticum*. Data showing risks for foetal loss are not available for any of these. *Ureaplasma urealyticum* is most frequently implicated in repetitive abortion, for which some data are available.

Stray-Pedersen *et al.* (1978) studied 46 women with histories of three or more consecutive losses of unknown aetiology. Endometrial *Ureaplasma* colonization proved significantly more frequent among women with repetitive abortions (28 per cent) than among female controls (7 per cent). Of 43 women in the former group, 13 harboured *Ureaplasma* in both cervix and endometrium. In 12 patients, the organism was found only in the cervix, a circumstance less plausibly likely to cause abortions because *Ureaplasma* is ordinarily ubiquitous in the vagina. The 43 women and their husbands were then treated with doxycycline for 11 days, with subsequent cultures showing no *Ureaplasma*. Nineteen of the 43 women became pregnant after treatment. Of these 19 women, three experienced another spontaneous abortion, and 16 had normal full-term infants. Among 18 women with *Ureaplasma* who were not treated, there were five more abortions and five full-term pregnancies.

Antibiotic therapy regardless of culture results is suggested to be of benefit to couples experiencing repetitive spontaneous abortions. In a study of pregnancy outcome by Toth *et al.* (1986), only 10 per cent of patients who were treated with tetracycline for four weeks and who became pregnant experienced another spontaneous abortion. By contrast, 38 per cent of patients who did not choose to take antibiotics and who later became pregnant had another spontaneous abortion. Because antibiotics were or were not given in accordance to the patients' desires the validity of the 'control' group is arguable. On the basis of this study, it is therefore difficult to draw any firm conclusion about the relationship of infectious processes and repetitive spontaneous abortion, although it does seem reasonable to conclude that *Ureaplasma urealyticum* could cause foetal losses.

Auto-immune Disease

That perturbations of the immunological system can be responsible for foetal wastage is intuitively obvious. The human rejects transplanted foreign organs, and the foetus is foreign. However, the nature of the immunological process responsible for maintaining pregnancy has proved to be very complex.

One well known example of an immunological mechanism causing foetal wastage is Rhesus sensitization. Mid- or late gestational foetal loss is well documented in Rh-negative (D negative) women having anti-D antibodies. Another example involves anti-P antibodies (Levine, 1978). Most individuals are genotype Pp or pp. However, an occasional female is homozygous for P (pp). If the mother develops anti-P antibodies, Pp foetuses will be rejected early in gestation.

More recently, it has been shown that individuals having lupus anticoagulant (LAC) have an increased likelihood of foetal wastage. *In vitro*, LAC is an anticoagulant; *in vivo* it paradoxically increases the likelihood of thrombosis (Gastineau *et al.*, 1985). Lupus anticoagulant (LAC) has been associated with sub-placental clotting and foetal losses in all trimesters, as well as with poor reproductive history in general (Elias and Eldor, 1984). Because only 5–10 per cent of patients with systemic lupus erythematosis (SLE) have LAC, individuals with positive antinuclear antibodies (ANA) may or may not have LAC (Exner *et al.*, 1987). Similarly, not all patients with LAC will have SLE. Therefore,

LAC but not necessarily ANA should be sought in couples having repeated reproductive losses. The general phenomenon is rare but worth taking into account in studies of mid-trimester losses.

Shared Parental Histocompatibility

During pregnancy, the foetal allograft is protected. It has long been suggested that the maternal immune system is regulated by a blocking or suppressive factor that protects the foetus from rejection. This blocking antibody seems paradoxically to be stimulated by maternal–foetal histoincompatibility, which enhances implantation and facilitates pregnancy maintenance (Fig. 17.5). Thus, greater than expected sharing of histocompatibility antigens between mother and father and, hence, mother and foetus appears deleterious due to the lack of stimulation of the blocking factor. Experimental support for a beneficial effect of maternal–foetal incompatibility includes: (1) increased placental size in mouse foetuses that result from matings in which paternally

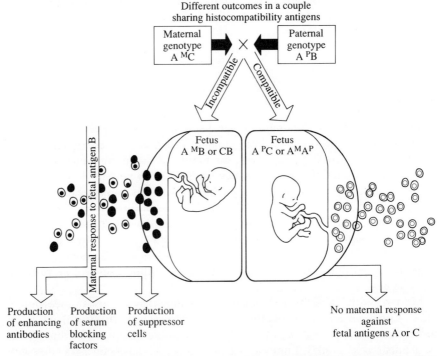

A, B, C Antigens of Histocompatibility Locus   • Maternal cells carrying Antigens A and C
A^M Antigen A Maternal Origin   • Fetal cells carrying Antigens B and A or C
A^P Antigen A Paternal Origin   • Fetal cells carrying Antigens A or C

Source: Simpson, 1986.

Fig. 17.5   Schematic diagram of the immunological responses operating in normal pregnancies

derived histocompatibility antigens differ from maternal antigens; (2) higher implantation frequencies in histoincompatible murine zygotes; and (3) maintenance of genetic polymorphisms at major histocompatibility loci despite over 70 generations of brother–sister mating in rats (Beer and Billingham, 1976).

Support for parental histoincompatibility being beneficial in humans can be deduced by comparing immunological variables in women achieving and not achieving successful pregnancies. The incidence of anti-paternal-leukocy-toxic antibodies in multiparous women is 64 per cent, compared to only 20 per cent in primiparous women and only 16.6 per cent in women who have multiple abortions (Gill and Repetti, 1979; Beard *et al.*, 1983). However, these antibodies may develop only late in pregnancy, so lack of antibodies does not reflect the inability to become pregnant *per se* (Regan and Braude, 1987). Similarly, 50 per cent of women with three or more recurrent abortions fail to demonstrate a mixed lymphocyte reaction when their lymphocytes are exposed to their spouse's lymphocytes (Beer *et al.*, 1987).

If histocompatible human foetuses are at selective disadvantage during early pregnancy, it follows that couples sharing HLA (human lymphocyte antigens) antigens should show poorer reproductive outcomes than couples not sharing antigens. In such cases, mother and foetus may fail to differ at some HLA loci (A, B, C, or D/DR). That is, the father may transmit to the foetus an antigen already possessed by the mother. Indeed, couples experiencing repetitive spontaneous abortions in early gestation are usually reported to share HLA antigens more often than controls (Schacter *et al.*, 1984). Of course, one would also wish to know whether the foetus actually inherited the paternal antigen shared by its mother and father. Unfortunately, HLA data on abortuses are not available.

The association between the sharing of HLA by parents and abortion seems greatest if there are no living children, if abortion occurs between 6 and 9 weeks' gestation, if two or more antigens are shared, and if a DR antigen is shared. HLA sharing may also be associated with a depressed mixed lymphocyte response (MLR) between maternal and paternal cells, and with blunted maternal blocking antibody (BA) responses. These data support the postulate that the mechanism making HLA sharing deleterious is the failure to initiate maternal blocking antibodies.

On the other hand, some couples sharing HLA-DR antigens have shown no spontaneous abortions, despite ten or more pregnancies. Moreover, other investigators have not observed increased HLA sharing, depressed MLR, or decreased blocking antibodies (Oksenberg *et al.*, 1984). The ostensible discrepancies between the various studies are difficult to reconcile. However, experimental designs have varied widely, and selection biases have not been evaluated adequately.

Ober *et al.* (1983) attacked the criticism that identifying a phenomenon in an abnormal (aborters) population does not prove cause and effect. Those investigators prospectively studied a fertile population (the Hutterites) not selected on the basis of prior knowledge of reproductive outcome. They first observed small yet consistent differences among Hutterite couples sharing HLA-DR antigen. Such couples were found to have longer intervals between births and smaller completed family sizes than couples not sharing HLA-DR antigens. The findings are consistent with the hypothesis that shared HLA antigens do indeed affect reproductive outcome deleteriously.

That some but not all couples sharing HLA antigens show deleterious effects could be reconciled readily by postulating that normal pregnancy requires maternal–foetal histocompatibility not for HLA-DR, but rather for another closely linked locus. This hypothesis is not only consistent with HLA antigens failing to be expressed on the trophoblast but is supported as well by direct data. Specifically, the blocking antibody (BA) present in normal pregnancies, but absent in women experiencing spontaneous abortion, is directed against neither HLA-A, B, C or DR (Power *et al.*, 1983).

Faulk and McIntyre (1981) have recently suggested that immune regulation is stimulated by a series of antigens on the placenta, so-called trophoblast lymphocyte cross-reactive (TLX) antigens. This group claims to have isolated three TLX antigens. They further claim that couples experiencing repetitive spontaneous abortions are more likely to share 'TLX antigens' than those couples without pregnancy wastage (McIntyre *et al.*, 1986).

Although parental antigen sharing can be plausibly expected to result in immunological perturbations leading to repetitive abortion, it is also possible to explain the same data on the basis of purely genetic factors. Closely linked to the mouse histocompatibility (H2) complex is locus T/t. Embryos homozygous for certain alleles at this locus die at various stages of embryogenesis. If a T/t-like complex exists in humans, it may also be linked to the human histocompatibility locus (HLS) on chromosome 6. If so, histocompatibility between a mother and her foetus (and her spouse) could merely secondarily reflect homozygosity for lethal alleles at the T/t locus. In fact, evidence for such an effect has been offered by Schacter *et al.* (1984).

Given the uncertainty concerning the role of immunological factors in repetitive abortions, it is difficult to determine whether such factors should be taken into account in epidemiological studies. However, merely determining HLA status alone is clearly not sufficient. Taking more complete immunological factors into account is, unfortunately, impractical.

Irradiation and Anti-Neoplastic Agent

X-irradiation and anti-neoplastic agents are accepted abortifacients, attesting that exogenous factors during embryogenesis can cause foetal loss. However, therapeutic X-rays or chemotherapeutic drugs are administered during pregnancy only to seriously ill women whose pregnancies are not of paramount concern. In diagnostic dosage, X-rays have not been proved to cause foetal demise. However, it would be prudent to consider X-rays as a potential confounding variable. Even relatively low doses of anti-metabolites (e.g. methotrexate) should, on the other hand, be considered abortifacients, judged by the success of such agents in management of ectopic gestations.

Cigarette Smoking

Smoking during pregnancy has been positively correlated with spontaneous abortion. Kline *et al.* (1980) found increased abortion rates in smokers, independent of maternal age and independent of alcohol consumption. A positive dose response curve was also observed. Alberman *et al.* (1976) also reported that smokers showed a higher (albeit not significantly higher) proportion of abortuses with normal karyotypes, an observation that if verified would suggest that smoking affects the conceptus directly.

It is difficult to assess the possibility that smoking and other toxins may exert deleterious effects only on susceptible hosts. It can be deduced that genetic susceptibility exists, however, on the basis of most exposed pregnancies ending normally. None the less, smoking is an important confounding variable in determining foetal loss rates.

Alcohol

Several studies have reported an association between foetal loss and alcohol consumption, making the latter another important variable. In one study, 616 women experiencing spontaneous abortions were compared with 632 women delivering at 28 gestational weeks or more (Kline *et al.*, 1980). Among women whose pregnancies ended in spontaneous abortion, 17 per cent drank at least twice per week; 8.1 per cent of controls drank similar quantities. After adjusting for other potential confounding factors (e.g. smoking, age, prior abortions), the association between alcohol and abortion remained significant. Harlap and Shiono (1980) also found a slightly increased risk for abortion in women who drank in the first trimester. The increase failed to reach statistical significance, but it could not be explained on the basis of smoking, prior abortion, age, or other known risk factors.

In aggregate, then, data suggest that alcohol, perhaps even in modest quantities, increases the risk of spontaneous abortion. Again, a susceptible host may be necessary for an effect to be exerted.

Other Environmental Chemicals

A few chemical agents have been claimed to show an association with foetal losses. These chemicals include anaesthetic gases, arsenic aniline, benzene, ethylene oxide, formaldehyde, and lead (Fija-Talamanaca and Settimi, 1984; Barlow and Sullivan, 1982). Although many environmental toxicologists accept these agents as proved, evidence is far from convincing at low-level exposures.

Many other factors, for example visual display units and altering shift work, have been implicated but with even less definitive data. (More details of the effects of toxic substances on pregnancy outcome are given in Chapter 18, below.)

Actually, there is a paucity of data for several understandable reasons. First, corporations naturally attempt to limit the exposure of women in the reproductive age-group to potentially dangerous chemicals. Thus, most exposures are unwitting and, hence, poorly documented. Second, pregnant workers are usually exposed to many agents concurrently, making it difficult to determine the effects of any specific agent. Third, pregnancy among workers is a difficult outcome to monitor because health-care authorities are not always notified. For these and other well-known (memory, recall) biases, the case-control design has even more pitfalls than usual in investigating the effect of environmental chemicals.

Intra-uterine Devices and other Contraceptive Agents

Conception with an intra-uterine device *in situ* markedly increases the risk of foetal loss. The presumed pathogenesis is infection. However, exposure to an IUD prior to pregnancy does not increase the risk of foetal loss.

Use of other contraceptives, before and during pregnancy, is not associated consistently with foetal loss. In particular, several studies have shown that women who discontinue oral contraceptives before conception are at no significantly increased risk of foetal loss. Spermicide exposure, either prior to or after conception, likewise does not appear to increase the rate of spontaneous abortion, despite earlier claims to the contrary (Mills *et al.*, 1985).

Trauma

Women commonly attribute pregnancy losses to trauma, such as a fall or blow to the abdomen. However, foetuses are actually well protected from external trauma by intervening maternal structures and amniotic fluid. Witness, for example, the relative safety of amniocentesis and chorionic villus sampling. Trauma probably need not be taken into account as a confounding variable.

Psychological Factors

That impaired psychological well-being predisposes to early foetal losses has been claimed but not proved. Neurotic or mentally ill women abort, but whether the frequency of losses is higher than in normal women is unknown. Confounding factors have not been excluded in studies claiming a relationship.

One of the more frequently cited studies is that by Stray-Pedersen *et al.* (1984). Women having experienced repetitive abortions received increased attention ('tender loving care'), but no specific medical therapy. Such women were more likely to complete their pregnancy than were women not provided with such care. Unfortunately, a major deficiency in study design was that only women living 'close' to the university were eligible for the increased attention. Women living farther away served as 'controls'. Of course, the 'controls' may have differed in other ways as well.

We suspect that any ostensible beneficial effect of psychological well-being is probably either more apparent than real or merely secondary to other factors. At any rate, probes to monitor this potential confounder would not be easy to construct; thus, this factor probably need not routinely be taken into account.

Severe Maternal Illness

Many maternal diseases have been implicated in spontaneous abortion. Pathogenesis is not necessarily independent of endocrinological, immunological, or infectious mechanisms. An example already cited is lupus erythematosus, a disorder in which affected individuals may show lupus anticoagulant antibody (LAC).

Maternal diseases not previously mentioned that may be associated with foetal wastage include Wilson disease, maternal phenylketonuria, cardiac disease (e.g. anomalies), and haematological disorders (e.g. haemoglobinopathies or aplastic anaemia). In fact, any life-threatening disease would be expected to be associated with increased abortion rates. Seriously ill women rarely become pregnant, but in some cases the disease process may deteriorate after the onset of pregnancy. Overall, only a small fraction of all foetal losses can be attributable to severe maternal disease. Thus, general probes for maternal health should be sought, but detailed disease-by-disease assessment is probably unnecessary.

Other Confounding Variables

It is obvious that a host of confounding variables influence the likelihood of foetal loss. Not all these variables are mutually exclusive, nor necessarily independent of those cited above. This statement is especially applicable to two variables: maternal age and number of prior losses. For this reason, we briefly discuss these and other factors separately from those cited in the previous section.

Maternal age. Women aged 40–4 have approximately twice the likelihood of foetal loss than that incurred by women two decades younger. This risk holds for both trisomic as well as euploid abortuses (Stein *et al.*, 1980). Possible explanations include cumulative exposure to toxins, greater opportunity to acquire chronic infections, diminished luteal response, and poorly vascularized endometria.

A maternal-age effect is difficult to assess because: (1) women with repetitive losses may continue to attempt pregnancy longer than women who successfully complete pregnancies earlier in life; and (2) higher gravidity is also associated with advanced maternal age. Indeed, there have also been claims of a relationship between foetal losses and gravidity (Roman and Alberman, 1980). The apparent association with gravidity is, however, probably only a secondary effect of maternal age. In addition, compensation for prior adverse pregnancy outcomes surely occurs. Paternal age does not seem important, although an increase in fresh dominant mutations occurs with advanced paternal age.

Prior losses.   For decades obstetricians subscribed to the concept of 'habitual abortion'. After three but not fewer foetal losses, the risk of subsequent losses was believed to rise sharply. This belief was based on calculations by Malpas (1938), who concluded that following three abortions the likelihood of a subsequent loss was 80–90 per cent. By contrast, a couple experiencing one or two spontaneous abortions was believed to have only a slightly increased recurrence risk compared to couples never experiencing a spontaneous abortion. Occurrence of three consecutive spontaneous abortions was said to confer upon a woman the designation of 'habitual aborter'. Unfortunately, these risk figures were not only later proved incorrect, but were used as 'controls' for clinical trials evaluating various treatment plans. This inevitably led to unwarranted acceptance of many treatment regimes, a famous example of which is diethylstilbestrol (DES).

In 1964, Warburton and Fraser (1964) studied a sample of Canadian women having at least one liveborn infant. The likelihood of recurrent abortion proved to be only 25–30 per cent, irrespective of whether a woman had previously experienced one, two, three, or even four spontaneous abortions. Thus, the concept of a discrete subclass of habitual aborters (i.e. women with three prior abortions) was refuted.

Because the study by Warburton and Fraser was limited to women having liveborn infants, analysis of other samples was necessary. Poland *et al.* (1977) calculated that the likelihood of foetal loss was 46 per cent if a woman had experienced at least one loss (spontaneous abortion, stillborn infant, or early neonatal death) without having had a liveborn infant. Women having at least one liveborn infant had a lower risk of abortion, as was evident from comparison to the data of Warburton and Fraser. Later studies showed recurrence risks to be slightly higher following cytogenetically normal abortuses (Boué *et al.*, 1975).

In aggregate, it is usually appropriate to offer recurrence risks of 25–30 per cent to couples having at least one liveborn and 40 per cent if they have none. The risk may be slightly higher if the complement of the previous abortus was normal.

References

Alberman, E. D. (1981), 'The Abortus as a Predictor of Future Trisomy 21', in F. F. De la Cruz, and P. S. Gerald (eds.), *Trisomy 21 (Down's Syndrome)*: 69, University Park Press, Baltimore, Md.

—— Creasy, M., Elliott, M., and Spicer, C. (1976), 'Maternal Effects Associated with Foetal Chromosomal Anomalies in Spontaneous Abortions', *British Journal of Obstetrics and Gynaecology* 83: 621.

Angell, R. R., Aitken, J. R., van-Look, P. F. A., Lumsden, M. A., and Templeton, A. A. (1983), 'Chromosome Abnormalities in Human Embryos After In Vitro Fertilization', *Nature* 303: 336.

Barlow, S., and Sullivan, F. M. (1982), *Reproductive Hazards of Industrial Chemicals: An Evaluation of Animal and Human Data*, Academic Press, New York.

Beard, R. W., Braude, P., Mowbray, J. F., and Underwood, J. L. (1983), 'Protective Antibodies and Spontaneous Abortion', *Lancet* 2: 1090.

Beer, A. E., and Billingham, R. F. (1976), *The Immunology of Mammalian Reproduction*, Prentice-Hall, Englewood Cliffs, NJ.

—— Quebbeman, J. F., and Semprini, A. E. (1987), 'Immuno-pathological Factors Contributing to Recurrent and Spontaneous Abortion in Humans', in M. J. Bennet and D. K. Edmonds (eds.), *Spontaneous and Recurrent Abortions*: 90, Blackwell, Oxford.

Boué, A., and Gallano, P. (1984), 'A Collaborative Study of the Segregation of Inherited Chromosome Structural Arrangements in 1356 Prenatal Diagnoses', *Prenatal Diagnosis* 4: 45.

Boué, J., Boué, A., and Lazar, P. (1975), 'Retrospective and Prospective Epidemiological Studies of 1500 Karyotyped Spontaneous Human Abortions', *Teratology* 12: 11.

—— Phillippe, E., Giroud A., and Boué A. (1976), 'Phenotypic Expression of Lethal Chromosomal Anomalies in Human Abortuses', *Teratology* 14: 3.

Carson, S. A., and Simpson, J. L. (1990), 'Spontaneous Abortion', in R. D. Eden and F. H. Boehm (eds.), *Fetal Assessment: Physiological, Clinical and Medico-Legal Principles*: 559–74, Appleton–Century–Crofts, Norwalk, Conn.

Cashner, K. A., Christopher, C. R., and Dysert, G. A. (1987), 'Spontaneous Fetal Loss after Demonstration of a Live Fetus in the First Trimester', *Obstetrics and Gynecology* 70: 827.

Chandley, A. C. (1987), 'The Origin of Chromosomal Aberrations in Man and their Potential for Survival and Reproduction in the Adult Human Populations', *Annals of Genetics* 24: 5.

Christiaens, G. C. M. L., and Stoutenbeek, P. H. (1984), 'Spontaneous Abortion in Proven Intact Pregnancies', *Lancet* 2: 572.

Daly, D. C., Walters, C. A., Soto-Albers, C. E., and Riddick, D. H. (1983), 'Endometrial Biopsy during Treatment of Luteal Phase Defects is Predictive of Therapeutic Outcome', *Fertility and Sterility* 40: 305.

Edmonds, D. K., Lindsay, K. S., Miller, J. R., Williamson, E., and Wood, P. J. (1982), 'Early Embryonic Mortality in Women', *Fertility and Sterility* 38: 447.

Elias, M., and Eldor, A. (1984), 'Thromboembolism in Patients with "Lupus" Type Circulating Anticoagulant', *Archives of Internal Medicine* 144: 510–5.

Exner, T., Richard, K. A., and Kronenberg, H. (1987), 'A Sensitive Test Demonstrating LAC and its Behavioural Patterns', *British Journal of Haematology* 40: 143.

Faulk, W. P., and McIntyre, J. A. (1981), 'Trophoblast Survival', *Transplantation* 32: 1.

Fija-Talamanaca, I., and Settimi, L. (1984), 'Occupational Factors and Reproductive Outcome', in E. S. E. Hafez (ed.), *Spontaneous Abortion*: 61, MTP Press, Lancaster, UK.

Gastineau, D. A., Kazimier, F. J., Nichols, W. L., and Bowie, E. J. (1985), 'Lupus Anticoagulant: An Analysis of the Clinical and Laboratory Features of 219 Cases', *American Journal of Hematology* 19: 265.

Gerbie, A., and Simpson, J. L. (1976), 'Antenatal Detection of Genetic Disorders', *Postgraduate Medical Journal* 59: 129.

Gill, T. J., and Repetti, C. F. (1979), 'Immunologic and Genetic Factors Influencing Reproduction', *American Journal of Pathology* 95: 464.

Gilmore, D. H., and McNay, M. B. (1985), 'Spontaneous Fetal Loss Rate in Early Pregnancy', *Lancet* 1: 107.

Gropp, A. (1973), 'Fetal Mortality due to Aneuploidy and Irregular Meiotic Segregation in the Mouse', in A. Boué and C. Thibault (eds.), *Les Accidents Chromosiques de la Reproduction*: 225, INSERM, Paris.

—— (1975), 'Chromosomal Animal Model of Human Disease: Fetal Trisomy and Development Failure', in L. Berry and D. E. Poswillo (eds.), *Teratology*: 17–35 Springer-Verlag, Berlin.

Guerneri, S., Bettio, D., Simoni, G., Brambati, B., Lanzani, A., and Fraccaro, M. (1987), 'Prevalence and Distribution of Chromosome Abnormalities in a Sample of First Trimester Internal Abortions', *Human Reproduction* 2: 735–9.

Harlap, S., and Shiono, P. H. (1980), 'Alcohol, Smoking and Incidence of Spontaneous Abortions in the First and Second Trimester', *Lancet* 2: 173.

Hassold, T. (1980), 'A Cytogenetic Study of Repeated Spontaneous Abortions', *American Journal of Human Genetics* 32: 723.

Heinonen, P., Saarikoski, S., and Pystynen, P. (1982), 'Reproductive Performance of Women with Uterine Anomalies: An Evaluation of 182 Cases', *Acta Obstetrica Gynecologica Scandinavica* 61: 157.

Hertig, A. T., and Rock, J. (1973), 'Searching for Early Human Ova', *Gynecological Investigations* 4: 121.

—— —— and Adams, E. C. (1956), 'Description of Human Ova Within the First 17 Days of Development', *American Journal of Anatomy* 98: 435.

—— —— —— Menkin, M. C. (1959), 'Thirty-four Fertilized Human Ova, Good, Bad and Indifferent, Recovered from 210 Women of Known Fertility: A Study of Biologic Wastage in Early Human Pregnancy', *Pediatrics* 25: 202.

Honoré, L. H., Dill, F. J., and Poland, B. J. (1976), 'Placental Morphology in Spontaneous Human Abortuses with Normal and Abnormal Karyotypes', *Teratology* 14: 151.

Kline, J., Shrout, P., Stein, Z. A., Susser, M., and Warburton, D. (1980), 'Drinking during Pregnancy and Spontaneous Abortion', *Lancet* 2: 176.

Kuleshov, N. P. (1976), 'Chromosome Anomalies of Infants Dying during the Perinatal Period and Premature Newborn', *Human Genetics* 34: 151.

Levine, P. (1978), 'ABO, P and MN Blood Group Determinants in Neoplasm Foreign to the Host', *Seminars in Oncology* 5: 25.

McCleod, P. M., Dill, F., and Hardwick, D. F. (1979), 'Chromosomes, Syndromes and Perinatal Deaths: The Genetic Counselling Value of Making a Diagnosis in a Malformed Abortus, Stillborn, and Deceased Newborns', *Birth Defects* 15(5A): 105.

McIntyre, J. A., Faulk, W. P., Nichols-Johnson, V. R., and Taylor, C. G. (1986), 'Immunologic Testing and Immunotherapy in Recurrent Spontaneous Abortion', *Obstetrics and Gynecology* 67: 169–75.

Malpas, P. (1938), 'A Study of Abortion Sequences', *Journal of Obstetrics and Gynecology of the British Commonwealth* 45: 931.

Martin, A. O., Simpson, J. L., Deddish, R. B., and Elias, S. (1983), 'Clinical Implications of Chromosomal Inversions: A Pericentric Inversion in No. 18 Segregating in a Family Ascertained Through an Abnormal Proband', *American Journal of Perinatology* 1: 81.

Michelman, H. W., Bonhoff, A., and Mettler, L. (1986), 'Chromosome Analysis in Polypoid Human Embryos', *Human Reproduction* 1: 243.

Miller, J. F., Williamson, E., Glue, J., Gordon, Y. B., Grudzinskas, J. G., and Sykes, A. (1980), 'Fetal Loss After Implantation: A Prospective Study', *Lancet* 2: 554.

Mills, J. L., Reed, G. F., Nugent, R. P., Harley, E. E., and Berendes, H. W. (1985), 'Are There Adverse Effects of Peri-conceptual Spermicide Use?' *Fertility and Sterility* 43: 442–6.

—— Simpson, J. L., Driscoll, S. G., Jovanovic-Peterson, L., Van Allen, M., Aarons, J. H., Metzger, B., Bieber, F. R., Knopp, R. H., Holmes, L. B., Peterson, C. M., Witham-Wilson, M., Brown, Z. A., Ober, C., Harley, E., McPherson, T. A., Duckles, A., Mueller-Heubach, E., and the National Institute of Child Health and Human Development, Diabetes in Early Pregnancy Study (1988), 'Incidence of Spontaneous Abortion Among Normal Women and Insulin-Dependent Diabetic Women whose Pregnancies were Identified within 21 Days of Conception', *New England Journal of Medicine* 319: 1617–23.

Mueller, R. F., Sybert, V. P., Johnson, J., Brown, Z. A., and Chen, W. J. (1983), 'Evaluation of a Protocol for Postmortem Examination of Still-Births', *New England Journal of Medicine* 309: 586–90.

Ober, C. L., Simpson, J. L., Hauck, W. W., Amos, D. B., Kostyu, D. D., Fotino, M., and Allen, F. H. (1983), 'Shared HLA Antigens and Reproductive Performance Among Hutterites', *American Journal of Human Genetics* 35: 994–1004.

Oksenberg, J. R., Persitz, E., Amar, A., and Brautbar, C. (1984), 'Maternal–Paternal Histocompatibility: Lack of Association with Habitual Abortion', *Fertility Sterility* 42: 389–95.

Plachot, M., Junca, A. M., and Mandelbaum, J. (1987), 'Chromosome Investigations in Early Life, II: Human Preimplantation Embryos', *Human Reproduction* 2: 29.

Poland, B. J., Miller, J. R., Jones, D. C., and Trimble, B. K. (1977), 'Reproductive Counseling in Patients Who Have Had a Spontaneous Abortion', *American Journal of Obstetrics and Gynceology* 127: 685–91.

Power, D. A., Catto, G. R., Mason, R. J., McLeod, A. M., Stewart, G. M., Stewart, K. N., and Shewan, W. G. (1983), 'The Fetus as an Allograft: Evidence for Protective Antibodies to HLA-linked Paternal Antigens', *Lancet* 2: 701–4.

Regan, L., and Braude, P. R. (1987), 'Is Antipaternal Cytotoxic Antibody a Valid Marker in the Management of Recurrent Abortion?' *Lancet* 2: 1280.

Rock, J., and Jones, H. W., Jr. (1977), 'The Clinical Management of the Double Uterus', *Fertility and Sterility* 28: 789.

Roman, E., and Alberman, E. (1980), 'Spontaneous Abortion, Gravidity, Pregnancy Order, Age and Pregnancy Interval', in I. H. Porter and E. B. Hook (eds.), *Human Embryonic and Fetal Death*: 129, Academic Press, New York.

Rudak, E., Dor, J., Mashiach, S., Nobel, L., and Goldman, B. (1985), 'Chromosome Analysis of Human Oocytes and Embryos Fertilized In Vitro', *Annals of the New York Academy of Sciences* 442: 476–86.

Ruzicska, P., and Cziezel, A. (1971), 'Cytogenetic Studies on Midtrimester Abortuses', *Humangenetik* 10: 273.

Schacter, B., Weitkamp, L. R., and Johnson, W. E. (1984), 'Paternal HLA Compatibility, Fetal Wastage, and Neural Tube Defects: Evidence for a T/t-like Locus in Humans', *American Journal of Human Genetics* 36: 1082.

Simpson, J. L. (1976), *Disorders of Sex Differentiation: Etiology and Clinical Delineation*, Academic Press, New York.

—— (1986), 'Repetitive Spontaneous Abortions', in I. H. Porter, N. H. Hatcher, and A. M. Wiley (eds.), *Perinatal Genetics: Diagnosis and Treatment*: 41, Academic Press, Orlando, Fla.

—— and LeBeau, M. M. (1981), 'Gonadal and Statural Determinants on the X Chromosome and their Relationship to in Vitro Studies Showing Prolonged Cell Cycles in 45,X; 46,X,del(X)-(p11); 46,X,del(X)(q13) and 46,X,del(X)(q22) Fibroblasts', *American Journal of Obstetrics and Gynecology* 141: 930.

—— and Mills, J. L. (1986), 'Methodologic Problems in Determining Fetal Loss Rates', in B. Brambati, G. Simoni, and S. Fabro (eds.), *Chorionic Villus Sampling: Fetal Diagnosis of Genetic Diseases in the First Trimester*: 227, Marcel Dekker, New York and Basel.

—— and Bombard, A. T. (1987), 'Chromosomal Abnormalities in Spontaneous Abortions: Frequency, Pathology and Genetic Counselling', in K. Edmonds and M. J. Bennett (eds.), *Spontaneous Abortion*: 51, Blackwell, Oxford.

—— Elias, S., and Martin, A. O. (1981), 'Parental Chromosomal Rearrangements Associated with Repetitive Spontaneous Abortions', *Fertility and Sterility* 36: 584.

—— Mills, J. L., Holmes, L. B., Ober, C. L., Aarons, J., Jovanovic, L., and Knopp, R. H. (1987), 'Low Fetal Loss Rates After Ultrasound-Proved Viability in Early Pregnancy', *Journal of the American Medical Association* 258: 2555.

—— Meyers, C., Martin, A. O., Elias, S., and Ober, C. (1989), 'Translocations are Infrequent among Couples having Repeated Spontaneous Abortions', *Fertility and Sterility* 51: 811–14.

—— Golbus, M. S., Martin, A. O., and Sarto, G. E. (1982), *Genetics in Obstetrics and Gynecology*: 126, Grune and Stratton, New York.

Southerland, G. R., Bauld, R., and Bain, A. D. (1974), 'Chromosome Abnormality and Perinatal Death', *Lancet* 1: 752.

Stein, Z., Kline, J., Susser, E., Shrout, P., Warburton, D., and Susser, M. (1980), 'Maternal Age and Spontaneous Abortion', in I. H. Porter and E. B. Hood (eds.), *Human Embryonic and Fetal Death*: 107–27, Academic Press, New York.

Stevenson, A. C., Dudgeon, M. Y., and McClure, H. I. (1959), 'Observations on the Results of Pregnancies in Women Resident in Belfast, II: Abortions, Hydatidiform Moles, and Ectopic Pregnancies', *Annals of Human Genetics* 23: 395.

Stray-Pederson, B., and Stray-Pedersen, S. (1984), 'Etiologic Factors and Subsequential Reproductive Performance in 195 Couples with a Prior History of Habitual Abortion', *American Journal of Obstetrics and Gynecology* 148: 140.

—— Eng, J., and Reikvan, R. M. (1978), 'Uterine T-mycoplasma Colonization in Reproductive Failure', *American Journal of Obstetrics and Gynecology* 130: 307.

Sutherland, G. R., Gardiner, A. J., and Carter, R. F. (1976), 'Familial Pericentric Inversion of Chromosome 19 Inv (19)(p13q13) with a Note on Genetic Counseling of Pericentric Inversion Carriers', *Clinical Genetics* 10: 53.

Tabor, A., Philip, J., Madsen, M., Bang, J., Obel, E. B., and Nrgaard-Pedersen, B. (1986), 'Randomized Controlled Trial of Genetic Amniocentesis in 4606 Low-Risk Women', *Lancet* 1: 1287–93.

Tho, P. T., Byrd, J. R., and McDonough, P. C. (1979), 'Etiologies and Subsequent Reproductive Performance of 100 Couples with Recurrent Abortions', *Fertility and Sterility* 32: 389.

Toth, A., Lesser, M. L., Brooks-Toth, C. W., and Feiner, C. (1986), 'Outcome of Subsequent Pregnancies Following Antibiotic Therapy After Primary or Multiple Spontaneous Abortions', *Gynecology and Obstetrics* 163: 243–50.

Vlaanderen, W., and Treffers, P. E. (1987), 'Prognosis of Subsequent Pregnancies After Recurrent Spontaneous Abortion in First Trimester', *British Medical Journal* 295: 92.

Warburton, D., and Fraser, F. C. (1964), 'Spontaneous Abortion Risks in Man: Data from Reproductive Histories Collected in a Medical Genetics Unit', *American Journal of Human Genetics* 16: 1–25.

—— Kline, J., Stein, Z., Hutzler, M., Chin, A., and Hassold, T. (1987), 'Does the Karyotype of a Spontaneous Abortion Predict the Karyotype of a Subsequent Abortion? Evidence from 273 Women with Two Karyotyped Spontaneous Abortions', *American Journal of Human Genetics* 41: 465–83.

—— Stein, Z., Kline, J., Susser, M. (1980), 'Chromosome Abnormalities in Spontaneous Abortion: Data from the New York City Study', in I. H. Porter and E. B. Hook (eds.), *Human Embryonic and Fetal Death*: 261–87, Academic Press, Orlando, Fla.

Watt, J. L., Templeton, A. A., Messinis, I., Bell, L., Cunningham, P., and Duncan, R. O. (1987), 'Trisomy I in an Eight Cell Human Pre-Embryo', *Journal of Medical Genetics* 24: 60–4.

Wentz, A. C., Martens, P., and Wilroy, R. S., Jr. (1984), 'Luteal Phase Inadequacy and a Chromosomal Anomaly in Recurrent Abortions', *Fertility and Sterility* 41: 142.

Whittaker, P. G., Taylor, A., and Lind, T. (1983), 'Unsuspected Pregnancy Loss in Healthy Women', *Lancet* 1: 1126.

Wilson, R. D., Kendrick, V., Wittman, B. K., and McGilliuray, B. C. (1984), 'Risk of Spontaneous Abortion in Ultrasonographically Normal Pregnancies', *Lancet* 2: 920–1.

Working Party on Amniocentesis (1978), 'An Assessment of the Hazards of Amniocentesis', *British Journal of Obstetrics and Gynecology* 85 (supplement): 1.

Zenzes, M. T., Belkien, L., Bordt, J., Kan, I., Schneider, H. P., and Nieschlag, E. (1985), 'Cytologic Investigation of Human in Vitro Fertilization Failures', *Fertility and Sterility* 43: 883.

18 Endocrine Detection of Conception and Early Foetal Loss

ALLEN J. WILCOX

CLARICE R. WEINBERG

DONNA D. BAIRD

ROBERT E. CANFIELD

At least 95 per cent of the menstrual cycles of healthy, reproductive-aged women are ovulatory (Vollman, 1977). However, for the average non-contracepting couple, there is only about a 25 per cent chance that an ovum will produce a recognized pregnancy (Leridon, 1977). This gap between the number of available ova and the much smaller number of observed pregnancies presumably reflects some mixture of failure to conceive and early death of the conceptus. The rate of fertilization in humans is unknown, because we have no method to detect the event of fertilization. That, in turn, makes us unable to measure the proportion of fertilized ova lost before pregnancy becomes clinically apparent. In principle, the risk of early loss could range from zero (assuming that 25 per cent of ova are fertilized and all survive) to nearly 75 per cent (assuming that every egg is fertilized but only 25 per cent survive).

Actual estimates of early pregnancy loss have nearly spanned that range: the lowest is 8 per cent (Whittaker *et al.*, 1983) and the highest is 57 per cent (Edmonds *et al.*, 1982). In this paper we discuss methodological problems in the detection of very early pregnancy and the ways in which those problems may contribute to disparities among estimates of early loss. We will also describe our experience with the detection of early pregnancy loss through the measurement of urinary human chorionic gonadotrophin (hCG).

Methods for the Detection of Early Pregnancy

Ovulation in humans usually occurs about 15 days (8 to 24 days) after the onset of the most recent menses (Lenton *et al.*, 1984*a*). Ovulation itself triggers a tightly-paced sequence of events that starts with the conversion of the ovarian follicle into a corpus luteum. If there is no pregnancy, the corpus luteum regresses, and menses begins about 14 days (10 to 18 days) after ovulation (Lenton *et al.*, 1984*b*).

A fertilized óvum quickly begins cell division and development into a blastocyst. The blasotocyst usually starts to attach to the lining of the uterus within 7 to 9 days after fertilization. Around the time of implantation, the blastocyst begins to produce the hormone hCG (human chorionic gonado-trophin). HCG stimulates and maintains the function of the corpus luteum. This, in turn, prolongs the production of progesterone by the corpus luteum and prevents the onset of menses. During this time, the conceptus is able to attach to the uterine wall, gaining access to nourishment from maternal blood.

For most women the first indication of pregnancy is the absence of a menstrual period. Symptoms of pregnancy are typically (but not invariably) experienced around this time, two to three weeks after conception. A pregnancy that is lost before two weeks is probably undetectable by the woman. A loss that occurs two to three weeks after conception can still easily be mistaken for a menstrual period. Pregnancies that end even as late as eleven weeks after the previous menses have sometimes been unrecognized by women or their physicians (Braunstein *et al.*, 1977). Thus, in order to measure pregnancy loss reliably, some biological marker of early pregnancy is required. Several biochemical substances have been proposed as markers of early pregnancy. These are early pregnancy factor (EPF), placental proteins, the steroid hormones oestrogen and progesterone, and hCG.

Early Pregnancy Factor

Early pregnancy factor is a protein reported to be detectable in the serum of mice, sheep, pigs, and humans within 24 hours of fertilization (Morton *et al.*, 1977, 1982, 1983; Smart *et al.*, 1981a, 1981b; Chen *et al.*, 1985). This protein is thought to contribute to immunosuppression during pregnancy (Noonan *et al.*, 1979; Shaw and Morton, 1980). No previously available method of pregnancy detection has been able to identify pregnancies before the time of implantation. As a result, there has been widespread interest in EPF as a factor which would come close to being a marker of conception itself. Smart and her colleagues (1982) reported that among 21 cycles of healthy women attempting pregnancy, EPF was detected in 14 cycles, of which 8 cycles eventually produced clinically apparent pregnancies. Using the same assay, Rolfe (1982) reported positive EPF in 18 of 28 cycles, of which 4 went on to be clinically apparent pregnancies.

However, some doubts have been raised about the specificity of EPF for pregnancy (Grudzinskas and Nysenbaum, 1985). In addition, despite a decade of work, there remain mechanical problems in the measurement of EPF. The only way EPF can be measured at present is by rosette inhibition using blood cells, which is a difficult assay to establish (Chen *et al.*, 1985). The development of a radio-immunoassay for EPF, particularly one that uses urine rather than serum, would be an important step. Until a urine assay is established, it is unlikely that EPF could be useful for epidemiological studies. The same would apply to any other marker, such as the factor responsible for early pregnancy-associated thrombocytopenia (EPAT), suggested as a possible sign of early pregnancy (Roberts *et al.*, 1987).

Oestrogen and Progesterone

Oestrogen and progesterone are steroid hormones produced by the ovary in every fertile menstrual cycle. In non-conception cycles, these hormones drop in the late luteal phase prior to menses. Under the stimulus of conception, levels of oestrogen and progesterone increase rather than decrease. Lasley *et al.* (1985: 866) have proposed that the late luteal increase of urinary concentrations of oestrogen and progesterone metabolites can be early markers of pregnancy and may 'prove valuable in detecting transient or "occult" pregnancies'.

However, this conclusion is based on comparisons of the steroid assays with a relatively insensitive assay for hCG. We have made similar comparisons of urinary steroids and hCG using a more sensitive hCG assay (described below). We find clear examples of early loss that occur without apparent effects on patterns of steroid excretion. Fig. 18.1 shows data from several hormone assays performed on daily urine specimens collected from a healthy woman attempting pregnancy. Shaded bars indicate days of menstrual bleeding. This woman did not achieve a clinical pregnancy until her sixth cycle. HCG results are shown in the bottom panel. There is biochemical evidence of early pregnancy loss in the third and fifth cycles, losses that were unrecognized by the woman herself. The top panel shows daily urine concentrations of oestrone-3-glucuronide and pregnanediol, which are metabolites of oestradiol and progesterone. (Assay methods have been described in Wilcox *et al.*, 1985.) The patterns of urinary steroid excretion are not obviously altered in the two cycles with early pregnancy loss. This suggests that urinary steroids are not as sensitive as hCG for the detection of very early pregnancy.

Placental Proteins

The placenta produces several proteins in addition to hCG (discussed separately below) that have been suggested as markers of pregnancy. Most of these, such as PAPP-A and PP5, do not appear until relatively late (about four weeks after conception) and so are not useful for measuring early loss (Grudzinskas and Nysenbaum, 1985). The Schwangerschaftsprotein 1 (SP1) is detectable earlier in pregnancy, but apparently it is not completely specific to pregnancy. The SP1 immunoassay cross-reacts with a substance around the time of ovulation (i.e. before pregnancy), creating the possibility of false-positive results (Ahmed and Klopper, 1985). Also, the SP1 does not appear more sensitive than routinely available hCG assays in the detection of early pregnancy.

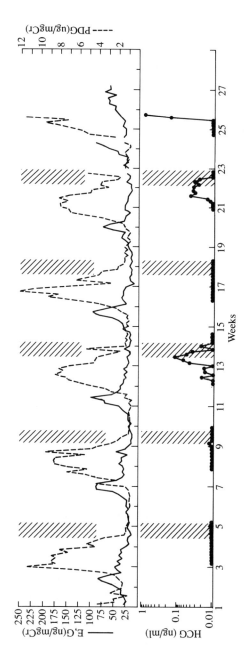

The hormones measured are oestrome-one-glucuronide (solid line), pregnanediol (dashed line), and hCG (lower panel). Shaded bars indicate menses.
Fig. 18.1   Three hormones measured in daily urines from a woman with two early pregnancy losses followed by a clinically recognized pregnancy

Human Chorionic Gonadotrophin

HCG was first identified 65 years ago as a biologically active substance excreted in large quantities in the urine of pregnant women (Aschheim and Zondek, 1927). HCG is produced by the trophoblast (the part of the conceptus which eventually forms the placenta). This hormone is detectable as early as one week after conception. Fishel and his colleagues (1984) assayed culture media from two plates in which fertilized human ova were being grown for embryo transfer. HCG was detected beginning on day 7 in one plate and day 8 in the other.

This is consistent with our data from daily urine specimens collected from women attempting pregnancy. We calculated the time from the ovulatory surge of luteinizing hormone (LH) to the first detectable hCG for 20 pregnancies that ended in live births. (The serum LH peak precedes ovulation by less than 24 hours, and fertilization is thought to occur within 24 hours of ovulation.) Mean time from urinary LH peak to hCG detection was 8.4 days, with a range of 5 to 13 days. For 17 of the 20 pregnancies, hCG was detected between 7 to 10 days after the LH peak. Thus, hCG begins to be detected around the time of implantation and provides a means of estimating post-implantation pregnancy loss.

HCG is one of a family of four glycoprotein hormones found in humans. The other three (follicle-stimulating hormone, thyroid-stimulating hormone, and luteinizing hormone) are pituitary hormones found in both men and women. The three pituitary hormones and hCG share a basic structure: each is made up of two chains, an alpha and a beta. The alpha chain is virtually identical in all four hormones. The beta chains differ, although in the case of hCG and luteinizing hormone, 82 per cent of the protein sequences in the beta chain are identical (Fiddes and Talmadge, 1984).

The structural similarity of hCG and luteinizing hormone (LH) is key to both the biological purpose of hCG and the difficulties in its measurement. HCG is produced by the conceptus as a substance that mimics LH; the hormone acts at the same receptor sites as LH. By prolonging the life of the corpus luteum, hCG leads to extended production of progesterone and to continued support of the uterine lining. This clear biological function of hCG in early pregnancy, together with its specifically-characterized molecular structure, have led hCG to be regarded as the cornerstone of the biochemical diagnosis of pregnancy (Grudzinskas and Nysenbaum, 1985).

The history of hCG measurement is largely a story of constantly improving techniques for discriminating between hCG and LH. The development of hCG radio-immunoassays in the 1970s allowed hCG to be detected with improved sensitivity, but not without persistent immunological cross-reactivity between LH and hCG. This has been true even for the so-called 'beta-chain specific' hCG radio-immunoassays. Truly specific assays for hCG were not possible until an antibody to a unique portion of the beta chain of the hCG molecule was produced. Such an antibody was not easy to develop because the unique portions of the hCG molecule are not highly antigenic. When a specific antibody finally became available, there was rapid progress in the development of sensitive and specific hCG assays.

In 1981 Wehmann *et al.*, using an antibody specific to the carboxyterminal peptide region of hCG, reported an hCG assay that was sensitive to urinary concentrations as low as 0.4 ng/ml, with virtually no cross-reactivity to LH. This represented at least a ten-fold increase in sensitivity over conventional hCG kits. In 1984 Armstrong *et al.* described an immuno-radiometric assay that was sensitive to hCG as low as 0.01 ng/ml, which is sensitive enough to detect hCG at the trace physiological levels sometimes found in healthy men and non-pregnant women (Borkowski and Muquardt, 1979). Most recently, researchers at the University of Utah reported an hCG serum assay sensitive to 4 pg/ml (0.004 ng/ml), which was able to detect trace amounts of hCG in every person, man or woman, who was studied (Odell and Griffin, 1987).

The first report of a sub-clinical pregnancy loss detected by an hCG assay was published more than twenty years ago (Morris and Udry, 1967). Since then there have been a number of reports, mostly case-series or small samples (Udry, 1971; Bloch, 1976; Braunstein *et al.*, 1977; Chartier *et al.*, 1979; Lenton *et al.*, 1982; Overstreet, 1984; Lippman and Farookhi, 1986; Ellish *et al.*, 1986).

In 1980 Miller and his colleagues published results from the first study intended to estimate the incidence of unrecognized early pregnancy loss. In their study of 197 women, a chemically-recognized pregnancy had a 33 per cent chance of ending before it was clinically recognized. Edmonds *et al.* (1982) published results from a study of 82 women, similarly designed but using a different assay for hCG. Their study showed a loss rate of 57 per cent. In 1983 Whittaker *et al.* reported a loss rate of 8 per cent among 91 women. The discrepancies among these three studies, all based on hCG detection of early pregnancy, warrant closer inspection.

Each of these studies was composed of clinic-based groups of women who were trying to become pregnant. Miller *et al.* and Edmonds *et al.* collected urine specimens starting around day 21 of a woman's cycle and then every other day until the onset of her menses. Miller assayed those urine specimens for hCG using a commercial kit. Edmonds measured urinary hCG with a radio-immunoassay based on the SB6 antibody. (The SB6 antibody is the basis for a serum assay that has been widely used in hCG research (Vaitukaitis *et al.*, 1972).) In the third study, Whittaker and his colleagues used a commercial kit to assay single blood specimens drawn from each woman during the luteal phase of her cycle. None of the assays used in these studies was completely specific to hCG in the presence of LH. In all of these studies, the authors regarded one day's elevation of hCG as a sufficient criterion for pregnancy.

The low incidence of loss found by Whittaker might easily be an underestimate, since only one specimen was collected in each cycle. The results of Miller and Edmonds could either be underestimates due to the relative insensitivity of their assays, or overestimates due to the possibility of cross-reaction with LH. Edmonds reports that the pregnancies detected earliest in the cycle were the ones most likely to be lost. The same appearance could be given by a late ovulation, in which a surge of LH after day 20 of the cycle was detected by their hCG assay. Sharp and colleagues (1986), using the same methods as Miller and Edmonds, speculate that late ovulations may in fact contribute to apparent 'early losses' seen with this approach.

We compared the ability of several hCG assays to detect early pregnancy loss (Wilcox *et al.*, 1985). Daily urine specimens were collected from 28 healthy women who had stopped using birth control in order to become pregnant. These women provided specimens for a total of 89 cycles. We analysed every urine for hCG using three assays: the SB6 assay used by Edmonds, the radio-immunoassay (RIA) used by Wehmann, and the immuno-radiometric assay (IRMA) used by Armstrong. In addition, we analysed these urines for LH using an RIA developed by Wehmann (Wilcox *et al.*, 1987).

Fig. 18.2 shows an example of these data for a woman who conceived a successful pregnancy in her second cycle. Note that the SB6 hCG assay cross-reacts in both cycles with the LH surge produced around the time of ovulation. Even while detecting the LH peaks, the SB6 assay is still too insensitive to detect the apparent pregnancy and early loss during the first cycle shown by the immuno-radiometric assay. The IRMA detected four early losses among these 28 women. Only one of those losses produced hCG in sufficient quantities to be detected by the SB6 assay.

Each of the IRMA-detected early pregnancy losses in our study occurred with vaginal bleeding. We found no instance of an hCG elevation in mid-cycle separated from bleeding. This differs from the large number of isolated mid-cycle elevations reported by Edmonds, which lends further support to the possibility that cross-reactivity with LH contributed to the incidence of early loss in Edmonds' data.

Baker and colleagues (1987) report similar findings in a study that compared Edmonds' assay with a more specific hCG assay. Urine specimens had been collected from 36 women attempting pregnancy. Baker concluded that Edmonds' SB6 assay was reactive to non-hCG substances in the urine produced during mid-cycle, while the more specific hCG assay did not detect those substances.

Results from the National Institute of Environmental Health Science (NIEHS) Early Pregnancy Study

We continued observations of early pregnancy by enrolling 200 additional women for study. Women were recruited from local communities and enrolled

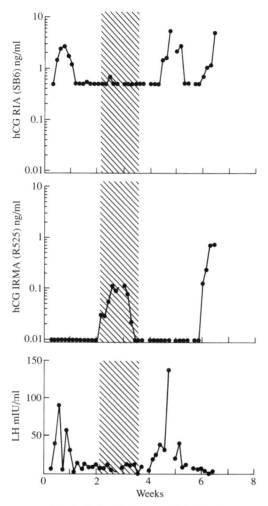

The hormones were measured by both the SB6 assay and the IRMA.

Source: Adapted from Wilcox *et al.*, 1985. Reproduced with permission of the publisher, the American Fertility Society.

Fig. 18.2   Luteinizing hormone and hCG measurements for a woman with an early pregnancy loss followed by a clinically recognized pregnancy

at the time they stopped using birth control in order to become pregnant. These women were required to have no known or suspected fertility problems and no chronic disease. Volunteers were asked to collect daily first-morning urine specimens until at least 8 weeks after their last menstrual period if they became clinically pregnant, or for 6 months if no pregnancy occurred.

Urine specimens were frozen at home at the time of collection and picked up by study personnel on a regular basis. Women were paid 10 dollars a week for the collection and storage of these specimens. Frozen specimens were shipped to Columbia University where they were assayed for hCG using the IRMA. Data from a total of 221 women were available for analysis. Further details of protocol and results have been published (Wilcox *et al.*, 1985, 1987, 1988).

In order to distinguish hCG in early pregnancy from low levels of hCG found in non-pregnant women, we also enrolled a group of 31 women with tubal ligations. These women were asked to collect daily urine specimens for three cycles each. Compliance was high in all groups: women collected urine specimens for 98 per cent of their days in the study.

We developed a criterion of three consecutive days of urinary hCG concentration above 0.025 ng/ml to define an early pregnancy. When we consider only the first pregnancy of each woman during the study, there were 171 pregnancies detected by urinary assay. Forty-one of these (or 24 per cent) ended before being clinically recognized. The remaining 130 pregnancies survived to become clinically diagnosed; of these, 14 ended in spontaneous abortion (11 per cent). Thus, total detected pregnancy loss (considering one pregnancy per woman) was 55/171 or 32 per cent. Many women with an early loss went on to conceive a second time during the study. When all pregnancies are included, results are unchanged. A total of 199 pregnancies were identified in the study, with 44 (22 per cent) ending in an unrecognized loss. Including the spontaneous abortions occurring to recognized pregnancies, total loss was 32 per cent.

The hormone events that we counted as very early losses covered a wide spectrum, ranging from those with only a few days of hCG production to some that produced large quantities of hCG over several weeks. Fig. 18.3 shows five typical examples of the hCG profile seen with early pregnancy loss. None of these losses was clinically recognized, even though the largest of these produced a pattern of hCG similar to that seen with the earliest clinically-recognized spontaneous abortions (Wilcox *et al.*, 1985). (Additional examples of hCG profiles of early losses are provided in Wilcox *et al.*, 1985, 1988.)

In conclusion, our data suggest that the occurrence of early loss is much less than the theoretical maximum and less than some estimates from other studies based on urinary hCG. We have discussed differences in results among previous studies, differences which reflect a lack of both sensitivity and specificity in the assays used to define early loss. Using a very sensitive and specific assay for hCG, we found that a relatively small number of 'non-conception' cycles could be explained by the occurrence of unrecognized pregnancy loss. Among 552 cycles with no clinical pregnancy there were only 44 early losses identified by assay, accounting for only 8 per cent of the apparently non-pregnant cycles. This suggests that the vast majority of 'non-conception' cycles represent either the failure of the ovum to be fertilized or the loss of the fertilized ovum before the time that hCG can be detected in the mother's urine.

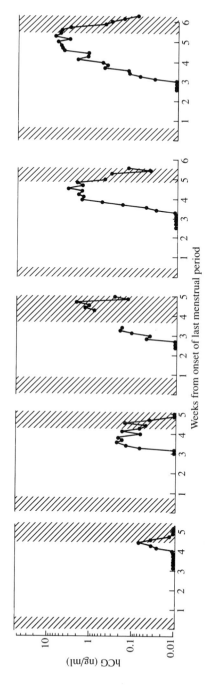

Fig. 18.3   Urinary hCG concentrations for five typical examples of early pregnancy loss from five different women

References

Ahmed, A. G., and Klopper, A. (1985), 'Serum Concentration of Placental Proteins in Non-pregnant and Pregnant Subjects', *Archives of Gynecology* 237: 41–9.

Armstrong, E. G., Ehrlich, P. H., Birken, S., Schlatterer, J. P., Siris, E., Hembree, W. C., and Canfield, R. E. (1984), 'Use of a Highly Sensitive and Specific Immuno-radiometric Assay for Detection of Human Chorionic Gonadotropin in Urine of Normal, Non-Pregnant and Pregnant Individuals', *Journal of Clinical Endocrinology and Metabolism* 59: 867–74.

Aschheim, S., and Zondek, B. (1927), 'Hypophysenvorderlappenhormon und Ovarial-hormon im Harn von Schwangeren', *Klinische Wochchenschrift* 6: 1322.

Baker, H. W. G., Kovacs, G. T., and Burger, H. G. (1987), 'Failure of Daily Measurements of hCH in Urine to Demonstrate a High Mortality', *Clinical Reproduction and Fertility* 5: 15–20.

Bloch, S. K. (1976), 'Occult Pregnancy: A Pilot Study', *Obstetrics and Gynecology* 48: 365–8.

Borkowski, A., and Muquardt, C. (1979), 'Human Chorionic Gonadtropin in the Plasma of Normal, Nonpregnant Subjects', *New England Journal of Medicine* 301: 298–302.

Braunstein, G. D., Karow, W. G., Gentry, W. D., and Wade, M. D. (1977), 'Subclinical Spontaneous Abortion', *Obstetrics and Gynecology* 50 (supplement): 41s–44s.

Chartier, M., Roger, M., Barrat, J., and Mickelon, B. (1979), 'Measurement of Plasma Human Chorionic Gonadotropin (hCG) and b-hCG Activities in the Late Luteal Phase: Evidence of the Occurrence of Spontaneous Menstrual Abortions in Infertile Women', *Fertility and Sterility* 31: 134–7.

Chen, C., Jones, W. R., Bastin, F., and Forde, C. (1985), 'Monitoring Embryos After in vitro Fertilization Using Early Pregnancy Factor', *Annals of the New York Academy of Science* 442: 420–8.

Edmonds, D. K., Lindsay, K. S., Miller, J. F., Williamson, E., and Wood, P. J. (1982), 'Early Embryonic Mortality in Women', *Fertility and Sterility* 38: 447–53.

Ellish, N. J., Chen, H.-C., Jason, C., and Janerick, D. T. (1986), 'Pilot Study to Detect Early Pregnancy and Early Fetal Loss', *Journal of Occupational Medicine* 28: 1069–73.

Fiddes, J. C., and Talmadge, K. (1984), 'Structure, Expression, and Evolution of the Genes for the Human Glycoprotein Hormones', *Recent Progress in Hormone Research* 40: 43–78.

Fishel, S. B., Edwards, R. G., and Evans, C. J. (1984), 'Human Chorionic Gonadotropin Secreted by Preimplantation Embryos Cultured in vitro', *Science* 223: 816–18.

Grudzinskas, J. G., and Nysenbaum, A. M. (1985), 'Failure of Human Pregnancy After Implantation', in: *In Vitro Fertilization and Embryo Transfer, Annals of the New York Academy of Science*, 442: 38–44.

Lasley, B. L., Stabenfeldt, G. H., Overstreet, J. W., Hanson, F. W., Czekala, N., and Munro, C. (1985), 'Urinary Hormone Levels at the Time of Ovulation and Implantation', *Fertility and Sterility* 43: 861–7.

Lenton, E. A., Neal, L. M., and Sulaiman, R. (1982), 'Plasma Concentrations of Human Chorionic Gonadotropin From the Time of Implantation Until the Second Week of Pregnancy', *Fertility and Sterility* 37: 773–8.

Lenton, E. A., Landgren, B.-M., Sexton, L., and Harper, R. (1984*a*), 'Normal Variation in the Length of the Follicular Phase of the Menstrual Cycle: Effect of Chronological Age', *British Journal of Obstetrics and Gynaecology* 91: 681–4.

—— —— —— (1984*b*), 'Normal Variation in the Length of the Luteal Phase of the Menstrual Cycle: Identification of the Short Luteal Phase', *British Journal of Obstetrics and Gynaecology* 91: 685–9.

Leridon, H. (1977), *Human Fertility: The Basic Components*, Chicago University Press, Chicago.

Lippman, A., and Farookhi, R. (1986), 'The Montreal Pregnancy Study: An Investigation of Very Early Pregnancies', *Canadian Journal of Public Health* 77 (supplement 1): 157–63.

Miller, J. F., Williamson, E., Glue, J., Gordon, Y. B., Grudzinskas, J. G., and Sykes, A. (1980), 'Fetal Loss After Implantation: A Prospective Study', *Lancet* 2: 554–6.

Morris, N. M., and Udry, J. R. (1967), 'Daily Immunologic Pregnancy Testing of Initially Non-Pregnant Women', *American Journal of Obstetrics and Gynecology* 98: 1148–50.

Morton, H., Morton, D. J., and Ellendorff, F. (1983), 'The Appearance and Characteristics of Early Pregnancy Factor in the Pig', *Journal of Reproduction and Fertility* 68: 437–46.

—— Rolfe, B., Clunie, G. J. A., Anderson, M. J., and Morrison, J. (1977), 'An Early Pregnancy Factor Detected in Human Serum by the Rosette Inhibition Test', *Lancet* 1: 394–7.

Tinneberg, H.-R., Rolfe, B., Wolf, M., and Mettler, L. (1982), 'Rosette Inhibition Test: A Multicentre Investigation of Early Pregnancy Factor in Humans', *Journal of Reproductive Immunology* 4: 251–61.

Noonan, F. P., Halliday, W. J., Morton, H., and Clunie, G. J. A. (1979), 'Early Pregnancy Factor is Immunosuppressive', *Nature* 278: 649–51.

Odell, W. D., and Griffin, J. (1987), 'Pulsatile Secretion of Human Chorionic Gonadotropin in Normal Adults', *New England Journal of Medicine* 317: 1688–91.

Overstreet, J. (1984), 'Assessment of Disorders of Spermatogenesis', in J. E. Lockey, G. K. Lemasters, and W. R. Keye (eds.), *Reproduction: The New Frontier in Occupational and Environmental Health Research*: (RMCOEH 5th Occupational and Environmental Health Conference, 1983, Park City, Utah) Alan R. Liss, New York: 275–92.

Roberts, T. K., Adamson, L. M., Smart, Y. C., Stanger, J. D., and Murdoch, R. N. (1987), 'An Evaluation of Peripheral Blood Platelet Enumeration as a Monitor of Fertilization and Early Pregnancy', *Fertility and Sterility* 47: 848–54.

Rolfe, B. E. (1982), 'Detection of Fetal Wastage', *Fertility and Sterility* 37: 655–60.

Sharp, N. C., Anthony, F., Miller, J. F., and Masson, G. M. (1986), 'Early Conceptual Loss in Subfertile Patients', *British Journal of Obstetrics and Gynaecology* 93: 1072–7.

Shaw, F. D., and Morton, H. (1980), 'The Immunological Approach to Pregnancy Diagnosis: A Review', *Veterinary Record* 106: 268–9.

Smart, Y. C., Roberts, T. K., Cancy, R. L., and Cripps, A. W. (1981*a*), 'Early Pregnancy Factor: It's a Role in Mammalian Reproduction—Research Review', *Fertility and Sterility* 35: 397–402.

—— Fraser, I. S., Roberts, T. K., Clancy, R. L., and Cripps, A. W. (1982), 'Fertilization and Early Pregnancy Loss in Healthy Women Attempting Conception', *Clinical Reproduction and Fertility* 1: 177–84.

Smart, Y. C., Cripps, A. W., Clancy, R. L., Roberts, T. K., Lopata, A., and Shutt, D. A. (1981*b*), 'Detection of an Immunosuppressive Factor in Human Preimplantation Embryo Cultures', *Medical Journal of Australia* 1: 78–9.

Udry, J. R. (1971), 'Pregnancy Testing as a Fertility Measurement Technique: A Preliminary Report on Field Results', *American Journal of Public Health* 61: 344.

Vaitukaitis, J. L., Braunstein, G. D., and Ross, G. T. (1972), 'A Radioimmunoassay which Specifically Measures Human Chorionic Gonadotropin in the Presence of Human Luteinizing Hormone', *American Journal of Obstetrics and Gynecology* 113: 751–8.

Vollman, R. F. (1977), *The Menstrual Cycle*, Saunders, Philadelphia, Pa.

Wehmann, R. E., Harman, S. M., Birken, S., Canfield, R. E., and Nisula, B. C. (1981), 'Convenient Radioimmunoassay that Measures Urinary Human Choriogonadotropin in the Presence of Urinary Human Lutropin', *Clinical Chemistry* 27: 1997–2001.

Whittaker, P. G., Taylor, A., and Lind, T. (1983), 'Unsuspected Pregnancy Loss in Healthy Women', *Lancet* 1: 1126–7.

Wilcox, A. J., Weinberg, C. R., Armstrong, E. G., Canfield, R. E., Nisula, B. C. (1985), 'Measuring Early Pregnancy Loss: Laboratory and Field Methods', *Fertility and Sterility* 44: 366–74.

—— Baird, D. D., Weinberg, C. R., Armstrong, E. G., Musey, P. I., Wehman, R. E., and Canfield, R. E. (1987), 'The Use of Biochemical Assays in Epidemiologic Studies of Reproduction', *Environmental Health Perspectives* 75: 29–35.

—— Weinberg, C. R., O'Connor, J. F., Baird, D. D., Schlatterer, J. P., Canfield, R. E., Armstrong, E. G., and Nisula, B. C. (1988), 'Incidence of Early Pregnancy Loss', *New England Journal of Medicine* 319: 189–94.

19 The Relationship Between Reduced Fecundability and Subsequent Foetal Loss*

DONNA D. BAIRD

N. BETH RAGAN

ALLEN J. WILCOX

CLARICE R. WEINBERG

Understanding the relationships among reproductive outcomes is important in both clinical and regulatory settings. In clinical settings, couples who have one reproductive problem may want to know whether they are at higher risk of others. In making regulatory decisions, it would be convenient to know if environmental or occupational exposures generally cause an array of reproductive problems. Then we could study a single outcome (the most convenient or the most sensitive). If, however, exposures are generally so specific in their biological effects that a given exposure affects only a specific outcome, a broader range of reproductive endpoints must be evaluated in order to assess the safety of exposures.

We are developing epidemiological methods for studying fecundability, the monthly probability of pregnancy for non-contracepting couples, in exposed and unexposed populations. We are particularly interested in the relationship between this reproductive outcome and others. In this paper we will describe the methods we have developed for measuring fecundability. Then we present a brief conceptual framework for generating hypotheses regarding the relationships between fecundability and foetal loss and summarize the existing literature. Data from the Collaborative Perinatal Project and the Early Pregnancy Study are used to evaluate the relationship in two very different data-sets.

Measuring Fecundability

Within a population of non-contracepting couples, the monthly probability of pregnancy ranges from zero for sterile couples to nearly one for the very fecund. Biological problems such as blocked tubes or hormonal imbalances that reduce fecundability have been identified in couples seeking medical

* We thank Dr Joseph Drage for giving us access to the NINCDS data tape of the Collaborative Perinatal Project.

treatment for infertility, and presumably these same sorts of biological problems contribute to the observed variations in fecundability among fertile couples. Tubal infections are known to reduce fecundability, but other causes are largely unknown. Little research has been conducted to investigate the possible influences of environmental and occupational factors.

A convenient way to measure fecundability is to collect data on time to pregnancy, that is, the number of non-contracepting months couples require to conceive. In order to evaluate the potential use of retrospectively collected time-to-pregnancy data, we conducted a study in Minnesota of married women who are pregnant with planned pregnancies. The study was designed to determine whether or not we could collect good time-to-pregnancy data, to identify important potentially confounding variables, to develop tools for analysis, and to estimate statistical power for study populations of various sizes (Baird and Wilcox, 1985; Baird *et al.*, 1986).

We found that most of the volunteers could provide data on time to pregnancy for their current pregnancies. Of the 762 women interviewed by phone, only three were unable to provide information. However, discontinuing contraception in order to get pregnant was not clearly defined for all of them. Unambiguous time-to-pregnancy data require that each couple uses effective birth control until the end of a given menstrual cycle, then remains at risk of pregnancy each cycle thereafter until pregnancy is achieved. Many couples do not behave in such an orderly fashion. 11 per cent of the 678 women for whom we collected complete data had used birth control sporadically for at least 2 months before discontinuing birth control completely. As an arbitrary way of including this time, the months of sporadic use were counted as half-months.

We could not evaluate the validity of our time-to-pregnancy data directly because alternative sources of accurate data were not available. Therefore, we used two indirect approaches to assess validity. First, we compared our data to similar data collected prospectively (Tietze, 1968). Cumulative times to pregnancy from our data and from Tietze's prospective data are shown in Fig. 19.1. Our data on the current pregnancies of Minnesota women, adjusted for menstrual cycle length and sporadic use of birth control, are quite similar to the prospective data. Second, we examined our data for digit preference. No statistically significant digit preference was observed in the time-to-pregnancy data on current pregnancies, but there was a significant preference for intervals of a half-year or a year in data on past pregnancies.

To identify potential confounders of time-to-pregnancy data, we collected information on factors that might influence fecundability. The factors most strongly associated with an increase in time to pregnancy were low frequency of sexual intercourse, recent oral contraceptive use, cigarette smoking, and recent pregnancy or nursing. Other factors associated with reduced fecundability in other populations, such as reported history of pelvic inflammatory disease (reviewed in Baird *et al.*, 1986), were not important in our group of women.

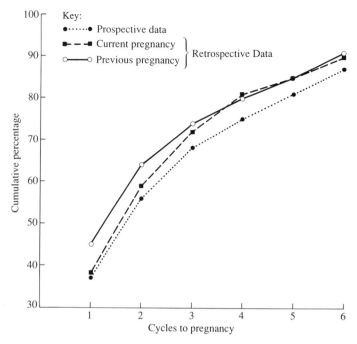

Sources: Prospective data from Tietze, 1968; retrospective data from Baird *et al.*, 1986.

Fig. 19.1 Comparison of data on time to pregnancy collected prospectively and retrospectively on current and past pregnancies

Data on time to pregnancy can be analysed in several ways that allow for simultaneous adjustment of variables. The most widely used survivorship model, the Cox proportional hazards model (Cox, 1972), can be used to estimate a relative fecundability associated with each factor of interest, controlling for all other factors. For example, the relative fecundability for smokers compared with non-smokers in the Minnesota population was 0.72, i.e. there was nearly a 30 per cent reduction in fecundability associated with smoking. Software for this model is widely available, and the measure is familiar to readers, but two problems arise in applying it to these data. Time-to-pregnancy data are discrete rather than continuous as assumed in the model (this results in many ties in the outcome), and subgroups may not show a fixed proportional probability of pregnancy over time. The latter is particularly problematic when recent pill users are included in the analysis, because the effects of oral contraceptives are transient.

To solve these problems, a discrete-time analogue of the Cox model can be applied using macros developed by Wacholder (1986). This model estimates the probability of conception for each menstrual cycle, assuming discrete data. Pill-users can be analysed with non-pill-users by including interaction terms 'pill by cycle' for each of the cycles (see Baird *et al.*, 1987 for an example).

Alternative methods of analysis, one based on the beta distribution (Weinberg and Gladen, 1986) and one using logistic analysis, can also be used to analyse time-to-pregnancy data. In the analyses we have done, results of each of these models, including the Cox model, are very similar despite the differences in model assumptions. The discrete-time analogue of the Cox model is our chosen analysis for most data because model assumptions are most clearly met.

One of the more advantageous aspects of time-to-pregnancy data for studying environmental or occupational hazards is the sensitivity of this measure. The power to detect significant differences between exposed and unexposed populations is relatively high. An exposure that causes a one-third reduction in fecundability can be detected over 80 per cent of the time with a population of 300 pregnant women, half of whom are exposed (Baird *et al.*, 1986).

We have used time-to-pregnancy data to study the influence on fecundability of a variety of common exposures, including cigarette smoking and prenatal exposure to cigarette smoking (Baird and Wilcox, 1985; Baird and Wilcox, 1986*a*; Baird *et al.*, 1987; Weinberg *et al.*, forthcoming; Wilcox *et al.*, 1991). We are currently studying time to pregnancy in dental assistants to examine the effect of their occupational exposures on fecundability.

Further methodological questions are being pursued with the population of dental assistants. We will be comparing data on time to pregnancy collected by asking a few simple questions with very detailed data that demands much more interview time and interviewer training. We also will be able to learn more about possible biases that arise from studying only planned pregnancies and excluding sterile couples, because some data are being collected from women with unplanned pregnancies and women trying to conceive.

Conceptual Framework

Evaluating the relationship between fecundability and the risk of foetal loss in populations is limited both by our lack of knowledge about the complex biological processes involved in reproduction and by the inadequacy of measurement tools for detecting reproductive loss. Fecundability must be measured by the ability to achieve a detectable pregnancy, and foetal loss must be measured by the loss of an already detected pregnancy. Because fecundability measurements depend on maintaining pregnancy to the time when it can be detected by widely available pregnancy tests, it involves three primary events: (1) ovulation, which is dependent on hormonal interactions of the ovary, hypothalamus, and pituitary; (2) tubal transport mechanisms, which allow sperm to reach the egg and the fertilized egg to reach the uterus in timely fashion; and (3) implantation, which is dependent on the development and responses of uterine tissue. Just as important, the egg must be fertilizable, the sperm able to fertilize, and the fertilized ova must remain viable through successive cell divisions. This requires adequate genetic potential and maternal environment. Once the pregnancy is recognized, its maintenance to delivery involves further adaptations of maternal physiology as well as adequate genetic potential of the embryo for continued growth and development.

The relationship between fecundability and risk of foetal loss depends on both the degree to which these two sets of biological processes overlap and whether or not factors that adversely affect one set also adversely affect the other set. Considering all reproductive loss from the failure of ovum development to late foetal loss, most occurs before pregnancy is detected (Fig. 19.2). Losses that occur about the time of detection will sometimes be interpreted as foetal loss and sometimes as reduced fecundability, yet they are not different events biologically. Another connection between the two outcomes involves biological processes required for both the attainment and maintenance of pregnancy. For example, an exposure that reduces progesterone production will affect both fecundability and foetal loss. If most reproductive toxins interfere with biological processes important for both achieving and maintaining

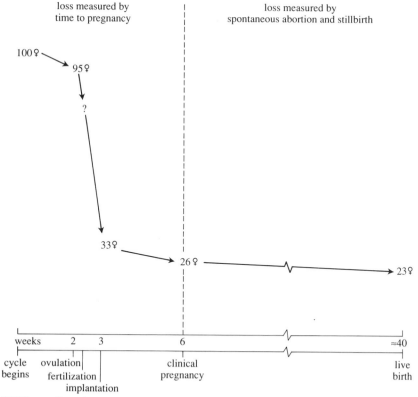

Of 100 sexually active women who start a non-contracepting cycle, approximately 95 will ovulate, but only 26 will achieve a clinically detected pregnancy. Relatively little loss occurs thereafter.

Source: Adapted from Fig. 1 in Baird *et al.*, 1986.

Fig. 19.2   Time-line of reproductive loss

detectable pregnancies or if the two sets of biological processes are highly interdependent, pregnancies that are more difficult to conceive will also be more likely to be lost.

Because the timing of pregnancy detection will affect the classification of reproductive loss, this can bias the measured relationship between fecundability and foetal loss in a population. If a pregnancy lasts long enough to be detected but is then lost, it will be considered a foetal loss. If the pregnancy is lost before a clinical pregnancy test has been done, the woman has menstrual bleeding and that cycle is added to her time to pregnancy. She then appears less fecund. Women with early positive pregnancy tests will tend to have a higher foetal loss rate and a shorter average time to pregnancy than women who wait longer to have a pregnancy test (Fig. 19.3). The foetal loss rate changes from an estimated 20 per cent if all pregnancies are detected at time of first missed period, to less than 10 per cent if women wait until the second missed period to have pregnancy tests done. If this shift in classification is not taken into account by controlling for gestational age at time of pregnancy test, a relationship between reduced fecundability and increased foetal loss will be underestimated or even appear negative.

Literature Review: Fecundability and Foetal Loss

Although spontaneous abortion has been studied extensively and reduced fecundability is a major clinical specialization, the relationship between these

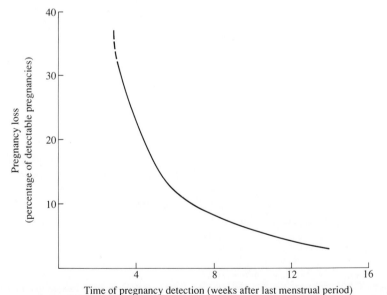

Fig. 19.3   Measured rate of pregnancy loss as a function of gestational age at time of pregnancy detection

two outcomes has seldom been examined. In an early paper, Tietze *et al.* (1950) noted that among nearly 1500 planned pregnancies, the pregnancies that took longer to conceive were more likely to be lost in spontaneous abortions. Women who took over six months to conceive were 2.2 times more likely to have a spontaneous abortion than women who conceived within the first six months. Age accounted for some of this association, but a significant relationship remained after controlling for age. In a stratified random sample of Danish women aged 25–45, Rachootin and Olsen (1982) reported that women with a history of lower fecundability were more likely to have had a spontaneous abortion. However, this study did not evaluate the relationship in a given pregnancy, i.e. the risk of spontaneous abortion following a longer or shorter time to pregnancy. Using data from a New York City case-control study of spontaneous abortion, Strobino *et al.* (1980) reported that 111 recurrent aborters had a longer time to pregnancy on average than either women with only one spontaneous abortion (n = 424) or women with all live births (n = 200).

Several other studies describe high spontaneous abortion rates in infertility patients. Jansen (1982) reviewed many of these reports and concluded that patients seeing physicians for infertility problems experience higher spontaneous abortion rates than the general public. Notable exceptions were women with hyperprolactinemia treated with bromocriptine, women receiving artificial insemination with donor semen because their partners had azoospermia, and women who had had surgical treatment for endometriosis.

Baird and Wilcox (1986*b*) reviewed toxicological data on mice and rats to evaluate whether substances tested for reproductive toxicity had adverse effects on both fecundability and foetal loss. Of the 36 studies showing some reproductive toxicity, 27 showed adverse effects on both outcomes. This suggests that many toxic substances adversely affect more than one of the biological processes involved in reproduction or cause any of several genetic defects that can interfere with development at different stages. Few data are available on the effects of toxic substances on multiple aspects of human reproduction, but those available suggest similar findings (Barlow and Sullivan, 1982; Kharrazi *et al.*, 1980; Schrag and Dixon, 1985; Wilcox *et al.*, 1989).

Analysis of Data

We are able to examine the relationship of fecundability and subsequent foetal loss in two very different data-sets. The first database we examined is the Collaborative Perinatal Project of the National Institute of Neurological and Communicative Disorders and Stroke, designed to investigate developmental consequences of pregnancy complications. Spontaneous abortion was ascertained in the usual fashion in these data, reported by either the woman or the physician, and gestational age at the time pregnancy was detected is not known. Thus, these data are subject to the bias discussed above. The second data-set, the Early Pregnancy Study (Wilcox *et al.*, 1985; Wilcox *et al.*, 1988), provides a special opportunity to look at the relationship in a population with very early pregnancy detection. Daily urines collected from the time a woman stopped contracepting were examined for human chorionic gonadotrophin (hCG). Pregnancy was defined by a very sensitive hCG assay that detected pregnancies soon after implantation. Most of the pregnancy loss reported in this study occurred sub-clinically, so this database allows us to examine the relationship between fecundability, as defined by ability to maintain pregnancy to implantation, and very early pregnancy loss. The literature suggests that we will find an association between reduced fecundability and foetal loss in both data-sets, but the relationship should be stronger in the data from the Early Pregnancy Study because the data are controlled for the time when pregnancy was detected.

The Collaborative Perinatal Project

Pregnant women enrolled in the study between 1959 and 1965, and data were collected by interview and examination (see Broman, 1984, for an overview of recruitment and data-collection methods). A total of 55 043 pregnancies were followed; however, data on time to pregnancy, outcome of pregnancy, and several covariates were available only for a small subset of the study subjects. We excluded unmarried women, women less than 18 years of age, and women with medical problems that might increase abortion risk. Data for a total of 1701 white and black women who enrolled by the end of their first trimester were analysed. Only women's first study pregnancies were included.

Characteristics of the 1701 women included in the analysis sample are shown in Table 19.1. The overall percentage of women experiencing a spontaneous abortion in the index pregnancy, slightly over 6 per cent, is low because women entered the study at different times during their first trimester. Those enrolling late were at a much reduced risk of subsequent foetal loss. A history of spontaneous abortion was relatively common. Of the 58 per cent of women with one or more previous pregnancies, 37 per cent had at least one spontaneous abortion.

The relationship between time to pregnancy and subsequent foetal loss was examined by logistic regression, with foetal loss as the outcome variable. All analyses of the relationship between time to pregnancy and foetal loss are controlled for gestational age at enrolment. Table 19.2 shows the relationships between the two outcomes with adjustments in some models for maternal age and smoking. As hypothesized, those with longer times to pregnancy were significantly more likely to experience a spontaneous abortion in that pregnancy. The relationship was relatively weak (OR = 1.18, 95 per cent CI = 1.06, 1.32). A 12-month delay in conception was associated with an 18 per cent increase in the odds of spontaneous abortion. Much of the increased risk could be explained by factors expected to affect both outcomes: increased maternal

TABLE 19.1. *Descriptive characteristics of the 1701 women of the Collaborative Perinatal Project*

Characteristic	Percentage
Age	
18–24 years	48.8
25–29 years	33.0
30–44 years	18.2
Race	
White	89.7
Black	10.3
Gravidity	
1st pregnancy	42.3
2nd pregnancy	28.5
> 2nd pregnancy	29.2
Education	
< 12 years	21.6
12 years	41.0
> 12 years	37.4
Gestational age at entry	
≤ 6 weeks	4.8
7–8 weeks	22.9
9–10 weeks	40.2
11–12 weeks	32.1
Smoking status	
smoker	41.8
non-smoker	58.2
Time to pregnancy	
1 month	29.9
2 months	15.2
3 months	9.4
4–6 months	16.6
7–12 months	13.6
13–98 months	15.3
Age at menarche	
< 12 years	21.2
12–14 years	70.1
> 14 years	8.7
Quetelet's index (weight/height^2)	
low	12.6
normal	76.0
high	11.4

Source: Broman, 1984.

age and cigarette smoking. The remaining association, an estimated 11 per cent increase in the odds, is no longer statistically significant (see Table 19.2). None of the other variables for which we had data affected the relationship.

The Early Pregnancy Study

Women enrolled in the study at the time they began trying to become pregnant (Wilcox *et al.*, 1985). The population has been described elsewhere (Wilcox *et al.*, 1988). Time to pregnancy was ascertained prospectively. Of the 221 women in the study, 171 conceived within the 6-month period of daily hCG surveillance. Of these women, 54 experienced pregnancy loss, 74 per cent of which was sub-clinical, identified only by hCG rise and fall. Among these women there is no relationship between time to pregnancy and pregnancy loss. Of those who conceived during the first cycle, 31 per cent experienced a loss. This percentage of loss remains quite stable regardless of the time to pregnancy (Table 19.3). Removing recognized spontaneous abortions from the analysis does not change the relationship. The number of women having recognized spontaneous abortions in this study is too small to evaluate the relationship between the risk of early unrecognized loss and later recognized loss.

Discussion

As suggested by the literature, reduced fecundability was associated with increased risk of spontaneous abortion in the subsequent pregnancy within the

TABLE 19.2. *Relationship between fecundability and spontaneous abortion among women in the Collaborative Perinatal Project*

Model	Variables	Relative odds of spontaneous abortion (95% confidence interval)
I	Time to pregnancy (12-month increase)	1.18 (1.06, 1.32)
II	Time to pregnancy	1.14 (1.02, 1.29)
	Maternal age (5-year increase)	1.15 (0.93, 1.43)
III	Time to pregnancy	1.14 (1.03, 1.29)
	Cigarette smoking	1.73 (1.16, 2.59)
IV	Time to pregnancy	1.11 (0.98, 1.25)
	Maternal age	1.20 (0.96, 1.49)
	Cigarette smoking	1.81 (1.20, 2.71)

Note: Models show different levels of adjustment for potential causes of reproductive loss.

TABLE 19.3. *Frequency of foetal loss in relation to fecundability among participants in the Early Pregnancy Study*

Cycles to pregnancy	Pregnancy loss (%)
1	21/67 (31)
2	14/45 (31)
3	11/33 (33)
4	3/12 (25)
5–7	5/16 (36)

Collaborative Perinatal Project sample. In this group nearly half the increased risk of spontaneous abortion associated with reduced fecundability could be accounted for by factors already identified as common 'causes' of both outcomes. Increased maternal age and cigarette smoking were about equally important. The remaining unexplained association was very small and not statistically significant.

The Early Pregnancy Study sample is a small group, but it provided unique data. Time to pregnancy was ascertained prospectively, and pregnancy loss includes all loss detectable by very sensitive measures of hCG. This eliminates the inherent bias in most populations from normal variability in gestational age at the time of pregnancy detection. Therefore, we expected a stronger association between outcomes in this population, and the lack of association was surprising. It suggests that the biological processes required for very early post-implantation development and those involved with achieving conception and implantation are not highly interdependent. It also raises the question of whether or not the associations observed in the Collaborative Perinatal Project data and in the literature could be due largely to bias. If women who require a long time to conceive tend to be more anxious about getting an early pregnancy test, these women will be more likely to have a spontaneous abortion identified. A woman who goes for a very early pregnancy test and has her pregnancy ascertained at 4 weeks after her last menstrual period will have an estimated risk of spontaneous abortion twice as high as a woman whose pregnancy was ascertained 4 weeks later, based on data from Harlap *et al.* (1980). This potential bias could be controlled in future retrospective studies by collecting data on gestational age at the time of the first positive pregnancy test.

Alternatively, it is possible that the Early Pregnancy Study showed no relationship between fecundability and foetal loss because this group of women were exceptionally free of adverse exposures. The women were generally well educated and health conscious. The known common 'causes', like smoking and increased maternal age, are not prevalent in this population. Only eleven of the 171 women who conceived in the study were smokers, and only seven were over 35 years of age. However, overall reproductive loss among the Early

Pregnancy Study women is not particularly low, suggesting that this population does not have exceptional reproductive success due to healthy living.

Finally, it is possible that the reported relationship between low fecundability and increased foetal loss is due primarily to an association between sub-clinical post-implantation loss and clinical spontaneous abortion. If so, once sub-clinical post-implantation loss is removed from the measure of fecundability, the two outcomes would become independent.

Taken together, the data-sets raise serious questions about the strength of a relationship between fecundability and foetal loss. It is possible that specific occupational or environmental exposures will affect both outcomes, but common exposures found in a volunteer population do not appear to be strongly related to both outcomes. At this point there is no good evidence that studying any one outcome will be sufficient to detect a problem in another outcome. The only safe approach to the study of potential environmental or occupational hazards is to examine a series of reproductive outcomes within each exposed population.

References

Baird, D. D., and Wilcox, A. J. (1985), 'Cigarette Smoking Associated with Delayed Conception', *Journal of the American Medical Association* 253: 2979–83.
—— —— (1986a), 'Future Fertility After Prenatal Exposure to Smoke', *Fertility and Sterility* 46: 368–72.
—— —— (1986b), 'Effects of Occupational Exposures on the Fertility of Couples', *Occupational Medicine: State of the Art Reviews* 1: 361–74.
—— —— and Weinberg, C. R. (1986), 'Use of Time to Pregnancy to Study Environmental Exposures', *American Journal of Epidemiology* 124: 470–80.
—— —— —— and Daling, J. (1987), 'More Evidence for Reduced Fertility among Women who Smoke Cigarettes' (abstract), *American Journal of Epidemiology* 126: 780.
Barlow, S. M., and Sullivan, F. M. (1982), 'Reproductive Hazards of Industrial Chemicals', Academic Press, London.
Broman S. (1984), 'The Collaborative Perinatal Project: An Overview', in S. A. Mednick, M. Harway, and K. M. Finello (eds.), *Handbook of Longitudinal Research*: 185–215, Praeger, New York.
Cox, D. R. (1972), 'Regression Models and Life-Tables', *Royal Statistical Society Journal (B)* 34: 187–220.
Harlap, S., Shiono, P. H., and Ramcharan, S. (1980), 'A Life Table of Spontaneous Abortions and the Effects of Age, Parity, and Other Variables', in I. H. Porter, and E. B. Hook (eds.), *Human Embryonic and Fetal Death*: 145–58, Academic Press, New York.
Jansen, R. P. S. (1982), 'Spontaneous Abortion Incidence in the Treatment of Infertility', *American Journal of Obstetrics and Gynecology* 143: 451–73.
Kharrazi, M., Potashnik, G., and Goldsmith, J. R. (1980), 'Reproductive Effects of Dibromochloropropane', *Israeli Journal of Medical Science* 16: 403–6.

Rachootin, P., and Olsen, J. (1982), 'Prevalence and Socioeconomic Correlates of Subfecundity and Spontaneous Abortion in Denmark', *International Journal of Epidemiology* 11: 245–9.

Schrag, S. D., and Dixon, R. L. (1985), 'Occupational Exposures Associated with Male Reproductive Dysfunction', *Annual Review of Pharmacology and Toxicology* 25: 567–92.

Strobino, B. R., Kline, J., Shrout, P., Stein, Z., Susser, M., and Warburton, D. (1980), 'Recurrent Spontaneous Abortion: Definition of a Syndrome', in I. H. Porter and E. B. Hook (eds.), *Human Embryonic and Fetal Death*: 315–30, Academic Press, New York.

Tietze, C. (1968), 'Fertility after Discontinuation of Intrauterine and Oral Contraception', *International Journal of Fertility* 13: 385–9.

—— Guttmacher, A. F., and Rubin, S. (1950), 'Unintentional Abortion in 1,497 Planned Pregnancies', *Journal of the American Medical Association* 142: 1348–50.

Wacholder, S. (1986), 'Binomial Regression in GLIM: Estimating Risk Ratios and Risk Differences', *American Journal of Epidemiology* 123: 174–84.

Weinberg, C. R., and Gladen, B. C. (1986), 'The Beta-Geometric Distribution Applied to Comparative Fecundability Studies', *Biometrics* 42: 547–60.

—— Wilcox, A. J., and Baird, D. D. (1991), 'Common Exposures and Fecundity: Results from a Prospective Study in North Carolina', forthcoming.

Wilcox A. J., Weinberg, C. R., O'Conner, J. R., Baird, D. D., Schlatterer, J. P., Canfield, R. E., Armstrong, E. G., and Nisula, B. C. (1988), 'Incidence of Early Loss of Pregnancies', *New England Journal of Medicine* 319: 189–94.

—— Baird, D. D., and Weinberg, C. R. (1989), 'Do Women with Childhood Exposure to Cigarette Smoking Have Increased Fecundability', *American Journal of Epidemiology* 129: 1079–83.

—— Weinberg, C. R., Wehmann, R. E., Armstrong, E. G., Canfield, R. E., and Nisula, B. C. (1985), 'Measuring Early Pregnancy Loss: Laboratory and Field Methods', *Fertility and Sterility* 44: 366–74.

Part VII

Post-Partum Infecundability and the Role of Lactation

20 Fecundability and Post-Partum Sterility: An Insuperable Interaction?

HENRI LERIDON

Introduction

The recent increase of interest in the 'intermediate variables' of fertility (a concept already used by Davis and Blake in 1955 and by the first modellers of the reproductive process such as Henry, Potter, and Sheps) has led to an intense scrutiny of birth intervals and their components. Attention has first been focused on the duration of the non-susceptible period, which is equated to the duration of post-partum amenorrhoea, especially in relation to breastfeeding, which is acknowledged to be its main determinant. But there are other ingredients contributing to the size of birth intervals, namely the duration of pregnancy (almost constant, at least for live births), the time lost by unreported or undetected abortions, and the waiting time to conception.

From the distribution of the delays before conception, it is possible to estimate the monthly risk of conception (fecundability) and its distribution among couples. Usually this research looks at the interval between marriage and first conception, because the date of marriage can usually be regarded as coinciding with the beginning of sexual relations or, at least, regular sexual relations. However, critics have objected that the first months of marriage may be characterized by an unusually high frequency of intercourse, thus leading to an upward bias in estimates of fecundability. In addition, the mean age of the newly married is, by definition, lower than the mean age at successive births, and the biological parameters influencing fecundability may vary with age. This latter objection can be overcome in part by tabulating the time to conception by age at marriage, but there still remains the risk of a temporarily high frequency of intercourse.

It is thus quite logical to think that we should get a more accurate view of the reproductive process by also estimating fecundability during subsequent birth intervals together with the non-susceptible period. In this paper, I will review the various techniques that have been used for this purpose and discuss their shortcomings. I will first review the indirect techniques that have been used to estimate the components of birth intervals without actually measuring each of them; then, we will examine methods using information on the duration of breastfeeding, which is, as already mentioned, a major determinant of the birth interval; and, finally, we will see what can be gained from information on the actual duration of amenorrhoea after the last birth.

Indirect Estimates of the Components

Methods Based on Dates of Marriage and Live-Births

When the only information recorded consists of the dates of marriage and births, the first step is to estimate fecundability from the distribution of the time between marriage and first conception, the first conception presumably occurring nine months before the first live birth. The next step is to compare this interval with the first inter-birth interval to get an estimate of the post-partum period of infecundity, which is included in the second interval but not the first. The first step of this procedure has been widely used: for a review of the results and a discussion of some of the problems encountered, see Leridon (1973) and Goldman, Westoff, and Paul (1985). The second step has been carried out more rarely, probably because it seems somewhat artificial to mix information from two different sources, especially if we assume that fecundability does vary with duration of marriage. As a first rough estimate of an invisible component of the interval, however, it must not be neglected.

Use of Information on Infant Deaths

In most cases, another piece of information is available: the date of the child's death. When the child dies early, the mother stops lactating and is likely to resume menstruation soon afterwards. By comparing the length of the interval for surviving children, on the one hand, and for children who die soon after birth, on the other hand, we can estimate the extent to which lactation lengthens the interval (for an example, see Cantrelle and Leridon, 1971). The main objection to this technique is that the probability of the child's death might be related to some characteristics of the mother which are not independent of her own fecundity: for example, severe malnutrition can lead to a higher risk of mortality for the child and to a lower fecundability or a longer period of anovulation for the mother. The situation could be clarified by getting some information on the major causes of infant death in the population: some causes may be strictly specific to the children and independent of the characteristics of the mothers, while others may not comply with these conditions.

Use of Models

The delay between a birth and the next conception is the net result of the combination of two distributions: one for the infecund period and one for the time to conception. It is thus tempting to formulate some hypotheses for the mathematical forms of these distributions and then estimate both of them simultaneously from the distribution of intervals (e.g. D'Souza, 1973). However, the major problem here is that the theoretical distribution of amenorrhoea is poorly known and, from what we do know, seems rather complex: sometimes unimodal, more often bimodal (Lesthaeghe and Page, 1980; Potter and Kobrin, 1981; Ford and Kim, 1987). Ford and Kim, for instance, use a model with five parameters, which can be useful for adjusting a crude distribution, but cannot realistically be used as an input to a model of indirect estimation.

Methods Using Information on Breastfeeding

Interval with or without Breastfeeding

When a child is weaned very early, the situation may seem similar to the sudden death of the child: in both cases, breastfeeding stops, and ovulation can be supposed to resume soon after. However, while some infant deaths are fully independent of the personal characteristics of the mother, early weaning or the full absence of lactation is quite unusual in a traditional society and is likely to be the result of an abnormal situation either for the mother or for the child. In addition, the specificity of such a situation makes it a rare event in non-contracepting populations (while the death of a child during the first months of life is, unfortunately, not infrequent), and any estimate derived from such limited cases may be unreliable. When mean waiting times to conception are computed for non-lactating women, they appear to be severely biased upwards. In the next section, we will examine how data on duration of breastfeeding can be more fruitfully used.

Regressing the Interval Between Birth and Next Conception by Duration of Breastfeeding

The length of the birth interval (or of the interval between birth and next conception) appears to be a rather simple function of the duration of breast-feeding; in fact, a simple linear regression often fits the cross-tabulated data reasonably well, except for the extreme values. It is thus logical to substitute for the observed value for non-lactating women (or for women with very short durations of breastfeeding), a value estimated from the regression line. Gold-man, Westoff, and Paul (1987) have successfully applied this technique to twenty WFS (World Fertility Survey) surveys from Asia, Latin America, and Africa, and their procedures yielded estimates of median waiting times to conception without breastfeeding on the order of 7 to 8 months. The definition of 'waiting time to conception' in this context must not be misunderstood: it is the time elapsed between the last delivery and the next conception leading to a live birth, not the time elapsed since the end of the sterile period. In other words, it includes the period of post-partum anovulation which lasts at least one to three months in the absence of breastfeeding. The authors also mention that this estimate of the delay to conception is slightly higher than the one they calculated in their earlier analysis of first intervals (between marriage and first birth) and is significantly lower than the figure derived from actual durations of amenorrhoea. This last point will be discussed in the third part of this paper. The first point could be explained by a decline in coital frequency as the duration of marriage increases: the median delay to conception is extended by roughly 2 months when the duration of marriage increases by 5 years.

Use of Hazards Models with Breastfeeding as a Time-Dependent Covariate

Proportional hazards models have been invading the demographic literature in recent years, especially for the analysis of birth intervals. The monthly risk of conception can be considered a perfect example of a 'hazard risk' depending on a set of covariates, either fixed or time-varying or with time-dependent effects. From individual data on the duration of breastfeeding or post-partum sterility and the time of next conception, this kind of model can provide estimates of the monthly rates of conception for all values of the covariates. I have used the word rate, and not risk, because the notion of risk is only an abstraction behind the model. The model is fed with data on events, and its only power is to convert a set of observed rates for various durations and various subgroups (in fact, it uses the crude individual data) into a well-structured set, according to the kind of dependences that have been assumed. The problem of properly interpreting the results begins when it is not obvious that the rates computed by the programme are real proxies of the underlying risks.

To be more specific, I suggest that this model fails to estimate properly the risk of conception for exposed women when data on breastfeeding is the only information available and is used as an indicator of the women's exposure status. In a thorough analysis of the determinants of birth intervals in three Asian countries, Trussell *et al.* (1985) computed the hazard rates for sections of birth intervals by breastfeeding status within each section (contraceptive status is also used, but I will restrict my discussion to non-contracepting women). For instance, the monthly rate for the period 18–23 months after birth is computed for women still lactating during this sub-interval and for women who stopped lactating before the 18th month. The latter are supposed to have resumed ovulation and to be at risk of conception during the whole sub-interval. This assumption is quite realistic. The problem results from the fact that they may already have been exposed for a long period of time: first, because lactation ended any time before the beginning of the sub-interval and, second, because ovulation usually resumes before the end of breastfeeding. If fecundability is not identical for all women, which is highly probable, a selection process will be operating, leaving women who are less and less fertile still at risk as the duration elapsed since the return of ovulation increases. Furthermore, the situation is exacerbated if the sub-intervals are rather long (6 or 12 months in the paper under discussion). This can result in a severe underestimation of fecundability.

Trussell *et al.* derived hazard rates for the Philippines as low as .022 for months 0–2 after birth, with a maximum value of .077 for months 18–23. (For the two other surveys, the maximum values were even lower.) In their discussion of these results, the authors acknowledged the possibility of a bias due to the above-mentioned selection, but they did not try to estimate its extent. I will try to make such an estimate in the next section.

The Selection of the Less Fecund

I will illustrate the selective process with data from the Philippines. The preliminary tables prepared by Singh and Ferry (1984) provide distributions of the duration of breastfeeding and post-partum amenorrhoea on a monthly basis. From these marginal distributions, I have derived a two-way table of combined durations for both events. After resumption of menstruation, the monthly rate of conception will be determined by the level of fecundability, which is assumed to be distributed among women according to a beta-distribution with parameters a and b. This means that after N months of exposure, the mean rate of conception is $a/(a + b + N)$. With $a = 3$ and $b = 12$, the initial mean fecundability (rate for month 0) is equal to 0.2.

Duration since last birth is broken into the same periods as in the Trussell study: 0–2, 3–5, 6–11, 12–17, 18–23, 24–35, and 36–47 months. For each month M, the number of women at risk is defined according to the same rules: if month M belongs to the period beginning with month K, women at risk are those who have stopped breastfeeding before month K and have not conceived before month M. Rates are computed per month and are also averaged over successive periods. Finally, a direct calculation has.been performed, using the distribution of the time of the return of menses as a starting date for exposure to conception.

Taking this last event as duration 0 for all women makes it easy to forecast monthly rates: the rate is 0.2 for the first month and then decreases by virtue of the selection of the less fecund. It is, however, unlikely that fecundability immediately comes back to its normal level during the first menstrual cycle; I have assumed that the rate of conception is only half its normal value during this first month and then 25 per cent below its normal value during the second month.

Table 20.1 shows the conception rate per 1000 women for each of the first 36 months following a live birth, calculated both from the 'actual values' (based on the duration of amenorrhoea) and from the 'Hazard simulation' (based on the duration of breastfeeding). This table suggests that:

1. Because of the selection process, the rate never exceeds 0.13, although the mean fecundability of the population was set equal to 0.20;

TABLE 20.1. *Monthly conception rates for the first 3 years following a live birth (per 1000): a model for the Philippines*

Years	Months since live birth											
	1	2	3	4	5	6	7	8	9	10	11	12
	Actual values											
1	50	59	75	98	119	129	131	130	129	127	126	124
2	123	123	122	122	121	121	120	119	118	117	117	117
3	116	113	108	104	100	96	92	89	86	83	81	78
	Hazard simulation											
1	9	48	91	114	130	133	121	82	73	65	57	50
2	81	35	31	27	23	20	58	23	20	17	15	13
3	40	13	11	10	9	8	7	6	5	5	4	4

2. The rate first increases, as the number of newly exposed women rises, and then it decreases slowly as the selection process overcomes the previous effect;

3. The hazard procedure severely distorts the profile of the rates: the maximum rate is still 0.13, but it declines rapidly after month 6 to very low values, with rather erratic fluctuations due to the use of 3-, 6-, and 12-month periods.

In Table 20.2, the conception rates are shown by periods, so they can be compared with the results of the hazard model used by Trussell and colleagues. The trend of these last results agrees better with our 'actual' values than with our simulation of the hazard computation; the mean level, however, is substantially lower (at least, by half). Thus, we could conclude that our simulation assumed too high a level of fecundability and that the hazard analysis does suggest a low level of fecundability for the Philippines population. Unfortunately, this conclusion is contradicted by the estimates of the mean time to conception derived from the conception rates (more precisely the trimean):

TABLE 20.2. *Monthly conception rates for the first 3 years following a live birth, by period (per 1000): a model for the Philippines*

	Months since live birth						Trimean of time to conception
	0–2	3–5	6–11	12–17	18–23	24–35	
Actual values	68	116	128	122	118	100	12.2
Hazard simulation	49	125	75	33	21	9	14.5
Hazard actual values	22	47	42	56	77	58	15.1

the result of the simulation (14.5 months) is in close agreement with the hazard analysis (15.1 months) and not much higher than the actual value (12.2). We must therefore conclude that our model failed to reproduce the exact conditions of the Philippines study, the reality being even more complex than our attempted simulation. For instance, coital frequency could be dependent on lactation status or age of the child, thus distorting the estimation of 'normal' fecundability for couples really exposed. In sum, more than one selection process must be operating, and the net result is somewhat unpredictable.

Methods Using Information on Amenorrhoea

When does Exposure to Conception Begin?

The most usual indicator of the end of the sterile period is the return of the first menstruation after delivery. Though this event is not strictly linked to the time of the first ovulation, 'it now appears that ovulation and menstruation following amenorrhea begin at roughly the same time' (John *et al.*, 1987: 434). It does not follow, however, that fecundity will immediately regain its maximum value: the first cycles may be longer than usual and/or of greater variance, and some may be anovulatory. As a matter of fact, the study by John and colleagues shows that breastfeeding has an effect after the end of amenorrhoea, probably by increasing the frequency of anovulatory cycles.

Apart from this problem, it appears that we may have been too confident in our use of data on amenorrhoea. Is the return of menses such a clear-cut event, especially for women who are undernourished or in poor health? Spotting and other bleeding episodes can be confused with the return of regular menses. It may well be impossible to determine a specific time for the return of fertility if the transition from sterility to normal fecundability is a continuous process. Leaving this problem aside, we shall now consider how data on the duration of post-partum amenorrhoea can be used.

The Fertility Exposure Analysis

Hobcraft and Little (1984) have recently developed an analytical technique based on previous work by Gaslonde (Gaslonde and Bocaz, 1970). This method demands a large quantity of data, but some surveys carried out within the WFS programme provide a fair amount of the necessary information. The principle is quite simple (but the practice is not): for some period of time before the survey, e.g. five years, women are allocated to one of a set of states for each month. A typical set of states is: not in union (or abstaining from sexual relations), post-partum infecund (while lactating or not), contracepting, pregnant, and at risk of conception, which includes any remaining women.

For practical reasons, computations are made over periods of 12 months or more, so we are faced with a problem of selection similar to the one discussed above when estimating the monthly risk of conception during periods of exposure. Furthermore, Hobcraft and Little did not use information on duration of amenorrhoea in their case-study of the Dominican Republic. Instead, women were allocated to two states of post-partum sterility according to the length of time they breastfed during the birth interval. This time-period has been converted into a period of 'post-partum infecundity' (without lactation) and a period of 'lactational infecundity' (during breastfeeding). The conversion used standard tables derived from the Philippines Survey. It follows that the method is an indirect one, according to our terminology, but it should be possible to make use of data on post-partum sterility and so make a more direct estimation.

Mean fecundability, defined as the ratio of the proportion of months with a conception to the proportion of months at risk, was about 0.14 for women aged 20 to 29 years and 0.08 for women aged 30 to 39 years (these estimates are based on months 10–21 before the survey). The authors found these results 'surprisingly reasonable', but their actual judgement was not based on these levels of fecundability but on the mean delay to conception taken as the reciprocal of fecundability (respectively, 7.1 months and 12.7 months). These last estimates are, indeed, comparable to those derived from intervals to first birth. However, the mean delay to conception is not correctly determined by the reciprocal of fecundability when the risk is not identical for all women (because a harmonic mean is not equal to the reciprocal of the arithmetic mean), and the actual value is always greater than this estimate. Looking back to the estimated values of fecundability, we can confirm that they are rather low, a plausible explanation being, once again, that post-partum sterility is not measured directly.

Use of Hazard Models with Data on Amenorrhoea

Most of the objections that I raised to the analysis by Trussell and colleagues have been overcome in a more recent analysis of the Matlab data by John and Colleagues (1987). The hazard risk here is computed only for the menstruating portion of the birth interval, based on data from an intensive prospective study with monthly visits to sample households. The status in a given month is thus always the current status for a month of observation, which should guarantee a more reliable estimation of the situation. A logistic formulation of the model is used, with fixed covariates (age, religion, husband's occupation, height, season of resumption of menses, etc.) and time-varying covariates (number of months since resumption of menses, breastfeeding pattern, separation, and nutritional status).

These data from the Matlab study, in a rural zone of Bangladesh, have already been used intensively. One of the most striking results is the very low estimate of fecundability in this population: even after various corrections (e.g. for seasonal variations of various factors), the mean value does not exceed 0.10 (Menken, 1975). The hazard analysis confirms this peculiar situation once again: during the first months of the menstruating interval, the average risk of conception does not exceed 0.06 with the simplest models. When breastfeeding status is included, an interesting result emerges: the risk is lower than 0.01 for women still fully breastfeeding, about 0.06–0.10 for partially breastfeeding women, and as high as 0.19 for women who have weaned their children in the preceding 4 months. Such a wide variation might illustrate the continuing effect of breastfeeding even after the end of amenorrhoea, but alternative interpretations can be suggested.

The authors report (John *et al.*, 1987: 436) that 'previous studies have shown an inverse relationship between the duration of postpartum amenorrhea and the subsequent waiting time to conception', citing Delgado *et al.* (1982). Such a relation does exist for the Matlab data, as will be shown in the next section.

A Reconsideration of Matlab Data on Time to Conception

In the early phases of an analysis of seasonal patterns of reproduction in Bangladesh (Becker *et al.*, 1986), Becker made available data on the distribution of time to conception by duration of amenorrhoea. More precisely, he computed a life-table analysis of time to conception, month by month, for intervals between a live birth and resumption of menses equal to 0–4, 4–7, 8–11, 12–15, 16–19, 20–23, and 24 or more months. The 'survivors' (Lx) of these tables have been taken as input for a computation of 3-month probabilities of conception (Qx) in Table 20.3, and these rates are also shown in Fig. 20.1.

For durations of amenorrhoea greater than one year, the trend of the rates is more or less as expected: they decrease as the time elapsed since the return of menses increases. The value for the first trimester is still not very high, hardly exceeding 0.3, which is equivalent to an average monthly value of 0.112. But for shorter durations of post-partum sterility, the picture is quite different: rates steadily rise as time passes, starting below 0.07 (monthly equivalent: 0.024), reaching a value close to 0.2 after two years, and possibly rising to 0.3 after three years.

Three central indicators of these distributions are shown in Fig. 20.2: the median, the trimean, and an estimate of the mean. A typical value for the time to conception when menses returned within 12 months is 20 months; in contrast, when amenorrhoea lasted more than 15 months, the typical value is half that: 10 months or less. When we look at the crude distribution of the duration of amenorrhoea, shown in Fig. 20.3, it appears bimodal: the first peak, at 3–4 months, is unexpected for a population where virtually all women breastfed their children, where the median duration of breastfeeding is 32 months, and where the median duration of full breastfeeding exceeds 6 months (see Huffman *et al.*, 1987; in passing, Fig. 4 of their paper shows the probability

TABLE 20.3. *Time to conception by duration of previous amenorrhoea, Matlab Study, 1975–9*

Months since resumption of menses (x)	Duration of amenorrhoea (months)													
	0–3		4–7		8–11		12–15		16–19		20–23		24+	
	Lx	Qx	Lx	Qx	Lx	Qx	Lx	Qx	Lx	Qx	Lx	Qx	Lx	Qx
0	1000	.066	1000	.042	1000	.063	1000	.216	1000	.339	1000	.275	1000	.351
3	934	.078	958	.074	937	.105	784	.147	661	.265	725	.274	649	.197
6	861	.024	887	.089	839	.163	669	.184	486	.267	526	.201	521	.301
9	840	.085	808	.177	702	.147	546	.114	356	.031	420	.176	364	.0
12	769	.150	665	.147	599	.080	484	.205	345	.133	346	.130	364	.107
15	654	.205	567	.136	551	.129	385	.239	299	.157	301	.223	325	.181
18	520	.108	490	.194	480	.167	293	.164	252	.079	234	.120	266	.0
21	464	.155	395	.127	400	.100	245	.106	232	.108	206	.0		
24	392	.166	345	.246	360	.075	219	.0	207	.0				
27	327	.376	260	.165	333	.0								
30	204	.266	217	.0										
33	158	.247	217	.313										
36	119	.407	149	.0										
39	071	.0												
Median	19.1		17.6		17.2		11.2		5.8		6.7		6.4	
Trimean	19.9		18.3		17.9		11.2		8.0		8.4		9.2	
Mean[a]	21.4		21.7		20.0		14.4		12.0		12.1		12.7	
No. obs.[b]	108		145		113		152		152		144		107	

[a] Estimation. Mean duration for values 21 and more (last two columns) is set at 30 months; for values 24 and more (three central rows) at 31 months.

[b] Initial number of women (radix of the table).

Notes: Lx is the proportion of women without conception at duration x.
Qx is the 3-month probability of conception.

Source: Derived from Becker *et al.*, 1986.

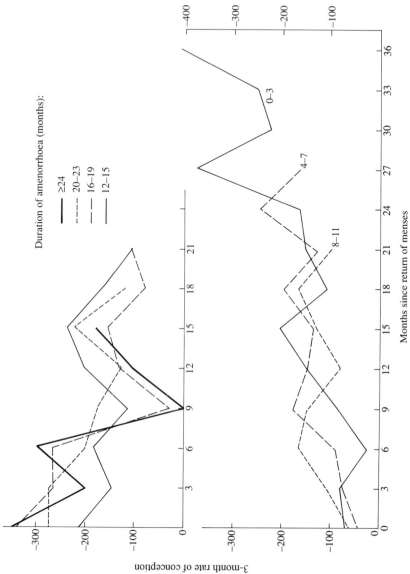

Fig. 20.1 Rate of conception, by months since return of menses, Matlab, Bangladesh

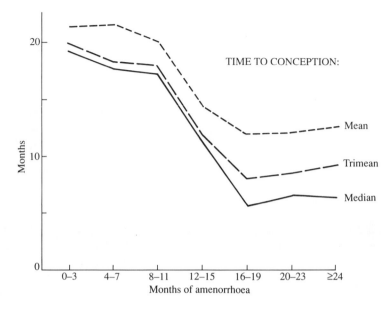

Fig. 20.2   Time to conception, by duration of amenorrhoea, Matlab, Bangladesh

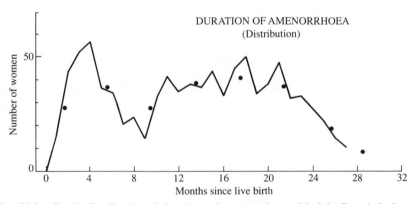

Fig. 20.3   Crude distribution of duration of amenorrhoea, Matlab, Bangladesh

of resuming menstruation during each post-partum month, in close agreement with the data in Fig. 20.3). There is a dip in the distribution for durations of 5–9 months and then a plateau for durations of 11–23 months. This leads us to question the accuracy of the data regarding the time of first menses after delivery: the inverse relationship between the duration of post-partum amenorrhoea and the menstruating interval may be a statistical artefact (John *et al.*, 1987). If that were the case, then estimates of fecundability derived from these data might be severely biased.

I agree that this is not the last word and that alternative explanations might still be considered: for example, a direct effect of breastfeeding on both amenorrhoeic and menstruating intervals, or coital patterns dependent upon either lactation or time elapsed since the last birth. If this last point were of great significance one might be led to question what 'normal' fecundability actually is. Are we trying to estimate the risk of conception when coital frequency is back, more or less, to its maximum, perhaps one year after birth? Or do we measure actual risks of conception, even as they vary with duration? In both cases, we will need accurate data on sexual behaviour.

Conclusion

These analyses suggest that it remains difficult to disentangle the components of birth intervals. Indirect techniques combining distributions of waiting time to conception and durations of post-partum amenorrhoea are limited by uncertainties about the shape of the second distribution. Methods using information on breastfeeding to compute monthly rates of conception after the supposed return of menses have severe biases, because the duration of breastfeeding is a very poor proxy for the duration of amenorrhoea and because of the heterogeneity of fecundability. Finally, even when data on amenorrhoea are available, we encounter the paradox of an apparent correlation between the duration of the non-susceptible period and the waiting time to conception that follows. If this relation is not an artefact, it means that fecundability does vary within the birth interval for some reason (physiological or behavioural) and that estimating such an unpredictable variable is indeed an insuperable challenge.

References

Becker, S., Chowdhury, A., and Leridon, H. (1986), 'Seasonal Patterns of Reproduction in Matlab, Bangladesh', *Population Studies* 40: 457–72.

Cantrelle, P., and Leridon, H. (1971), 'Breastfeeding, Mortality in Childhood and Fertility in a Rural Zone of Senegal', *Population Studies* 25: 505–33.

Delgado, H., Martorell, R., and Klein, R. (1982), 'Nutrition, Lactation and Birth Interval Components in Rural Guatemala', *American Journal of Clinical Nutrition* 35: 1468–76.

D'Souza, S. (1973), *Interlive-Birth Intervals of Non-Contracepting Populations: A Data Analytic Survey*, Sterling Publishing, New Delhi.

Ford, K., and Kim, Y. (1987), 'Distributions of Postpartum Amenorrhea: Some New Evidence', *Demography* 24: 413–30.

Gaslonde, S., and Bocaz, A. (1970), *Metodo para Medir Variaciones en el Nivel de Fecundidad*, Centro Latino Americano de Demografia (CELADE), series A., no. 107.

Goldman, N., Westoff, C. F., and Paul, L. (1985), 'Estimation of Fecundability from Survey Data', *Studies in Family Planning* 16: 252–9.

358   *Post-Partum Infecundability and Lactation*

Goldman, N., Westoff, C. F., and Paul, L. (1987), 'Variations in Natural Fertility: The Effect of Lactation and Other Determinants', *Population Studies* 41: 127–46.

Hobcraft, J., and Little, R. J. (1984), 'Fertility Exposure Analysis: A New Method for Assessing the Contribution of Proximate Determinants to Fertility Differentials', *Population Studies* 38: 21–45.

Huffman, S. L., Ford, K., Allen, H. A., and Streble, P. (1987), 'Nutrition and Fertility in Bangladesh: Breastfeeding and Postpartum Amenorrhea', *Population Studies* 41: 447–62.

John, A. M., Menken, J. A., and Chowdhury, A. (1987), 'The Effects of Breastfeeding and Nutrition on Fecundability in Rural Bangladesh', *Population Studies* 41: 433–46.

Leridon, H. (1973), *Human Fertility: The Basic Components*, University of Chicago Press, Chicago.

Lesthaeghe, R., and Page, H. J. (1980), 'The Postpartum Non-Susceptible Period: Development and Application of Model Schedules', *Population Studies* 34: 143–70.

Menken, J. (1975), *Estimating Fecundability*, Ph.D. dissertation, Princeton University, Princeton, NJ.

Potter, R. G., and Kobrin, F. E. (1981), 'Distributions of Amenorrhea and Anovulation', *Population Studies* 35: 85–99.

Singh, S., and Ferry, B. (1984), *Biological and Traditional Factors that Influence Fertility: Results from WFS Surveys* (Preliminary Tables), WFS Comparative Studies no. 40: 7–102.

Trussell, J., Martin, L. G., Feldman, R., Palmore, J. A., Conception, M., and Abu Bakar, D. (1985), 'Determinants of Birth-Interval Length in the Philippines, Malaysia and Indonesia: A Hazard-Model Analysis', *Demography* 22: 145–68.

21 Demographic Research on Lactational Amenorrhoea

KATHLEEN FORD

YOUNG J. KIM

The importance of lactational amenorrhoea as a determinant of fertility levels has long been recognized in demographic research. Breastfeeding practices vary widely across and within countries, and there is evidence of change in the extent of breastfeeding in several areas. Much work has been conducted in this area, including examination of data and measurement problems in population surveys, modelling of lactational amenorrhoea, and studies of its determinants.

A sample of the range of international variation in the length of breastfeeding and post-partum amenorrhoea that has been found in demographic and epidemiological studies is shown in Table 21.1. The shortest mean or median length of post-partum amenorrhoea (1.8 months) occurred in Taiwan among women who did not lactate, while the longest lengths of post-partum amenorrhoea (14–15 months) were recorded where breastfeeding is prolonged: in Bangladesh and Guatemala. There is considerable variation within each geographical region shown in the table. These data are mainly from less developed countries. In more developed countries, the lengths of breastfeeding and amenorrhoea tend to be much shorter.

This paper describes the approaches that demographers have taken toward collecting data on lactational amenorrhoea and modelling its determinants. The first section of the paper describes approaches to data collection and attempts to model the distribution of amenorrhoea; the second section discusses demographic models of the determinants of amenorrhoea.

Data and Measurement Problems

Researchers have attempted to measure the length of post-partum amenorrhoea in population surveys in a number of different ways using a variety of data-collection systems. The problems with data on amenorrhoea vary with the type of data-collection system used (Lesthaeghe and Page, 1980). Most data on amenorrhoea are from retrospective studies. When data are collected retrospectively, that is, when women are asked how long after the birth of their last child they resumed menstruation, the data often have large concentrations at

TABLE 21.1. *Duration of breastfeeding and post-partum amenorrhoea in selected populations (months)*

Population	Mean (median) duration of breastfeeding	Mean (median) duration of amenorrhoea
I. USA (Boston)	1.5	2.3
Colombia and Venezuela (cities)	6.0	2.9
Thailand (cities)	8.0	4.3
Turkey	9.0	3.7
Fiji[a]	9.4	4.6
Egypt (cities)	11.0	5.2
Syria[a]	11.2	6.6
Philippines (rural)	11.9	5.2
Nigeria (Lagos)	12.2	8.1
Philippines[a] (urban)	12.6	8.0
Tunisia[a]	14.0	6.9
Zaïre (Bukavu)	15.5	9.0
Mauritania[a]	15.6	8.8
Sudan[a]	15.8	10.8
Taiwan	16.1	10.1
Egypt[a]	16.3	8.9
India (Bombay)	16.5	11.9
Kenya[a]	16.9	9.9
Ivory Coast[a]	17.5	10.4
Cameroon[a]	17.5	11.8
Ghana[a]	17.9	12.4
Senegal (Pikine)	18.4	12.8
Zaïre (Ngweshe)	18.8	13.8
Benin[a]	19.2	11.9
Guatemala (rural)	19.2	14.8
India (Khanna)	21.0	10.6
Zaïre (Idjiwi)	21.8	17.9
Korea	23.0	13.5
Bangladesh (Matlab)	24.0	18.9
Senegal (rural)	24.3	14.7
Zaïre (rural)	26.0	20.0
Bangladesh[a]	26.5	14.6
II. Taiwan	0	1.8
	1–6	2.8
	7–12	5.2
	13–18	11.8
	19–24	13.5
	25+	14.8

Sources: Figures for countries marked [a] are from Singh and Ferry (1984) and represent mean durations; the other figures come from Bongaarts and Potter (1983) who combined means and medians.

preferred durations (typically 3, 6, 12, 18 or 20, and 24 months). Heaping is evident in these data. Some of this heaping may reflect the true distribution of the return of menstruation; however, if this were true, these extreme patterns should appear in data collected in different ways from the same population. Lesthaeghe and Page (1980) have presented some evidence that the heaping is not necessarily genuine.

A second approach to the collection of data on amenorrhoea relies on 'current status' data. With this method, durations of amenorrhoea are estimated from the proportions of women who are not menstruating at the time of the interview, tabulated by length of time since the last birth. While the problem of heaping on preferred digits is not excessive with this type of data, sampling fluctuations often create irregularities in the data. Furthermore, Bracher and Santow (1981) have shown that data on current status overestimate the duration of amenorrhoea, since women who discontinue breastfeeding early and so resume menstruation early are underrepresented. However, if fertility histories are available, this problem can be overcome by including all women with a birth *n* months ago in the calculation of the proportion not yet menstruating *n* months after the last birth.

Prospective studies, that is, studies where the data are collected at short time-intervals from the same women over a long period of time, offer the best possibility for producing data of good quality. However, to produce good data, these studies need to involve a large number of women, and the interviews have to be repeated at frequent intervals. Because of the great expense involved in collecting data in this way, such studies are rare. Researchers have collected data from five large prospective studies conducted in India, Bangladesh, and Guatemala (Chen *et al.*, 1974; Delgado *et al.*, 1978; Ford and Kim, 1987; Potter *et al.*, 1965).

Estimation of Duration of Amenorrhoea

Empirical estimates of the mean length of amenorrhoea have been made from large-scale surveys using both classical life-table procedures and a prevalence–incidence method borrowed from epidemiology (Ferry and Page, 1984; Knodel and Lewis, 1984; Singh and Ferry, 1984). The name 'prevalence–incidence mean' refers to the fact that it has been used in epidemiology to estimate the mean duration of a condition (Ferry and Page, 1984: 51). The mean can be estimated by:

Mean of amenorrhoea = Prevalence/Incidence,

where

Prevalence = number of women still in post-partum amenorrhoea
Incidence = average number of births per month.

Several efforts have also been made to model the distribution of post-partum amenorrhoea in a more formal way. A modified Pascal distribution, developed by Barrett (1969), has been used extensively in reproductive models. One of the advantages of this distribution is that it generates conditional monthly probabilities of resuming ovulation that increase with the period elapsed since childbirth. This rise is in keeping with insights into the mechanisms relating the length of post-partum amenorrhoea to lactational behaviour which imply a weakening inhibition of ovulation as the mother passes from more intensive breastfeeding to less intensive breastfeeding. This model is also compatible with Markov processes and Monte Carlo simulation, the two forms commonly taken by family-planning models. However, existing data on post-partum amenorrhoea, which correlates highly with post-partum anovulation, do not fit Barrett's distribution very well (Potter and Kobrin, 1981). Barrett's distribution is unimodal, and in many populations bimodal distributions are typical. Furthermore, in populations with long amenorrhoea, the distribution produces excessive variances (Potter and Kobrin, 1981).

Potter and Kobrin proposed a mixed geometric, negative binomial model which produced reasonable numbers resuming menstruation after a short period of time and less positive skewness. However, although they experienced some success in fitting the mixed distributions to available published data, lack of detail about the proportions lactating and the timing of infant deaths prevented them from drawing any strong conclusions about the appropriateness of the model.

Ford and Kim (1987) evaluated the fit of several models to longitudinal data collected from India and Bangladesh. They eliminated Barrett's model from consideration due to its excessive variances. Potter and Kobrin's mixed distribution was eliminated, since the distribution should begin with a small hill, not a sloping line. They recommended the use of a mixture of two Type 1 extreme value distributions for use with data on post-partum amenorrhoea. The Type 1 extreme value distribution is sometimes called the Gumbel distribution (Johnson and Kotz, 1970) and its distribution is given by

$$F(x) = \exp\left\{-\exp\left[-\left(\frac{x-\xi}{\theta}\right)\right]\right\}$$

Its density function is given by

$$f(x) = \frac{1}{\theta} \exp\left\{-\left(\frac{x-\xi}{\theta}\right) - \exp\left[-\left(\frac{x-\xi}{\theta}\right)\right]\right\}.$$

The mixture of the two distributions may be written as

$$f(x) = k\, f_1,\, (x) + (1-k)\, f_2\, (x)$$

where $f_1(x)$ has the parameters ξ_1 and θ_1, and $f_2(x)$ has the parameters ξ_2 and θ_2.

The parameters of the mixed distribution have demographic meanings. The model assumes that the population is made of two subgroups: one group with a short and the other with a long duration of amenorrhoea. The first parameter k indicates the proportion of women with short amenorrhoea, while $(1 - k)$ indicates the proportion of women with long amenorrhoea. The remaining parameters, (ξ_1, θ_1) and (ξ_2, θ_2), reflect the means and variances of the distributions of amenorrhoea for women with short and long durations. The parameters were estimated by minimizing the sum of squares of deviations for $f(x)$ or $F(x)$ (a least squares fit) and by minimizing the sum of squared deviations divided by the function (minimum chi-square).

Lesthaeghe and Page (1980) found that data on amenorrhoea from a large number of samples revealed bimodality and a large amount of heaping on multiples of 6 months. To cope with this, Lesthaeghe and Page developed a relational model based on the logit transformation. Their procedure is as follows:

1. Administer a three-point average to smooth the data
2. Convert the resulting proportions still amenorrhoeic into logits using the formula:

$$Y(d) = \text{logit } P(d) = (1/2)\ln \{P(d) / [1 - P(d)]\}.$$

3. Linearly regress the set of logits $Y(d)$ on a set of standard logits $Y(d)$ generated by Lesthaeghe and Page on the basis of Guatemalan data:

$$Y(d) = a + b \, Y(d).$$

4. Estimate the proportions still amenorrhoeic by the inverse transformation:

$$P(d) = \exp[2Y(d)] / \{1 + 1 + \exp[2Y(d)]\}.$$

This system smoothes the data while ensuring that the proportion remains greater than or equal to zero and less than or equal to one. This method can also produce unimodal and bimodal distributions of amenorrhoea. Distributions smoothed in this manner have a negative skewness when the series is of intermediate length and a positive skewness when the series is very short or very long (Potter and Kobrin, 1981). Data to show whether or not this series is real or is an artefact of the smoothing process have been hard to find.

Model Fitting

Ford and Kim (1987) evaluated the mixture model by fitting it to data from India and Bangladesh. In general the mixed distribution was able to reproduce the empirical distributions well. They also used the model to produce a pattern of the length of post-partum amenorrhoea by age and parity.

Fig. 21.1 shows the empirical density function (the probability of resuming menses in a given month) and model estimates for data from a large prospective study in Bangladesh. The empirical density function was calculated by the life-table method to take care of censored observations. The first figure includes

TABLE 21.2. *Parameter estimates for the mixed distribution of Type I distributions*

	k	ε_1	σ_1	ε_2	σ_2
Bangladesh					
Total sample	.26	2.86	1.56	15.73	6.54
Infant deaths removed	.24	3.33	1.91	16.27	6.29
Narangwal					
Total sample	.36	2.58	1.31	10.40	5.04
Infant deaths removed	.35	2.61	1.49	10.67	5.03
Bangladesh					
By age					
<25	.26	2.60	1.43	11.24	5.64
25–9	.31	2.88	1.49	15.83	6.36
30–4	.19	3.86	2.03	16.94	5.71
35+	.44	8.19	5.35	19.63	4.58
By parity					
1–2	.29	2.87	1.45	12.85	6.52
3–4	.21	3.25	1.91	17.24	6.15
5+	.26	5.29	3.50	18.02	5.11

data for all births. Parameter estimates for this model and models shown in the following figures are shown in Table 21.2. Fig. 21.2 shows the empirical density and model estimate for Bangladesh when cases with child deaths were removed. In this case the initial peak is much smaller, since women whose children die and who have much shorter periods of amenorrhoea are removed.

Figs. 21.3 and 21.4 show similar data from a longitudinal study conducted in Narangwal, India. Fig. 21.3 includes the empirical density and model estimate for all births, and Fig. 21.4 includes the empirical density and model estimate for all surviving births. The Narangwal population had a shorter length of breastfeeding than the Bangladesh population with much earlier supplementation. This is reflected in the shorter duration of amenorrhoea.

Figs. 21.5 and 21.6 show data by age and parity for Bangladesh. As can be seen from the graphs and the parameter estimates (Table 21.2), as age or parity increase, the distributions become longer.

Ford and Kim (1987) also evaluated the fit of the logit relational model to the data-sets from India and Bangladesh. They found that the model, using the original standard, did not fit the data very well. As with logit models of mortality, a good fit of the logit model for amenorrhoea may depend upon the use of an appropriate standard. They suggested the use of an additional standard, the smoothed Bangladesh data, for use with populations with long amenorrhoea and bimodal distributions.

In all of these modelling efforts, the question has often been raised of

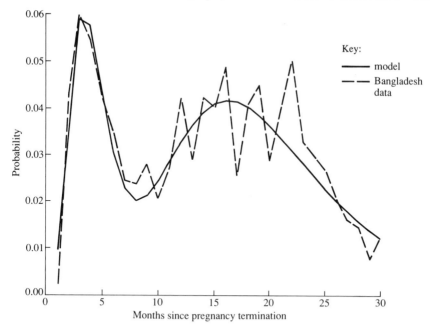

Fig. 21.1   Empirical density and model estimate for all births, Bangladesh

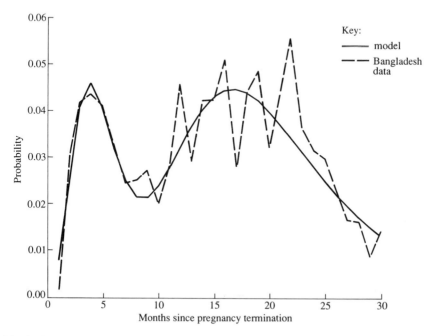

Fig. 21.2   Empirical density and model estimates for surviving births only, Bangladesh

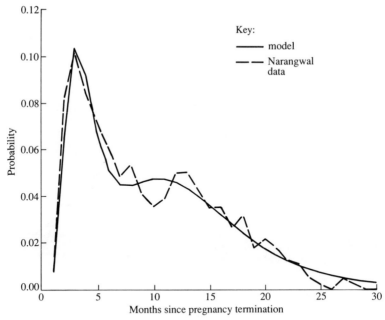

Fig. 21.3   Empirical density and model estimate for all births, Narangwal

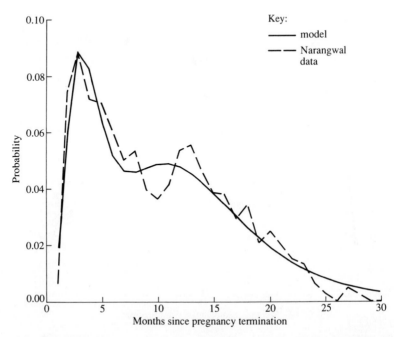

Fig. 21.4   Empirical density and model estimate for surviving births only, Narangwal

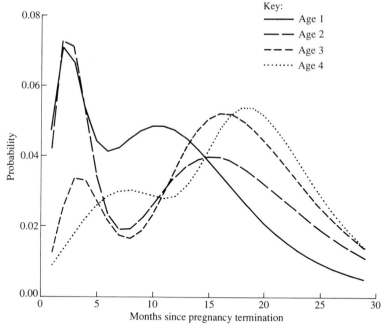

Fig. 21.5 Model density functions for age-groups, Bangladesh

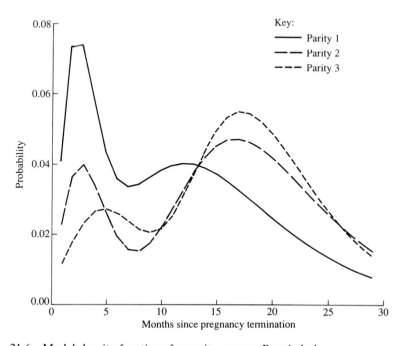

Fig. 21.6 Model density functions for parity groups, Bangladesh

whether the distribution of post-partum amenorrhoea should be unimodal or bimodal. Reviews of the research literature have provided evidence that the major determinant of prolonged anovulation is lactation (Billewicz, 1979; Habicht *et al.*, 1985; McNeilly, 1977; and others). The sucking stimulus of breastfeeding delays the return of menstruation and ovulation. The hazard rate of menstrual onset should be sensitive to the stage of lactation: full, partial, or none. Given this, Potter and Kobrin speculated that in a screened sample of women whose infants survive and who establish lactation, one expects a unimodal distribution of amenorrhoea characterized by a rising hazard rate as more and more members pass from demand feeding to less frequent, less intensive feeding and then cease nursing altogether. They did caution, however, that this model would not be appropriate if women vary in their menstrual response to breastfeeding.

In Potter and Kobrin's model, the degree of bimodality will depend on the weighting of (1) non-lactators, (2) infant deaths, (3) foetal losses and still-births, and (4) instances of post-partum bleeding being recorded as menstrual onset. In the samples from India and Bangladesh used by Ford and Kim (1987), the data had bimodal distributions with a small mode a few months after birth and a larger mode many months later. This bimodality remained even after known infant deaths, stillbirths, and foetal deaths were removed. The small mode within a few months after childbirth may be present either for substantive reasons, including heterogeneity in patterns of infant feeding and heterogeneity in the menstrual response to breastfeeding, and/or for errors in the data, such as undetected infant deaths and stillbirths or confusion between post-partum bleeding and menstruation.

In India and Bangladesh, where the studies used by Ford and Kim were conducted, long breastfeeding was the practice of most women. However, in Bangladesh there is evidence from other studies that there is heterogeneity in breastfeeding patterns (Huffman *et al.*, 1981, 1987). The first mode in these studies could be due to heterogeneity in breastfeeding patterns.

Heterogeneity of response to menstrual patterns is difficult to study due to lack of data. Habicht *et al.* (1985) reported data from Malaysia that showed some women (196 out of 5312) resuming menstruation 1–2 months post-partum while fully breastfeeding. Although prolonged breastfeeding may be the primary determinant of long periods of post-partum amenorrhoea, prediction of the timing of the return of fertility after childbirth is not an exact science, suggesting that there may be heterogeneity due to other variables (see Chapter 25, below). Nutrition is one such variable that has been identified (Frisch, 1978; Huffman *et al.*, 1987).

Certainly, without more biological data we cannot reject the hypothesis that the first mode in these samples is due to errors in the data due to undetected stillbirths, foetal losses, or infant deaths or due to confusion between menstruation and post-partum bleeding. However, given that the above considerations may provide a biological basis for an early mode and given that most researchers will be working with bimodal distributions due to likely heterogeneity in many samples and difficulty in separating out infant deaths and stillbirths, bimodal models of post-partum amenorrhoea are needed in many situations.

Modelling of the Determinants of Lactational Amenorrhoea

There have been many efforts to model the effects of lactation and other variables on the length of post-partum amenorrhoea. There are a number of issues that need to be resolved in this area. First, data on lactation share a number of measurement problems with post-partum amenorrhoea, including heaping, sampling error, and sample selection of data.

Beyond these problems with the measurement of the duration of lactation, there is recognition that not only the length of breastfeeding but also the pattern of breastfeeding should be included in the model. Data are needed on variables such as timing of liquid and solid supplementation and intensity of breastfeeding, including frequency and duration of suckling (Gray, 1987). Most surveys have collected data only on the number of months that a woman has breastfed her child.

The question of how to model the relationship is a third source of discussion. Many researchers have proceeded simply by presenting tables which cross-tabulate length of lactation by length of post-partum amenorrhoea. Others have used regression analysis to predict the length of amenorrhoea from the length of breastfeeding. Bongaarts and Potter (1983) fitted the mean duration of amenorrhoea by an exponent raised to quadratic power of breastfeeding,

$$A = 1.753^{0.1396B - 0.001872B^2}$$

with the population data presented in Table 20.1. Although this equation may be used to predict the mean length of amenorrhoea in a population where only breastfeeding data are available, the relationship cannot be used at the individual level.

A more elaborate model has been proposed by Habicht *et al.* (1985). They designed a three-equation model that estimates the impact of breastfeeding on the length of post-partum anovulation, depending on whether the woman was fully breastfeeding, partially breastfeeding, or not breastfeeding, as well as on her past breastfeeding activity. While this model pays closer attention to the underlying physiological processes than earlier models, there are still some aspects of the relationship that are not represented in the model. These may include heterogeneity of response to breastfeeding patterns possibly caused by differences in hormonal levels at different intensities of breastfeeding and differences in threshold levels of prolactin for the onset of menses.

Finally, proportional hazards models (Cox, 1972; Menken *et al.*, 1981) have been used to study the effects of lactation and other variables upon the resumption of menses (Huffman *et al.*, 1987; Ford and Kim, 1987; Santow,

1987). These models have the advantages of both permitting a regression analysis of censored data, including a time dimension in the analysis that allows for changes in breastfeeding patterns with post-partum duration and providing estimates of the relative magnitudes of the hazards to which different subgroups are subject. However, in most of these models measurement of the pattern of lactation has been limited.

Summary

Demographic research on lactational amenorrhoea has involved extensive data collection at the population level. Estimates of the length of post-partum amenorrhoea have been made for many countries in the world. Many problems have been encountered in collecting good quality data on lactational amenorrhoea, and prospective studies have yielded the most satisfactory results.

Several attempts have been made to model the distribution of post-partum amenorrhoea. Most recently, Ford and Kim (1987) have proposed a mixed distribution consisting of the sum of two Type 1 extreme value distributions. For a logit model developed by Lesthaeghe and Page (1980), which has been widely used, Ford and Kim suggest a new standard.

A debate persists over whether or not the distribution of lactational amenorrhoea should be unimodal or bimodal. While bimodal distributions turn up in most studies, in large-scale population surveys it is difficult to determine whether the first mode is due to undetected infant deaths and stillbirths and confusion with post-partum bleeding or whether it is due to heterogeneity in breastfeeding patterns and the menstrual response to those patterns. Large-scale studies with biomedical data that confirm the onset of fecundity will be needed to decide this issue.

A wide variety of techniques have been used to assess the effect of breastfeeding on amenorrhoea. Some investigators have presented very simple tables, while others have used much more elaborate models. Estimates of the effect of breastfeeding on amenorrhoea vary considerably in these studies. Further development of these models should incorporate more data on the pattern of breastfeeding as well as the possibility that the menstrual response to breastfeeding is heterogeneous.

References

Barrett, J. C. (1969), 'A Monte Carlo Simulation of Human Reproduction', *Genus* 25: 1–22.

Billewicz, W. C. (1979), 'The Timing of Postpartum Menstruation and Breastfeeding: A Simple Formula', *Journal of Biosocial Science* 11: 141–51.

Bongaarts, J., and Potter, R. G. (1983), *Fertility, Biology, and Behavior*, Academic Press, New York.

Bracher, M., and Santow, G. (1981), 'Some Methodological Considerations in the Analysis of Current Status Data', *Population Studies* 35: 425–38.

Chen, L. C., Ahmed, S., Gesche, M., and Mosley, W. H. (1974), 'A Prospective Study of Birth Interval Dynamics in Rural Bangladesh', *Population Studies* 28: 277–89.

Cox, D. R. (1972), 'Regression Models and Life Tables', *Journal of the Royal Statistical Society B* 34: 187–220.

Delgado, H., Lechtig, A., Breneman, E., Martorell, R., Yarbrough, C., and Klein, R. O. (1978), 'Nutrition and Birth Interval Components: The Guatemalan Experience', in W. H. Mosley (ed.), *Nutrition and Human Reproduction*: 385–99, Plenum, New York.

Ferry, B., and Page, H. J. (1984), 'The Proximate Determinants of Fertility and their Effect on Fertility Patterns: An Illustrative Analysis Applied to Kenya', *Scientific Reports*, no. 71, December, World Fertility Survey, London.

Ford, K., and Kim, Y. J. (1987), 'Distributions of Postpartum Amenorrhea: Some New Evidence', *Demography* 24: 413–30.

Frisch, R. E. (1978), 'Population, Food Intake, and Fertility', *Science* 199: 22–30.

Habicht, J. P., Davanzo, J., Butz, W. P., and Meyers, L. (1985), 'The Contraceptive Role of Breastfeeding', *Population Studies* 39: 213–32.

Huffman, S. L., Chowdhury, A. K. M. A., Chakraborty, J., and Simpson, N. (1981), 'Breastfeeding Patterns in Rural Bangladesh', *American Journal of Clinical Nutrition* 33: 144–53.

—— Ford, K., Allen, H., and Streble, P. (1987), 'Nutrition and Fertility in Bangladesh: Breastfeeding and Postpartum Amenorrhoea', *Population Studies* 41: 447–62.

Johnson, N. L., and Kotz, S. (1970), *Continuous Multivariate Distributions*, Wiley, New York.

Knodel, J., and Lewis, G. (1984), 'Postpartum Amenorrhea in Selected Developing Countries: Estimates from Contraceptive Prevalence Surveys', *Social Biology* 31: 308–20.

Lesthaeghe, R., and Page, H. J. (1980), 'The Postpartum Nonsusceptible Period: Development and Application of Model Schedules', *Population Studies* 34: 143–70.

McNeilly, A. S. (1977), 'Physiology of Lactation', *Journal of Biosocial Science* 4 (supplement): 5–21.

Menken, J., Trussell, J., Stempel, D., and Babakol, O. (1981), 'Proportional Hazards Life Table Models: An Illustrative Analysis of Sociodemographic Influences on Marriage Dissolution in the United States', *Demography* 18: 181–200.

Potter, R. G., and Kobrin, F. (1981), 'Distributions of Amenorrhea and Anovulation', *Population Studies* 35: 85–94.

—— Wyon, J. B., Parker, M., and Gordon, J. G. (1965), 'A Case Study of Birth Interval Dynamics', *Population Studies* 19: 81–96.

Santow, G. (1987), 'Reassessing the Contraceptive Effect of Breastfeeding', *Population Studies* 41: 147–60.

Singh, S., and Ferry, B. (1984), 'Biological and Traditional Factors that Influence Fertility: Results from WFS Surveys', *Comparative Studies* no. 40, December, World Fertility Survey, London.

22 Statistical Evidence of Links Between Maternal Nutrition and Post-Partum Infertility

A. MEREDITH JOHN

The question at hand is whether mild or moderate undernutrition affects the ability of a woman to reproduce, and, in particular, whether mild or moderate undernutrition affects the duration of post-partum infertility, either by affecting the duration of post-partum amenorrhoea or by affecting the subsequent waiting time to conception.

Simple comparisons of mean length of the birth interval, mean duration of post-partum amenorrhoea, or mean waiting time to conception among populations are uninformative: differences among populations may equally well be nutritional or behavioural. Intra-community variations in the duration of post-partum amenorrhoea or the waiting time to conception as a function of, for example, weight, are only slightly more informative, since women will still differ, in, say, the timing of the introduction of supplemental foods to their infants.

It is not quite clear what one is modelling when one posits a relationship between maternal nutritional status and post-partum infertility. It is possible that maternal nutritional status has a direct effect on the duration of post-partum amenorrhoea or the waiting time to conception. It is equally plausible, however, that maternal nutritional status plays an indirect role in determining the duration of post-partum infertility by influencing the woman's breastfeeding behaviour: for example, if the quality or quantity of milk produced by an undernourished woman is inadequate, her infant may suckle more frequently or more vigorously, thus increasing the fertility-inhibiting effects of lactation. Alternatively, the timing of the introduction of supplemental foods to the infant may depend upon maternal nutritional status. The only way to sort out the role played by maternal nutritional status on post-partum infertility is to consider it in conjunction with breastfeeding behaviour, rather than as a sole explanatory factor.

Indicators of Nutriture: Measurement of Nutritional Status

Nutrition is 'the process by which the organism uses food . . . for purposes of maintenance of life, growth, normal functioning of organs and the production of energy' (McLaren, 1976:3). Nutriture is 'the state resulting from the balance between supply of nutrition . . . and the expenditure of the organism' (ibid.). Nutritional status is 'the expression of nutriture in a specific variable; therefore one must always specify the variable or variables when referring to nutritional status (i.e., nutritional status as reflected in height)' (Habicht *et al.*, 1979: 366).

Malnutrition is an imbalance of specific nutrients in the diet: for example, the diet may be deficient in proteins, vitamins, or fats. Undernutrition, on the other hand, refers to the caloric inadequacy of a diet: the diet may be relatively well balanced, but there is simply not enough food. Thus, an individual may be both undernourished and malnourished, or overnourished but malnourished. In this paper, the nutritional status of an individual refers to the level of undernutrition rather than to malnutrition.

The nutriture of an individual cannot be directly measured in the field; hence, one must rely on measurements from which inferences about the individual's nutritional status can be made. Anthropometric measures are body measurements that can be used to assess or describe the nutritional status of individuals in a population (Habicht *et al.*, 1979; Zerfas, 1979).

In developing countries, skeletal measurements are often used to represent the past nutritional status of the individual, especially chronic undernutrition. In contrast, the degree of current wasting or acute nutritional deficiency can be assessed by such measures as weight, weight-for-height, weight-for-height squared, fatfold thickness, and arm circumference. In order to be useful in assessing changes in the degree of undernutrition in the individual, the anthropometric measure must not only be sufficiently sensitive to detect changes in nutritional status, but must also be insensitive to other influences: for example, weight is a sufficiently sensitive measure to reflect changes in nutritional status, but it is not a very specific indicator, since many factors other than nutrition will cause an individual's weight to change.

Measurement of skeletal size is often used as a way of assessing chronic malnutrition; it may be argued that those nutritional factors which led to the incomplete development of the skeletal system may have also led to the incomplete development of other systems, including the reproductive system. Height is the anthropometric indicator which is most closely linked to the socio-economic status of an individual during childhood and adolescence; other useful measures are biacromial (shoulder) and bicristal (hip) widths.

Measurements of weight, alone or in combination with height, are often used to assess recent, acute changes in the nutrition of an individual; variations in weight represent variations in labile tissues such as muscles and fat. However, this measure of undernutrition often proves unsatisfactory for several reasons: dehydration or overhydration will cause variations in weight; weight routinely displays significant diurnal variations, even in well-nourished and healthy individuals; and low weight may be misleading if the individual is also stunted or short. Thus, weight alone is not sufficiently specific for assessing changes in nutritional status.

The skinfold thickness (or more accurately, fatfold thickness) is a measure of the fatness of an individual. Fatfold thickness may be measured at the triceps, below the scapula, at the abdomen, at the hip, and at the lowest rib. Fatfold thicknesses are often much more useful in the assessment of obesity than in the assessment of undernutrition. The measurement of fatfold thickness requires the use of standardized calipers which pinch the fat at a specified pressure; the accuracy of fatfold thickness measurements taken by well-trained clinicians compares well with fatness measurements taken by ultrasound and electro-conductivity methods.

Mid-upper arm circumference can be used to assess protein deficiency. Arm circumference measurements, in combination with fatfold thickness data, may be used to calculate arm-muscle circumference which, in turn, serves as a measure of protein reserves. Mid-upper arm circumference may also be more specific than weight in detecting small variations in nutritional status, since arm circumference is less likely to fluctuate with liquid retention. A variation on mid-upper arm circumference measurement is the use of the QUAC measurement, which scales arm circumference to height.

All of these anthropometric measurements are, of course, subject to myriad errors in measurement. In measuring height, the individual may have bent knees, or an arched back. Weight measurements are plagued by scales which are not properly calibrated and inaccuracy in reading the scales. Fatfold thickness calipers may be applied to the wrong place on the body, the caliper may grasp muscle as well as fat, and the dial may be misread. Arm circumference measurements depend on the tape being positioned at the correct place on the arm, being drawn neither too tightly nor too loosely, and being accurately read.

Theoretical Models of the Relationship between Nutritional Status and Post-Partum Infertility

There are several ways in which one might model the relationship between the nutritional status of a woman and post-partum infertility, measured either in terms of post-partum amenorrhoea or the waiting time to conception. Three different approaches are presented here, each of which is consistent with a different hypothesis about how the nutritional status of a woman directly affects her post-partum infertility: the pre-ordination model, the threshold model, and the triggering model.

In the pre-ordination model of the relationship between nutritional status and post-partum infertility, it is hypothesized that a woman's characteristics at a given instant—typically at pregnancy termination, at resumption of menses, or at conception—determine the duration of post-partum amenorrhoea or the conception wait. Thus the duration of post-partum infertility is pre-ordained: breastfeeding behaviour or changes in nutritional status during the amenorrhoeic or during the fertile period have no impact on the duration of post-partum infertility. Suppose, for example, that a woman's post-partum infertility is modelled as a function of her weight at pregnancy termination; then whether she gained or lost weight during the subsequent amenorrhoeic period is, according to this model, irrelevant in determining the length of her post-partum infecundability. Such a theoretical model is implicit in statistical models of the duration of post-partum amenorrhoea or of the waiting time to conception based upon linear multiple regression models or upon life-tables.

In the second class of models, the threshold models, it is hypothesized that once the post-partum nutritional status of a woman reaches a certain level—a threshold level—she will resume menses or her menstrual cycles will become ovular. For example, one might hypothesize that women whose body composition includes at least 15 per cent fat will be fecund, while those with less than 15 per cent fat will not be fecund. Such a theoretical model is implicit in statistical models based upon linear multiple regression models which include as a covariate a binary variable indicating whether or not the woman had reached the hypothesized threshold at the resumption of menses or at conception. A variation on this theme employs hazard models in which the woman's nutritional status is treated as a time-varying covariate and is monitored throughout the infertile period; the model is interpreted as estimating the odds, or probability, that a woman will resume menses or conceive at any given duration post partum as a function of her nutritional status at that time.

The third class of models employs a triggering mechanism: duration of amenorrhoea or of the waiting time to conception is modelled as a function of changes in the nutritional status of the woman. For example, if the nutritional status of the woman changes markedly, as it might when she weans her infant and so no longer has lactation exacting a toll upon her nutritional reserves, then she might be more likely to resume menses than would a woman whose nutritional status is changing very slowly over the course of post-partum amenorrhoea. Such a theoretical model is implicit in statistical models based upon linear multiple regression models which include as a covariate the change in the woman's nutritional status during amenorrhoea or during the conception wait. This theoretical model is also implicit in life-table studies in which women are grouped according to the magnitude of the change in their nutritional status during the period in question. Alternatively, one might use hazard models in which changes in the woman's nutritional status are treated as time-varying covariates and monitored throughout the infertile period; the model is interpreted as estimating the odds, or probability, that a woman will resume menses or conceive at any given duration post partum as a function of changes in her nutritional status at that time.

Thus, there are at least three different ways of modelling the relationship between a woman's nutritional status and her post-partum infertility; the models differ in whether nutritional status plays a passive role, as in the pre-ordination model, or an active role, as in the triggering model. As described, however, none of these models can discern whether the nutritional status of a woman has a direct effect on her post-partum infertility or whether the effect is indirect, with nutritional status influencing breastfeeding behaviour, which, in turn, controls post-partum infertility.

Statistical Models of the Relationship between Nutritional Status and Post-Partum Infertility

There are two types of statistical problems which arise in the modelling of the relationship between post-partum infertility and a woman's nutritional status. The first problem stems from the choice of the appropriate class of model to use in estimating the relationship: linear regression models, simple life-tables, or hazard models with time-varying covariates. The second problem stems from the fact that the nutritional status of a woman is denoted by a random variable, which is measured with error.

Multivariate linear regression models have often been used in the study of the duration of post-partum amenorrhoea or the waiting time to conception, but such models have several limitations. First, for models in which the duration of amenorrhoea or the waiting time to conception is used as the dependent variable, only observations of closed amenorrhoeic intervals or closed waits can be used: censored observations must be excluded since the dependent variable is undefined. This results in a downward bias in the estimated mean duration of amenorrhoea or of the menstruating interval. Second, the use of completed duration of lactation as an explanatory variable leads to other problems. The duration of lactation is often longer than the duration of post-partum amenorrhoea, thus making its interpretation in models of amenorrhoea difficult. The duration of lactation may not be independent of the duration of the menstruating interval, particularly in those societies, such as Bangladesh, where women tend to wean their children when they discover they are again pregnant: conception causes weaning rather than vice versa (Hobcraft and Guz, 1985). Yet another problem is introduced by the use of the duration of post-partum amenorrhoea as an explanatory variable in studies of the waiting time to conception: if weaning coincides with conception, then the duration of lactation simply equals the sum of the duration of post-partum amenorrhoea and the duration of the menstruating interval.

In addition, multivariate linear models cannot accommodate time-varying covariates: variables which change over the course of the study. For example, when a woman resumes menstruation, she may still be fully breastfeeding her infant; by the time she conceives, she may have completely weaned her child. In a model of the waiting time to conception, should she be considered lactating or not lactating?

Some of these problems—most notably, the biases stemming from the exclusion of censored observations—can be avoided by using life-tables, rather than regression models, to study fecundability. The techniques for including censored observations in life-tables are well established, and the inclusion of censored intervals results in an unbiased estimate of the life-table for inevitable events such as death. Unfortunately, the life-table for the duration of post-partum amenorrhoea or for the waiting time to conception is not unbiased, even when the censored intervals are included in the calculations.

Suppose that the survey collects information on the length of the menstruating interval. At the end of the survey, there will be some women who have not yet conceived and who are therefore censored. For example, a woman may be in the 18th month of her menstruating interval at the end of the survey. It is known that she did not conceive within 18 months of the resumption of menses and that she may conceive at some duration greater than 18 months, but it is not inevitable that she will conceive: she may bear no more children in her life. The inclusion in the table of women who will ultimately never again conceive biases the estimated mean conception wait towards infinity. The longer the survey period, the greater the bias, since the women who are destined never to conceive will appear as women still waiting to conceive at the longest durations of observation.

The problem in the life-table can be solved by constructing a new life-table, $1^*(t)$, devoid of the influence of the women who are destined never again to resume menses or to conceive (these women are identified as women who have not resumed menses or who have not conceived after a reasonable period, such as 48 months). The survival function for the new life table, $1^*(t)$, is

$$1^*(t) = 1 - \frac{1-1(t)}{1-1(48)}. \tag{1}$$

While such life-tables allow the use of both closed and censored observations, they are none the less rather limited models because they are essentially univariate in nature: it is relatively simple to compare the life-tables for, say, urban and rural women, but as the number of characteristics considered increases, the required number of life-tables escalates rapidly.

Some of the modelling limitations of multivariate linear models and of life-tables can be avoided by the use of hazard models, which can accommodate both time-varying covariates and censored observations (see, for example, Alison, 1983; Foster *et al.*, 1986; Menken *et al.*, 1981; Trussell and Hammer-slough, 1983). In a hazard model, the probability of resuming menses at time t for individual i, $2_i(t)$, is modelled as a multiplicative function of an underlying duration function $2(t)$ and a vector of covariates, z_i:

$$2_i(t) = 2(t)e^{\beta z_i} \tag{2}$$

where β is a vector of coefficients. Thus, in this model, the dependent variable is the rate at which women resume menses at each duration post partum, rather than the duration of the menstruating interval. A binary variable denoting whether or not the woman resumed menses in a given month is the dependent variable; the unit of observation is the woman-month of exposure to the risk of resuming menses. Since there is a separate observation for each month that a woman is exposed to the risk of resuming menses, the inclusion of time-varying covariates is simple. For example, if a woman weans her child in the 14th month post partum, she is classified as lactating in the first 13 monthly observations and as non-lactating in the remaining observations.

A completely different sort of statistical problem is introduced into the models of nutritional status and post-partum infertility by the use of anthropometric measures of nutritional status. In a standard, classical linear regression model, it is assumed that all the explanatory variables are measured without error. However, this is clearly not the case when one of the variables is an anthropometric indicator of nutritional status: as noted earlier, such measures are fraught with error. In such a case, the classical least squares estimate of a linear regression coefficient will be an underestimate of the true coefficient (Wald, 1940). A similar problem arises in hazard models and logistic regression models.

Statistical Studies of Nutritional Status and Post-Partum Infertility

In recent years, a great deal of attention has been focused on the determinants of post-partum amenorrhoea. A wide variety of studies have examined the roles played by the woman's nutritional status, breastfeeding patterns, personal characteristics, and socio-economic conditions in determining the length of post-partum amenorrhoea (Chen *et al.*, 1975; Chowdhury, 1978; Delgado *et al.*, 1978; Huffman *et al.*, 1978; Lunn *et al.*, 1984). In sharp contrast stands the relative dearth of information on the corresponding determinants of the waiting time to conception (Bongaarts, 1982; Chowdhury, 1978; Delgado *et al.*, 1978; Jain *et al.*, 1979). In both the cases of post-partum amenorrhoea and waiting time to conception, few of the studies attempt to investigate simultaneously the roles played by lactation and maternal nutritional status.

In an early study using monthly prospective survey data from Matlab Thana, Bangladesh, Chowdhury (1978) calculated the mean duration of post-partum amenorrhoea for three groups of women classified by weight; he failed to find statistically significant differences in the mean duration of post-partum amenorrhoea among the three groups and so concluded that there was no evidence that nutritional status as measured by weight was a determinant of the duration of amenorrhoea. In a subsequent study, also using data from Matlab Thana, women were divided into groups on the basis of weight-for-height; very small, but statistically significant differences were found in the duration of amenorrhoea, with the women with greatest weight-for-height having the shortest amenorrhoea (Huffman *et al.*, 1978).

These studies from Bangladesh do not control for the effect of lactation on the duration of post-partum amenorrhoea. Although, in Bangladesh, women tend to resume menses while still nursing their infants (complete weaning tends to coincide with the recognition of the next conception), the pattern of supplemental feeding and, therefore, the frequency and intensity of suckling varies among women; this effect is obscured in these studies.

Similar studies have been carried out using prospective survey data from Guatemala, collected fortnightly. In one study, women were divided into three groups on the basis of weight; small but statistically significant differences were found in the mean duration of post-partum amenorrhoea, with the heaviest group having a mean duration of amenorrhoea about 1.5 months shorter than that of the lightest group (Bongaarts and Delgado, 1979). In another study using the Guatemalan data, women were grouped according to their mean daily calorie intake and completed duration of lactation, and mean duration of post-partum amenorrhoea was calculated for each group. The researchers concluded that the influence of lactation was far stronger than the influence of nutritional status in determining the duration of post-partum amenorrhoea (Delgado *et al.*, 1977). However, it is difficult to interpret exactly what role is played by the duration of lactation, since many women resumed menses while still nursing, and breastfeeding after the resumption of menses cannot influence the timing of the resumption of menses.

Yet another study based on Guatemalan data used linear regression models to assess the relative influence of nutritional status and lactation on the duration of post-partum amenorrhoea. In these models, the dependent variable was the observed duration of post-partum amenorrhoea; the explanatory variables included the change in the woman's weight between the third and ninth months post partum, the daily frequency of suckling at 3, 6, 9, and 12 months post partum, and various socio-economic indicators. It was again found that the effect of nutritional status on the duration of post-partum amenorrhoea was small when compared to the effect of lactation (Wyon and Gordon, 1971). In addition, there seems to be indirect evidence in this study that women do not need to reach a certain threshold weight before resuming menses: most of the women studied lost weight during amenorrhoea.

The roles played by a woman's nutritional status and her breastfeeding practices in determining her fecundability are somewhat clearer. The extant field studies of fecundability tend to support the hypothesis that breastfeeding after the resumption of menses influences fecundability but that the woman's nutritional status does not.

In a study of Taiwanese women, Jain *et al.* (1979) found that women who had weaned infants before resumption of menses had a shorter waiting time to conception than did women who were still breastfeeding during menstruation; they made no attempt to control for the nutritional status of the women.

Among samples of women in the Punjab (Wyon and Gordon, 1971) and among Eskimo women (Berman *et al.*, 1972) there appeared to be no significant lactation effect on the waiting time to conception.

In conjunction with his study of post-partum amenorrhoea, Chowdhury (1978) examined the effect of the woman's nutritional status on her probability of conceiving within 12 months of the resumption of menses. He found no significant effect for either of two nutritional indicators: height and weight at the time of conception. Bongaarts and Delgado (1979) investigated the relationship between maternal nutritional status and fecundability in Guatemala using four different anthropometric indices of nutritional status. In their simple linear regression models, they found no significant relationship between nutritional status and waiting time to conception resulting in a live birth.

Delgado *et al.* (1982) examined the impact of nutritional intervention programme on the length of the menstruating interval among lactating women in rural Guatemala. Nutritional status, represented in the linear multiple regression models by anthropometric measurement and caloric intake, had no significant effect on the waiting time to conception; the duration of lactation was associated with a shorter conception wait. It was also found that the duration of post-partum amenorrhoea was inversely related to the length of the menstruating interval.

These studies, while quite useful, all suffer from similar limitations. None of the studies allows for changes in breastfeeding or nutritional status during amenorrhoea or during the menstruating interval: a shift from full breastfeeding to supplementation, or from supplementation to complete weaning, may well affect the timing of resumption of menses or of conception. Similarly, the timing of resumption of menses or of conception may be tied to variations in nutritional status: the evidence from Bangladesh indicates that women tend to resume menses and to conceive in those seasons when food is most plentiful.

In a hazard model study of the waiting time to conception among women in Bangladesh, the breastfeeding behaviour of women was treated as a time-varying covariate, taking a different value in each month of exposure to the risk of conception (John *et al.*, 1987). The nutritional status of the women (measured as weight/height-squared) was also used as a time-varying covariate, as were covariates representing the elapsed duration of the conception wait and the proportion of each month that the husband and wife were separated. In the hazard models, nutritional status played no role in determining the fecundability of the women, while the breastfeeding pattern—whether the woman was fully breastfeeding her child, had introduced supplemental foods, or had completely weaned the child—showed a clear effect: women who had been giving supplemental foods to their infants for several months were more likely to conceive than were those who had recently introduced supplemental foods to the child's diet or who had not yet done so.

Although many of the extant studies of the relationship between maternal

nutritional status and post-partum infertility are flawed, either methodologic-
ally or because they fail to consider nutritional status and breastfeeding
behaviour simultaneously, a general picture none the less emerges: the nutritional status of a woman may play a direct role in determining the length of
post-partum amenorrhoea, but such a role is small when compared to that
played by her breastfeeding behaviour. In contrast, there is no evidence that
maternal nutritional status has any effect on fecundability, while breastfeeding
beyond the resumption of menses does reduce fecundability.

References

Alison, P. (1982), 'Discrete Time Methods for Analysis of Event Histories', in *Sociology Methodology*: 61–98.

Berman, M., Hanson, K., and Hellman, I. (1972), 'Effect of Breast-feeding on Postpartum Menstruation, Ovulation and Pregnancy in Alaskan Eskimos', *American Journal of Obstetrics and Gynecology* 114: 524–6.

Bongaarts, J. (1982), 'Does Malnutrition Affect Fecundity? A Summary of the Evidence', *Science* 208: 564–9.

—— and Delgado, H. (1979), 'Effects of Nutritional Status on Fertility in Rural Guatemala', in H. Leridon and J. Menken (eds.), *Natural Fertility*, Ordina Editions, Liège, Belgium: 109–33.

Chen, L., Ahmed, A., Gesche, M., and Mosley, W. H. (1975), 'A Prospective Study of Birth Interval Dynamics in Rural Bangladesh', *Population Studies* 28: 277–97.

Chowdhury, A. K. M. A. (1978), 'Effect of Maternal Nutrition on Fertility in Rural Bangladesh', in W. H. Mosley (ed.), *Nutrition and Human Reproduction*, Plenum Press, New York: 404–10.

Delgado, H., Lechtig, A., Martorell, R., Brineman, E., and Klein, R. (1978), 'Nutrition, Lactation and Postpartum Amenorrhea', *American Journal of Clinical Nutrition* 31: 322–6.

—— Martorell, R., and Klein, R. (1982), 'Nutrition, Lactation and Birth Interval Components in Rural Guatemala', *American Journal of Clinical Nutrition* 35: 1468–76.

—— Lechtig, A., Brineman, E., Martorell, R., Yarbrough, C., and Klein, R. (1977), 'Nutrition and Birth Interval Components: The Guatemalan Experience', in W. H. Mosley (ed.), *Nutrition and Human Reproduction*: 385–99, Plenum Press, New York.

Foster, A., Menken, J. A., Chowdhury, A. K. M. A., and Trussell, J. (1986), 'Female Reproductive Development a Hazard Model Analysis', *Social Biology* 33: 183–98.

Habicht, J.-P., Yarbrough, C., and Martorell, R. (1979), 'Anthropometric Field Methods: Criteria for Selection', in D. B. Jelliffe and E. F. P. Jelliffe (eds.), *Human Nutrition: A Comprehensive Treatise*, ii. *Nutrition and Growth*: 365–87, Plenum Press, New York.

Hobcraft, J., and Guz, D. (1985), 'Lactation and Fertility: A Comparative Analysis', paper presented to the Population Association of America, Boston, Mass.

Huffman, S. L., Chowdhury, A. K. M. A., Chakraborty, J., and Mosley, W. H. (1978), 'Nutrition and Post-Partum Amenorrhoea in Rural Bangladesh', *Population Studies* 32: 251.

Jain, A., Hermalin, A., and Sun, T. (1979), 'Lactation and Natural Fertility', in H. Leridon and J. Menken (eds.), *Natural Fertility*, Ordina Editions, Liège, Belgium.

John, A. M., Menken, J. A., and Chowdhury, A. K. M. A. (1987), 'The Effects of Breastfeeding and Nutrition on Fecundability in Rural Bangladesh: A Hazards-Model Analysis', *Population Studies* 41: 433–46.

Lunn, P., Austin, S., Prentice, A., and Whitehead, R. (1984), 'The Effect of Improved Nutrition on Plasma Prolactin Concentrations and Postpartum Infertility in Lactating Gambian Women', *American Journal of Clinical Nutrition* 39: 227–35.

McLaren, D. S. (1976), *Nutrition in the Community*, Wiley, New York.

Menken, J. A., Trussell, J., and Watkins, S. C. (1981), 'The Nutrition–Fertility Link: An Evaluation of the Evidence', *Journal of Interdisciplinary History* 12: 425–41.

Trussell, J., and Hammerslough, C. (1983), 'A Hazards Model Analysis of the Covariates of Infant and Child Mortality in Sri Lanka', *Demography* 20: 1–26.

Wald (1940), 'The Fitting of Straight Lines if Both Variables are Subject to Error', *Annal of Mathematical Statistics* 11: 284–300.

Wyon, J., and Gordon, J. (1971), *The Khana Study: Population Problems in the Rural Punjab*, Harvard University Press, Cambridge, Mass.

Zerfas, A. J. (1979), 'Anthropometric Field Methods: General', in D. B. Jelliffe and E. F. P. Jelliffe (eds.), *Human Nutrition: A Comprehensive Treatise*, ii. *Nutrition and Growth*: 39–364, Plenum Press, New York.

23 Maternal Nutrition, Infant Feeding, and Post-Partum Amenorrhoea: Recent Evidence from Bangladesh*

KATHLEEN FORD

SANDRA L. HUFFMAN

Introduction

Post-partum amenorrhoea is the time from the end of a woman's pregnancy until the time that she begins to menstruate. In countries where women breastfeed their infants for long periods of time and levels of contraceptive practice are low, breastfeeding and the amenorrhoea related to breastfeeding are important determinants of fertility levels. The role of nutritional status in lengthening the duration of amenorrhoea has been the focus of research for several years. It has been hypothesized that nutrition may affect the length of post-partum amenorrhoea in two ways. First, inadequate nutrition may have a direct effect on the functioning of a woman's reproductive system and cause a delay in the return of menses. A second mechanism may be through the pattern of breastfeeding. Women with low levels of nutrition may have reduced milk output so that infants have to suckle more to obtain adequate nutrition. This more intensive suckling may delay the return of menses.

The objectives of this paper are to review studies of the effects of maternal nutrition and lactation on post-partum amenorrhoea and to present results from a recent study of a group of chronically malnourished women in a rural area of Bangladesh.

Previous Research

Several longitudinal studies have examined the relationship between maternal nutritional status and amenorrhoea. A longitudinal study conducted by INCAP (Instituto de Nutrición de Centro America y Panama) in Guatemala examined the duration of amenorrhoea of approximately 400 breastfeeding women in

* Support for this paper came from the Determinants of Natural Fertility Award, provided by the Population Council (CP 82.36A and CP 83.40A) through a contract with the Agency for International Development; and funding from the National Institutes of Child Health and Human Development (NICHD Grant R01-HD-17709-02).

relation to their nutritional status based on anthropometric measures averaged over the first 3 months after the birth of a child. The age-standardized duration of amenorrhoea was 14.8 months for women weighing 43.7 kg, compared to 13.2 months for those weighing 55.6 kg on average (Bongaarts and Delgado, 1979). The study also found a 1–2 month difference in the duration of amenorrhoea depending on the women's dietary intakes during pregnancy and lactation.

Researchers in the Gambia (Lunn *et al.*, 1981, 1984) also examined the association of maternal nutritional status with lactational amenorrhoea. These studies did not collect data on the duration of lactational infertility but instead examined the association of oestrogen and progesterone levels with prolactin levels. Compared to women who did not receive food supplements, women who were supplemented during pregnancy also resumed menstruation 5 months earlier. Women supplemented during both pregnancy and lactation resumed menstruation 9 months earlier than the unsupplemented group.

Although milk output did not increase with the food supplements, maternal weights improved slightly. The authors suggest that the association of supplementation with prolactin and oestrogen/progesterone levels may be related to frequency of suckling, which was not accurately measured in these studies. With the improvement in maternal nutritional status, milk production may not have increased, but infants may not have needed to suckle as much to obtain the same amount of milk when their mothers were supplemented. This may be the mechanism by which maternal nutritional status appeared to be correlated with prolactin levels. It may also be, however, that supplementation affected the mothers' activity patterns, which led them to suckle their infants less frequently. Milk production could have remained constant, but infants of unsupplemented mothers may have spent more time in non-nutritive suckling or have had more frequent feeds throughout the day, instead of longer feeds that may have been more suitable for the unsupplemented mother in her changed activity patterns.

Previous cross-sectional studies in Hyderabad, India have examined the relationship between nutritional status and post-partum amenorrhoea in low income, urban women (Prema *et al.*, 1981). For lactating women whose duration of lactation was held constant, the median duration of amenorrhoea decreased from 13.1 months among women weighing less than 40 kg to 8.2 months for those weighing more than 54 kg. This study, however, did not control for age, parity, or suckling patterns of the infants. In other studies conducted by Prema, the duration of unsupplemented lactation was correlated with the duration of amenorrhoea. Women who supplemented their infants' diets between 0 and 3 months of age had an average duration of amenorrhoea of 7.6 months, compared to an average duration of amenorrhoea of 20 months for those who did not supplement their infants' diets until they were over 2 years of age (Prema and Philip, 1980).

Researchers in developed countries have also examined the association of maternal nutritional status and supplementation practices with the duration of post-partum amenorrhoea. Elias *et al.* (1986) studied the association of lactation and amenorrhoea among women in Boston. They found that for La Lèche League women, who practise intensive breastfeeding, a high frequency of night feeds had a major effect on extending amenorrhoea. For women who breastfed less frequently, the introduction of supplements was the strongest predictor of the return of menstruation. The median duration of amenorrhoea was 13.3 months among La Lèche League women and 8.5 months among other women studied. This study also noted a significant difference in nutritional status between the two groups, with those with a shorter duration of amenorrhoea having a lower weight corrected for height than those with longer amenorrhoea. Another study conducted in Japan also noted that women who were obese had a delay in the onset of ovulation (Okai *et al.*, 1981).

In a study of La Lèche League women in Toronto, the introduction of supplements was not strongly correlated with duration of amenorrhoea (Knauer, 1985). The mean duration of breastfeeding in this study population was 23 months, and the average duration of amenorrhoea was 11.4 months. Factors that were associated with an earlier onset of menses included the time at which the child began to sleep through the night and the maximum interval between feedings during the first 3 months. Similar findings have also been reported within studies of lactation as a method of natural family planning in Australia (Gross, 1984).

Howie and McNeilly (1982) observed that the frequency of supplemental feeds was associated with the length of time before the first ovulation and also with the total duration of suckling in minutes per day. Basal prolactin levels were dependent upon the interval between suckling episodes. Shorter intervals were associated with higher basal levels. As women introduced supplements to their infants, the number of suckling episodes declined, as did basal prolactin levels (Howie *et al.*, 1981; Glasier *et al.*, 1984). These studies also found that prolactin concentrations were more likely to remain elevated if suckling took place after midday, which the authors suggest may help explain the importance of night feedings in the maintenance of amenorrhoea.

Results from Bangladesh

Because Bangladesh exhibits one of the longest durations of amenorrhoea and because the level of chronic malnutrition among women is high, it is an appropriate location to study the relationship between biological and behavioural variables and the patterns of resumption of post-partum menstruation. Some results of a longitudinal study in this area have recently been published (Huffman *et al.*, 1987; Ford and Huffman, 1988).

The data used in these analyses were collected in the Birth Interval Dynamics study conducted in Matlab, Bangladesh at a field research site operated by the

International Centre for Diarrheal Disease Research (ICDDR-B). Detailed information on the data-collection and editing procedures can be found in Huffman *et al.* (1987). A total of 2445 women were available for study at some point during the period from October 1975 to January 1980.

During the first two-and-a-half years women were interviewed each month; for the remainder of the study women were interviewed at bi-monthly intervals. At interview, women were asked whether they had experienced a change in their reproductive or breastfeeding status. Reproductive status included information on pregnancy terminations (including miscarriages, stillbirths, and live births), resumption of menses post partum, or onset of pregnancy. Breastfeeding status included information on when liquids were first fed to the infant, when solid supplements were first introduced, and when breastfeeding had terminated.

Precise definitions of the samples of women and variables used were presented in a previous paper (Huffman *et al.*, 1987). Since maternal weight is not a constant measure, it is necessary to select certain points in time to define maternal nutritional status. We have used weight at pregnancy termination as a measure of maternal nutritional status. Weight at pregnancy termination is defined as the average of the first three post-partum weights taken within the first 90 days post partum. There were 884 live births with weight at pregnancy termination available for analysis. Many live births were not available for analysis because data on nutritional status was collected only during the first two-and-a-half years of the study. The term 'supplementation' is used to indicate whether or not solid foods were being fed to the infant. This term is not used here to describe the mother's diet.

The average duration of amenorrhoea was 15.5 months for women who breastfed and 2.5 months for those not breastfeeding. Weight at pregnancy termination was consistently related to the duration of amenorrhoea: women with higher weights had a shorter duration of amenorrhoea (Table 23.1). Those who weighed more than 44 kg on average had a median duration of amenorrhoea of 13.6 months, compared to 15.9 months for those weighing 38 kg to 43.9 kg, and 17.6 months for those weighing less than 38 kg. This relationship remained even when supplementation practices were controlled.

The effect of full breastfeeding was of a similar magnitude. Those who fed any type of supplement to their infant prior to 4 months had a median duration of amenorrhoea of 14.6 months, compared to 15.3 months in those who first introduced supplements between 4 and 7 months and 16.1 months among those who fully breastfed for 7 months or more. Increases in maternal age and parity showed similar positive associations with extending the duration of amenorrhoea.

In this study, we have used a statistical model, called a hazard model, in which the monthly probability of return of menses is modelled as a multiplicative function of the duration of the amenorrhoeic interval and a set of covariates that influence the return of menstruation (Cox, 1972; Menken *et al.*, 1981).

TABLE 23.1. *Median duration of total and full breastfeeding and amenorrhoea by maternal and infant characteristics*

Variable	N	Median duration of breastfeeding (months)		N	Median duration of amenorrhoea (months)
		All breast-feeding	Full breast-feeding only		
Parity					
1–2	509	32.3	6.4	519	11.6
3–4	478	30.4	7.0	479	16.8
5+	692	33.5	6.6	701	17.5
Age					
13–19	195	31.3	6.2	199	11.0
20–4	493	31.0	6.9	499	13.7
25–9	363	31.0	7.0	365	16.6
30–4	316	32.7	6.2	319	17.9
35+	312	40.3	6.7	317	17.7
Weight at pregnancy termination (kgs)					
<38	207	34.0	5.6	213	17.6
38–43	439	32.8	6.4	441	15.9
44+	223	30.2	6.6	230	13.6
Duration of full breastfeeding (months)					
<4				598	14.6
4–6.9				371	15.3
7+				647	16.1

Source: Huffman *et al.*, 1987, Table 2, p. 453.

This model was chosen because multivariate linear models cannot handle censored observations and variables that change over the course of the study.

Using proportional hazard analyses, we were able to assess the relationship of several behavioural and biological factors with the probability of resuming menstruation. The relative risk of resuming menstruation associated with several variables is shown in Table 23.2. Parity, weight at pregnancy termination, and supplementation were significantly related to the risk of resuming menstruation. Increases in maternal parity (which also reflects increasing maternal age) were associated with a decreased risk of resuming menses even when nutritional status and supplementation practices were held constant. Maternal weight at pregnancy termination increased the risk of resuming menstruation, and delaying supplementation reduced the risk of resuming menstruation.

Results from the proportional hazard models were used to estimate the

TABLE 23.2. *Estimates from hazard models of the relative risk of resuming menstruation*[a]

Independent variable	Relative risk
Parity	.967[b]
Weight at pregnancy termination	1.033[c]
Age at supplementation (months)	
1–2.9	0.776[c]
3–5.9	0.798
6+	0.730[b]

[a] Education, religion, season of birth, and height were also included in the analysis.
[b] $p < .05$
[c] $p < .10$

median duration of amenorrhoea for specific weights at pregnancy termination. A 10 kg increase in maternal weight was associated with a 3-month decrease in amenorrhoea, other things being equal.

Summary and Discussion

The Bangladesh data showed independent effects of infant feeding and maternal nutrition upon the length of post-partum amenorrhoea. The effect of maternal nutrition on the length of post-partum amenorrhoea was small compared to the effect of the pattern of infant feeding. These results are in general agreement with those of other studies.

An earlier study in Bangladesh showed nutrition to have a smaller effect on amenorrhoea (Huffman *et al.*, 1978). In this cross-sectional study conducted in Matlab in 1975 and 1976, nearly 2000 women were divided into quartiles by nutritional status. Pregnant women were excluded because their weight would be different from normal. The exclusion of pregnant women may have influenced the results. Women who conceived may have been better nourished. This would help to explain the stronger association between mother's nutritional status and amenorrhoea in the present study. This study can account for the duration of amenorrhoea in a larger proportion of women.

Besides sample selection due to pregnancy status, the earlier study assessed nutritional status between November and January, a time when nutritional status improves and the frequency of suckling falls off (Huffman *et al.*, 1980; Brown *et al.*, 1985). The current study has a more representative distribution of the timing of nutritional status.

In 1974–5 a famine occurred in Bangladesh following severe floods. There was a slightly increased risk of resuming menses during the early months of the study, November and December 1975, and the risk of conception and live birth rates increased during 1976. No other difference related to year of pregnancy termination could be noted, since the duration of post-partum amenorrhoea was similar for pregnancies ending in 1976, 1977, and 1978. Given these results, the effects of famine on this study are likely to be minimal.

This study also found an association between mother's weight and amenorrhoea for women who experienced stillbirths and neonatal deaths. This suggests a direct effect of malnutrition on post-partum amenorrhoea, although the difference was quite small (0.005 per cent per kg of body weight). Maternal nutrition may also influence post-partum amenorrhoea through suckling patterns.

The information available from this study on infant supplementation is minimal. Future studies of the relationship between post-partum amenorrhoea and maternal nutrition should collect more detailed information on the pattern of breastfeeding and infant supplementation, including frequency and duration of feedings as well as the nutritional quality of food supplements.

References

Bongaarts, J., and Delgado, H. (1979), 'Effects of Nutritional Status on Fertility in Rural Guatemala', in H. Leridon and J. Menken (eds.), *Natural Fertility*, Ordina Editions, Liège, Belgium: 107–33.

Brown, K. H., Black, R. E., Robertson, A. D., and Becker, S. (1985), 'Effects of Season and Illness on the Dietary Intake of Weanlings during Longitudinal Studies in Rural Bangladesh', *American Journal of Clinical Nutrition* 41: 343–55.

Cox, D. R. (1972), 'Regression Models and Life Tables', *Journal of the Royal Statistical Society*, series B34: 187–220.

Elias, M. F., Teas, J., Johnston, J., and Bora, C. (1986), 'Effects of Maternal Care on Lactation Amenorrhea', *Journal of Biosocial Science* 18: 1–10.

Ford, K., and Huffman, S. L. (1988), 'Nutrition, Infant Feeding, and Post-Partum Amenorrhea in Bangladesh: Interactions with Season of Birth', *Journal of Biosocial Science* 20: 461–70.

Glasier, A., McNeilly, A. S., and Howie, P. W. (1984), 'The Prolactin Response to Suckling', *Clinical Endocrinology* 21: 109–16.

Gross, B. A. (1984), 'Breastfeeding and the Return to Fertility', *International Review of Natural Family Planning* 8(2): 102–20.

Howie, P. W., McNeilly, A. S., Houston, M. J., Cook, A., and Bayle, H. (1981), 'Effect of Supplementary Food on Suckling Patterns and Ovarian Activity during Lactation', *British Medical Journal* 283: 757–9.

Huffman, S., Chowdhury, A. K. M. A., Chakraborty, J., and Mosley, W. H. (1978), 'Nutrition and Postpartum Amenorrhea in Rural Bangladesh', *Population Studies* 32: 251–60.

—— —— —— and Simpson, N. (1980), 'Breastfeeding Patterns in Rural Bangladesh', *American Journal of Clinical Nutrition* 33: 144–53.

—— Ford, K., Allen, H. A., and Streble, P. (1987), 'Nutrition and Fertility in Bangladesh: Breastfeeding and Postpartum Amenorrhea', *Population Studies* 41: 447–92.

Knauer, M. (1985), 'Determinants and Correlates of the Return of Menstruation in Nursing Mothers Following "Natural Motherhood" ', in V. Hull and M. Simpson-Hebert (eds.), *Breastfeeding and Child Spacing: Anthropological Insights*, Croom-Helm, London: 187–212.

Lunn, P. G., Austin, S., Prentice, A. M., and Whitehead, R. G. (1984), 'The Effect of Improved Nutrition on Plasma Prolactin Concentrations and Postpartum Infertility in Lactating Gambian Women', *American Journal of Clinical Nutrition* 39: 227–35.

—— Watkinson, M., Prentice, A. M., Morrell, P., Austin, P., and Whitehead, R. G. (1981), 'Maternal Nutrition and Lactational Amenorrhea', *Lancet* 1: 1428–9.

Menken, J., Trussell, J., Stempel, D., and Babakol, O. (1981), 'Proportional Hazards Life Table Models: An Illustrative Analysis of Sociodemographic Influences on Marriage Dissolution in the United States', *Demography* 18: 181–200.

Okai, R., Fukuiya, T., Kanakura, Y., Morisuda, M., Kawakumi, S., Takahashi, T., and Iizuka, R. (1981), 'Study on the Onset of the First Ovulation during the Puerperium', in F. Mundo, E. Ines-Cuyegking, and D. M. Aviado (eds.), *Primary Maternal and Neonatal Health: A Global Concern*: 219–26, Plenum Press, New York.

Prema, K., and Philip, F. S. (1980), 'Lactational Amenorrhea Survey', *Indian Journal of Medical Research* 71: 538–46.

—— Nadamuni, A., Neelakumari, E., and Ramalakshimi, B. A. R. (1981), 'Nutrition–Fertility Interaction in Lactating Women of Low Income Groups', *British Journal of Nutrition* 45: 461–7.

24 Breastfeeding and Fertility

A. S. McNEILLEY

Introduction

Breastfeeding suppresses fertility for a period which varies considerably between individuals and among different societies. Until recently the reason for this variation in the duration of infertility was unclear, but it is now apparent that it depends on the strength of the suckling stimulus and its impact on prolactin and gonadotrophin secretion.

In a non-contracepting, breastfeeding woman, the interbirth interval can be divided into four major components: (1) the recovery of the hypothalamo–pituitary–ovarian axis from the suppressive effects of placental steroids during pregnancy (20 to 30 days); (2) the period of lactational amenorrhoea; (3) a period during which menstruation returns associated with inadequate or adequate corpus luteum function; and (4) pregnancy. Over the last few years we have investigated the relationship between suckling activity and the resumption of ovarian activity, concentrating on the underlying mechanisms involved.

Lactational Infertility

Recovery from Pregnancy

During pregnancy, the high circulating plasma levels of placental steroids suppress pituitary levels of both luteinizing hormone (LH) and follicle-stimulating hormone (FSH) to approximately 1 per cent of normal (see McNeilly, 1979), while the increased levels of oestrogen induce a substantial increase in the number of pituitary lactotrophes and the plasma levels of prolactin (Robyn and Meuris, 1982). After delivery and clearance of these steroids, which takes 2 to 4 days (West and McNeilly, 1979), plasma levels of FSH and LH increase and prolactin levels decline to normal limits over a 30-day period in non-breastfeeding women (Bonnar et al., 1975; Howie and McNeilly, 1982). This leads to a resumption of menstrual cycles, although first menstruation is usually preceded by an absent (20 per cent) or inadequate (80 per cent) luteal phase in terms of luteal progesterone or pregnanediol excretion (Howie et al., 1982; Poindexter et al., 1983). Normal ovulation has resumed by the second and subsequent cycles between 45 and 120 days post partum. It can be assumed, therefore, that in the presence of suckling, recovery from pregnancy will account for up to 50 days of the initial period of lactational infertility. Thereafter, it is dependent on suckling.

Suckling-Induced Suppression of Ovarian Activity

Studies in Scotland, Denmark, Africa, Australia, the USA, Mexico, Egypt, and Thailand, where ovarian activity has been monitored directly by measurement of either plasma or urinary levels of ovarian steroids, have confirmed that ovulation rarely occurs during lactational amenorrhoea (Anderson and Schioler, 1985; Brown *et al.*, 1985; Hennart *et al.*, 1985; Duchen and McNeilly, 1980; McNeilly *et al.*, 1980; Konner and Worthman, 1980; Gross and Eastman, 1985; Lunn, 1985; Rivero *et al.*, 1985; Wood *et al.*, 1985). These studies also show that in the majority of cases (60–70 per cent) follicular development is suppressed, assessed both in terms of plasma and urinary oestrogens (Fig. 24.1)

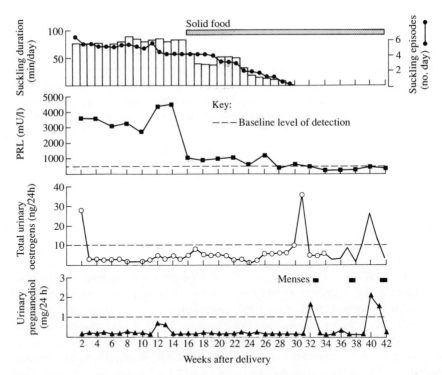

Source: Howie *et al.*, 1982.

Fig. 24.1   Infant feeding patterns, basal prolactin levels, menstruation, and suppression of urinary steroid excretion in a breastfeeding mother with amenorrhoea during lactation and ovulation before first menses, during the post-partum period (see McNeilly, 1984; McNeilly *et al.*, 1980 and 1982; Brown *et al.*, 1985; Gross and Eastman, 1985) and by ultrasound visualization of follicles within the ovary (Glasier *et al.*, 1986). However, in some 30 per cent of cases, ovarian oestrogen secretion indicative of follicular development does occur (Fig. 24.2) (Brown *et al.*, 1985; Howie *et al.*, 1982; McNeilly *et al.*, 1982, 1983*a*). These levels of oestrogen do not increase to those seen in the normal pre-ovulatory phase of the menstrual cycle, indicating that follicular development, if it occurs, is not sustained throughout lactational amenorrhoea.

The duration of lactational amenorrhoea is extremely variable and depends upon the pattern of suckling. Intense suckling can delay the onset of menses for 1 to 2 years (Howie and McNeilly, 1982; Hennart *et al.*, 1985; Brown *et al.*, 1985; Stern *et al.*, 1986). In our own studies of Scottish women, we reported that those who ovulated while breastfeeding had reduced suckling frequency to less than six times/day and reduced suckling duration to less than 60 min/day at the time of first ovulation (Howie *et al.*, 1982; McNeilly *et al.*, 1983*a*). This was not stated as a reliable minimum for all breastfeeding women and should not be taken as such. Nevertheless, Anderson and Schioler (1982) suggested a

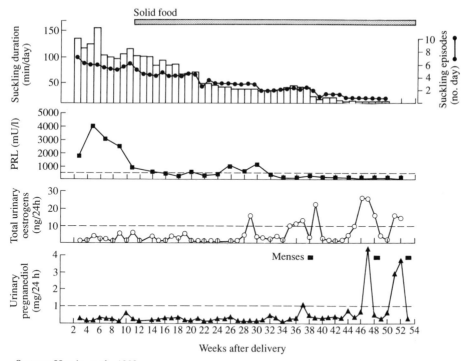

Source: Howie *et al.*, 1982.

Fig. 24.2 Infant feeding patterns, basal prolactin levels, menstruation, and suppression of urinary steroid excretion in a breastfeeding mother with menses during lactation and ovulation before first menses, during the post-partum period

similar figure of five feeds per day as a minimum required to reliably protect against pregnancy. More recently figures of 80 minutes of nursing per day, in conjunction with a minimum of six nursing episodes, were highly predictive for the maintenance of amenorrhoea for up to 18 months post partum in a study of American women (Stern *et al.*, 1986). The suckling pattern can apparently consist of fewer, longer episodes (for example, 0.9 episodes per hour,each lasting approximately 11 minutes) or more numerous, but shorter episodes (for example, around five episodes per hour, each lasting approximately 3 minutes) (Stern *et al.*, 1986). These results (from US and !Kung women, respectively) emphasize the major difficulty in deriving a universal minimum frequency and duration of suckling which will guarantee the maintenance of infertility in all societies. The pattern of suckling in relation to amenorrhoea must be established for each society; amenorrhoea can be maintained with a high number of suckling episodes of short duration each day or lower number of episodes of short duration each day or a lower number of episodes, each of a longer duration. We have previously suggested that total suckling duration per day becomes more important as suckling frequency declines (McNeilly *et al.*, 1985).

Resumption of Ovarian Activity, Ovulation, and Menstruation

Longitudinal studies have now confirmed that the resumption of ovarian activity is associated with a decrease in suckling frequency and/or duration (Howie *et al.*, 1981; Howie and McNeilly, 1982; Andersen and Schioler, 1982; Gross and Eastman, 1985; Brown *et al.*, 1985; Stern *et al.*, 1986; Hennart *et al.*, 1985). In our own studies the introduction of supplementary food was associated with a significant decline in suckling duration, an effect which passed unnoticed by most women unless accomplished by a reduction in suckling frequency (Fig. 24.3) (Howie *et al.*, 1981).

The impact of supplements depends on the effect on suckling activity. If the impact is small and suckling declines only gradually, then menses is preceded by a normal luteal phase in only about 30 per cent of cycles, the remainder of the luteal phases being deficient (30 per cent) or absent (42 per cent) (Howie *et al.*, 1982; McNeilly *et al.*, 1982; Glasier *et al.*, 1983). Luteal function improves with each successive menstrual period as suckling declines (Fig. 24.1 and 24.2). A similar sequence of events has been observed in studies in Zaïre (Delvoye *et al.*, 1980; Hennart *et al.*, 1985) and Australia (Brown *et al.*, 1985; Gross and Eastman, 1985), and it is similar to the pattern of return of luteal function post partum in bottle-feeding women (McNeilly *et al.*, 1980; Howie *et al.*, 1982; Poindexter *et al.*, 1983) and during menarche (Brown *et al.*, 1985).

If supplementation results in a rapid decline in suckling, then there is an increased probability that a normal luteal phase will precede menses (Brown *et al.*, 1985; McNeilly *et al.*, 1982). Indeed, conception can occur before menses, but in our limited experience this only happens when there has been a rapid

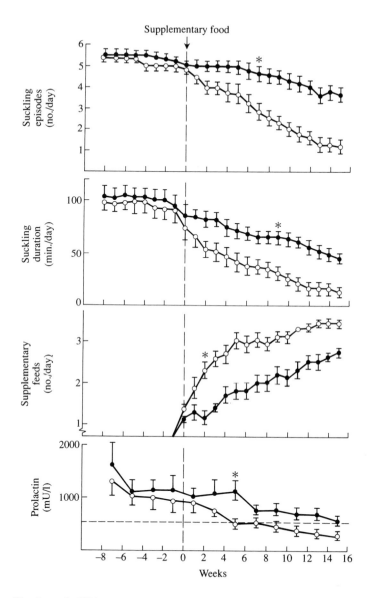

Source: Howie *et al.*, 1981.

Fig. 24.3 Comparison of suckling episodes, suckling duration, supplementary feeds, and basal prolactin in breastfeeding mothers who ovulated (o–o) or continued to suppress ovulation (●–●) after the introduction of supplementary feeds

reduction in suckling frequency and duration (Fig. 24.4) (McNeilly *et al.*, 1983*a*).

Ovulation with normal luteal function can occur during full breastfeeding, although this appears to be a relatively infrequent occurrence. In our own studies, this has occurred when suckling frequencies are maintained but suckling duration falls below 40 minutes per day (A. Glasier and A. S. McNeilly, unpublished observations).

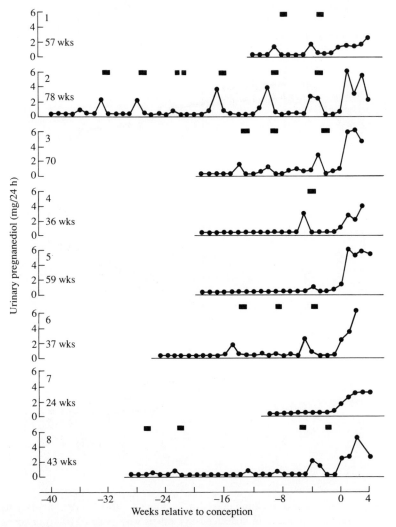

The time of conception in weeks post partum is indicated.

Source: McNeilly *et al.*, 1983*a*.

Fig. 24.4   Changes in urinary levels of pregnanediol glucuronide (●–●) and menses (■) prior to conception in seven breastfeeding women

These results emphasize that it is changes in the suckling stimulus, and not maternal or infant body weight, that is the important factor maintaining infertility. It is clear that the longer first menses is delayed during lactation, the more likely it is to be preceded by ovulation (Howie and McNeilly, 1982; Brown *et al.*, 1985; Rivero *et al.*, 1985). Nevertheless, conception rates in menstruating, breastfeeding women are only around 30 per cent of those in non-breastfeeding women (see Howie and McNeilly 1982; Brown *et al.*, 1985; Rivero *et al.*, 1985). The probable explanation for this is that a substantial number of menstrual periods are preceded by inadequate luteal function, which would not be capable of supporting a pregnancy (McNeilly *et al.*, 1983*a*).

Mechanisms Controlling Lactational Infertility

Gonadotrophins

Ovarian follicle growth, ovulation, and corpus luteum function are dependent on an adequate supply of both FSH, to sustain follicle growth, and LH (released as pulses of short duration) to maintain steroidogenesis within the follicle. LH stimulates the release of androgens from the theca of the follicle, and these androgens are converted to oestradiol via an active aromatase enzyme within the granulosa cells of the developing follicle. During the menstrual cycle, LH pulse frequency increases, stimulating an increase in plasma levels of oestradiol which, on reaching a critical level as the pre-ovulatory follicle matures, triggers the mid-cycle surge of LH (positive feedback) causing ovulation and the formation of the corpus luteum.

Each pulse of LH occurs as a result of the pulsatile release of gonadotrophin-releasing hormone (GnRH) from the hypothalamus. During the menstrual cycle, oestradiol appears to increase the frequency of GnRH and, hence, LH pulses, whereas luteal phase progesterone and oestradiol from the corpus luteum suppress the frequency of these pulses. The drop in frequency appears to result from an increase in opiate activity within the hypothalamus, which reduces the secretory activity of GnRH neurons (Crowley *et al.*, 1985; Lincoln *et al.*, 1985). The importance of the pulsatile release of LH in maintaining ovarian activity has been established in cases of primary and secondary amenorrhoea (e.g. Crowley *et al.*, 1985). It has been shown that an inadequate frequency of pulses or an inability to sustain a high pulse frequency is associated with failure or inadequacy of follicle growth.

By 4 weeks post partum, plasma levels of FSH increase to within the normal menstrual cycle range, while LH levels increase to and remain at the lower limit of normal (Reyes *et al.*, 1972; Bonnar *et al.*, 1975; Rolland *et al.*, 1975; Delvoye *et al.*, 1978; Duchen and McNeilly, 1980; Glasier *et al.*, 1983; Gross and Eastman, 1985). In our own studies, mean basal levels of LH did not change significantly after 4 weeks post partum until normal ovulatory cycles had resumed (Glasier *et al.*, 1983). Although overall basal levels were low, it was evident that in around 30 per cent of women levels of LH were within the normal range or even slightly higher, even though there was no evidence of major follicular development (Glasier *et al.*, 1983). Indeed, we have failed to show any significant difference in basal levels of LH or FSH at the time when ovarian follicular development resumes during breastfeeding (McNeilly *et al.*, 1980; Glasier *et al.*, 1983, 1984*b*), an observation recently confirmed by Gross and Eastman (1985). It was apparent, however, that mean basal levels of LH did increase gradually with time post partum (Glasier *et al.*, 1983, 1984*b*), and we have recently confirmed this by measuring LH in urine specimens collected daily throughout breastfeeding (A. S. McNeilly and A. Glasier, unpublished observations).

The failure to show any major change in LH during the period of ovarian suppression and the resumption of ovarian activity is related to the pulsatile nature of LH release. We have now established that the pulsatile release of LH is suppressed for 70 per cent of the time during breastfeeding-induced ovarian inactivity (Fig. 24.5) (Glasier *et al.*, 1984*b*) with LH pulses of low frequency and low amplitude being observed (Madden *et al.*, 1978; Tyson *et al.*, 1978; Glasier *et al.*, 1984*b*).

These results suggest that ovarian inactivity during breastfeeding is related to a suppression of the pulsatile release of LH, presumably as a result of the reduced secretion of GnRH from the hypothalamus. This is further implied by the inability of oestrogen to induce a positive feedback release of LH as normally seen in the menstrual cycle (Baird *et al.*, 1979; Glass *et al.*, 1981; Vermer and Rolland, 1982). Indeed, not only is positive feedback suppressed, but the negative feedback effect of oestrogen appears to be enhanced (Baird *et al.*, 1979).

In 30 per cent of observation periods during ovarian inactivity, pulsatile release of LH was observed, and in some instances both pulse frequency and amplitude was similar to that in the normal menstrual cycle (Glasier *et al.*, 1984*b*). Although limited follicle growth in terms of oestrogen secretion was observed, this was not sustained, and a state of ovarian inactivity returned while breastfeeding continued at a sufficient level.

Sustained ovarian follicular development resumed only when suckling decreased (Delvoye *et al.*, 1978; McNeilly *et al.*, 1980; Howie *et al.*, 1981, 1982; Glasier *et al.*, 1983, 1984*b*), related to an ability to sustain an increase in the frequency of pulsatile LH secretion (McNeilly *et al.*, 1985; A. S. McNeilly and A. Glasier, unpublished observations).

These observations have led us to suggest that the maintenance of ovarian inactivity caused by breastfeeding is due to the ability of low levels of oestrogen, produced by any developing follicles, in response to an increase in the pulsatile secretion of hypothalamic GnRH and hence pituitary LH, to inhibit further secretion of GnRH (Fig. 24.6). Follicular development is therefore attenuated until the suckling input has reduced sufficiently to allow

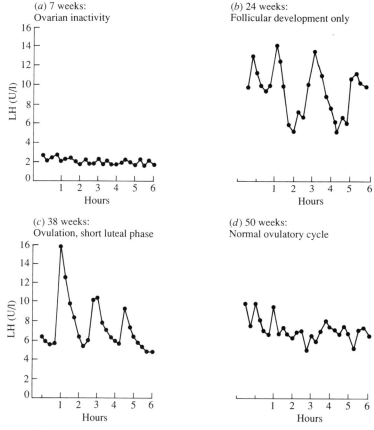

(*a*) 7 weeks:
Ovarian inactivity

(*b*) 24 weeks:
Follicular development only

(*c*) 38 weeks:
Ovulation, short luteal phase

(*d*) 50 weeks:
Normal ovulatory cycle

Note that the pattern of LH secretion is similar at both 24 and 38 weeks post partum, although ovulation did not occur until 32 weeks.

Source: Glasier *et al.*, 1984*b*.

Fig. 24.5   Changes in the pulsatile secretion of LH in relation to the return of ovarian activity

the hypothalamic GnRH neurons to withstand an increase in levels of oestrogen from developing follicles and so to allow the pulsatile secretion of GnRH and LH to continue promoting follicular development and ovulation (McNeilly *et al.*, 1985).

We have recently shown that sustained follicular development and ovulation can be induced in breastfeeding mothers by the pulsatile infusion of GnRH in a manner which will induce ovulation in non-breastfeeding women (Fig. 24.7) (Glasier *et al.*, 1986). Once the pulsatile infusion was stopped, all women returned to a state of ovarian inactivity if breastfeeding continued.

The occurrence of inadequate corpus luteum function in many of the first menstrual cycles following lactational amenorrhoea in particular, if breastfeeding

LACTATION

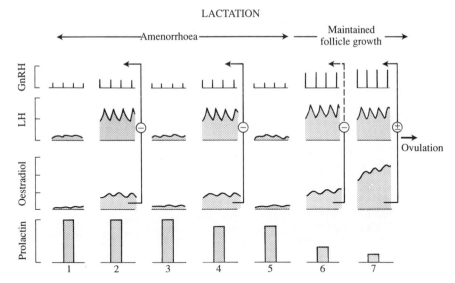

Suckling causes a decrease in hypothalamic capacity to release GnRH with a subsequent reduction in the pulsatile release of LH (1). If pulsatile release of LH occurs during lactational amenorrhoea (up to 30 per cent of the time), the resulting increase in oestrogen secretion (2) acts to inhibit further release of GnRH due to the suckling-induced increase in sensitivity to the negative feedback effects of oestrogen (3). Such a situation continues (4, 5) until suckling declines, resulting in a decrease in prolactin (6) when the hypothalamic sensitivity to the negative feedback of oestrogen is reduced and the hypothalamic capacity to release GnRH returns to normal with normal negative/positive feedback action of oestrogen (6,7). This results in the maintenance of pulsatile LH secretion, sustained follicular growth, and ovulation.

Source: McNeilly, 1984.

Fig. 24.6   Diagrammatic representation of the control of gonadotrophin secretion and its interaction with prolactin during lactational amenorrhoea and the resumption of follicle growth and ovulation in breastfeeding women

continues, also suggests a continued impairment of ovarian function. Inadequate corpus luteum function in non-breastfeeding women post partum (Howie and McNeilly, 1982) is associated with a pre-ovulatory LH surge of reduced amplitude and duration (Poindexter *et al.*, 1983). A similar situation appears to occur in breastfeeding women: the amount of LH released during the pre-ovulatory surge is reduced, compared to normal, if the woman continues to breastfeed (Fig. 24.8) (McNeilly *et al.*, 1985).

It is clear that the reduction in ovarian follicular development is related to a suppression of the normal pulsatile pattern of LH secretion. This implies a suckling-induced suppression of the pulsatile release of GnRH from the hypothalamus, which also results in the inability of oestrogen to induce a positive feedback release of LH; hence, the pre-ovulatory surge mechanism fails. Thus, even if follicle growth did occur, ovulation would not take place until suckling reduced sufficiently to allow sustained GnRH release from the hypothalamus.

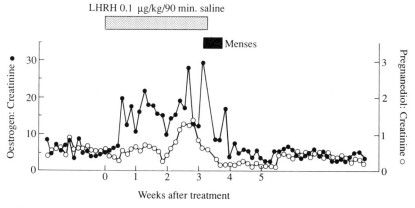

Note that ovarian steroid secretion before and after treatment was suppressed.
Source: Glasier *et al.*, 1986.

Fig. 24.7   Induction of ovulation in a breastfeeding woman by the pulsatile infusion of LHRH (GnRH) starting at 6 weeks post partum

The precise mechanism whereby suckling suppresses GnRH release remains unclear. Recent evidence in animals suggests that suckling may increase hypothalamic opiate activity which, in turn, suppresses GnRH release (Sirinathsinghji and Martini, 1984; Mattoli *et al.*, 1986). Indeed, an increase in the hypothalamic secretion of β-endorphin into the hyopophyseal portal blood in response to suckling has now been shown in lactating ewes (Gordon *et al.*, 1987). While there is no direct evidence for a similar mechanism in women, heroin will cause suppression of gonadotrophin and an increase in prolactin secretion similar to that seen in lactation (Pelosi *et al.*, 1974).

These preliminary observations suggest that the suckling-induced release of opioids within the hypothalamus may be the principal mediator of the suppression of LH release during lactation.

Prolactin

The role of prolactin in lactational amenorrhoea cannot be ignored. Prolactin is released in response to suckling throughout lactation and is essential for maintaining milk production (see McNeilly, 1977, 1984). Prolactin levels are high during the first 3 to 4 months post partum and the gradual decline throughout lactation is parallel with the decline in suckling (Delvoye *et al.*, 1978; Tyson *et al.*, 1978; Madden *et al.*, 1978; Glasier *et al.*, 1983; Howie *et al.*, 1981; Gross and Eastman, 1983, 1985; Anderson and Schioler, 1982; Lunn *et al.*, 1980; Hennart *et al.*, 1985; Stern *et al.*, 1986). An increase in prolactin concentrations induced by metoclopramide (Kauppila *et al.*, 1984) or sulpiride (Aono *et al.*, 1982; Ylikorkala and Kauppila, 1981) improves inadequate lactation, confirming a direct relationship between prolactin and milk yield

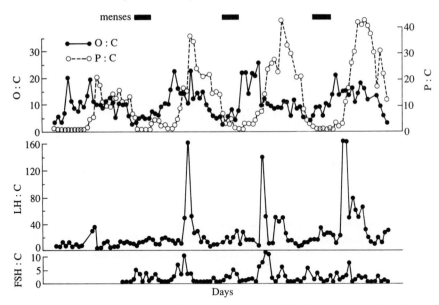

Sample collection was started on day 136 post partum when suckling frequency was three times per day and suckling duration was 37 min per day. The baby was weaned after the second menstrual period when suckling had declined to one 13-minute feed per day. Note that there is a progressive improvement of luteal function as suckling decreases. This increase in luteal pregnanediol levels is associated with an increase in the amount of LH released at mid-cycle.

Source: A. S. McNeilly and A. Glasier, unpublished observations.

Fig. 24.8   Changes in urinary oestrogen (O:C), pregnanediol (P:C), LH (LH:C), and FSH (FSH:C) in early morning specimens collected daily throughout consecutive menstrual cycles during the transition from lactational amenorrhoea to normal luteal function

during established lactation. The prolactin response to suckling appears to be greater in the afternoon and evening, as compared to the morning (Fig. 24.9) (Glasier *et al.*, 1984*a*; Gross and Eastman, 1985; Stern *et al.*, 1986), although milk production is similar (Glasier *et al.*, 1984*a*). This suggests that there is not a direct relationship between the amount of prolactin released and the amount of milk produced during each suckling episode. This is particularly the case in the early post-partum period when basal levels are very high (Howie *et al.*, 1982). In prolonged lactation, daily milk yields may be correlated to basal prolactin levels (Hennart *et al.*, 1981).

There is no doubt that suckling is the principal mediator of prolactin release in lactation, and there is a close correlation between the basal levels of prolactin throughout lactation and suckling frequency in many studies (Hennart *et al.*, 1981, 1985; Gross and Eastman, 1985; McNeilly *et al.*, 1980; Howie *et al.*, 1980; Stern *et al.*, 1986). There is also a direct relationship between the duration of lactational amenorrhoea and the degree of hyperprolactinaemia (Delvoye *et al.*, 1978; Duchen and McNeilly, 1980; Howie *et al.*, 1981, 1982;

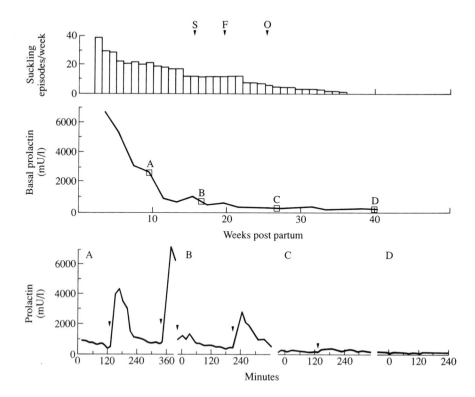

The times of introduction of supplements (S), follicular development (F), and ovulation (O) are indicated. Note that the prolactin response to suckling is greater in the afternoon than the morning, although suckling time and feed volume are similar. The symbols A, B, C, and D indicate the time post partum at which the timed prolactin responses in the lower panel were measured. The time post partum in the middle panel at which the lower measurements were made are as follows:

A = prolactin response at *c*.10 weeks; B = *c*.17 weeks; C = *c*.26 weeks; D = *c*.40 weeks.

Source: Glasier *et al.*, 1984*a*.

Fig. 24.9   Changes in suckling frequency, basal prolactin levels, and the prolactin response to suckling, with time post partum

Gross and Eastman, 1985; Stern *et al.*, 1986). This, together with the link between hyperprolactinaemia and amenorrhoea in a proportion of women with non-lactational, secondary amenorrhoea, has led many to suggest that the suppression of ovarian activity during breastfeeding is directly related to the high circulating levels of prolactin. This has been discussed in detail previously (McNeilly, 1979, 1985, 1987; McNeilly *et al.*, 1983*c*; Robyn and Meuris, 1982).

Prolactin may act directly at the hypothalamus to inhibit GnRH release or at the ovary to reduce ovarian sensitivity to gonadotrophin stimulation. While there is limited evidence in animals that prolactin may interfere directly at the ovary (see McNeilly, 1979, 1985), follicular development and ovulation can be induced in the face of high circulating levels of prolactin by pulsatile GnRH therapy in breastfeeding women (Glasier *et al.*, 1986) and women with hyperprolactinaemic amenorrhoea (Gindoff *et al.*, 1986; Bergh *et al.*, 1984). These results support the concept that an alteration in the pulsatile secretion of GnRH/LH is of principal importance in lactational infertility.

Could prolactin act directly at the hypothalamic level to impair gonadotrophin secretion? The resumption of ovulatory cycles is associated with an increase in LH and a decrease in mean basal levels of prolactin. In all individuals, basal prolactin levels at the time of resumption of ovarian activity decrease from those during ovarian inactivity (Howie and McNeilly, 1982; Gross and Eastman, 1985; Stern *et al.*, 1986). However, the level of prolactin at which resumption of activity occurs varies widely, and in some women ovulatory cycles have been observed when prolactin levels are four to five times the upper limit seen during normal menstrual cycles (Howie *et al.*, 1982; Hennart *et al.*, 1985; Stern *et al.*, 1986). The close association between suckling and prolactin makes it difficult to accept conclusively that prolactin itself is the mediator of the inhibition of GnRH release.

Induction of hyperprolactinaemia in normally cyclic women using dopamine antagonists may lead to a disruption of follicular development if hyperprolactinaemia is induced in the early follicular development, but not the late follicular or luteal, phases of the cycle (see McNeilly, 1985; Kauppila *et al.*, 1984; Payne *et al.*, 1985; Sowa *et al.*, 1986). Relatively high doses of dopamine antagonists were used in the majority of these studies (McMurdo *et al.*, 1987), and a direct effect of the drug alone on GnRH and LH secretion, independent of the effect on prolactin, cannot be ruled out (Payne *et al.*, 1985). Indeed, women with normoprolactinaemic, functional hypóthalamic amenorrhoea show an increase in LH and FSH secretion and the stimulation of ovarian activity when treated with the same dopamine antagonists that cause significant hyperprolactinaemia (Djursing *et al.*, 1986).

In the rat, hyperprolactinaemia causes a suppression of gonadotrophin release (see Adler, 1986 for review), apparently by increasing sensitivity to the negative feedback effects of gonadal steroid (McNeilly *et al.*, 1983*b*). An increase in the peripheral concentration of prolactin leads to an increase in hypothalamic dopamine turnover, the auto-regulatory control of prolactin secretion (see Leong *et al.*, 1983; Moore and Demarest, 1982). Since dopamine can directly inhibit GnRH and LH secretion (Leblanc *et al.*, 1976; Huseman *et al.*, 1980), principally by acting through dopamine D-1 receptors (Fuxe *et al.*, 1980; Wilson *et al.*, 1985), it has been suggested that the increase in prolactin associated with breastfeeding results in an increase in hypothalamic dopamine turnover which causes the suppression in GnRH/LH release (see McNeilly, 1984, 1987 for discussion). However, this link remains unproven in women or any other species. An increase in hypothalamic dopamine turnover may not occur during lactation even in the rat (Demarest *et al.*, 1983; Selmanoff and Wise, 1981), while a prolactin-induced increase in hypothalamic dopamine turnover is associated with an increase in LH and FSH secretion in the mouse and hamster (Shrenker and Burtke, 1987).

Thus, the role, if any, of prolactin in maintaining ovarian inactivity during breastfeeding remains unclear. While hypothalamic opiates may be involved in maintaining the elevated levels of prolactin associated with suckling in animals (see e.g. Sirinathsinghji and Martini, 1984; Mattioli *et al.*, 1986; Gordon *et al.*, 1987), this may not be the case in breastfeeding women (Lodico *et al.*, 1983; Cholst *et al.*, 1984). Clearly the link between suckling, prolactin, and gonado-trophin release requires further investigation.

Effects of Nutrition on Lactational Amenorrhoea

It has been suggested that nutrition may play a major role in maintaining lactational amenorrhoea and infertility. The metabolic drain of milk production may directly suppress gonadotrophin secretion in a situation analogous to that of training-induced amenorrhoea in athletes (see Frisch, 1985 and Chapter 9, above). However, recent studies suggest that this is not the case. Maternal nutritional status in the absence of alterations in suckling pattern did not explain the prolonged duration of lactational amenorrhoea in women in Africa compared to European counterparts (Hennart *et al.*, 1985; Lunn, 1985). In addition, it is now clear that, while the resting metabolic rate is the same in breastfeeding and non-breastfeeding women, the response to a metabolic challenge is greatly reduced in women during breastfeeding who, therefore, show an enhanced metabolic efficiency during lactation (Illingworth *et al.*, 1986).

Studies in red deer have suggested that poor maternal nutrition leads to a reduced milk production (Loudon *et al.*, 1983). This results in an increase in the suckling activity of the young in order to maintain the required milk input per day, and this, in turn leads to the prolongation of lactational anoestrus. A similar situation is thought to occur in breastfeeding women (Lunn, 1985) and could occur if maternal water intake was restricted as this, presumably, would also lead to a reduction in milk production.

The effects of reduced milk supply may not necessarily be seen in an increase in suckling frequency or duration. Instead, the pattern of suckling during a period of suckling may be altered, with greater suckling activity resulting if milk flow is reduced (Bowen-Jones *et al.*, 1982). Since it is the strength of suckling-dependent stimulation of the neurons in the nipple which is ultimately responsible for the suppression of fertility and the release of prolactin and oxytocin during lactation, an alteration in suckling pattern may prove to be of vital importance.

Contraception

Because of the variability in the duration of lactational infertility, there is a definite need to provide contraceptives suitable for the breastfeeding mother. In terms of breastfeeding, guidelines for suckling frequencies and durations which will maintain infertility can be determined for individual societies, but these do not, and have never been claimed to, guarantee complete protection from conception. Such guidelines must be established for each society only after sufficient data has been collected.

The combined oral contraceptive is contra-indicated for breastfeeding mothers as it appears to suppress milk production. Thus, most nursing mothers who wish to use a steroidal contraceptive use the progestogen-only formulation. Its major disadvantage is frequent episodes of vaginal bleeding (WHO Task Force on Oral Contraceptives, 1987), similar to those seen in non-breastfeeding women using the same formulations (Rice-Wray *et al.*, 1972). Sulpiride, a dopaminergic antagonist, in combination with the progestogen-only pill, markedly improved the efficiency of the progestogen (Payne *et al.*, 1985). The prolactin-releasing properties of sulpiride should also improve lactation, offering a dual targeted contraceptive suitable for breastfeeding women.

Highly potent GnRH agonists paradoxically suppress gonadotrophin secretion in non-lactating women (Fraser, 1982). These agonists have now been shown to be an excellent contraceptive in breastfeeding mothers. The small amount of agonist which passes through into the milk has no effect on the suckling infant, since GnRH agonists are orally inactive except in excessively large doses (Dewart *et al.*, 1986).

Thus, two new safe contraceptives should soon be available for breastfeeding mothers, both of which will complement the natural anti-fertility effect of breastfeeding.

Conclusions

Breastfeeding provides a period of ovarian inactivity and infertility of variable duration. The suckling stimulus itself is the key factor in controlling the duration of infertility. While guidelines can be defined for the frequency and duration of episodes of breastfeeding which will maintain infertility, these are not 100 per cent effective and will vary with the pattern of suckling behaviour both within and between different societies. It is unlikely that universal guidelines can be established.

Suckling appears to suppress gonadotrophin, principally LH secretion, by reducing the pulsatile release of GnRH from the hypothalamus. The exact mechanisms involved remain to be elucidated but may include a suckling-induced activation of a hypothalamic opioid pathway. The role of prolactin in lactational infertility, other than being essential for the maintenance of milk production and thereby influencing suckling activity, remains unresolved. Recent studies do not suggest a major role for prolactin *per se*.

In spite of the relative unpredictability of the duration of lactation infertility, breastfeeding continues to be of major importance in prolonging the inter-birth interval worldwide.

References

Adler, R. A. (1986), 'The Anterior Pituitary-Grafted Rat: A Valid Model of Chronic Hyperprolactinaemia', *Endocrine Reviews* 7: 302–13.

Anderson, A. N., and Schioler, V. (1982), 'Influence of Breastfeeding Pattern on Pituitary–Ovarian Axis of Women in an Industrialized Community', *American Journal of Obstetrics and Gynecology* 143: 673–7.

Aono, T., Aki, T., Koike, K., and Kurachi, K. (1982), 'Effect of Sulpiride on Poor Lactation', *American Journal of Obstetrics and Gynecology* 143: 927–32.

Baird, D. T., McNeilly, A. S., Sawers, R. S., and Sharpe, R. M. (1979), 'Failure of Estrogen Induced Discharge of Luteinizing Hormone in Lactating Women', *Journal of Clinical Endocrinology and Metabolism* 49: 500–9.

Bergh, T., Skarin, G., Nillius, S. J., and Wide, L. (1984), 'Pulsatile LHRH Administration to Women with Bromocriptine-Resistant Hyperprolactinaemia', in S. W. Lamberts, F. H. J. Tilders, E. A. van der Veen, and J. Assiers (eds.), *Trends in Diagnosis and Treatment of Pituitary Adenomas*: 195–8, Free University Press, Amsterdam.

Bonnar, J., Franklin, M., Nott, P. N., and McNeilly, A. S. (1975), 'Effect of Breastfeeding on Pituitary–Ovarian Function After Childbirth', *British Medical Journal* 4: 82–4.

Bowen-Jones, A., Thompson, C., and Drewett, R. F. (1982), 'Milk Flow and Suckling Rates During Breast Feeding', *Developments in Medical Child Neurology* 24: 626–33.

Brown, J. B., Harrison, P., and Smith, M. A. (1985), 'A Study of Returning Fertility after Childbirth and during Lactation by Measurement of Urinary Oestrogen and Pregnanediol Secretion and Cervical Mucus Production', *Journal of Biosocial Science*, supplement 9: 5–23.

Cholst, I. N., Wardlaw, S. L., Newman, C. B., and Frantz, A. G. (1984), 'Prolactin Response to Breast Stimulation in Lactating Women is Not Mediated by Endogenous Opiods', *American Journal of Obstetrics and Gynecology* 150: 558–61.

Crowley, W. F., Jr., Filicori, M., Spratt, D. I., and Santoro, N. F. (1985), 'The

Physiology of Gonadotrophin-Releasing Hormone (GnRH) Secretion in Men and Women', *Recent Progress in Hormone Research* 41: 473–526.

Delvoye, P., Delogne-Desnoeck, J., and Robyn, C. (1980), 'Hyperprolactinaemia during Prolonged Lactation: Evidence for Anovulatory Cycles and Inadequate Corpus Luteum', *Clinical Endocrinology* 13: 243–7.

—— Badawi, M., Demaegd, M., and Robyn, C. (1978), 'Serum Prolactin, Gonado-trophins and Estradiol in Menstruating and Amenorrhoeic Women During Two Years of Lactation', *American Journal of Obstetrics and Gynecology* 130: 635–40.

Demarest, K. T., McKay, D. W., Riegle, G. D., and Moore, K. E. (1983), 'Biochemical Indices of Tuberoinfundibular Dopaminergic Neuronal Activity During Lactation: A Lack of Response to Prolactin', *Neuroendocrinology* 36: 130–7.

Dewart, P. J., McNeilly, A. S., Smith, S. K., Sandow, J., and Fraser, H. M. (1987), 'LHRH Agonist Buserelin as a Post-Partum Contraceptive: Lack of Biological Activity of Buserelin in Breast Milk', *Acta Endocrinologica* 114(2): 185–92.

Djursing, H., Hagen, C., Andersen, A. N., Nyholm, H. C., and Petersen, K. (1986), 'Prolonged Dopamine Receptor Blocker in Normoprolactinaemic Amenorrhoea: A Double-Blind Placebo Study', *Fertility and Sterility* 46: 840–5.

Duchen, M. R., and McNeilly, A. S. (1980), 'Hyperprolactinaemia and Long-Term Lactational Amenorrhoea', *Clinical Endocrinology* 12: 621–7.

Fraser, H. M. (1982), 'New Prospects for Luteinizing Hormone Releasing Hormone as a Contraceptive and Therapeutic Agent', *British Medical Journal* 285: 990–1.

Frisch, R. E. (1985), 'Maternal Nutrition and Lactational Amenorrhoea: Perceiving the Metabolic Costs', in J. Dobbing (ed.), *Maternal Nutrition and Lactational Infertility*: 65–78, Vevey/Raven Press, New York.

Fuxe, K., Anderson, L., Ferland, R., Hokfelt, T., Eneroth, P., and Gustafsson, J. A. (1980), 'Hypothalamic Monoamine Pathways and their Possible Role in Disturb-ances of the Secretion of Hormones from the Anterior Pituitary Gland', in G. Fagha, M. A. Giovanelli, and R. M. McLeod (eds.), *Pituitary Microadenomas*: 15–35, Academic Press, New York.

Gindorff, P. R., Loucopoulos, A., and Jewelewicz, R. (1986), 'Treatment of Hyper-prolactinaemic Amenorrhoea with Pulsatile Gonadotropin-Releasing Hormone Therapy', *Fertility and Sterility* 46: 1156–8.

Glasier, A., McNeilly, A. S., and Howie, P. W. (1983), 'Fertility After Childbirth: Changes in Serum Gonadotrophin Levels in Bottle and Breastfeeding Women', *Clinical Endocrinology* 24: 243–52.

—— —— —— (1984a), 'The Prolactin Response to Suckling', *Clinical Endocrinology* 21: 109–16.

—— —— —— (1984b), 'Pulsatile Secretion of LH in Relation to the Resumption of Ovarian Activity Post Partum', *Clinical Endocrinology* 19: 493–501.

—— —— and Baird, D. T. (1986), 'Induction of Ovarian Activity by Pulsatile Infusion LHRH in Women with Lactational Amenorrhoea', *Clinical Endocrinology* 24: 243–52.

Glass, M. R., Rudd, B. T., Lynch, S. S., and Butt, W. R. (1981), 'Estrogen-Gonadotrophin Feedback Mechanisms in the Puerperium', *Clinical Endocrinology* 14: 257–67.

Gordon, K., Renfree, M. B., Short, R. V., and Clarke, I. J. (1987), 'Hypothalamo–Pituitary Portal Blood Concentration of B-Endorphin During Suckling in the Ewe', *Journal of Reproduction and Fertility* 79: 397–408.

Gross, B. A., and Eastman, C. J. (1983), 'Effect of Breastfeeding Status on Prolactin Secretion and Resumption of Menses', *Medical Journal of Australia* 1: 313–20.

—— —— (1985), 'Prolactin and the Return of Ovulation in Breastfeeding Women', *Journal of Biosocial Science*, supplement 9: 25–42.

Hennart, P., Delogue-Desnoeck, J., Vis, H., and Robyn, C. (1981), 'Serum Levels of Prolactin and Milk Production in Women During a Lactation Period of Thirty Months', *Clinical Endocrinology* 14: 349–53.

—— Hofvander, Y., Vis, H., and Robyn, C. (1985), 'Comparative Study of Nursing Mothers in Africa (Zaïre) and in Europe (Sweden): Breastfeeding Behaviour, Nutritional Status, Lactational Hyperprolactinaemia and Status of the Menstrual Cycle', *Clinical Endocrinology* 22: 179–87.

Howie, P. W., and McNeilly, A. S. (1982), 'Effect of Breastfeeding Patterns on Human Birth Intervals', *Journal of Reproduction and Fertility* 65: 545–57.

—— —— McArdle, T., Smart, L., and Houston, M. J. (1980), 'The Relationship Between Suckling-Induced Prolactin Response and Lactogenesis', *Journal of Clinical Endocrinology and Metabolism* 50: 670–3.

—— —— Houston, M. J., Cook, A., and Boyle, H. (1981), 'Effect of Supplementary Food on Suckling Patterns and Ovarian Activity during Lactation', *British Medical Journal* 283: 757–9.

—— —— —— —— —— (1982), 'Fertility After Childbirth: Postpartum Ovulation and Menstruation in Bottle and Breastfeeding Mothers', *Clinical Endocrinology* 17: 323–34.

Huseman, C. A., Kugler, J. A., and Schneider, I. G. (1980), 'Mechanism of Dopaminergic Suppression of Gonadotropin Secretion in Men', *Journal of Clinical Endocrinology and Metabolism* 51: 209–14.

Illingworth, P. J., Jung, R. T., Howie, P. W., Leslie, P., and Isles, T. E. (1986), 'Diminution in Energy Expenditure During Lactation', *British Medical Journal* 292: 437–41.

Kauppila, A., Kirkinen, P., Orava, M., and Vihko, R. (1984), 'Effects of Metoclopramide-Induced Hyperprolactinaemia during Early Follicular Development on Human Ovarian Function', *Journal of Clinical Endocrinology and Metabolism* 59: 875–81.

Konner, M., and Worthman, C. (1980), 'Nursing Frequency, Gonadal Function and Birth Spacing Among !Kung Hunter Gatherers', *Science* 207: 788–91.

LeBlanc, H., Lachelin, G. C. L., Abu-Fadil, S., and Yen, S. S. C. (1976), 'Effects of Dopamine Infusion on Pituitary Hormone Secretion in Humans', *Journal of Clinical Endocrinology and Metabolism* 43: 668–74.

Leong, D. A., Rawley, L. S., and Neill, J. D. (1983), 'Neuroendocrine Control of Prolactin Secretion', *Annual Review of Physiology* 45: 109–27.

Lincoln, D. W., Fraser, H. M., Lincoln, G. A., Martin, G. B., and McNeilly, A. S. (1985), 'Hypothalamic Pulse Generators', *Recent Progress in Hormone Research* 41: 369–411.

Lodico, G., Stopelli, I., Delitala, G., and Mattoli, M. (1983), 'Effects of Naloxone Infusion on Basal and Breast-Stimulated Prolactin Secretion in Puerperal Women', *Fertility and Sterility* 40(5): 600–3.

Loudon, A. I., McNeilly, A. S., and Milne, J. A. (1983), 'Nutrition and Lactational Control of Fertility in Red Deer', *Nature* 302: 145–7.

Lunn, P. G. (1985), 'Maternal Nutrition and Lactational Infertility: The Baby in the

Driving Seat', in J. Dobbing (ed.), *Maternal Nutrition and Lactational Infertility*: 41–53, Vevey/Raven Press, New York.

Lunn, P. G., Prentice, A. M., Austin, S., and Whitehead, R. G. (1980), 'Influence of Maternal Diet on Plasma-Prolactin Levels During Lactation', *Lancet* 1: 623–5.

McMurdo, M. E. T., Howie, P. W., Lewis, M., Marnie, M., McEwen, J., and McNeilly, A. S. (1987), 'Prolactin Response to Low Dose Sulpiride', *British Journal of Clinical Pharmacology* 24(2): 133–7.

McNeilly, A. S. (1977), 'Physiology of Human Lactation', *Journal of Biosocial Science* supplement 4: 5–21.

—— (1979), 'Effects of Lactation on Fertility', *British Medical Bulletin* 35: 151–4.

—— (1984), 'Prolactin and Ovarian Function', in E. E. Miller and R. M. McLeod (eds.), *Neuroendocrine Perspectives* iii: 279–316, Elsevier Biomedical Press, Amsterdam.

—— (1985), 'Prolactin and the Corpus Luteum', in S. L. Jeffcoate (ed.), *The Luteal Phase*: 71–87, Wiley, Chichester.

—— (1987), 'Suckling and the Control of Gonadotropin Secretion', in E. Knobil and J. D. Neill (eds.), *The Physiology of Reproduction*: 2323–49, Raven Press, New York.

—— Howie, P. W., and Houston, M. J. (1980), 'Relationships of Feeding Patterns, Prolactin and Resumption of Ovulation Post Partum', in G. I. Zatuchni, M. H. Labbok, and J. J. Sciarra (eds.), *Research Frontiers in Fertility Regulation*: 102–16, Harper and Row, New York.

—— Sharpe, R. M., and Fraser, H. M. (1983*b*), 'Increased Sensitivity Negative Feedback Effects of Testosterone Induced by Hyperprolactinaemia in the Adult Male Rat', *Endocrinology* 112: 22–8.

—— Glasier, A., and Howie, P. W. (1985), 'Endocrine Control of Lactational Infertility', in J. Dobbing (ed.), *Maternal Nutrition and Lactational Infertility*: 1–16, Vevey/Raven Press, New York.

—— —— Swanston, I. and Djahanbakhch, O. (1983*c*), 'Prolactin and the Human Ovary', in G. Tolis (ed.), *Prolactin and Prolactinomas*: 173–8, Raven Press, New York.

—— Howie, P. W., Houston, M. J., Cook, A., and Boyle, H. (1982), 'Fertility after Childbirth: Adequacy of Post-Partum Luteal Phases', *Clinical Endocrinology* 17: 609–15.

—— Glasier, A., Howie, P. W., Houston, M. J., Cook, A., and Boyle, H. (1983*a*), 'Fertility After Childbirth: Pregnancy Associated with Breast Feeding', *Clinical Endocrinology* 19: 167–74.

Madden, J. D., Boyar, R. M., MacDonald, P. C., and Porter, J. C. (1978), 'Analysis of Secretory Patterns of Prolactin and Gonadotrophins During 24 Hours in a Lactating Woman Before and After Resumption of Menses', *American Journal of Obstetrics and Gynecology* 132: 436–41.

Mattoli, M., Conte, F., Graleati, G., and Seren, E. (1986), 'Effect of Naloxone on Plasma Concentrations of Prolactin and LH in Lactating Sows', *Journal of Reproduction and Fertility* 76: 167–73.

Moore, K. E., and Demarest, K. T. (1982), 'Tuberoinfundibular and Tuberohyphyseal Dopaminergic Neurons', in L. Martini and W. F. Ganong (ed.), *Frontiers in Neuroendocrinology* vii: 161–90, Raven Press, New York.

Payne, M. R., Howie, P. W., Cooper, W., Marnie, M., Kidd, L., and McNeilly, A. S.

(1985), 'Sulpiride and the Potentiation of Progestogen-only Contraception', *British Medical Journal* 291: 559–61.

Pelosi, M. A., Sama, J. C., Caterini, H., and Kaminetzky, H. A. (1974), 'Galactorrhoea–Amenorrhoea Syndrome Associated with Heroin Addiction', *American Journal of Obstetrics and Gynecology*, 118: 966–70.

Poindexter, A. N., Ritter, M. B., and Besch, P. K. (1983), 'The Recovery of Normal Plasma Progesterone Levels in the Post-Partum Female', *Fertility and Sterility* 39: 494–8.

Reyes, F. I., Winter, J. S. D., and Faiman, C. (1972), 'Pituitary–Ovarian Interrelationships During the Puerperium', *American Journal of Obstetrics and Gynecology* 114: 589–94.

Rice-Wray, E., Beristain, I. I., and Cervantes, A. (1972), 'Clinical Study of a Continuous Daily Micro-Dose Progestogen Contraceptive-d-norgestrel', *Contraception* 5: 279–94.

Rivero, R., Ortiz, E., Barrera, M., Kennedy, K., and Bhiwandiwala, P. (1985), 'Preliminary Observations on the Return of Ovarian Function Among Breast Feeding and Post-Partum Non-Breast Feeding Women in a Rural Area of Mexico', *Journal of Biosocial Science* supplement 9: 127–36.

Robyn, C., and Meuris, S. (1982), 'Pituitary Prolactin, Lactational Performance and Puerperal Infertility', *Seminars in Perinatology* 6: 254–64.

Rolland, R., Leouin, R. M., Schellekens, L. A., and DeJong, F. H. (1975), 'The Role of Prolactin in Restoration of Ovarian Function During the Early Post-Partum Period in the Human Female, I: A Study During Physiological Lactation', *Clinical Endocrinology* 4: 15–25.

Selmanoff, M., and Wise, P. M. (1981), 'Decreased Dopamine Turnover in the Median Eminence in Response to Suckling in the Lactating Rat', *Brain Research* 212: 101–16.

Shrenker, P., and Burtke, A. (1987), 'Effects of Hyperprolactinaemia on Male Sexual Behaviour in the Golden Hamster and Mouse', *Journal of Endocrinology* 112: 221–8.

Sirinathsinghji, D. J. S., and Martini, L. (1984), 'Effects of Bromocriptine and Naloxone on Plasma Levels of Prolactin, LH and FSH During Suckling in the Female Rat: Responses to Gonadotrophin Releasing Hormone', *Journal of Endocrinology* 100: 175–82.

Sowa, M., Rsuji, K., and Nakano, R. (1986), 'Effects of Sulpiride-Induced Hyperprolactinemia on Human Ovarian Follicles During the Late Follicular Phase', *Fertility and Sterility* 46(6): 1032–6.

Stern, J. M., Konner, M., Herman, T. N., and Reichlin, S. (1986), 'Nursing Behaviour, Prolactin and Post-Partum Amenorrhoea During Prolonged Lactation in American and !Kung Mothers', *Clinical Endocrinology* 25: 247–58.

Tyson, J. E., Carter, J. N., Andreassen, B., Hugh, J., and Smith, B. (1978), 'Nursing-Mediated Prolactic and Luteinizing Hormone Secretion During Puerperal Lactation', *Fertility and Sterility* 30: 154–62.

Vermer, H. M., and Rolland, R. (1982), 'The Influence of Exogenous Oestradiol Benzoate on the Pituitary Responsiveness to LHRH during the Puerperium in Women', *Clinical Endocrinology* 16: 251–8.

West, C. and McNeilly, A. S. (1979), 'Hormonal Profiles in Lactating and non-Lactating Women Immediately After Delivery and Their Relationship to Breast Engorgement', *British Journal of Obstetrics and Gynaecology* 86: 501–6.

WHO Task Force on Oral Contraceptives (1987), 'Contraception during the Postpartum Period and during Lactation: The Effects on Women's Health', *International Journal of Gynaecology and Obstetrics* 25: 13–26.

Wilson, C. A., MacKenzie, F. J., and James, M. D. (1985), 'The Effect of Selective D1 and D2 Agonists and Antagonists Injected into the Zona Incerta on Ovulation and LH Release', *Journal of Endocrinological Investigation* (supplement 3), 8: 85–90.

Wood, J. W., Lai, D., Johnson, P. L., Campbell, K. L., and Maslar, I. A. (1985), 'Lactation and Birth Spacing in Highland New Guinea', *Journal of Biosocial Science* supplement 9: 159–73.

Ylikorkala, O., and Kauppila, A. (1981), 'The Effects on the Ovulatory Cycle of Metoclopramide-Induced Increased Prolactin Levels during Follicular Development', *Fertility and Sterility* 35: 588–9.

25 Breastfeeding and the Length of Post-Partum Amenorrhoea: A Hazards Model Approach

GERMÁN RODRIGUEZ

SOLEDAD DIAZ

Introduction

It is now widely accepted that breastfeeding is associated with longer periods of post-partum amenorrhoea, a delay in the return of ovulation, and therefore longer birth ·intervals; see, for example, Van Ginneken (1977), Simpson-Hebert and Huffman (1981), Howie and McNeilly (1982) and Diaz et al. (1982). Breastfeeding is also associated with reduced fecundability after the return of menses and ovulation (see McNeilly et al., 1982; John et al., 1987). There is also evidence that the effect of breastfeeding is substantially weakened with the introduction of food supplements (see, for example, Prema and Ravindranath, 1982). A key factor mediating the effect of breastfeeding on the length of post-partum amenorrhoea is the frequency of suckling through the day and night, as shown, for example, by Howie et al. (1982). Indeed, the apparent effect of the introduction of supplements could well be a consequence of a decrease in the frequency or intensity of suckling.

The physiological mechanisms by which breastfeeding affects menstruation, ovulation, and fertility remain to be fully specified. It is known that lactation is associated with high levels of prolactin, low levels of oestradiol and progesterone, and normal or slightly sub-normal levels of gonadotrophins (Howie et al., 1982). The increased production of prolactin is clearly related to suckling by the infant, which stimulates receptors in the nipple, thus sending a signal to the hypothalamus, which, in turn, signals the pituitary to increase the production of prolactin. It is also known that prolactin inhibits ovulation, but the exact mechanism has not been isolated. It is important to note that this theory identifies nipple stimulation as the key factor in maintaining anovulation (Bongaarts and Potter, 1983: 27–8). A reduction in the frequency or intensity of breastfeeding, whether related to the introduction of supplements or to other behavioural changes, would be expected to lead to a reduction in levels of prolactin and eventually to the return of menses and ovulation.

Although there is widespread agreement on the nature of the effects of breastfeeding on the reproductive process, progress in the quantification of the effects has been stymied by the use of inappropriate statistical procedures. Many demographers and other analysts have relied on highly aggregate cross-sectional data linking the mean duration of breastfeeding to the mean duration of post-partum amenorrhoea (see, for example, Bongaarts and Potter, 1983: 25). These data are subject to biases arising from the fact that breastfeeding may be prolonged past the return of menses, when it is no longer relevant, or may be interrupted by conception (see Smith, 1985). A further and perhaps more serious drawback of this type of data, however, is that distinctions between full and partial breastfeeding are rarely made; as a result the averages, which combine the experience of women with different types of breastfeeding patterns, often hide more than they reveal.

On the other hand, biomedical researchers and other analysts with access to longitudinal data tend to adopt a retrospective stance and compare character-istics of women who have recovered menstruation or ovulation during follow-up with those who have not, sometimes classified by duration and often using simple t-tests (see, for example, Howie *et al.*, 1982). While generally valid, these tests fail to take into proper account the nature of the events studied, which take place over time. Some of these comparisons may be subject to the same biases as the aggregate analyses described above. Moreover, knowing that women who ovulate at later rather than earlier durations tend to have longer durations of breastfeeding tells us little about the magnitude of the underlying effect.

A third approach is illustrated by the work of Habicht *et al.* (1985), who developed a model of the underlying physiology assuming the existence of a key hormone whose concentration declines linearly over time, with the slope depending on breastfeeding practices. These authors use data from Malaysia to estimate the slopes for full and partial breastfeeding as well as for weaned children, using an *ad hoc* least-squares procedure. The model is purely deterministic, although a vague distinction is made between individual and population levels; as long as systematic and random components are not clearly specified, the use of least squares (or any statistical estimation technique) is highly questionable. Furthermore, the assumptions about unobservable hor-mone levels are, as stated, clearly unverifiable. Lastly, none of the approaches described so far can easily take into account the multivariate nature of the problem, that is, the multiplicity of factors which affect the length of amenor-rhoea and the anovulatory period.

Yet appropriate statistical procedures, which are consistent with the nature of the underlying processes as well as the types of data collected, do exist and have been available for a relatively long time. We refer here to older procedures such as the Kaplan–Meier (1959) product-limit estimate of a life-table and the Mantel–Haenszel test (Mantel 1966) for comparing two or more survival curves, as well as relatively more recent contributions by Cox (1972) and others in the development of hazard-rate models and methods for the analysis of life-tables with covariates. While extremely popular in the analysis of the remission of cancer and other events which take place over time, these techniques have largely been ignored in the analysis of the effects of breast-feeding on human reproduction.

Notable exceptions to the general trend are a study of birth intervals in the Philippines, Malaysia, and Indonesia by Trussell *et al.* (1985), which treats breastfeeding status (breastfeeding versus weaned) as a time-varying covariate affecting the probability of conception, and a study by John *et al.* (1987) on the effect of nutrition on fecundability, which treats the length of breastfeeding before the return of menses as a covariate affecting the probability of conception in subsequent months. Both studies focus on the effect of breastfeeding on the risk of conception in the post-partum period, although they take different starting-points. We are not aware of any study applying hazard-rate models to the study of the effect of breastfeeding on the length of post-partum amenor-rhoea and the length of the anovulatory period.

The main purpose of this paper is to provide an illustrative analysis which will fill this gap. We describe a small data-set arising from a longitudinal study and then proceed to explain in some detail a simple approach to the construction of life-tables and hazard models involving fixed as well as time-varying covariates.

The Data

The data for this analysis come from a longitudinal study undertaken in Santiago, Chile. The subjects were recruited among post-partum women who had delivered a child at the Paula Jaraquemada Hospital in Santiago. They were all healthy women in a normal nutritional state, aged 18–35 and with 1–3 children, who had a normal pregnancy ending in the vaginal delivery of a healthy child of normal birth-weight. All women were willing to breastfeed the child for as long as possible, had no permanent job nor intentions of seeking employment, and were regularly cohabiting with their partners.

Follow-up took place at a Family Planning Clinic affiliated to the Chilean Institute of Reproductive Medicine. Initial appointments were scheduled at 7, 20, and 30 days post partum and were used for clinical evaluation, reinforce-ment of breastfeeding instructions, and provision of information on contra-ceptive choices. All women received a general physical, pelvic, and breast examination, as well as a Pap smear and haemoglobin test at the completion of the first month post partum. Further follow-up visits took place at monthly intervals throughout the first year, although participants were encouraged to attend the clinic at any time if they felt it necessary. At each visit the mother was weighed and received a physical examination of the abdomen, pelvis, and breasts, while children were measured and weighed. All intercurrent diseases were recorded.

The subjects received instructions to breastfeed their infants on demand.

They were encouraged to give the baby no food, liquid or solid, and to use the breast as the only source of water and nutrients, except for vitamin drops. Milk supplements were indicated only when milk output was deemed inadequate in the light of insufficient infant weight gain (less than 20 g per day, unless the child continued to weigh more than expected for the age and length), mother's perception of child's satisfaction, her report of breastfeeding practices, the characteristics of the infant's stools, and a breast examination. Solid supplements consisting of non-dairy foods were routinely recommended after the sixth month post partum. All women received a monthly calendar to register the number of breastfeeding episodes each day and night, as well as all days of bleeding or spotting.

During follow-up the sample was divided into three different groups, determined partly by their choice of contraception. Group A consisted of 236 women who relied initially on lactational infertility but later adopted hormonal contraception. Data from these women may be used to study both the length of amenorrhoea and the risk of conception up to the date when they started contraception. Group B consisted of 440 women who selected an IUD, which was inserted at durations 30 to 60 days post partum. Data from these women may be used to study the length of amenorrhoea throughout the follow-up period and the risk of conception only up to the date of IUD insertion (which is so early as to be uninformative). Finally, Group C consisted of 50 women who remained amenorrhoeic and in full nursing at durations 60 to 90 days post partum and were then chosen to participate in a study of hormonal profiles, which involved taking blood samples fortnightly during the first three months following delivery and twice a week thereafter, up to the second menstruation post partum. Data from this group may be used to study the return of menses and ovulation.

This paper will deal only with data from Group C. Note how the selection criteria affect the type of phenomena that can be investigated using the various data-sets; in particular, Group C can only be used to study the length of amenorrhoea conditional on its exceeding at least 60 days. Fortunately, the risk of menstruation in full nursing women during the first 60 days post partum is sufficiently small that it can safely be neglected.

Methodology: Hazard Models

We assume that at each duration of amenorrhoea t a woman is subject to an instantaneous risk $\lambda(t)$ of experiencing the first post-partum menses. The function $\lambda(t)$ is called the hazard function and is analogous to the force of mortality. The hazard is closely related to the more familiar survival function $S(t)$ or probability of remaining in amenorrhoea at duration t: integrating the hazard from 0 to t gives the cumulative hazard $\Lambda(t)$, and changing signs and exponentiating gives the survival probability

$$S(t) = \exp[-\Lambda(t)],$$

a well-known result from life-table analysis. For estimation purposes we will partition duration of exposure into intervals, such that we may assume with some confidence that the risk of first menstruation is constant within each interval. Under this assumption the risk λ_i in the i-th interval may be estimated as the ratio of the number of events to total exposure time in the interval (see Holford, 1976).

So far we have assumed that women are homogeneous in the sense that they are all subject to the same risks λ_i. We now relax this assumption by letting the hazard depend on one or more covariates representing breastfeeding patterns and other characteristics of the women. Following Holford (1980), we will group duration into discrete intervals indexed by i, and we will assume that the covariates of interest permit classifying the women into subgroups or categories indexed by j, so that λ_{ij} represents the risk at duration i for women in the j-th category. Possible models of interest for the λ_{ij} are best expressed in terms of the logarithm of the risk and include the null model where the risk is constant over time for all women ($\log\lambda_{ij} = \alpha$); the duration model where the risk varies over time but is the same for all women ($\log\lambda_{ij} = \alpha_i$), a model where the risk is constant at all durations but its value depends on characteristics of the women ($\log\lambda_{ij} = \alpha + \beta_j$); and the proportional hazards model, developed by Cox (1972), where the risk may be factored into a component which depends on duration and another which depends on the characteristics of the women ($\log\lambda_{ij} = \alpha_i + \beta_j$). Further discussion of these models and their interpretation will follow below.

An important feature of these models, noted by Holford (1980) and Laird and Oliver (1981), is that they are equivalent to log-linear models for simple counts of events (first menstruations) classified by duration of exposure and categories of the covariates. Log-linear models, in turn, may be fitted to data using existing software packages such as GLIM (Baker and Nelder, 1978). Specifically, if m_{ij} and E_{ij} denote the number of first menstruations and total days of exposure in duration interval i for category j of the covariates, the equivalence involves treating the m_{ij} as Poisson random variables with means $\lambda_{ij}E_{ij}$, where λ_{ij} is the risk of menstruation in duration interval i for category j of the covariates and fitting log-linear models to the m_{ij} using the logarithm of exposure as an offset. The procedures may be applied to covariates which remain fixed for each individual over the follow-up period and to covariates that vary over time, such as breastfeeding status.

The Length of Post-Partum Amenorrhoea

We start our discussion of results with a description of the length of post-partum amenorrhoea for the total sample of nursing women. The variable of interest is the time from delivery to first menstruation, but some of the observations are censored because the women continued to be amenorrhoeic at the time of their last follow-up visit. To estimate the risk and survival using the procedure outlined above, we will use 30-day intervals. A woman who first menstruates or is last seen 45 days after delivery, for example, contributes 30 days of exposure to the first interval and 15 days to the second interval. If she menstruates at duration 45 days, she contributes one event to the second interval. The results of tabulating events and exposure for our sample appear in Table 25.1 (see columns 3 and 4). Note that 47 out of the 50 women in the sample experienced the return of menstruation during follow-up. Column 5 shows the estimated monthly risk of first menstruation, calculated as 30 times the ratio of events to days of exposure. Adding up the monthly risks, we obtain cumulative risks up to the end of each month, and, exponentiating minus the cumulative risk, we obtain the estimates of the survival probabilities up to the end of each month shown in column 6.[1]

The estimates of survival probabilities in Table 25.1 are practically identical to estimates based on the product-limit method of Kaplan and Meier (1959) applied to the same data (not shown), indicating that not much information is lost by grouping the data in single months. An advantage of the present approach is that we obtain estimates of the risks of first menstruation month by month. As may be appreciated from column 5 of Table 25.1, the risk is initially low[2] but rises over time to reach 0.67 by the end of the first post-partum year.

TABLE 25.1. *First menstrual events and women days of exposure for the total sample and estimated risk of first menses and survival in amenorrhoeic state*

Month i	Interval (days)	Menstrual events	Women days of exposure	Monthly risk of first menstruation	Survival
(1)	(2)	(3)	(4)	(5)	(6)
1	1–30	—	1500	—	1.0000
2	31–60	—	1500	—	1.0000
3	61–90	6	1442	.1248	.8826
4	91–120	5	1260	.1190	.7836
5	121–50	5	1050	.1429	.6793
6	151–80	5	919	.1632	.5770
7	181–210	6	738	.2439	.4521
8	211–40	3	614	.1466	.3905
9	241–70	5	442	.3394	.2781
10	271–300	6	295	.6102	.1511
11	301–30	3	173	.5202	.0898
12	331–60	2	89	.6742	.0458

[1] For example, the cumulative risk in the first 120 days is 0.1248 + 0.1190 = 0.2438, and the probability of surviving in amenorrhoea for 120 days is exp(−0.2438) = 0.7836 or 78.4 per cent.

[2] Recall that the design of the sample is such that the risk is forced to be zero in the first two months.

The latter figure means that we expect about two-thirds of the women who enter the twelfth post-partum month in amenorrhoea to experience their first menses that month. The monotonic nature of the increase suggests that we might have achieved greater parsimony of description modelling the logarithm of the risk as a linear function of duration.

Time-varying Covariates

Supplementation

We now consider the effect of breastfeeding on post-partum amenorrhoea, treating breastfeeding status as a time-varying covariate. Information available in the data-set includes the dates of milk supplementation, introduction of foods, and weaning, where applicable. In principle, it is possible to distinguish five different statuses: full breastfeeding, liquid supplementation only, solid supplementation only, both liquid and solid supplements, and weaned; and initially we tabulate events and exposure for all five categories. Calculations are tedious but relatively straightforward. All women start contributing days of exposure to the full breastfeeding category until they introduce supplements, wean the child, or reach the end of follow-up, whichever comes first. If exposure ends with the return of menstruation they also contribute an event to whichever category corresponds to their status at the time. Table 25.2 shows our basic tally of events and exposure. From now on we ignore the first two months, which have no events.

TABLE 25.2. *Tabulation of menstrual events and women days of exposure by duration post-partum and breastfeeding status*

Month	Breastfeeding status									
	Full		Solid supplements		Liquid supplements		Solid and liquid supplements		Weaned	
	m	E	m	E	m	E	m	E	m	E
3	6	1395			0	47				
4	3	1050			2	210				
5	2	789			3	218	0	38	0	5
6	1	584	0	6	1	158	2	150	1	21
7	0	122	2	343	0	20	4	249	0	4
8	0	19	2	237			1	238	0	30
9	0	16	2	215			2	209	1	2
10	0	5	3	137			3	153		
11	0	22	1	73			2	78		
12			1	28			1	61		

Note: m = first menses; E = woman days of exposure in the interval.

The first thing to note from the table is that practically all exposure in the first couple of months corresponds to full breastfeeding; liquid supplements occur early, solid supplements occur later, and there is practically no exposure following weaning. A preliminary fitting showed that duration effects varied rather slowly over time, a fact which led us to further group duration into 60-day categories in order to obtain slightly more precision in our estimates of the effects of breastfeeding. Table 25.3 shows goodness of fit chi-square statistics for the four possible models of interest.

TABLE 25.3. *Goodness of fit statistics for models involving breastfeeding status*

Model	Chi-square	d.f.
Null	32.28	18
Duration	18.74	14
Breastfeeding	11.88	14
Duration + breastfeeding	6.76	10

The null model assumes a constant risk over duration and across breastfeeding practices and is clearly inadequate. Allowing for an effect of duration improves the fit, as does introducing breastfeeding status as a time-varying covariate. The best fit is obtained when allowance is made for both duration and breastfeeding status in a proportional hazards framework. The chi-square of 6.76 on ten degrees of freedom indicates a good fit. Adding breastfeeding status to duration reduces chi-square by 11.98 (from 18.74 to 6.76) at the expense of four degrees of freedom; this result indicates a significant net effect of breastfeeding status even after allowance is made for duration effects. The estimates of the parameters for the proportional hazards model appear in Table 25.4.

The final model is of the form

$$\log \Lambda_{ij} = \mu + \alpha_i + \beta_j,$$

where the α_i are duration effects and the β_j are effects of breastfeeding status. We adopt the convention that $\alpha_1 = 0$ and $\beta_1 = 0$, so that the first category of each factor serves as a reference group. The estimate of -5.7 is thus the log risk at durations 3–4 months for women in full breastfeeding. The next four values down the table show how the baseline risk dips and then increases over time. The effects of breastfeeding status show that women in partial breastfeeding have a risk between three and five times[3] the risk of a woman in full breastfeeding at the same post-partum duration. Note that there is little difference according to whether supplementation is solid, liquid, or both. Finally, we note that women who have weaned their children have a risk of first menstruation 16

---

[3] Calculated as $\exp(1.186) = 3.274$ and $\exp(1.608) = 4.993$, respectively.

TABLE 25.4. *Parameter estimates for model with proportional effect of breastfeeding status*

Parameter	Estimate	Standard error
Constant duration		
(3–4)	−5.700	.3287
5–6	−.2897	.4959
7–8	−.8026	.7637
9–10	−.0150	.7755
11–12	.2710	.8349
Breastfeeding status		
(full)		
Solid	1.433	.7533
Liquid	1.186	.5112
Both	1.608	.6790
Weaned	2.791	.8622

times the risk of a woman in full breastfeeding. Although there is no question of the effect of breastfeeding status, the estimates just quoted should be taken with caution because they have rather large standard errors.

Frequency of Suckling

We now consider the number of breastfeeding episodes during the day and at night as two additional time-varying covariates. The information recorded for each follow-up visit is the 'average' frequency of breastfeeding in the period since the previous control. The controls are unequally spaced, with some only a week apart and others somewhat longer than a month apart. For the purposes of the present analysis, we took the 'average' number of episodes to represent the actual frequency at the midpoint of the reporting period. Linear interpolation was then used to estimate the frequency of suckling on any day during follow-up. The information is necessarily of an approximate nature, but is believed to be reasonably accurate.

Note that frequency of suckling during the day or at night is a covariate which can change values at any time, but accumulation of events and exposure proceeds along familiar lines: each woman contributes each day of post-partum exposure to whatever category corresponds to her frequency of breastfeeding that day or night, as determined by the interpolation procedure described earlier. Calculations are tedious but easily implemented by computer. Following preliminary examination of counts of events and exposure, we decided to group day and night frequency initially as follows:

day: 0, 1–3, 4, 5, 6, 7, 8, or more
night: 0, 1, 2, 3, 4, or more.

These categories were chosen to retain as much initial detail as was feasible, yet have at least three events in each category. In addition we retained a three-fold classification of breastfeeding status. The final table involving five categories of duration and all three covariates has 5 by 3 by 7 by 5 = 375 possible cells, but only 185 contained some exposure. Table 25.5 shows goodness of fit chi-square statistics for various models of interest.

TABLE 25.5. *Goodness of fit statistics for models with frequency of suckling during the day and night*

Model	Chi-square	d.f.
Null	128.4	184
Duration	114.9	180
Day	111.7	178
Night	125.7	180
Duration + day	101.3	174
Duration + night	111.4	176
Duration + day + night	98.4	170
Duration + day . night	81.6	148

We start with the null model postulating a constant risk, which has a chi-square of 128.4. Taking into account frequency of suckling during the day reduces chi-square by 16.7 at the expense of six degrees of freedom, a significant gain. Of course, high frequencies tend to be concentrated early in the post-partum period, when the risk is low anyway. A better assessment of the effect of frequency of suckling requires allowing for duration effects. If we start with the model involving duration only, which has a chi-square of 114.9, we note that adding duration reduces chi-square by 13.6 using six degrees of freedom, still a significant effect. Parameter estimates for this model are given in Table 25.6.

Two aspects of interest in this table are as follows. Firstly, the duration effects are clearly monotonic and show a substantial increase in risk for the last two categories. Secondly, the effects of frequency of suckling during the day fail to exceed their standard errors except for a frequency of eight or more times.

A similar analysis for frequency of breastfeeding at night shows no significant effect whatsoever. Starting from the null model, frequency at night reduces chi-square by 2.7 at the expense of four degrees of freedom. Starting from the model with duration effects, adding night-time frequency reduces chi-square by 3.5 again using four degrees of freedom. The lack of an effect is confirmed by the parameter estimates in Table 25.7, which fail to exceed their standard errors; although the effects are at least in the correct direction, with lower risk of menstruation at higher frequencies of suckling. Of course, lack of significance should not be taken too seriously in a very small sample, where power considerations imply that only very large effects can be detected.

TABLE 25.6. *Parameter estimates for model with
a proportional effect of frequency of
suckling during the day*

Parameter	Estimate	Standard error
Constant duration		
(3–4)	−4.960	.6655
5–6	.2114	.4385
7–8	.2344	.4622
9–10	1.109	.4432
11–12	1.529	.5677
Daytime frequency		
(0)		
1–3	−.8195	.8215
4	.4600	.6813
5	−.1681	.6694
6	−.2659	.6585
7	−.4484	.7081
8+	−1.449	.7375

TABLE 25.7. *Parameter estimates for model with
a proportional effect of frequency of
suckling during the night*

Parameter	Estimate	Standard error
Constant duration		
(3–4)	−5.417	.5057
5–6	.2121	.4365
7–8	.4906	.4548
9–10	1.341	.4337
11–12	1.597	.5423
Night-time frequency		
(0)		
1	.2667	.5275
2	−.0471	.4866
3	−.1365	.5189
4+	−.6965	.6080

The next model of interest in Table 25.5 involves proportional effects of frequency of suckling during the day and at night. The goodness of fit statistics indicate that daytime frequency has an effect net of night-time frequency, reducing chi-square by 13 points (from 111.4 to 98.4), but night-time frequency has no effect net of daytime frequency, with a chi-square reduction of only 2.9

(from 101.3 to 98.4). The last model listed in Table 25.5 allows for an inter-action effect of daytime and night-time frequency, but the reduction in chi-square does not match the expense in degrees of freedom.

In order to be able to have a better look at the joint effects of daytime and night-time frequency of suckling, we further grouped the data using only three categories for each variable. Daytime frequency was grouped into 0–4, 5–7, and 7+, while night-time frequency was collapsed into 0–1, 2, and 3+. Parameter estimates for the model with the combination of daytime and night-time frequencies are shown in Table 25.8.

It is highly suggestive that the only three negative estimates occur in a corner of the table, where daytime frequency is at least seven and night-time frequency is at least three, for a combined total of ten or more episodes in 24 hours. If we create a new variable to contrast this extreme category versus the rest, we obtain a chi-square of 108.5 with 179 degrees of freedom, which captures most of the effects of suckling during the day and at night. The parameter estimates appear in Table 25.9.

TABLE 25.8. *Parameter estimates for model with a proportional effect of the combination of daytime and night-time frequency of suckling*

Day	Night		
	0–1	2	3+
0–4	(base)	.1960	.6412
5–6	.4348	.6708	−.3378
7+	.1591	−.8367	−.4753

TABLE 25.9. *Parameter estimates for model with a combined frequency of suckling of at least seven daytime and three night-time episodes*

Parameter	Estimate	Standard error
Constant duration		
(3–4)	−4.973	.3531
5–6	.1906	.4361
7–8	.2872	.4563
9–10	1.097	.4337
11–12	1.399	.5424
Frequency		
(low)		
high	−.7689	.3045

Exponentiating the estimate for high frequency we note that the effect of a pattern of at least seven episodes during the day and three at night is to halve the risk of menstruation at any given duration.

Supplementation and Frequency of Suckling

Our final analysis treats both breastfeeding and frequency of suckling as time-varying covariates. The main question to be addressed is whether the effect of supplementation may be attributed to differences in suckling frequency between infants in full and partial breastfeeding. A first approximation to the answer is obtained by fitting a model with duration, a proportional effect of the combination of daytime and night-time frequencies (grouped into three categories each), and a separate effect of supplementation. The chi-square goodness of fit statistic for this model is 93.3 with 170 degrees of freedom, compared to 103 with 172 degrees of freedom for the model without the supplementation covariate. The difference of 9.7 on 2 degrees of freedom is highly significant, and the parameter estimates for the effect of supplementation are barely attenuated from the values noted above.

A second approach to the problem is to ascertain whether the effect of high frequency as defined above is observed both under full and partial breastfeeding. To investigate this question we fitted a model involving the effects of duration, breastfeeding status (full or partial), frequency of suckling (contrasting 7 plus 3 episodes versus the rest), and an interaction between breastfeeding status and frequency of suckling. The model has a goodness of fit chi-square of 101.1 with 177 degrees of freedom, and represents the most parsimonious fit so far. Parameter estimates are given in Table 25.10.

TABLE 25.10. *Parameter estimates for proportional hazards model with an interaction effect of supplementation and frequency of suckling*

Parameter	Estimate	Standard error
Constant duration		
(3–4)	−5.310	.5188
5–6	−.1934	.4658
7–8	−.6552	.5515
9–10	.1026	.5387
11–12	.4729	.6275
Breastfeeding status		
(full) partial	1.316	.6357
Frequency		
(low) high/full	−.5818	.6107
high/partial	−.6849	.3554

The final estimates show several points of interest: (1) the effects of duration are now fairly modest, indicating that we have captured most of the effect of duration in terms of breastfeeding patterns; (2) partial breastfeeding represents a substantial increase in risk relative to full breastfeeding, even adjusting for frequency of suckling; and (3) a high frequency of suckling reduces the risk both under full and partial breastfeeding, but while the magnitude of the effects appears similar, only the effect under partial breast-feeding is significant. This last result is suggestive of a compensation mechanism. Our interpretation of this finding is that supplementation is probably related to intensity of suckling and thus has an effect over and above frequency of suckling.

References

Baker, R. J., and Nelder, J. A. (1978), *General Linear Interactive Modelling (GLIM)*, release 3, Numerical Algorithms Group, Oxford, England.

Bongaarts, J., and Potter, R. (1983), *Fertility, Biology and Behavior: An Analysis of the Proximate Determinants*, Academic Press, New York.

Cox, D. R. (1972), 'Regression Models and Life Tables (with discussion)', *Journal of the Royal Statistical Society, Series B* 34: 187–202.

Diaz, S., Peralta, O., Juez, G., Salvatierra, A. M., Casado, M. E., Durán, E., and Croxatto, H. B. (1982), 'Fertility Regulation in Nursing Women, I: The Probability of Conception in Full Nursing Women Living in an Urban Setting', *Journal of Biosocial Science* 14: 329–41.

Habicht, J.-P., DaVanzo, J., Butz, W. P., and Meyers, L. (1985), 'The Contraceptive Effect of Breastfeeding', *Population Studies* 39: 213–32.

Holford, T. R. (1976), 'Life Tables with Concomitant Information', *Biometrics* 32: 587–98.

—— (1980), 'The Analysis of Rates and Survivorship Using Log-Linear Models', *Biometrics* 36: 299–306.

Howie, P. W., and McNeilly, A. S. (1982), 'Effect of Breast-Feeding Patterns on Human Birth Intervals', *Journal of Reproductive Fertility* 65: 545–57.

—— —— Houston, M. J., Cook, A., and Boyle, H. (1981), 'Effect of Supplementary Food on Suckling Patterns and Ovarian Activity during Lactation', *British Medical Journal* 283: 757–63.

—— —— —— —— —— (1982), 'Fertility after Childbirth: Post-Partum Ovulation and Menstruation in Bottle and Breast Feeding Mothers', *Clinical Endocrinology* 17: 323–32.

John, A. M., Menken, J. A., and Chowdhury, A. K. M. A. (1987), 'The Effects of Breastfeeding and Nutrition on Fecundability in Rural Bangladesh: A Hazards Model Analysis', *Population Studies* 41: 433–46.

Kaplan, E. L., and Meier, P. (1959), 'Non-Parametric Estimation from Incomplete Observations', *Journal of the American Statistical Association* 53: 457–81.

Laird, N., and Oliver, D. (1981), 'Covariance Analysis of Censored Survival Data using Log-linear Analysis Techniques', *Journal of the American Statistical Association* 76: 231–40.

McNeilly, A. S., Howie, P. W., Houston, M. J., Cook, A., and Boyle, H. (1982), 'Fertility After Childbirth: Adequacy of Post-Partum Luteal Phases', *Clinical Endocrinology* 17: 609–15.

Prema, K., and Ravindranath, M. (1982), 'The Effect of Breastfeeding Supplements on the Return of Fertility', *Studies in Family Planning* 13: 293–6.

Simpson-Hebert, M., and Huffman, S. L. (1981), 'The Contraceptive Effect of Breastfeeding', *Studies in Family Planning* 12: 125–32.

Smith, D. P. (1985), 'Breastfeeding, Contraception and Birth Intervals in Developing Countries', *Studies in Family Planning* 16: 154–63.

Trussell, J., Martin, L. G., Feldman, R., Palmore, J. A., Concepcion, M., and Abu Bakar, D. (1985), 'Determinants of Birth-Interval Length in the Philippines, Malaysia, and Indonesia: A Hazard-Model Analysis', *Demography* 22(2): 145–68.

Mantel, N. (1966), 'Evaluation of Survival Data and Two New Rank Order Statistics Arising in Consideration', *Cancer Chemotherapy Reports* 50: 163–70.

Van Ginneken, J. K. (1977), 'The Chance of Conception During Lactation', *Journal of Biosocial Science* supplement 44: 41–54.

26 The Return of Ovarian Function during Lactation: Results of Studies from the United States and the Philippines*

RONALD H. GRAY

OONA CAMPBELL

SUSAN ESLAMI

HOWARD ZACUR

MIRIAM LABBOK

RUBEN APELO

Introduction

Demographers and biomedical scientists have long been interested in the return of fecundity during lactation. For demographers, this interest largely focuses on the length of the post-partum infertile period, which is a major determinant of birth intervals. But because post-partum infertility cannot be directly measured in most demographic surveys, the duration of lactational amenorrhoea has generally been used as a proxy. There is, however, concern that amenorrhoea may not be a satisfactory proxy measure, both because pregnancy may occur in amenorrhoeic women and because there is evidence that fecundability is suppressed in breastfeeding women even after the resumption of menstruation. Moreover, numerous retrospective, cross-sectional, and prospective demographic studies of the duration of lactational amenorrhoea suggest serious data problems due to recall error, digit preference, and marked heaping of menstrual return around 6 and 12 months post partum. In addition, there are limitations to the measurement of lactational status, with often crude categorization of women into full or partial breastfeeding groups (Lesthage and Page, 1980; Hobcraft and Guz, 1985; Ford and Kim, 1987).

Biomedical scientists have focused on the endocrine mechanisms underlying lactational amenorrhoea and on the behavioural or nutritional factors that modulate the endocrine milieu. It has been clearly shown that the suckling

* This paper is based on collaborative studies involving the Johns Hopkins University, Baltimore, and the Fabella Memorial Hospital in Manila. The studies were supported by grants from NICHD (R01-HD-16879-01), The Population Council (CP83-58A), and the Institute for International Studies in Natural Family Planning at Georgetown University (U/BR-US-002).

stimulus, mediated through neuronal pathways, causes the release of prolactin from the pituitary gland and directly or indirectly suppresses the release of the gonadotrophin hormones, FSH and LH, which are required for the initiation of ovarian activity and for ovulation. There is also evidence that poor maternal nutritional status may reinforce the suppressive effects of suckling (McNeilly *et al.*, 1982; Glasier *et al.*, 1983; Gross and Eastman, 1985).

A number of epidemiological studies have attempted to evaluate the relationship between breastfeeding patterns and ovarian function, but these have been constrained by difficulties in measuring feeding behaviour, detecting ovarian activity and ovulation, and assessing the adequacy of the luteal phase in ovulatory cycles. Investigators have used basal body temperature (BBT), repeat endometrial biopsy, weekly measurements of hormonal metabolites in 24-hour urine samples, or single measurements of hormones in blood and saliva (see Table 26.7 for references). Information on breastfeeding intensity and the introduction of supplementary foods has been obtained from maternal interviews, observational studies, and feeding diaries completed by the mother. It is inherently difficult to measure both the breastfeeding stimulus and the endocrine response in sufficiently large populations over the long periods of time required to quantify the relationships between these factors clearly and to determine the change in stimulus/response that may occur with the passage of time post partum. Furthermore, because of the variation in intensity and duration of breastfeeding between populations, it has been difficult to generalize results.

The present study was designed to assess predictors of ovulation in breastfeeding women, because this is of programmatic importance to policies on contraceptive introduction during lactation. However, we also wished to advance our understanding of the relationship between breastfeeding and the return of ovarian activity by using more refined research measures applied in an identical manner to populations with widely divergent patterns of feeding, socio-economic conditions, and maternal nutritional status. Therefore, the following investigations were conducted with lactating women in Manila, the Philippines, and in Baltimore, USA.

Research Methods and Study Populations

The study subjects were breastfeeding women who delivered normal singleton infants at the Dr Jose Fabella Memorial Hospital in Manila (N = 40) and the St Agnes or Sinai Hospitals in Baltimore (N = 60). In addition, we conducted preliminary studies to establish the research methodology in 16 non-post-partum women with regular cycles and 22 non-breastfeeding post-partum women in Baltimore.

Women recorded the number and timing of breast feeds or other forms of infant feeding on a daily diary sheet. They were interviewed at weekly intervals to determine whether they experienced menses, used contraception, or had an illness, and questions were asked about the average duration of suckling episodes. The analysis of feeding patterns is complex because the numerous potential measures are highly correlated. The most useful measures were the number of feeding episodes, the intervals between breastfeeding episodes, the length of suckling episodes, and the total duration of suckling (episode length × number of episodes), the introduction of supplementary feeds, and the percentage of all feeds contributed by breast milk. These measures were tabulated for weekly intervals of time post partum. In addition, the diurnal patterns of breastfeeding were examined.

Ovarian activity was determined by assay of two ovarian steroid hormone metabolites, pregnanediol-3-α-glucuronide (PdG) and oestradiol-17β-glucuronide (E2G), and of pituitary LH using early morning urine samples collected daily. The assay procedures have been described previously (Gray *et al.*, 1987), and all assays were performed at the Reproductive Endocrinology Laboratory at the Johns Hopkins University. Other investigators and our own preliminary studies have shown that urinary concentrations of these hormones are highly correlated with serum levels, that the early morning urine samples adequately reflect 24-hour urinary metabolite excretion, and that the hormone concentrations in frozen urine samples are stable over time. Cost and logistic constraints precluded assay of all samples, so one sample in three was screened to detect a rise in PdG indicative of ovulation. If evidence of ovulation was detected on these screening assays or if a woman reported menses, all samples for the estimated duration of the cycle were assayed for E2G and PdG, and then mid-cycle samples were assayed to determine the timing of the LH surge. Ovulation was detected by a mid-cycle LH peak, a significant rise in PdG, and a reversal of the E2G:PdG ratio. We also examined the timing of ovulation in relation to the timing of menstruation to determine the frequency of anovular cycles (i.e. cycles in which menses was not preceded by ovulation). The luteal phase was evaluated both for length (from estimated time of ovulation to onset of menses) and for the level of progesterone production (as reflected in the quantity of PdG excreted in the urine). Abnormally short luteal phases were defined as 8 days or less in duration, and deficiencies in PdG excretion were defined by two measures: the mean peak level of urinary PdG and the area under the luteal phase PdG curve. We conducted preliminary studies in women with regular cycles and non-breastfeeding post-partum women to assess the adequacy of the luteal phase using urinary hormones. In our laboratory a mean peak of PdG production less than 4 ng/ml and an area under the luteal phase curve less than 20 ng/ml were found to differentiate clearly between normal and deficient luteal phases, with very few equivocal cycles (Campbell, 1987; Gray *et al.*, 1987). Fig. 26.1 shows the daily luteal phase PdG levels for normal and abnormal cycles, and it is clear that there are two distinct and significantly different distributions.

The study protocol required that women withdraw after experiencing two normal ovulations, and the duration of observation was determined by the

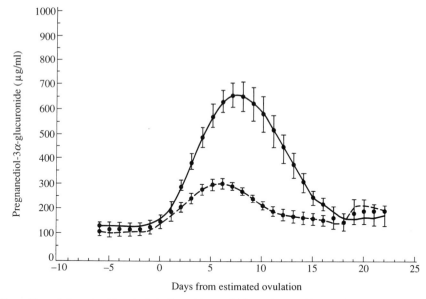

Normal luteal phase for 17 cycles is indicated by a solid line; abnormal luteal phase for 10 cycles is indicated by a dashed line. The mean is ±S.E.; measurements are from first morning urine samples.

Fig. 26.1   Mean daily luteal phase urinary Pd-G excretion comparing cycles with normal and abnormal luteal phases

timing of these events. However, some women withdrew without experiencing ovulation and/or menses. Thus the length of observation is truncated in some cases and varies between individuals.

The patterns of breastfeeding in relation to the onset of menses and return of ovarian activity were examined by univariate statistics to determine which feeding patterns were associated with the onset of ovarian activity, and from this preliminary analysis we selected the independent variables for inclusion in multivariate models. Logistic regression was used when the study population could be dichotomized (e.g. into women experiencing early or late ovulation), and proportional hazards models were used to determine the effects of time-varying covariates, such as breastfeeding or menses, on the probability of ovulation (Miller, 1981). Because the breastfeeding measures (e.g. frequency and interval) are highly correlated, a step-up procedure was employed to determine which measures of breastfeeding or supplementation had the strongest associations with the dependent variables. The final models incorporated those variables which were consistently significant and provided the best statistical fit.

Results

Table 26.1 shows the socio-demographic characteristics and prior reproductive history of the women, as well as the birth-weights of their infants. Compared to

TABLE 26.1. *Characteristics of the study populations in Baltimore and Manila*

	Baltimore (n = 60)	Manila (n = 40)
Mean age	28.4	24.2
Mean parity	1.8	3.0
Mean birth-weight of infant (g)	3557	2920
Married (%)	97	100
Years of Education (%)		
0–12	22	97.5
12+	78	2.5
Occupation (%)		
housewife	52	100
non-professional	21	0
professional	27	0
Sex of Infant		
female	55	40
male	45	60

women in Manila, the women in Baltimore were older, more educated, more frequently employed, and had fewer children. The US-born infants had substantially higher birth-weights than the infants in Manila, despite the predominance of male births in the latter population. Maternal post-partum body weight was not available for the majority of Baltimore women, although the mean weight for those mothers with measurements was 65 kg. The average maternal post-partum body weight was 50.1 kg in Manila with a range from 36 to 75 kg. During the course of the study, over 90 per cent of women experienced either ovulation or menstruation. There were 55 women in Baltimore and 36 women in Manila who experienced either or both of these events (Table 26.2).

The mean frequencies of breast and supplementary feeding per week for the two study populations are shown in Figs. 26.2 and 26.3. It must be noted that these graphs represent changing cohorts over time, because the duration of observation varied between individual subjects and women who experienced early events discontinued from the study. Nevertheless, it is clear that the women in Manila breastfed more frequently than the women in Baltimore. For example, at 10 weeks post partum the women in Manila had an average of 11.4 breast feeds per day, compared to 7.1 in Baltimore, and these differentials persisted throughout most of the first year of observation. Also, the

TABLE 26.2. *Number of women experiencing events during the study*

	Baltimore		Manila	
	N	%	N	%
Total number of women in the study	60		40	
Women experiencing any event	55	91.7	36	90.0
Censored information	5	8.3	4	10.0
Women who ovulated	49	81.7	32	80.0
Women who menstruated	55	91.7	33	82.5
Women who ovulated and menstruated	49	81.7	29	72.5

women in Baltimore tended to decrease suckling frequency as they introduced supplemental foods (i.e. they substituted supplemental foods for breast milk), and this substitution effect was most pronounced with bottle feeds. Figs. 26.4 and 26.5 show that the frequency of suckling episodes declined as the number of bottle feeds increased, whereas no clear relationship was observed between breastfeeding and the introduction of foods given by cup or spoon.

The mean durations of amenorrhoea were 26.3 and 31.7 weeks and the mean delays prior to first ovulation were 27 and 38 weeks in Baltimore and Manila, respectively. Almost half the women in Baltimore had ovulated by 6 months post partum, whereas in Manila only 31 per cent had ovulated by this time. To determine whether menses was predictive of ovulation, we examined the relative timing of first ovulation and first menstruation (Table 26.3). Ovulation prior to first menstruation was more frequently observed among women in Baltimore, particularly during the first 6 months post partum, when 58.6 per cent of Baltimore women had an ovulatory first menses as compared to 38.9 per cent of women from Manila. It is clear from Table 26.3 that menses is a poor predictor of incipient ovulation, because in the majority of cases the first menses is preceded by ovulation. Also, among those women who menstruated prior to ovulation, the mean delay between first anovular menses and first subsequent ovulation was 80.5 days in the Baltimore women and around 84 days in Manila women. Thus, demographic studies that use the duration of amenorrhoea as a proxy for post-partum infecundity may underestimate the duration of lactational infertility. The prolonged interval between an initial anovulatory menses and first ovulation might, in part, explain the reduced fecundability after first menstruation reported in some demographic studies (Jain and Bongaarts, 1979; Hobcraft and Guz, 1985).

In Manila there was a bimodal distribution of the return to ovulation (Fig. 26.6), with one cluster of 11 women who experienced ovulation 'early' (at a

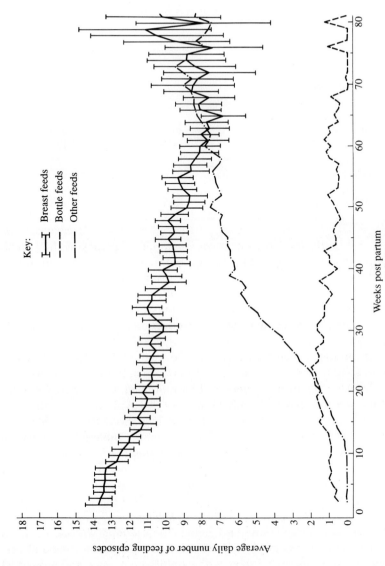

Key:

⊢—I   Breast feeds
– – –   Bottle feeds
—·—   Other feeds

Fig. 26.2   Average daily breast, bottle, and other feeding episodes by week post partum, Manila

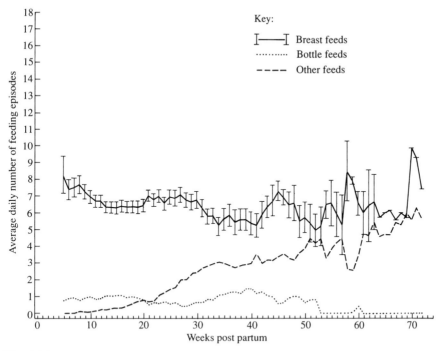

Fig. 26.3   Average daily breast, bottle, and other feeding episodes by week post partum, Baltimore

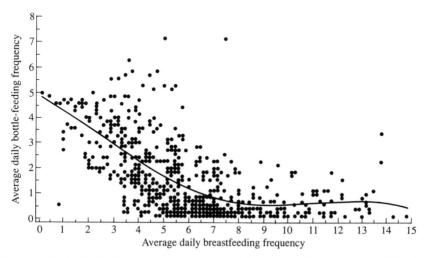

Average daily bottle-feeding frequency by average daily breastfeeding frequency: cubic spine fitting.

Fig. 26.4   Relationship between breastfeeding frequency and the use of bottle feeds in Baltimore women

TABLE 26.3. *Number and percentage of women who ovulated prior to first menses,*
by time post partum

Weeks post partum	Baltimore			Manila		
	Ovulation prior to first menstruation		Number menstruating in each interval	Ovulation prior to first menstruation		Number menstruating in each interval
	N	%		N	%	
0–24	17	58.6	29	7	38.9	18
25–52	15	75.0	20	9	64.3	14
>52	6	100.0	6	3	75.0	4
	38	69.1	55	19	52.8	36

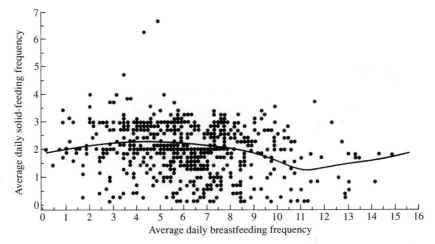

Average daily solid-feeding frequency by average daily breastfeeding frequency: cubic spine
fitting.

Fig. 26.5   Relationship between breastfeeding frequency and the use of solid feeds in
Baltimore women

median time of 15 weeks post partum) and a second cluster of 21 women who
experienced 'late' ovulation (at a median time of 48 weeks post partum). A
similar, though less pronounced, bimodal pattern was observed in the timing of
first menstruation. However, no bimodality in the timing of ovulation or
menstruation was apparent in the Baltimore population (Fig. 26.7). These
results are analogous to those reported by some demographic studies of the
duration of amenorrhoea, in which both bimodal and diffuse distributions have
been observed in different populations (Ford and Kim, 1987).

Table 26.4 shows the endocrine characteristics of the first menstrual episodes,

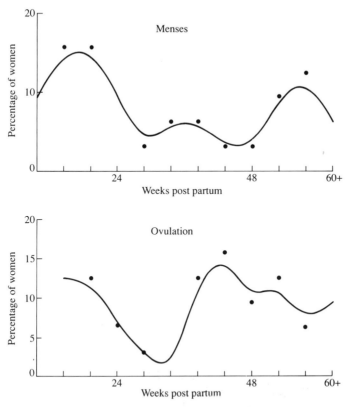

Fig. 26.6 Timing of first menses and ovulation in Manila women

TABLE 26.4. *Characteristics of the first menstrual episode*

	Baltimore		Manila	
	N	%	N	%
All cycles	55	100.0	36	100.0
Anovulatory cycles	17	30.9	17	47.2
Ovulatory cycles	38	69.1	19	52.8
Cycles in which luteal phase could be assessed	36	100.0	14	100.0
Normal luteal phase	19	52.8	9	64.3
Abnormal luteal phase	17	47.2	4	28.6
Equivocal luteal phase	0	0	1	7.1

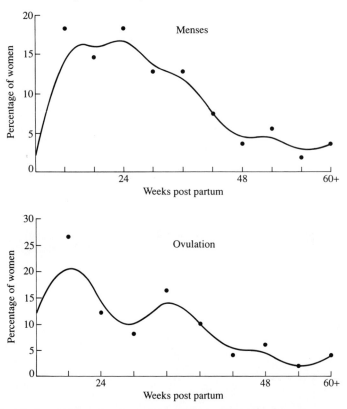

Fig. 26.7   Timing of first menses and ovulation in Baltimore women

irrespective of time post partum. The frequency of anovular first menses was higher in Manila (47.2 per cent) than in Baltimore (30.9 per cent). During the second menstrual episode the proportion of anovulatory cycles declined to 35.7 per cent in Manila and 15 per cent in Baltimore. Among those first ovulatory cycles in which the luteal phase could be assessed, there were slightly more abnormal luteal phases in the Baltimore subjects (47.2 per cent) than in Manila subjects (28.6 per cent). The predominant type of luteal phase defect was a deficiency in PdG excretion, rather than a reduction of luteal phase length. Deficient PdG excretion with luteal phases of normal length was observed in 70.6 per cent of abnormal first cycle luteal phases in Baltimore; in Manila the proportion was 60 per cent. With regimens employing less frequent sampling and assays, these luteal phase defects might not be detected and could be misinterpreted as anovulatory cycles.

Detailed feeding and endocrine results cannot be presented due to limitations of space. However, examples of individual results for two women from Manila are given in Figs. 26.8 and 26.9. Subject *A*, who was observed for 35 weeks, showed a declining frequency of breastfeeding and early introduction of bottle

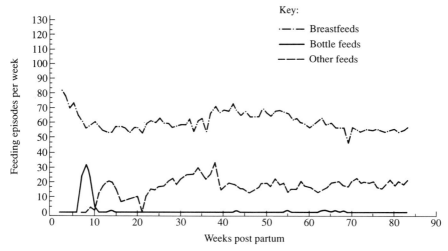

Feeding episodes by weeks post partum

Set Bottom Panel: Daily pregnanediol and oestradiol levels

Fig. 26.8   Feeding frequency and resumption of ovulation for subject *A*, who gave early supplementary feeds

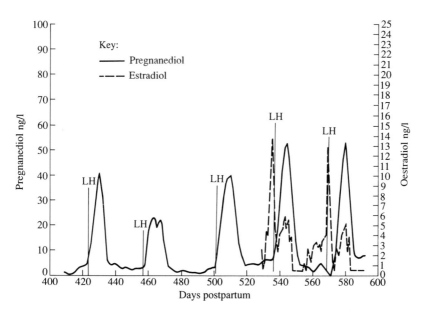

Feeding episodes by weeks post partum

Set Bottom Panel: Daily pregnanediol and oestradiol levels

Fig. 26.9   Feeding frequency and resumption of ovulation for subject *B*, who maintained a high frequency of breastfeeding with only modest supplementation

and other supplementary feeds (Fig. 26.8). She had an anovulatory menses on day 130 and ovulated around 148 days post partum, with a normal luteal phase. In contrast, subject *B* was observed for around 85 weeks. She maintained a high frequency of breastfeeding with modest supplementation and first ovulated at 422 days post partum (Fig. 26.9).

Univariate survival analyses showed that many of the measures of breastfeeding such as the number of episodes, the interval between episodes, the proportion of all feeds contributed by breast feeds, and the duration of suckling were associated with the resumption of ovulation or menstruation. Since these are all highly correlated, multivariate analyses were used to determine which measures provided the strongest association between breastfeeding patterns and resumption of ovarian activity. In the Baltimore data-set, the proportional hazards analysis showed that the frequency of breast feeds and the average duration of suckling episodes during the two weeks preceding ovulation were the best and most parsimonious predictors of ovulation return (Table 26.5). These variables remained significant in all models, whereas other measures either dropped out or were not consistent in their effects. In Manila the strongest predictor was the percentage of all feeds contributed by breast feeds (PctBF) during the weeks before ovulation (Table 26.6). This variable was statistically significant in all models, whereas no other feeding parameters were significant in models which incorporated the PctBF variable. Tables 26.5 and 26.6 present these results as relative risks of ovulation at specified levels of

TABLE 26.5. *Relative risk of ovulation in relation to breastfeeding frequency, Baltimore*

Average number of feeds per day	Relative risk
0	1.0
1	0.62
2	0.43
3	0.28
4	0.19
5	0.12
6	0.08
7	0.05
8	0.04
9	0.02
10	0.01

Model:

Breast feeds per day prior to ovulation	$B_1 = -0.4207$ $p < 0.0001$	
Average duration of suckling episodes per day	$B_2 = -0.6566$ $p = 0.0071$	$\xi^2 = 36.05$ 2 d.f.

TABLE 26.6. *Relative risk of ovulation in relation to the percentage of all feeds contributed by breast feeds, Manila*

Percentage of all feeds provided by breast feeds	Relative risk
0	1.0
10	0.80
20	0.64
30	0.50
40	0.40
50	0.32
60	0.26
70	0.21
80	0.17
90	0.14
100	0.11

Model:
Percentage of all feeds that are breast feeds for weeks prior to ovulation (x_i) $B = -0.02197$ $MLL = -171$
   $p < 0.05$

feeding frequency for the Baltimore population and at specified proportions of breast feeds to total feeds for the Manila women. The risk of ovulation in the absence of breastfeeding is set at 1.

In the Baltimore women, the relative risk of ovulation decreased markedly with increasing frequency of breastfeeding, and the risk was negligible with ten or more feeds per day. In Manila, the risk of ovulation declined as the proportion of breast to total feeds increased, but even with full breastfeeding the risk of ovulation was not negligible.

Because there was a bimodal distribution of the resumption of ovulation among the women in Manila, we also performed a logistic analysis with the dependent variable defined as membership in the 'early' ovulation cluster (first ovulation before 26 weeks post partum) or the 'late' ovulation cluster (first ovulation after 36 weeks post partum). The percentage of all feeds contributed by breast feeds was again the strongest and most consistent variable associated with early ovulation along with the average duration of suckling episodes.

Discussion

It is difficult to compare the results of the present study with those of previous investigators, because of differences in the levels and patterns of infant feeding and in the methods used to detect ovulation or to assess the adequacy of the luteal phase. It must be noted that no previous study has examined the return of ovarian activity in two populations with such divergent feeding behaviours, using daily measures of both feeding frequencies and endocrine status. Table 26.7 attempts to summarize the main findings with regard to anovulatory first menses and the proportion of abnormal luteal phases among ovulatory first cycles. The frequencies of anovulatory cycles observed in the present studies are within the range reported by other researchers. However, the proportion of ovulatory cycles with luteal phase abnormalities is higher in the current investigations, and we believe this is because daily hormonal assays provide more sensitive measures of luteal phase adequacy.

TABLE 26.7. *Percentage of anovulatory cycles in first menstrual episodes and percentage of ovulatory cycles which are normal among breastfeeders in 12 studies*

Study	N	Anovulatory cycles (%)	Normal ovulations (%)
Rolland et al., 1975[a]	7	0.0	28.6
Gross and Eastman, 1985[b]	34	10.0	33.0
Perez et al., 1971[c]	200	22.0	—
Parrenteau-Carreau, 1984[d]	54	35.0	—
Brown et al., 1985[b]	32	40.0	15.8
McNeilly et al., 1982[b]	27	42.0	46.4
Elsner[e]			
(cited in Perez, 1971)	60	42.0	—
Pascal, 1969[f]	509	43.0	49.0
Glasier et al., 1983[b]	24	45.0	32.0
Rivera et al., 1985[b]	20	50.0	—
Current Baltimore study[g]	60	30.9	52.8
Current Manila study[g]	40	47.2	64.3

Method of detecting ovulation:
 [a] Biopsy and weekly RIA
 [b] Weekly RIA, 24-hour urines
 [c] Biopsy and BBT
 [d] BBT and cervical mucus
 [e] Biopsy
 [f] BBT
 [g] Daily RIA, early morning urines

The proportional hazards analyses indicated that the frequency of breast-feeding was the variable most strongly and consistently associated with return of ovulation among the Baltimore sample, but the percentage of all feeds contributed by breast feeds was the dominant variable in the Manila data (Tables 26.5 and 26.6). The differences in the predictors of ovulation for these two populations are probably attributable to several factors related to the nature of the proportional hazards model, variation in feeding practices, and changing relationships between feeding patterns and ovarian activity over time.

1. The proportional hazards model essentially compares a covariate (e.g. feeding frequency) in a woman who experiences an event to the level of that covariate in all other women who have not experienced the event up to that point in time. Thus, the level and degree of heterogeneity of the covariate in the population will influence the strength of the association as measured by the beta-coefficients. If the level and distribution of the covariates differ between populations, it is to be expected that the betas will differ from one population to the next. Also, the beta-coefficient of a proportional hazards model provides a single summary estimate of the association between a covariate and the dependent variable over the whole duration of observation, and a single beta cannot indicate a changing relationship over time.

2. Compared to the women in Manila, the women in Baltimore breastfed less often (Figs. 26.2 and 26.3). We believe that the frequency of suckling episodes was most strongly associated with ovulation in the Baltimore population because even modest declines in the initially low frequency of breastfeeding were sufficient to initiate the return of ovarian activity. Also, since most Baltimore women used some supplemental foods, measures of supplementation such as the percentage of all feeds contributed by breast milk were only weakly associated with the return of ovulation. Many women in Manila practised prolonged, exclusive breastfeeding, and they often maintained a high frequency of suckling even when they introduced other foods. Thus, the frequency of breastfeeding episodes provided less discrimination in this population, but supplementation (as measured by the PctBF variable) affected the risk of ovulation, probably through a modest reduction in suckling frequency and a shorter duration of suckling episodes.

3. The relationship between suckling frequency and the resumption of ovarian activity may well vary over time post partum (Gross and Eastman, 1985). Women who ovulated prior to 6 months post partum frequently exhibited substantial declines in breastfeeding, whereas after more prolonged periods of lactation, relatively minor alterations in breastfeeding patterns appeared to evoke ovulation (Figs. 26.8 and 26.9). In this regard, it is noteworthy that there were similarities in the breastfeeding patterns of the Baltimore and Manila women who ovulated during the first 6 months after delivery. However, 49 per cent of the Baltimore women as compared to 31 per cent of the Manila women ovulated before 6 months post partum, so the results of the proportional hazards analysis for the Baltimore subjects were more heavily weighted by these early events.

Previous studies have suggested that relatively simple measures of breastfeeding level can be used to predict when a woman is at risk of ovulation. For example, it has been proposed that the number of daily feeds—6.1 in Edinburgh (McNeilly *et al.*, 1982), 8 in Boston (Elias *et al.*, 1986), and 10 in rural Mexico (Rivera *et al.*, 1985)—provides adequate warning of incipient ovulation.

However, these estimates are not based on rigorous statistical analyses, and the success of the proposed cut-off levels is determined by applying them to the population from which they are derived. The latter is something of a tautology, and since the cut-off levels have not been tested in other populations, there is no evidence of external validity. The results of the present study suggest that the situation is more complex and that it may not be possible to devise simple algorithms to predict ovulation in individual women, particularly in populations with disparate feeding practices.

We intend to merge these two data-sets together with additional data from 22 non-lactating post-partum women to provide information on the resumption of ovarian activity in 122 women with widely divergent levels and patterns of infant feeding. This enlarged data-set may provide more insight into the relationship between breastfeeding and the return of ovulation, particularly with regard to factors associated with early ovulation during the first 6 months after delivery. If it were possible to identify the characteristics of women at high risk of early ovulation, we could devise more rational guidelines for the timely introduction of contraception after childbirth. Such an approach to high risk group identification may be more appropriate than attempts to predict individual risks.

References

Brown, J. B., Harrisson, P., and Smith, M. A. (1985), 'A Study of Returning Fertility after Childbirth and during Lactation by Measurement of Urinary Oestrogen and Pregnanediol Excretion and Cervical Mucus Production', *Journal of Biosocial Science* supplement 9: 5–23.

Campbell, O. M. R. (1987), 'A Prospective Study of Breastfeeding Patterns and the Resumption of Ovarian Activity Postpartum', Ph.D. dissertation, Johns Hopkins University, School of Hygiene and Public Health, Baltimore, Md.

Elias, M. F., Teas, J., Johnston, J., and Bora, C. (1986), 'Nursing Practices and Lactational Amenorrhea', *Journal of Biosocial Science* 18: 1–10.

Ford, K., and Kim, Y. (1987), 'Distributions of Postpartum Amenorrhea: Some New Evidence', *Demography* 24(3): 413–30.

Glasier, A., McNeilly, A. S., and Howie, P. W. (1983), 'Fertility after Childbirth: Changes in Serum Gonadotrophin Levels in Bottle and Breast Feeding Women', *Clinical Endocrinology* 19: 493–501.

Gray, R. H., Campbell, O. M., Zacur, H. L., Labbok, M. H., and MacRae, S. L. (1987), 'Postpartum Return of Ovarian Activity in Non-Breastfeeding Women Monitored by Urinary Assays', *Journal of Clinical Endocrinology* 64(4): 645–50.

Gross, B. A., and Eastman, C. J. (1985), 'Prolactin and the Return of Ovulation in Breast-feeding Women', *Journal of Biosocial Science* supplement 9: 25–42.

Hobcraft, J., and Guz, D. (1985), 'Lactation and Fertility: A Comparative Analysis', paper presented at the Population Association of America Annual Meeting, Boston.

Jain, A. K., and Bongaarts, J. (1979), 'Breastfeeding: Patterns, Correlates and Fertility Effects', *Studies in Family Planning* 12(3): 79–99.

Lesthage, R., and Page, H. J. (1980), 'The Postpartum Nonsusceptible Period: Development and Application of Model Schedules', *Population Studies* 34: 143–70.

McNeilly, A. S., Howie, P. W., Houston, M. J., Cook, A., and Boyle, H. (1982), 'Fertility after Childbirth: Adequacy of Post-Partum Luteal Phases', *Clinical Endocrinology* 17: 609–15.

Miller, R. G. (1981), *Survival Analysis*, Wiley, New York.

Parenteau-Carreau, S. (1984), 'The Return of Fertility in Breastfeeding Women', *International Review of Natural Family Planning* 8: 34–43.

Pascal, J. (1969), 'Analyse d'une thèse pour le doctorat en medecine', Université de Nancy, France; data cited in H. Leridon (1972), 'Nouvelles donnés biometriques sur la postpartum', *Population* 27(1): 117–20.

Perez, A., Vela, P., Potter, R., and Masnick, G. S. (1971), 'Timing and Sequence of Resuming Ovulation and Menstruation after Childbirth', *Population Studies* 25(3): 491–503.

Rivera, R., Ortiz, E., and Barrera, M. (1985), 'Preliminary Observations on the Return of Ovarian Function among Breastfeeding and Postpartum Non-breast-feeding Women in a Rural Area of Mexico', *Journal of Biosocial Science* supplement 9: 127–36.

Rolland, R., Lequin, R. M., Schellekens, L. A., and DeJong, F. H. (1975), 'The Role of Prolactin in the Restoration of Ovarian Function during the Early Postpartum Period in the Human Female: A Study during Physiological Lactation', *Clinical Endocrinology* 4: 15–25.

27 Post-Partum Sexual Abstinence in Tropical Africa

ETIENNE VAN DE WALLE

FRANCINE VAN DE WALLE

> I order all women who are breastfeeding babies to abstain completely from sex relations. For menstruation is provoked by intercourse, and the milk no longer remains sweet. Moreover some women become pregnant, than which nothing could be worse for the suckling infant. For in this case the best of the blood goes to the fetus.
>
> (Galen AD 131–200)

Post-partum taboos on sexual intercourse have been encountered in many countries throughout history. They were once advocated by medical authorities in Europe. The Greek and Roman doctors of antiquity were opposed to sexual relations during nursing, and their opinions were quoted until the nineteenth century. Galen (1951 edn.: 29) thought that the milk of the nursing mother would be spoiled because of the admixture of sperm in the mother's blood. Soranos and Hippocrates believed that coitus and passionate behaviour provided the stimulus that reactivated menstruation. Prior to the eighteenth century, there was no medical knowledge of the biological effect of breastfeeding on amenorrhoea. Sexual abstinence, not the action of breastfeeding, was thought to delay the return of the menses. This interpretation was still widely held in Europe in the eighteenth century (see, for example, Roussel, 1813, a medical textbook with multiple editions).

The existence of sexual taboos linked to breastfeeding are quoted in contemporary lay writings in Europe up to the late nineteenth century. In his novel *Fecondité*, Émile Zola (1903) associates the prolonged lactation taboo with normal and happy conjugal behaviour. It is, of course, impossible to verify whether the average nineteenth-century woman abided by the rules, but the literature is explicit on the subject. In France, it appears that the upper classes attempted to impose sexual continence on the wet nurses whom they employed to raise their children (van de Walle and van de Walle, 1972).

Today, sexual abstinence is best known in the context of the sub-Saharan African countries, where it is widespread. It is also common, however, in traditional societies elsewhere. In contemporary Java, for example, sexual relations are proscribed during the entire period of breastfeeding. People believe that the man's semen spoils the quality of the mother's milk, a belief the Javanese share with many peoples of tropical Africa (Bracher and Santow, 1982). M. Singarimbun and C. Manning (1976) found a post-partum abstinence of 23.4 months in the village of Mojolama in central Java. Varying lengths of post-partum abstinence have been reported in other Asian countries. The World Fertility Survey found an average period of abstinence of 8 months in Haiti (United Nations, 1985). This paper will, however, deal only with sub-Saharan Africa.

Birth Spacing in Sub-Saharan Africa

The first fact about Africa south of the Sahara is that there are usually strong public and private norms about birth spacing as a type of behaviour necessary for the health of the mother and the child. The following statement, by the head of the Federal Military Government of Nigeria, is representative of several made by African leaders in preparation for the 1984 World Population Conference in Mexico City:

[A population] policy should have as a main focus, guidance in fertility behaviour which will emphasize the health of both mother and child. This policy calls for the reorientation of mothers as to the benefits of adequate birth spacing, a practice which has long been embedded in the African tradition but which is being eroded by the influence of modernization (UNFPA, 1985: 120).

Maybe more than anywhere else, individual women in Africa have a clear notion of an ideal spacing between births. Survey questions on family size often leave African respondents puzzled, and many will answer that the number of children is 'up to God'. In contrast, a question on the optimum interval between births usually elicits a precise answer. The length of the ideal spacing may be stated to be from 2 to 5 years, depending on age, parity, local customs, and sometimes personal preferences. At any rate, public opinion universally approves of a reasonable interval between births.

Traditionally, spacing is seen as the most rational means to ensure the well-being of both the mother and the baby. People are convinced that a new pregnancy may have serious deleterious effects on the health of the suckling child. Spacing births is so inherent in African culture that there exists in most languages a name for the woman who becomes pregnant while still nursing. These names imply disapproval, mockery, and other negative connotations, such as bad luck in Senegal (Ferry, 1981). Similarly, in many sub-Saharan cultures, there is a name for the disease of the suckling child whose mother has sexual relations or is pregnant. For example, among the Havu of eastern Zaïre, the child removed too soon from the breast because his mother is pregnant will suffer from *bwaki*; among the Ganda, the baby will get *obwosi*; and among the Dioula and the Bambara of the Sahel, the child will have *sere*. Among the Ikale of Nigeria, the baby will suffer from a condition called *apa* (Adeokun, 1981).

Among the Ewondo of Cameroon, the child whose mother has sexual relations during breastfeeding will suffer from *agnos*. In short, spacing is the norm, and the woman who does not succeed is viewed negatively by the community. The medical term 'kwashiorkor' came originally from a Ghanaian language, in which the word refers to the disease of the child who has been weaned too soon and does not receive adequate food. Diseases such as kwashiorkor and marasmus, caused by protein or calorie deficiency, are often attributed in traditional lore to the quality of the mother's milk, which has been 'poisoned' by male sperm. Similarly, infant diarrhoea, which is especially frequent when mothers give supplementary food or when they wean a child, is often attributed by the community to the resumption of intercourse.

Post-Partum Sexual Abstinence

Until recently, demographers agreed that most couples were not efficient birth spacers. This generalization was based on fertility surveys in the Western world. Do we have to revise this view in the light of information on voluntary spacing behaviour in Africa? In order to do so, this spacing would have to be in excess of what is the normal result of breastfeeding.

The fact that African populations have traditional intercourse taboos has been well documented in the anthropological literature. After Frank Lorimer published his book on *Culture and Human Fertility* in 1954, it became an object of speculation among demographers that there might be populations in Africa that were spacing their births, if not consciously, at least in conformity with an implicit rationality recognized and enforced by the social system. For Lorimer, 'the cultural interdiction to impregnate a wet nurse is a customary way of fertility control which is very widespread in patriarchal African societies'. In Africa, 'abrupt weaning must often have been followed by the sickness and death of the child. Such association of events must have been a matter of common observation' (Lorimer, 1969: 87). Abstinence, then, allowed the mother to breastfeed the baby for a longer period of time, and according to Lorimer, 'motivation for fertility in all societies is toward children, not toward live births as statistics. A baby at the breast is worth more than one in the womb and one lying neglected on the ground' (Lorimer, 1969: 87).

Perhaps more than anybody else, the Caldwells (1977) helped establish the place of sexual abstinence in the study of the determinants of fertility in Africa. They showed that the Yoruba of Nigeria push the duration of the sexual interdiction to its maximum. In the Yoruba populations surveyed, taboos were almost universally observed and often lasted up to 3 years following the birth of a child. Typically, the sexual taboo was maintained for 6 months after the end of breastfeeding.

At the time, the Caldwells exaggerated both the prevalence of abstinence and its effect on fertility:

In Yoruba society, and in most of sub-Saharan Africa, fertility is reduced not by postpartum amenorrhea extended by prolonged lactation but by postpartum sexual abstinence which exceeds the period of lactation (Caldwell and Caldwell, 1977: 197).

A later study edited by Page and Lesthaeghe (1981) showed that the Yoruba were by no means representative of all Africa. Adeokun's survey (1987) has shown that the long post-partum taboo is not universal even among Yoruba populations. Below, we shall present evidence that breastfeeding remains the main determinant of fertility levels in the subcontinent.

World Fertility Survey data from Africa confirm that the post-partum sexual taboo is still very widespread, but large variations in its duration have been observed even inside the different countries surveyed. For example, in Cameroon and Ghana the gap between the minimum and maximum durations of abstinence, by region, is 10.6 and 23.5 months respectively (Table 27.1). The anthropological literature indicates that local customs and traditions are very diverse and evolve rapidly (Schoenmaeckers *et al.*, 1981). Wide differences between ethnic groups in the length of post-partum abstinence were reported in Ghana. Among the Ashanti of the Southern province, the woman is secluded for 40 days after childbirth and given 40 more days of recovery thereafter. She then returns to her husband, and normal sexual relations are resumed (Fortes, 1954, in Lorimer, 1969: 265). Among the Bono of Brong-Ahafo, where the woman must abstain for 6 months after the birth of the first child, Warren (1975) found that a period of 40 days' abstinence is sufficient for subsequent pregnancies. In contrast, the Lowilli of North Ghana, the Tallensi, and the Ewe of the Black Volta abide by a post-partum taboo of 2 to 3 years (Gaisie, 1981). In the Great Lakes region of eastern Africa, tradition compels spouses to have sexual relations within one week of delivery (for Rwanda, see Bonte and Van Balen, 1969; for Kivu, see Caraël, 1979: 86 and 1981: 278). The absence of a post-partum taboo among the Havu of the Kivu is not compensated by other deliberate child spacing practices: coitus interruptus is generally

TABLE 27.1. *Duration of post-partum abstinence, breastfeeding, and amenorrhoea: mean, minimum, and maximum by region of residence*

Country	Abstinence	Breestfeeding	Amenorrhoea
Ghana	12.4 (7.4–30.9)	20.2 (13.6–32.5)	14.6 (10.3–19.9)
Lesotho	18.0 (17.0–19.3)	21.8 (20.7–22.3)	11.4 (10.5–12.3)
Senegal	—	20.5 (18.0–22.9)	—
Benin	18.2 (12.3–23.0)	21.4 (17.3–23.1)	13.8 (9.6–16.5)
Cameroon	16.2 (11.3–21.9)	19.5 (13.7–22.9)	13.3 (7.9–15.5)
Kenya	4.1 (2.9–5.8)	17.8 (14.4–23.2)	11.7 (8.8–15.7)
Sudan	3.2 (2.5–3.9)	17.3 (17.1–20.0)	12.1 (9.7–14.7)
Ivory Coast	16.5 (14.2–20.2)	19.7 (16.8–22.6)	13.0 (10.2–15.9)

Source: Eelens and Donné, 1985.

viewed negatively, while abortion and infanticide are explicitly condemned (Caraël, 1979, 1981). The Banyankole of Uganda believe in the healing power of sperm, and customarily the man was enjoined to have intercourse with his wife four days after delivery; a recent survey shows that the timing is between 10 days and one month (John B. Kabera, personal communication).

Schoenmaeckers *et al.* (1981) have drawn maps of Africa where they distinguish three categories of post-partum abstinence of different duration. The first duration, 40 days or less, is increasingly observed among the followers of Islam, who interpret Koranic tradition in this way. Durations longer than 40 days but shorter than a year are observed in much of East Africa. Finally, durations of more than a year characterize, among others, non-Islamic Western and Central Africa. (For a map of Africa using this classification system, see Bongaarts *et al.*, 1984.)

The strength of the taboo may be being rapidly eroded. A mean of 12 months of abstinence has been reported in contemporary South Togo (Locoh, 1984) and in Bobo-Dioulasso, Burkina Faso (F. van de Walle, 1987). It is likely that post-partum sexual taboos were of longer duration in the past, if one trusts the reports of earlier anthropologists. With the spread of Islam in Africa, lengthy periods of abstinence seem to have disappeared from some areas where they had been reported earlier. For example, Jean-Baptiste Durand had this to say about the populations of the coast of Senegal in 1802:

Women wean their children only when they are able to walk and bring a calabash full of water to their mother. They are promptly trained to do so, since during feeding, the spouses keep the laws of chastity, the infringement of which would be considered the weightier a crime, that it would be detrimental to the state of nursing mother and to the health of the child (225).

Henry, writing in 1910, and Tauxier, in 1927 (cited in Schoenmaeckers *et al.*, 1981), reported a sexual taboo upwards of 3 years among the Bambara of Mali. Today, however, the Islamic prohibition of intercourse during the 40 nights following a birth is almost universal in Senegal and Mali. F. van de Walle (1987) reported a mean length of abstinence of 3 months in the city of Bamako, Mali. Besides the influence of Islam, modernization, urbanization, and education are also whittling away at the custom of post-partum abstinence. The long taboo was usually associated with male dominance, polygyny, the early marriage of women, and large difference in ages between spouses. Saucier (1972) argues that female abstinence can be maintained more easily in a society that practises female circumcision. All these traits are fading among educated and urban populations.

The Different Functions of Abstinence

The long abstinence of the Yoruba of Nigeria has been attributed mostly to the preservation of the health of the baby, while a subsidiary motivation involved the mother's health. The Caldwells (1977: 198) specify that 'the main reason for ensuring the mother's health has been to ensure her capacity for further successful childbearing'. It appears clear here that the aim of abstinence is to space births in order to achieve a large family. For Locoh (1984) too, abstinence in South Togo is pro-natalist because it aims at keeping as many children as possible alive. We find it difficult to interpret the custom as a mechanism for limiting the size of the family or the growth of society.

Nevertheless, Orubuloye (1981: 53) notes that post-partum sexual abstinence has probably reduced the fertility of the Yoruba by one-fourth and believes that this custom will continue to be the most important way of controlling fertility among them. In an influential article, Lesthaeghe (1980) has compared the role of African post-partum taboos to that of the Western European pattern of marriage before the adoption of family limitation. Both, Lesthaeghe argues, were social mechanisms aimed at adapting populations to the available resources (see also Frank and McNicoll, 1987).

Although some form of post-partum abstinence exists in a majority of African societies, it should not be assumed a priori that the intent of intercourse taboos is always to ensure adequate birth spacing. In fact, a number of other reasons are given. Henry (1964: 485) used the term 'lactation taboo' as a general term covering African abstinence customs. The implication was that sexual relations were forbidden for the duration of breastfeeding. For the Caldwells (1981: 79), post-partum abstinence, though associated with breast-feeding, cannot be completely assimilated into a lactation taboo. Indeed, in many societies the post-partum taboo is shorter than the period of breastfeeding, while among the Yoruba it is longer.

Spacing as such is not necessarily a conscious objective when a woman refuses sexual relations because she believes that it will spoil her milk. The health of her child is the predominant concern. The Lowilli of northern Ghana believe that sexual relations during the nursing period will interrupt the flow of milk and that the child will not grow (Goody, 1955). Among the Yoruba (Caldwell and Caldwell, 1977: 199), as well as in other groups such as the Ewondo of Cameroon, there exists a strong belief that the man's sperm actually enters and poisons the milk which is being fed to the baby. The child's diarrhoeal episodes are interpreted as the result of this poisoning of the milk. Under the logic of this taboo, the woman who decides to resume sexual relations should wean her child. But in Africa, as in most other cultures, normative rules are full of contradictions and exceptions. It is perceived that the evil of combining sexual relations and breastfeeding is relatively tolerable, compared, for example, to resisting the husband's entreaties or running the risk of losing him to another, more available woman. Compromises and accommodations are possible. One such compromise is to have only intermit-tent sexual relations during the lactation period. Some women solve the problem by washing themselves and allowing time to elapse between intercourse and suckling. Abstinence is not always an 'all or nothing' type of behaviour, and it can still reduce fertility significantly after sexual relations have resumed at a reduced pace. Another compromise could consist of giving traditional or modern medicine to the child (or using contraception) to counteract the action of the sperm in the milk and so keep the baby healthy.

The list of motivations given for abstinence is long and complex. The shortest taboo, the one prescribed by Islam in a growing part of Africa, lasts 40 days. It is difficult to interpret it as a means to delay the arrival of the next child. What is involved here is more a notion that women are impure during menstruation, when Islam also prescribes sexual abstinence. In a comparable way, the Ikale, a Yoruba subgroup, invoke *agbon*, a bad body odour of the woman following parturition, to justify an abstinence of 2 to 9 months (Adeokun, 1981). For many observers, abstinence serves other purposes than the health of the mother and her children. Different authors have seen in sexual abstinence the objective of furthering social control and assuring the necessary effective distance between husband and wife. Societies based on the extended family recognize the danger of nucleation; the role of abstinence is to keep husband and wife remote from one another, and this is perceived as beneficial for society. The taboos also serve to maintain patriarchal authority over the younger generation and parental authority over children (Caraël, 1981: 278).

It is certain that the practice of abstinence is only possible in cultures where the conjugal link is weak, where polygamy exists, where a single wife is never sure to remain her husband's only partner, and mostly where the extended family prevails. Saucier (1972) emphasizes that the taboo is more frequent in gerontocratic societies and in patrilocal and patrilinear exogamies, where women are considered as outsiders and have little say.

In West Africa it is not unusual for the woman who gave birth to return home and visit her mother for a time. In Bobo-Dioulasso it is said that such a woman 'went to drink water at her mother's house'. Kumekpor (1975: 978) reports a similar custom among the Ewe of Togo and Ghana. In this case, the young woman stays with her parents or her in-laws until 'her child is weaned and she is ready to have another baby'. Similar practices exist in western Zaïre (Sala-Diakanda *et al.*, 1981) and in the Dagbon country in northern Ghana, where the young mother goes to live with her parents for 2 years after the birth of her first child (Oppong, 1973: 37).

More urbanized couples, who have increasingly adopted a Westernized view of the couple and the nuclear family, are rejecting the long abstinence period as inimical to happy conjugal relations. For the Caldwells (1987: 244):

a broader phenomenon which now affects the majority of Ibadan marriages . . . is the potential that the abstinence period possesses for destroying marriages. With increasing education and middle-class jobs for wives as well as husbands and with models provided by the media and church, there is a growing interest in, and expectation of, marital sex by husbands. Many of them do not expect to have to go outside to find their pleasures and many put increasing pressure on apprehensive and confused wives for an early resumption of sexual relations . . . Many of our respondents called this the 'fighting period' . . . The wife is afraid of alienating her husband's affection, of losing him altogether, or of his bringing home a new wife. These are new fears and new situations.

It is worth noting that post-partum abstinence is mostly a female responsibility. Male sexual behaviour is usually not strongly conditioned by a concern for birth spacing, or the quality of breast milk, or the diseases which the child may contract. It is unlikely, therefore, that men abstain from sexual relations to the same extent as their wives do.

In polygamous unions, it is unusual for all wives to be with child at the same time. Caldwell and Caldwell (1977: 202) report that, among the Yoruba in monogamous marriages, 31 per cent of husbands abstained from sexual relations during the period their wives were practicing post-partum abstinence, while the remainder had extra-marital relations. Among polygamous husbands, 8 per cent abstained, 88 per cent had sexual relations with other wives, and only 4 per cent had extra-marital relations. Polygamous men are less promiscuous than monogamous men, who look outside for partners during their wives' post-partum period.

Finally, the existence of terminal abstinence should be mentioned. Older women may decide, or be encouraged by custom, to abandon regular sexual relations with their husbands, either because they have reached a certain age or because their children have married and possibly become parents themselves. Terminal abstinence may occur at different ages, for different reasons, and according to different customs. The Caldwells identified the existence of the custom among the Yoruba and saw it as a potential exception to the generalization about the prevalence of natural fertility in Africa. In general, subsequent research, including the results of the World Fertility Survey, has not confirmed that terminal abstinence is very important anywhere (Cleland and Wilson, 1987: 14).

Is Abstinence an Important Factor in Spacing?

In much of contemporary sub-Saharan Africa, a long period of spacing between births is the combined result of extended post-partum amenorrhoea due to prolonged, demand breastfeeding and of sexual abstinence. These variables—breastfeeding, amenorrhoea, and abstinence—together determine the length of the protected or non-susceptible period following parturition (Henry, 1964; Bongaarts and Potter, 1983) and are themselves influenced by local customs and the environment. Variations in the length of breastfeeding and of abstinence seem to be the principal sources of the heterogeneity of levels of natural fertility that exist in Africa (Bongaarts *et al.*, 1984).

Spacing norms ingrained in African populations do not necessarily imply the conscious use of techniques, such as abstinence, aimed at avoiding the next birth. After all, long breastfeeding, which is still the rule in Africa (with a few exceptions among educated, urban women), is sufficient in itself to explain relatively long intervals between births (see Santow, 1987). Knowledge about the biological effect of prolonged breastfeeding on the post-partum period seems generally absent in African populations. What effect, then, does post-partum abstinence, often practised in connection with breastfeeding and linked with it in the mind of the nursing mother, have on the birth interval?

By providing empirical data on the subject, the World Fertility Survey has added greatly to our knowledge of the relationships among this complex of factors. On the basis of WFS data for seven countries, Eelens and Donné (1985) have compiled a convenient factbook, which includes summary measures of the duration of breastfeeding, of amenorrhoea, and of abstinence obtained from current status data by the prevalence–incidence ratio method. We use these data for several comparisons in the table and figures included in this report.

Although there are a priori reasons to believe that some populations may synchronize the time of weaning and the resumption of sexual relations, there is little visible relationship overall between the duration of breastfeeding and of abstinence. But the relationship between the duration of breastfeeding and the length of post-partum amenorrhoea has been found to conform to several formal expressions. Bongaarts and Potter (1983: 25) found that the curve best fitting the relationship between A, the duration of post-partum amenorrhoea in months, and B, the duration of breastfeeding, was provided by the following exponential:

$$A = 1.753e^{0.1396 \times B - 0.001872 \times B^2}$$

As a first approximation, Lesthaeghe *et al.* (1981: 7) describe the relationship as follows:

Postpartum amenorrhea lasts on average about 2 months for non-breastfeeding women and increases to roughly 60 to 75 percent of the average duration of breastfeeding in populations practising breastfeeding.

Although presumably more accurate, Bongaarts' formulation is less intuitively satisfying than Lesthaeghe's, which accentuates the essentially linear relation between the two variables. The WFS data for Africa confirm the linear relation: the coefficient of correlation between the duration of breastfeeding and the duration of amenorrhoea among the 48 observations is 0.80 (see Fig. 27.1). In a way, it is surprising that the link is so tight: after all, there is probably a great deal of cultural variability in the introduction of supplementary food and the intensity of feeding episodes and a great deal of ambiguity in the different definitions of weaning.

The relationship between amenorrhoea and the birth interval is fairly direct. The main problem, then, is assessing the effect of abstinence on the birth interval, since a substantial proportion of it occurs when the woman is amenorrhoeic and not at risk of conceiving. For individual women, only abstinence beyond

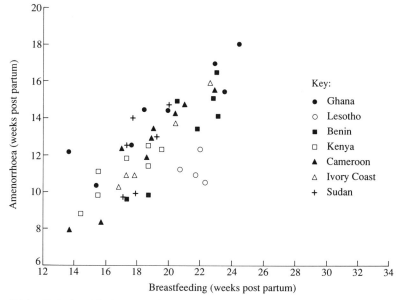

Fig. 27.1   Relationship between breastfeeding and amenorrhoea

the resumption of ovulation (which, for practical purposes, is signalled by the resumption of menstruation) will have an impact. The answer is not this simple, however, in a population where women have heterogeneous behaviour with respect to breastfeeding and abstinence and may resume ovulation at different times. It would not do to take the average duration of abstinence in the population and compare it to the average duration of amenorrhoea, since the averages conceal the heterogeneity. Assume, for example, two women: one does not breastfeed at all and abstains for 2 years; the other does not abstain, nurses her child for 2 years, and as a result prolongs amenorrhoea substantially. The average duration of abstinence and the average duration of breastfeeding for the two women will be 1 year each, but the average effect on the non-susceptible period (i.e. the joint effect of breastfeeding and abstinence) may be considerably longer, close to 2 years.

Fig. 27.2 (based on Eelens and Donné, 1985) shows that there is a linear relationship between the duration of abstinence and the length of time by which the non-susceptible period exceeds the period of post-partum amenorrhoea. The linear regression equation between abstinence, A, and the non-susceptible period, NSP, can be represented by the equation:

$$NSP = -1.12 + 0.389A$$

Thus, as a rule, the WFS data suggest that every 2.5 months of abstinence in a population prolongs the non-susceptible period by roughly 1 month over and above the period of amenorrhoea (see Fig. 27.2). In general, the effect of

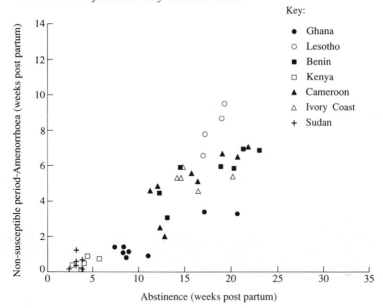

Fig. 27.2   Effect of abstinence on the non-susceptible period

abstinence beyond that of lactational amenorrhoea is, to use an expression of Lesthaeghe (1986: 221), no more than 'a bonus'. The abstinence bonus is, of course, increasingly significant when its duration extends past the average duration of post-partum amenorrhoea.

The Case of Bobo-Dioulasso

Through a combination of methodologies, we have investigated the operation of the proximate determinants of fertility in Bobo-Dioulasso, a town in Burkina Faso where the Sahel Institute and the National Institute of Statistics organized a multi-round infant and child mortality survey (van de Walle and Traoré, 1986; van de Walle, 1987). Starting at the time of birth, the survey collected prospective information on the birth-interval variables (resumption of intercourse and menstruation, supplementation and weaning, and new pregnancies) for each woman whose child was still alive. The observations were truncated either by the death of the child, the departure of the mother, or the second birthday of the child. The data were analysed in a series of hazard models. Additional qualitative information was collected in tape-recorded interviews with a small sample of women (Trussell *et al.*, 1987).

The qualitative survey revealed strong norms about spacing and strong desires among women to abstain from intercourse for an extended period, ideally until the child was weaned. A certain stage of physical maturity (teething, walking, ability to carry a pot of water) was indicative that the child could be weaned.

The actual behaviour of the women, as revealed in the prospective survey, was somewhat at variance with the stated norms. There was little statistical evidence of taboo on intercourse linked to lactation. Neither full nor partial breastfeeding had any effect on whether sexual relations were resumed. It is likely, however, that the intensity of sexual relations was considerably reduced by a nursing mother, and this seemed to contribute to the (not inconsiderable) apparent effect of supplemented breastfeeding on the rate of conception (50 per cent compared with 80 per cent for unsupplemented breastfeeding). Only full breastfeeding, however, provided any delay in the return of menses. Women seemed much more likely to resume sexual relations if they had resumed menstruation. The main reason to wean the child was the advent of another pregnancy.

The Bobo-Dioulasso data suggest that the interaction of breastfeeding, abstinence, and amenorrhoea may be more complex than it first appears. There may be many local combinations and adaptations. Retrospective statements made about the duration of abstinence may be normative in nature and reflect what women feel they should have done, rather than what they actually did. Breastfeeding with supplementation may not extend the duration of post-partum amenorrhoea, but it may none the less affect fertility by reducing the frequency of intercourse among women who are afraid of the effect of intercourse on the quality of their milk—a fear that is all too frequently reinforced by the repeated episodes of diarrhoea from which their children suffer.

Conclusion

One of the paradoxes of fertility regimes in Africa is that they place a strong emphasis on the advantages of spacing, but actually achieve a lengthy birth interval mostly by extended and intensive breastfeeding, even though the populations are not aware of the physiological effect of lactation on fertility. Abstinence, the one mechanism that could be volitional, is actually rather ineffective in attaining the goal of spacing. For the most part, abstinence takes place during the period of lactational amenorrhoea, when women are not at risk of conception. We have seen, however, that abstinence is often not perceived by African populations primarily as a spacing mechanism, but rather as a purification ritual or a means of preventing the pollution of the breast milk. The logic of this relationship was expressed by Galen more than a millennium and a half ago.

Intercourse taboos have been reduced in many parts of Africa, a fact which may have caused fertility to rise (for Kenya, see Frank and McNicoll, 1987). Some observers have predicted the disappearance of abstinence as a relevant proximate determinant of fertility in the near future (Lesthaeghe, 1986: 14). If couples continue to be conscious of the importance of spacing, they may increasingly substitute contraception for abstinence. But where abstinence has not been seen traditionally as a spacing mechanism, the prognosis is less favourable. The net result may hinge on the extent to which the population sees contraception as preventing the poisoning of the milk, for instance by preventing the mixing of the sperm and the woman's blood. Such an interpretation might well seem obvious in the case of barrier methods and might even appear attractive for hormonal methods of contraception.

References

Adeokun, L. A. (1981), 'The Next Child: Spacing Strategy in Yorubaland (with translations from taped interviews)', African Demography Working paper no. 8, Population Studies Center, University of Pennsylvania, Philadelphia: 183–214.

—— (1987), 'Explaining Sub-Ethnic Variations in Breastfeeding and Marital Sexual Relations among the Yoruba', in *The Cultural Roots of African Fertility Regimes*, proceedings of the Ife Conference, Obafemi Awolowo University, Ile-Ife and University of Pennsylvania, Philadelphia.

Bongaarts, J., and Potter, R. G. (1983), *Fertility, Biology and Behavior: An Analysis of the Proximate Determinants*, Academic Press, New York.

—— Frank, O., and Lesthaeghe, R. (1984), 'The Proximate Determinants of Fertility in Sub-Saharan Africa', *Population and Development Review* 10(3): 511–37.

Bonte, M., and Van Balen, H. (1969), 'Prolonged Lactation and Family Spacing in Rwanda', *Journal of Biosocial Science* 1: 97–100.

Bracher, M. D., and Santow, G. (1982), 'Breastfeeding in Central Java', *Population Studies* 36(3): 413–29.

Caldwell, J. C., and Caldwell, P. (1977), 'The Role of Marital Sexual Abstinence in Determining Fertility: A Study of the Yoruba in Nigeria', *Population Studies* 31(1): 193–215.

—— —— (1981), 'Cause and Sequence in the Reduction of Postnatal Abstinence in Ibadan City, Nigeria', in H. J. Page and R. Lesthaeghe (eds.), *Child Spacing in Tropical Africa, Traditions and Change*, Academic Press, London: 181–200.

Caldwell, P., and Caldwell, J. C. (1987), 'Fertility Control as Innovation: A Report on In-Depth Interviews in Ybadan, Nigeria', in *The Cultural Roots of African Fertility Regimes*, Proceedings of the Ife Conference, Obafemi Awolowo University, Ile-Ife and University of Pennsylvania, Philadelphia:

Caraël, M. (1979), 'Espacement des naissances, nutrition et écologie au Kivu (Zaïre)', *Population et Famille* 47(2): 81–99.

—— (1981), 'Child-spacing, Ecology and Nutrition in the Kivu Province of Zaïre', in H. J. Page and R. Lesthaeghe (eds.), *Child-Spacing in Tropical Africa: Traditions and Change*, Academic Press, London: 275–86.

Cleland, J., and Wilson, C. (1987), 'Demand Theories of the Fertility Transition: An Iconoclastic View', *Population Studies* 41(1): 5–30.

Durand, J. B. (1802), *Voyages au Sénégal*, Henri Agasse, Paris.

Eelens, F., and Donné, L. (1985), *The Proximate Determinants of Fertility in*

Sub-Saharan Africa: A Factbook Based on the Results of the World Fertility Survey, IPD-Working Paper 1985–3, Free University, Brussels.

Ferry, B. (1981), 'The Senegalese surveys', in H. J. Page and R. Lesthaeghe (eds.), *Child-Spacing in Tropical Africa: Traditions and Change*, Academic Press, London: 265–73.

Fortes, M. (1954), 'A Demographic Field Study in Ashanti', in F. Lorimer (ed.), *Culture and Human Fertility*, Greenwood Press, New York: 253–338.

Frank, O., and McNicoll, G. (1987), 'An Interpretation of Fertility and Population Policy in Kenya', Center for Policy Studies working paper 131, Population Council, New York.

Gaisie, S. K. (1981), 'Child Spacing Patterns and Fertility Differentials in Ghana', in H. J. Page and R. Lesthaeghe (eds.), *Child-Spacing in Tropical Africa: Traditions and Change*, Academic Press, London: 237–53.

Galen (1951 edn.), *De Sanitate Tuenda*, translated by Robert Montraville Green, Charles C. Thomas, Springfield, Ill.

Goody, J. R. (1955), *The Social Organization of the Lowilli*, London: HMSO.

Henry, L. (1964), 'Mesure du temps mort en fécondité naturelle', *Population* 19(3): 485–514.

Kumekpor, T. K. (1975), 'Togo', in J. C. Caldwell (ed.), *Croissance démographique et Évolution socio-économique en Afrique de l'ouest*, The Population Council, New York.

Lesthaeghe, R. (1980), 'On the Social Control of Human Reproduction', *Population and Development Review* 6(4): 527–48.

—— (1986), 'On the Adaptation of Sub-Saharan Systems of Reproduction', in D. Coleman and R. Schofield (eds.), *The State of Population Theory: Forward from Malthus*, Basil Blackwell, Oxford: 212–38.

—— Page, H. J., and Adegbola, O. (1981), 'Child-Spacing and Fertility in Sub-Saharan Africa: An Overview of Issues', in H. J. Page and R. Lesthaeghe (eds.), *Child-Spacing in Tropical Africa: Traditions and Change*: Academic Press, London: 147–80.

Locoh, T. (1984), *Fecondité et famille en Afrique de l'Ouest: Le Togo méridional contemporain*, Travaux et Documents, cahier no. 107, INED (Institut National d'Études Demographiques), Paris.

Lorimer, F. (1969) (ed.), *Culture and Human Fertility* , Greenwood Press, New York (orig. edn. 1954).

Oppong, C. (1973), *Growing Up in Dagbon*, Ghana Publishing Corporation, Accra-Tema.

Orubuloye, I. O. (1981), *Abstinence as a Method of Birth Control*, Changing African Family Project Series, monograph 8, Australian National University, Canberra.

Page, H. J., and Lesthaeghe, R. (eds.) (1981), *Child-Spacing in Tropical Africa: Traditions and Change*, Academic Press, London.

Roussel, P. (1813), *Système physique et moral de la femme*, Caille et Ravier, Paris.

Sala-Diakanda, M., Ngondo, A. P., Tabutin, D., and Vilquin, E. (1981), 'Fertility and Child-Spacing in Western Zaire', in H. J. Page and R. Lesthaeghe (eds.), *Child-Spacing in Tropical Africa: Traditions and Change*, Academic Press, London: 287–302.

Santow, G. (1987), 'Reassessing the Contraceptive Effect of Breastfeeding', *Population Studies* 41(1): 147–60.

Saucier, J. F. (1972), 'Correlates of the Long Postpartum Taboo: A Cross-Cultural Study', *Current Anthropology* 3(2): 238–49.

Schoenmaeckers, R., Shah, I. H., Lesthaeghe, R., and Tambashe, O. (1981), 'The Child Spacing Tradition and the Postpartum Taboo in Tropical Africa: Anthropological Evidence', in H. J. Page and R. Lesthaeghe (eds.), *Child-Spacing in Tropical Africa: Traditions and Change*, Academic Press, London: 25–71.

Singarimbun, M., and Manning, C. (1976), 'Breastfeeding, Amenorrhea and Abstinence in a Javanese Village: A Case Study of Mojolama', *Studies in Family Planning* 7(6): 175–9.

Trussell, J., van de Walle, E., and van de Walle, F. (1987), 'Norms and Behavior in Burkinabe Fertility', paper presented at the Population Association of America Meeting, Chicago.

United Nations (1985), *Breastfeeding and Related Aspects of Postpartum Reproductive Behaviour*, prepared by the Population Division, Department of International Economic and Social Affairs of the United Nations Secretariat, New York.

UNFPA (United Nations Fund for Population Activities) (1985), *Population Perspectives: Statements by World Leaders*, 2nd. edn., United Nations, New York.

van de Walle, E., and van de Walle, F. (1972), 'Allaitement, stérilité et contraception: Les opinions jusqu'au 19ème siècle', *Population* 27(4–5): 685–701.

—— and Traoré, B. (1986), 'Attitudes of Women and Men towards Contraception in Bobo-Dioulasso', African Demography Working Paper no. 13, Population Studies Center, University of Pennsylvania, Philadelphia.

van de Walle, F. (1987), 'The Diversity of Fertility Behavior: Bobo-Dioulasso, Bamako, Yaounde and Ngayokheme', in *The Cultural Roots of African Fertility Regimes*, Proceedings of the Ife Conference, Obafemi Awolowo University, Ile-Ife and University of Pennsylvania, Philadelphia: 215–23.

Warren, D. M. (1975), *The Techiman-Bono of Ghana: An Ethnography of the Akan Society*, Kendall-Hunt, Dubuque, Ia.

Zola, E. (1903), *Les Quatre Evangiles: Fecondité*, Les Œuvres Complètes, Eugène Fasquelle, Paris.

Index of Names

Adams, D. B. 91, 92
Adeokun, L. A. 449, 452
Adler, M. W. 104
Adler, R. A. 404
Ahlborg, G. 176
Ahmed, A. G. 318
Alberman, E. 279, 295, 307, 310
Alison, P. 377
Allen, I. 102
Anderson, A. N. 392, 393, 394, 401
Anderson, B. A. 81, 278
Anderson, J. L. 137
Anestad, G. 111, 112
Angell, R. R. 288
Ann, T. B. 29
Aono, T. 401
Apter, D. 53, 56, 60
Aral, S. O. 106, 107, 108, 115
Aravindakshan, S. T. K. 37 n.
Armstrong, B. G. 176
Armstrong, E. G. 321, 322
Aschheim, S. 320
Atallah, N. L. 27, 28
Avery, R. 183 n.

Baanders-Van Halewin, E. A. 139
Baird, D. 6, 330, 331, 332, 333 n., 335, 398
Baker, E. R. 137, 142, 143
Baker, H. W. G. 322
Baker, R. J. 417
Balasuriya, S. 29
Ballard, R. C. 109
Bancroft, J. 88
Bangham, C. R. M. 29
Barlow, S. 307, 335
Barrett, J. C. 79, 186, 187, 194, 196, 197, 198, 199, 235, 236 n., 362
Bartsch, W. 140
Bateman, B. G. 114
Battaglia, F. C. 56
Battin, D. A. 110
Baumann, G. 56
Beal, C. M. 29
Bean, J. A. 281
Beard, R. W. 305
Becker, S. 3, 51, 353, 354 n.
Beer, A. E. 305
Beitins, I. Z. 141
Belcastro, A. N. 136
Bell, T. A. 106
Bendel, J.-P. 201, 209

Bentzoin, M. 139
Bergh, T. 404
Bergman, P. 160
Bergstrom, R. 158, 159
Berman, M. 380
Bertrand, J. 140
Beumont, P. J. 141
Bhalla, M. 50
Bhatia, S. 37 n., 78, 79
Bhattacharya, B. N. 186, 187, 188, 189
Bidlingmaier, F. 140, 141
Bierman, J. M. 201
Billewicz, W. C. 368
Billewicz, W. S. 140
Billingham, R. F. 305
Blake, J. 21, 345
Bloch, S. K. 321
Blount, J. H. 115
Bocaz, A. 351
Bojilen, K. 139
Bombard, A. T. 291
Bonen, A. 134
Bongaarts, J. 3, 10, 12 n., 15 n., 37, 42, 52, 71, 73, 75, 79, 80 n., 184, 186, 187, 188, 189, 190, 191, 193, 194, 200, 201, 210, 360 n., 369, 370, 378, 379, 380, 384, 413, 414, 431, 450, 453, 454
Bonnar, J. 391, 397
Bonte, M. 449
Borgerhoff-Mulder, M. B. 51
Borkowski, A. 321
Borsos, A. 53
Boué, A. 291, 295, 310
Bourque-Scholl, N. 42
Bowen-Jones, A. 406
Bowie, W. R. 103, 104
Boyar, R. 141
Boyden, T. W. 137, 144, 145
Bracher, M. 361, 447
Bracken, M. B. 39, 54, 55, 61
Brass, W. 186
Braude, P. R. 305
Braunstein, G. D. 317, 321
Brihmer, C. 102
Brix, K. A. 177
Broman, S. 336, 337 n.
Brown, J. B. 33, 392, 393, 394, 397, 442
Brown, K. H. 388
Brown, L. 243
Brown, P. E. 138
Brundtland, G. H. 31

Brunham, R. C. 102, 103, 104, 105, 108, 110, 112, 113
Bryant, H. E. 177
Bullen, B. A. 132, 134
Burkman, R. T. 163
Burmeister, L. F. 56, 59
Burtke, A. 405
Butler, W. J. 177

Caldwell, J. C. 78, 79, 448, 451, 452
Caldwell, P. 78, 79, 448, 451, 452
Campbell, O. M. R. 430
Cantrelle, P. 346
Caraël, M. 449, 450, 452
Carfagna, M. 25
Carlberg, K. A. 142
Carr, D. B. 147
Carrasco, E. 37
Carson, S. 6
Carson, S. A. 287
Cartwright, A. 77 n.
Casagrande, J. T. 39, 54, 61
Cashner, K. A. 290
Cates, W. 4, 108, 115
Centulo, C. L. 173
Cevenini, R. 109
Chaden, B. C. 279
Chakravarty, I. 141
Chandley, A. C. 293
Chaning-Pearce, S. M. 27, 31
Channing, C. P. 263
Chaparro, M. V. 102
Chartier, M. 321
Chen, C. 317
Chen, L. C. 361, 378
Chen, R. S. 183 n., 192
Chiazze, L. 80
Chillik, C. R. 247
Cholst, I. N. 405
Chowdhury, A. K. M. A. 29, 31, 50, 52, 59, 60, 378, 380
Christiaens, G. C. M. L. 290
Chung, C. S. 158, 159
Clark, A. L. 95
Cleary, R. E. 104
Cleland, J. 14 n., 37, 453
Cliquet, R. L. 34, 52, 60
Coale, A. 67, 79, 201, 222 n.
Cohen, F. L. 278
Cohen, J. 238, 260 n., 274
Connell, E. B. 164
Conway, D. 110
Copeland, P. C. 144
Cox, D. R. 331, 369, 386, 414, 417
Cramer, D. W. 104, 107, 113, 164
Crawford, J. D. 141
Creasy, M. R. 81
Crick, F. 269
Crowley, W. F. 397

Cumming, D. C. 4, 136, 140, 142, 143, 144, 145, 146, 147, 148, 149
Cushman, S. 135, 137, 143
Cziezel, A. 293

Dacou-Voutetakis, C. 25
Dale, E. 135, 136, 137, 142, 143
Daling, J. R. 107, 113, 158, 159, 164, 165 n.
Daly, D. C. 299
Damon, A. 23, 139
Dann, T. C. 25, 31
Darroch-Forrest, J. 43
David, G. 231, 232, 237, 238, 239 n., 272
Davila, G. H. 57
Davis, K. J. 21, 345
Delgado, H. 353, 361, 378, 379, 380, 384
Delvoye, P. 394, 397, 398, 401, 402
Demarest, K. T. 405
Deuster, P. A. 136, 142, 143
de Ward, F. 139
Dewart, P. J. 406
Diaz, S. 7, 413
Dixon, G. 148
Dixon, R. L. 335
Djursing, H. 404
Donné, L. 449 n., 454, 455
Doring, G. K. 32-3, 42, 43, 80
Drage, J. 329 n.
Draper, D. L. 104, 105
Dreizen, S. 50, 57, 139
Drew, F. L. 135
Dryfoos, J. G. 28, 42
Dubey, A. K. 141
Ducharme, J. R. 140, 141
Duchen, M. R. 392, 397, 402
Duenholter, J. H. 56

Eastman, C. J. 392, 393, 394, 397, 398, 401, 402, 404, 429, 442, 443
Eaton, J. W. 279
Edlefsen, L. 17 n.
Edmonds, D. K. 38, 211, 287, 316, 321
Edwards, R. 243, 251
Eelens, F. 449 n., 454, 455
Eilard, T. 104
Eldor, A. 303
Elias, M. 303, 385, 443
Ellish, N. J. 321
Ellison, P. T. 51, 134
Emanuel, I. 158, 159
Emperaire, J. C. 237
Erkan, K. A. 56
Eschenbach, D. A. 102, 103, 104, 107, 113
Espenschade, A. 133
Eveleth, P. B. 23, 25, 26, 27, 28, 29, 50, 51
Exner, T. 303

Faiman, C. 141
Fakeye, O. 27

Falk, V. 108
Farid-Coupal, N. 27, 31
Farookhi, R. 321
Farrel, P. A. 147
Farris, E. J. 92, 195
Faulk, W. P. 306
Faulkner, W. L. 163
Feicht, C. B. 135, 137
Ferraretti, A. P. 262 n.
Ferry, B. 349, 350 n., 361, 447
Fiddes, J. C. 320
Fija-Talamanaca, I. 307
Fishel, S. B. 320
Fishman, J. 140
Ford, K. 6, 7, 347, 361, 363, 364, 368, 369, 370, 385, 428, 436
Forest, M. G. 140
Fortes, M. 449
Foster, A. 56, 61, 377
Fowler, R. E. 261
Frank, O. 451, 457
Fraser, F. C. 310
Fraser, H. M. 406
Frazier, T. M. 56
French, F. E. 201
Friday, P. 209 n.
Fries, H. 135, 142
Fries-Hansen, B. J. 139
Frisancho, A. R. 59, 60
Frisch, R. E. 31, 50, 51, 132, 139, 140, 142, 143, 368, 405
Fuxe, K. 405

Gaisie, S. K. 449
Galen 446, 457
Gallano, P. 295
Galle, P. C. 138
Gallo, P. G. 25
Garcia, C. R. 159, 160
Garcia, J. E. 264 n., 265 n.
Garfinkel, J. 211
Garn, S. M. 57, 59
Gaslonde, S. 351
Gastineau, D. A. 303
Gelphman, K. A. 113
Gerbie, A. 296 n.
Geronimus, A. T. 56
Gibbs, J. 16 n.
Gilbert, G. L. 111
Gill, T. J. 305
Gilmore, D. H. 290
Gindorff, P. R. 404
Gini, C. 185, 193, 209
Gjonnaess, H. 103, 104, 112
Gladen, B. C. 332
Glasier, A. 385, 394, 396, 397, 398, 399, 401, 402, 403 n., 404, 429, 442
Glass, D. V. 185, 194, 195, 199
Glass, M. R. 398

Glasser, J. H. 194, 197, 199, 214
Glenc, F. 157
Gold, A. R. 91
Golden, M. L. 5, 202
Goldhaber, M. K. 177
Goldman, N. 193, 194, 210, 346, 347
Goodman, M. 29
Goodrich, J. T. 113
Goody, J. R. 451
Gordon, J. 379, 380
Gordon, K. 401, 405
Goulet, L. 173
Grady, W. R. 40, 43 n.
Grainger, C. R. 27
Gray, R. H. 27, 28, 29, 42, 52, 65, 66 n., 67, 81, 369, 430
Grebenik, E. 185, 194, 195, 199
Gregg, C. R. 105
Griffin, J. 321
Grimes, D. A. 113
Gropp, A. 289, 291
Gross, B. A. 385, 392, 393, 394, 397, 398, 401, 402, 404, 429, 442, 443
Grossman, A. 146
Grudzinskas, J. G. 318, 320
Guderian, A. M. 111, 112
Guerneri, S. 293
Guerrero, R. 282
Gump, D. W. 112
Gupta, D. 140, 141
Guttmacher, A. F. 279
Guz, D. 376, 428, 433

Habicht, J.-P. 368, 369, 373, 414
Hadgu, A. 102
Hafez, E. S. E. 23
Hager, W. D. 101
Hallberg, T. 106
Hammerslough, C. 377
Hansen, J. W. 141
Harlap, S. 159, 211, 282, 307, 339
Hassold, T. 294
Hawes, L. A. 111
Hawkswell, J. 103, 104
Hayashi, M. 157
Hedricks, C. 92, 214
Heinonen, P. K. 102, 300
Hellighers, A. E. 56
Helm, P. 31
Helm, S. 31
Hendershot, G. E. 279
Hennart, P. 392, 393, 394, 401, 402, 404, 405
Henripin, J. 187
Henry, L. 9, 71, 73, 189, 345, 450, 451, 453
Henry-Suchet, J. 103, 104, 107, 109
Henshaw, S. K. 116
Hermon, D. 281
Hertig, A. T. 37, 42, 43 n., 267, 288
Hippocrates 446

Hirsch, M. B. 107
Hobcraft, J. 14 n., 351, 352, 376, 428, 433
Hodgen, G. D. 5, 243
Hodgson, M. 16 n.
Hogue, C. J. R. 158
Holford, T. R. 417
Holmes, K. K. 106, 107
Honoré, L. H. 293
Hoshi, H. 28, 31
Howell, N. 28
Howie, P. W. 385, 391, 392 n., 393, 394,
    395 n., 397, 398, 400, 401, 402, 404, 413
Hua, C.-I. 201, 209
Huffman, S. L. 7, 353, 368, 369, 378, 379,
    385, 386, 387 n., 388, 413
Huggins, G. 5
Hull, M. G. 114, 279
Huseman, C. A. 405
Hutton, E. M. 278

Illingworth, P. J. 405
Irwin, K. L. 126, 127
Israel, R. 160

Jacobs, P. A. 211, 291
Jacobson, L. 102, 163
Jain, A. 378, 379, 433
James, W. H. 31, 37, 88, 91, 186, 187, 191,
    210, 211, 213 n., 220, 224, 278
Jasso, G. 87, 211
Jelovsek, F. R. 173
Jenner, M. R. 141
John, A. M. 7, 351, 352, 353, 356, 415
Johnson, L. 278
Johnson, N. L. 220, 362
Johnson, P. 209 n.
Johnston, F. E. 31, 140
Jones, E. F. 34, 37, 43
Jones, G. S. 252, 254 n., 256 n., 257 n.
Jones, H. 103, 104
Jones, H. W. 244, 246 n., 247 n., 266 n.,
    302
Jones, R. B. 104, 109
Juberg, R. C. 280

Kabera, J. B. 450
Kabule-Sabiti, I. 37 n.
Kahn, J. R. 87
Kaku, M. 140
Kane, J. L. 110
Kannel, W. B. 65
Kantner, J. F. 42, 43
Kaplan, E. L. 414, 418
Kapoor, I. 37 n.
Karim, A. 66
Kauppila, A. 401, 404
Keith, L. G. 106
Kelch, R. P. 141
Kelver, M. E. 110

Kenigsberg, D. 258 n., 259 n.
Kennedy, G. C. 139, 142
Keyfitz, N. 186
Kharrazi, M. 335
Kim, Y. J. 6, 347, 361, 363, 364, 368, 369,
    370, 428, 436
Kinsey, A. C. 35, 86, 87 n., 88, 212 n.,
    217 n., 218
Kirkwood, R. F. 138
Klein, S. M. 159, 160
Klibanski, A. 141
Kline, J. 307
Klopper, A. 318
Knapp, J. S. 105
Knodel, J. 70, 79, 361
Kobrin, F. E. 347, 362, 363, 368
Kolmorgen, U. K. 102
Konner, M. 392
Kotz, S. 220, 362
Kouchi, M. 28, 31
Kramer, D. G. 106
Kremer, J. 75
Kuleshov, N. P. 294
Kulin, H. E. 57, 141
Kumekpor, T. K. 452
Kurzel, R. B. 173

Lachenbruch, P. A. 85, 189, 191, 194, 195,
    196, 197, 199, 214
Lactot, C. A. 282
Lager, C. 134
Laird, N. 417
Lansic, J. 5
Larsen, S. A. 127, 129
Larsen, U. 67, 68 n., 72, 73, 74 n., 75, 76 n.
Larsson-Cohn, U. 161
Laska-Mierzejewska, T. 25
Lasley, B. L. 318
Lazar, P. 81, 279, 280
Lean, T. H. 158
LeBeau, M. M. 293
LeBlanc, H. 405
Lee, N. C. 106
Lee, P. 23, 141
Lejarraga, H. 27
LeLannou, D. 238, 239 n.
Leong, D. A. 405
Leridon, H. 6, 9, 14 n., 15 n., 28, 38, 42,
    44, 72, 73, 81, 94, 190, 198, 201, 213, 316,
    346
Lerner, R. C. 158, 159
Lesthaeghe, R. 347, 359, 361, 363, 370, 428,
    449, 451, 454, 456, 458
Levine, H. S. 135, 136, 142, 143
Levine, P. 303
Lewis, G. 361
Lewitt, S. 164
Liestol, K. 38, 54, 61
Lincoln, D. W. 397

Lindquist, O. 65
Linhares, E. D. R. 26
Linn, S. 160
Lippman, A. 321
Little, R. J. 351, 352
Livson, N. 23, 133, 139
Locoh, T. 450, 451
Lodico, G. 405
Logrillo, V. M. 158, 159
Lorimer, F. 448, 449
Loudon, A. I. 405
Love, E. J. 177
Low, W. D. 28, 31
Lucky, A. W. 141
Lunn, P. 378, 384, 392, 401, 405
Lutter, J. M. 135, 137, 143

Mabey, D. C. W. 108, 110
McAnarney, E. R. 56
McArthur, J. W. 148
McDonald, A. D. 176, 177
MacDonald, P. K. 12 n., 140
McIntyre, J. A. 306
Mackenzie, J. A. 33, 34 n., 42
McKinlay, S. M. 65, 66 n., 67
McLaren, D. S. 373
McLeod, P. M. 294
MacMahon, B. 66
McMurdo, M. E. T. 404
McNay, M. B. 290
McNeil, D. R. 201, 222
McNeill, D. 23, 133, 139
McNeilly, A. S. 7, 368, 385, 391, 392, 393,
    394, 396, 397, 398, 399, 400, 401, 402,
    404, 405, 413, 429, 442, 443
McNicoll, G. 451, 457
Madden, J. D. 398, 401
Mahadevan, M. M. 238
Mahlstedt, P. T. 114
Majumdar, H. 189, 190, 191, 192
Makinson, C. 56
Malcolm, L. A. 53
Malina, R. M. 31, 50, 132
Malpas, P. 310
Mamelle, N. 176
Mangold, W. D. 56
Manning, C. 447
March, C. M. 160
Marchbanks, P. A. 107, 108 n., 127, 130
Mardh, P.-A. 103, 104
Marshall, J. C. 79, 145, 194, 196, 197, 198,
    199, 235, 236 n.
Marshall, W. A. 50, 51, 56, 57
Martin, A. O. 297 n.
Martini, L. 401, 405
Mascie-Taylor, C. G. N. 25, 26
Mattei, A. 238, 239 n.
Mattioli, M. 405
Mauger, S. 56

Mayaux, M. J. 210, 223, 237, 238 n.
Mayer, A. J. 279
Meier, P. 414, 418
Meirik, O. 158, 159
Menken, J. A. 4, 10, 32, 33, 56, 67, 68 n.,
    72, 73, 74 n., 75, 76 n., 183 n., 188, 189,
    192, 193, 209 n., 210, 213 n., 353, 369,
    377, 386
Menken, O. R. 4
Merriam, G. R. 148
Metcalf, M. G. 33, 34 n., 42
Method, M. W. 101
Meuris, S. 391, 404
Michelman, H. W. 288
Miller, J. F. 38, 211, 287, 288, 322
Miller, R. G. 431
Millman, S. R. 5, 185, 194, 198, 199, 202, 281
Mills, J. L. 288, 289, 299, 308
Mineau, G. 67, 69 n., 70 n., 81
Mishell, D. R. 106, 162
Moll, G. W. 140
Moller, B. R. 103, 104, 108, 111
Momose, K. 157
Moor, R. M. 261
Moore, D. E. 109
Moore, K. E. 405
Morera, A. M. 140, 141
Morgan, W. P. 138
Morris, L. 34
Morris, N. M. 87, 90, 91, 94, 195, 211, 321
Morton, H. 317
Mosher, W. E. 107, 116
Moss, T. R. 103, 104
Mouzon, J. B.-A. de 240, 279
Muasher, S. 248
Mueller, R. F. 294
Muquardt, C. 321

Naeye, R. L. 56, 59
Nag, M. 77, 78 n., 79
Nair, N. 55
Nakamura, I. 50
Nakao, K. 147
Nath, D. C. 186, 187
Naylor, A. F. 81
Nelder, J. A. 417
Newton, W. 106
Neyzi, O. 28
Noonan, F. P. 317
Nysenbaum, A. M. 318, 320

Obel, E. 158
Ober, C. L. 305
Oberle, M. W. 4, 126, 127, 129, 130
Odell, W. D. 321
Okai, R. 385
Okorafar, A. E. 27
Oksenberg, J. R. 305
Oliver, D. 417

Olsen, J. 335
Opler, J. 77
Oppong, C. 452
O'Reilly, K. R. 106
Orr, M. T. 116
Orubuloye, I. O. 451
Ory, H. W. 163
Osler, D. C. 141
Osser, S. 104
Overstreet, J. 321

Paavonen, J. 102, 104
Padjen, A. 110
Page, H. J. 347, 359, 361, 363, 370, 428, 449
Palmer, J. D. 90
Parker, M. P. 189, 190, 194
Parrenteau-Carreau, S. 442
Pascal, J. 442
Pasteur, L. 269
Pastides, H. 173
Patton, D. L. 112
Paul, L. 346, 347
Payne, M. R. 404, 406
Pebley, A. R. 55
Pelosi, M. A. 401
Pena, G. 160
Perez, A. 442
Persson, K. 104
Petterson, F. 135, 161
Philip, F. S. 384
Pineda, M. A. 37 n.
Plachot, M. 288
Platt, R. 103, 115
Plummer, F. 108, 113
Plymate, S. R. 140
Poindexter, A. N. 391, 394, 400
Poland, B. J. 310
Potter, R. G. 10, 12 n., 15 n., 37, 42,
    183 n., 185, 189, 190, 194, 198, 199, 200,
    201, 281, 345, 347, 360 n., 361, 362, 363,
    368, 369, 413, 414, 453, 454
Power, D. A. 306
Prakash, S. 29
Pratt, W. F. 42, 86
Prema, K. 384, 413
Price, W. S. 232, 238
Prior, J. C. 132, 134, 136, 137, 144, 145
Punnonen, R. 109

Quinn, P. A. 111

Rachootin, P. 335
Raman, L. 51
Ramirez, J. A. 127
Rana, T. 50
Rand, W. M. 57
Rapoport, S. I. 147
Ravindranath, M. 413
Rebar, R. W. 136, 140, 142, 143, 148, 149

Redwine, D. B. 135, 137, 142
Reeves, J. 140
Regan, L. 305
Reid, R. L. 147
Reiter, E. O. 141
Repetti, C. F. 305
Revelle, R. 139, 140
Reyes, F. I. 397
Rice-Wray, E. 160, 406
Ridley, J. C. 186
Riley, A. P. 3, 57, 58 n., 59
Rimer, B. A. 56
Ripa, K. T. 104
Rivero, R. 392, 397, 442
Roberts, D. F. 25, 31
Roberts, T. K. 318
Robertson, J. N. 108
Robyn, C. 391, 404
Roche, A. F. 57
Rock, J. 288, 302
Rodriguez, G. 7, 222 n.
Rolfe, B. E. 317
Rolland, R. 397, 398, 442
Roman, E. 38, 310
Ronkainen, H. 145, 148
Rosenberg, M. J. 5, 171, 172 n., 173, 176
Rosenfeld, R. L. 140
Rosero-Bixby, L. 126, 127, 130
Roussel, P. 446
Royston, J. P. 201, 216 n.
Rudak, E. 288
Ruder, A. 278
Russell, J. B. 137, 146, 147 n., 148
Ruzicka, L. T. 37 n., 78, 79
Ruzicska, P. 293
Ryder, N. B. 34

Sacherer, J. M. 29
Saez, J. M. 140, 141
Sala-Diakanda, M. 452
Sandler, D. P. 39, 52, 55, 56, 60, 61
Santow, G. 361, 369, 370, 447, 454
Saucier, J. F. 450, 452
Saxen, L. 280
Schachter, J. 112
Schacter, B. 305, 306
Schioler, V. 392, 393, 394, 401
Schlesselman, J. J. 178
Schoemaker, J. 263
Schoenmaeckers, R. 449, 450
Schrag, S. D. 335
Schwartz, B. 136, 137, 138, 142, 143, 144
Schwartz, D. 194, 197, 198, 210, 223, 224,
    225 n., 236, 278
Scott, A. 51
Scragg, R. F. R. 66
Sellors, J. W. 111
Selmanoff, M. 405
Selvin, S. 211

Senanayake, P. 106
Settimi, L. 307
Shangold, M. M. 134, 135, 136, 142, 143
Shapiro, S. 81
Sharp, N. C. 322
Shaw, F. D. 317
Shearman, B. M. 160, 161
Sheps, M. C. 32, 188, 189, 190, 191, 192,
  193, 194, 213, 222, 345
Sher, N. 135
Sherman, K. J. 107, 108
Shiono, P. H. 307
Shoon, M. G. 102
Shrenker, P. 405
Shrivatava, J. R. 50
Shy, K. K. 162
Simpson. J. L. 6, 287, 289, 290, 291, 293,
  294, 295, 296 n., 300, 301 n., 304 n.
Simpson-Hebert, M. 413
Singarimbun, M. 447
Singh, K. K. 186, 188, 189
Singh, S. 321, 349, 350 n., 361
Sirinathsinghji, D. J. S. 401, 405
Sitteri, P. K. 140
Skakkebaek, N. 88
Smart, Y. C. 317
Smith, D. P. 414
Solomon, L. 31
Soranos 446
D'Souza, S. 192, 193, 347
Sowa, M. 404
Speroff, L. 135, 137, 142
Spira, A. 6, 214 n., 272, 279
Spira, N. 273
Stacey, C. M. 104
Stamm, W. E. 103
Stanley, F. J. 56
Stein, Z. A. 139, 211, 279, 280, 309
Steiner, R. A. 141
Steptoe, P. 243, 251
Stern, J. M. 393, 394, 401, 402, 404
Stevenson, A. C. 38, 289
Stine, O. C. 56
Stone, K. M. 106
Stoutenbeek, P. H. 290
Stray-Pedersen, B. 302, 308
Strobino, B. R. 335
Stubbs, W. A. 147
Suchindran, C. M. 191
Sullivan, F. M. 307, 335
Susser, M. 139
Sutherland, G. R. 294
Svensson, L. 106, 107, 112
Swan, S. H. 177
Sweet, R. L. 102, 104, 105
Swenson, C. E. 112

Tabor, A. 290
Talbert, L. M. 33

Talmadge, K. 320
Tanner, J. M. 23, 25, 26, 27, 28, 29, 31, 50,
  51, 56, 57, 58, 138, 139, 144
Tatum, H. J. 162, 164
Taylor, E. S. 163
Teisala, K. 113
Theriault, G. 173
Tho, P. T. 299
Thompson, M. W. 278
Thompson, S. E. 103, 113
Tietze, C. 38 n., 42, 44, 164, 199, 279, 330,
  331 n., 335
Tijam, K. H. 108
Toth, A. 106, 303
Traoré, B. 456
Treffers, P. E. 299
Treloar, A. E. 53, 201, 210, 216 n., 281
Trichopolous, D. 157
Trobough, G. E. 111, 112
Trounson, A. O. 238, 253
Trussell, J. 37 n., 42, 67, 69 n., 70 n., 72,
  73, 74 n., 75, 76 n., 79, 81, 140, 194, 197,
  222 n., 348, 349, 350, 352, 377, 415, 456
Tyson, J. E. 398, 401

Uche, G. O. 27
Udo, A. A. 79
Udry, J. R. 4, 34, 36, 37 n., 52, 60, 86, 87,
  88, 89 n., 90, 91, 92, 94, 95, 195, 211,
  213 n., 221, 321

Vaessen, M. 72 n., 73, 126
Vaitukaitis, J. L. 321
Van Balen, H. 449
van de Walle, É. 8, 446, 456
van de Walle, F. 8, 446, 450, 456
Van der Spuy, Z. M. 50
Van Ginneken, J. K. 413
Van Keep, P. A. 67
Van Loon, G. R. 148
Varma, A. O. 158, 159
Veeck, L. L. 243, 261 n.
Veldhuis, J. D. 145
Vermer, H. M. 398
Vessey, M. P. 75, 106, 160
Vetter, K. M. 127, 129
Vigersky, R. A. 141
Vihko, R. 53, 56, 60
Vlaanderen, W. 299
Vollman, R. F. 201, 216 n., 281, 316

Wacholder, S. 331
Wakat, D. K. 132, 137
Wallin, P. 95
Warburton, D. 293, 294, 310
Ware, H. 77, 78
Warren, D. M. 449
Warren, M. P. 50, 132, 133, 138, 140, 142,
  144

Washington, A. E. 106, 115
Wasserheit, J. N. 102, 103, 104, 105, 106
Watson, J. 269
Watt, J. L. 291
Wehmann, R. E. 321, 322
Weinberg, C. R. 332
Weinstein, M. 185, 199, 200, 201, 203, 204, 211, 212 n., 214, 215, 225
Weir, J. 139
Weiss, E. 79
Wentz, A. C. 298
West, C. 391
Westoff, C. F. 23, 34, 37 n., 42, 88, 346, 347
Westrom, L. 102, 107, 108, 112, 113, 163
Wheeler, G. D. 146, 147
Whittaker, J. F. 211
Whittaker, P. G. 287, 316, 321, 322
Whittington, W. L. 108
Wilcox, A. J. 6, 42, 44, 54, 171, 211, 279, 322, 323 n., 324, 330, 332, 335, 336, 338
Wiler, J. C. 147
Wilson, C. 72, 73, 74 n., 75, 76 n. 453
Wilson, C. A. 405
Wilson, R. D. 290
Winter, J. S. D. 141

Wise, P. M. 405
Wishik, S. M. 140
Wolanski, N. 139
Wolner-Hanssen, P. 102, 104, 106
Wood, C. 253
Wood, J. W. 52, 53, 60, 160, 185, 199, 200, 201, 203, 204, 211, 212 n., 214, 215, 225, 392
Worcester, J. 66
Worthman, C. 392
Wrensch, M. 177
Wurtman, R. J. 26
Wyon, J. 379, 380
Wyshak, G. 26, 31, 38, 50, 54, 61

Yen, S. S. C. 145
Ylikorkala, O. 401

Zabin, L. S. 34
Zacharias, L. 26, 31, 57
Zelnik, M. 42, 43
Zenzes, M. T. 288
Zerfas, A. J. 373
Zlatnik, F. J. 56, 59
Zola, É. 446
Zondek, B. 320

Index of Subjects

abortifacients 306–7
abortions 3, 21, 23, 157–60, 301, 450
  aneuploid 295
  chromosomally abnormal 293
  chromosomally normal 279, 280
  clinically recognized 287, 290
  first-trimester 166, 300
  habitual 159, 310
  late 55, 198
  legal 38, 39
  missed 290, 293, 300
  multiple 305
  non-septic 166
  rates of 251, 309
  risk of 38, 61, 279, 282, 310, 339
  second-trimester 300, 302
  therapeutic 166
  trisomic 280
  unreported or undetected 345
  use of 40
  vacuum aspiration 158
  see also induced abortions; repetitive
    abortions; spontaneous abortions
achondroplasia 278
adenomas 161, 162
adhesions:
  bilateral intra-tubal 112
  intra-uterine (synechiae) 159, 300
  lysis of 300
  minor avascular 250
  pelvic 157, 162, 167
  peritoneal 240
adnexal tenderness 101
adolescents 88, 373
  fertility 21–44, 50–61
  growth spurt 53, 58–60, 140
  low marriage rates 34
  sexually active teenagers 34, 106
  sterility 3
  subfecundity 51, 52–3, 60
  subfertility 55, 56
  undernourished 50–61
  adrenarche 140, 144
aetiologies 107–12, 114, 254, 302
  microbial 102–3
Africa 3, 4, 14, 39, 81, 347, 405
  sub-Saharan 446–57
  see also under individual country names;
    also Bamako; Bantus; Dobe !Kung;
    Yoruba
agbon 452

age:
  gestational 176, 334, 336, 337, 339
  maternal 274–5, 278–9, 280, 309–10, 336–9
  paternal 75, 239, 274, 278, 280
  see also birth (first/last); coital frequency;
    coitus; fecundability; fertility; marriage;
    menarche; menopause; sterility
ageing of women 69, 75
agnos 448
AID (artificial insemination by donor) 5–6,
    272, 274–7, 279, 281–2, 335
  CECOS programme 5, 231–41
  fertilization 266
AIDS virus 232
alcohol 172, 173, 177, 307
alleles 306
alpha foetoprotein 269
aluteal cycle 53
amenorrhoea 40, 170, 351–7, 394
  diet/nutrition and 139, 141, 142, 149
  duration 361–70, 433, 436, 455; duration
    of abstinence shorter than 8;
    inconsistencies in data 6, 346, 348,
    352–4, 356; nutritional status and 7,
    375; temporary 65
  exercise-associated 144
  hyperprolactinaemia and 404
  hypothalamic 144, 146, 404
  post-abortal 160
  post-pill 160, 161, 167
  prevalence 137
  primary 144, 397
  secondary 40, 135–6, 144, 161, 397
  stress and 50
  theoretical distribution 347
  see also lactational amenorrhoea;
    post-partum amenorrhoea
American Fertility Society 323
amniocentesis 308
anaerobic flora 104, 105
anaesthetic gases 173, 174, 307
androgens 36, 88, 144, 397
  conversion to oestrogens 140
  declining testicular production 81
  male levels 278
androstenedione 143, 263
aneuploidy 291–5, 298
aniline 307
animals 172–6
anomalies 293, 300, 309
  congenital 280, 294

facial 291
anorexia nervosa 140, 149
anovulation 5, 134, 249, 346, 414, 415
  lactational 209
  nipple stimulation as key factor 413
  post-partum 348
  prolonged 368
anovulatory cycles 43, 53, 80, 225, 437
  frequency 201, 351, 430, 442
  luteal phase inadequacy and 134
  strenuous physical activity and 132
anthropometric measures 373, 374, 378, 380, 384
antibiotics 113, 303
antibodies 103, 106, 320–1
  anti-D/anti-P 303
  antinuclear 303, 304
  anti-sperm 248, 249
  blocking 304, 305, 306
  chlamydia 108, 129
  gonococcal 108
  immunoglobulin M 112
  lack of 305
antigens 105, 303, 304, 305, 306
anti-neoplastic agents 306–7
apa 447
Apert's syndrome 278
aplastic anaemia 309
arm circumference 373, 374
aromatase enzyme 397
arsenic 174, 307
artificial insemination 73, 74, 75, 210
  see also AID
Asherman's Syndrome 159–60, 166
ashrama 77
Asia 39, 194, 347, 348
aspirin 280
athletes 50, 149
  see also ballet dancers; joggers; runners
AUC analysis 258
Australia 23, 33, 252, 253, 385, 392, 394
autopsy 294
azoospermia 73, 232, 237, 238–40, 272

bacteria 103, 104, 105–6, 162, 163
ballet dancers 51, 132, 133, 138, 142
Baltimore 429–43
Bamako 450
Bangladesh 213 n., 368, 376, 380
  adolescent fertility 21, 30, 33, 56
  adolescent growth 57, 58
  age at marriage/age at menarche 52
  amenorrhoea 359–67 *passim*, 383, 385–90
  birth intervals 192
  coital frequency 78
  contraceptive use 71
  earlier menopause for thinner women 66
  interval between marriage and first birth 60–1

number of children ever born 16
risk of stillbirths and abortions 55
  see also Matlab
Bantus 65, 139
barrier contraceptives 4, 32, 106, 163, 167, 458
  see also condoms; spermicides
Bavaria 193
Belgium 34, 86
benzene 174, 307
bilateral oophorectomy 249
biological factors 3, 9–12, 15–16, 75, 80–1
biopsies 442
  endometrial 37, 134, 264, 298, 429; advanced 265; timed 248
birth 81, 186–9, 194, 272, 386
  control 330
  defects 171, 172, 176
  first: age at 51, 56, 59; marriage and 60–1; menarche and 52, 55–6
  last 346, 349; age at 69, 70
  multiple, cumulative damage of 75
  non-marital 34
  order 280
  pre-term 176
  rate 32, 43; estimated yearly 44
  risk of congenital defect at 280
  see also birth intervals; birth-weights; still-births
Birth Interval Dynamics study 385
birth intervals 9–10, 192–3, 202, 204, 216, 345, 348, 352, 357, 415
  determinants 8, 447–58
  first 190–1
  longer than average 16
  shorter 51
birth-weights 51, 415, 431, 432
  low 56, 60, 158, 171, 176
Black Volta 449
Blacks 89, 107
blastocysts 264, 317
bleeding episodes 318, 322, 334, 351, 368, 370, 406
Bobo-Dioulasso 450, 452, 456–7
body composition 138–43
Boston 385, 443
bottle feeds 394, 435, 438–40
breast development 51, 144
breastfeeding 8, 9, 11, 18, 140, 347–53 *passim*, 357, 364, 376
  absence of 441
  abstinence during/after 448, 449, 451, 457
  age 387
  behaviour 372, 381
  demand 453
  duration 17, 455; selected countries 360
  during menstruation 379
  extended 457

and fertility 391–407
frequency 432, 435, 442; declining 438; high 439, 440; increasing 441; low 443
intensive 362, 385, 457
intervals between episodes 430
long 453–4
ovulation and 393, 444
patterns 7, 17, 368, 369–70, 378, 431; and ovarian function 429
and post-partum amenorrhoea 345, 383, 386, 389, 413–26, 454, 457; selected countries 360
practices 359, 379
sexual taboos linked to 446
sucking stimulus and return of menses/ovulation 368
Britain, *see* United Kingdom
bromocriptine 335
Brong-Ahafo 449
Burkina Faso 450, 456
bwaki 447

Cameroon 73, 74, 448, 451
Canada 23, 34, 68, 187, 191, 310
cancer 269, 415
breast 54, 126
cervical 126
carcinoma 81
Caribbean islands 21
'catch-up puberty' 134
catecholamines 146
Caucasian women 65
cauterization 302
celioscopy 240
cells:
division 317, 332
granulosa 397
Leydig 81, 278
plasma, within the endometrium 102
Sertoli 278
vaginal 254
white blood 102
Census of Ireland (1911) 187
central nervous system 147, 294
centromere 295–7
cerebrospinal fluid 147
cervical mucus 105, 106, 233, 235, 240, 254
abundant 236, 241
excessive white blood cells in 102
cervicitis 102, 103
cervix 103, 233, 249, 301, 303
deformities 248
dilation 233, 235, 236; premature 302
ectopy 106
incompetent 157, 166, 291, 302
infections 104, 105, 106, 108
tenderness 101
see also cervical mucus
chemicals, *see* toxic substances

chemotherapeutic agents 173, 306
childbearing 76
completion of 70
delaying 75
early 59
expected rate 186
postponing 82, 157
successful, capacity for further 451
termination of 77, 187
see also birth
childhood malignancy 171
childlessness, *see* sterility
Chile 7, 415
Chlamydia 114, 115, 129
lower genital tract 106
trachomatis 102–5 *passim*, 108–12, 113, 116, 127, 232, 302
chorionic vesicles 291
chorionic villus sampling 293, 308
Christians 90
chromosomes 306
aberrations/abnormalities 6, 81, 82, 171, 211, 278–9, 288, 291–8
cigarette smoking 6, 164, 307, 330, 331, 332
maternal age and 336–9
cilia 104, 112
Clomid 161
clomiphene 161, 167
clomiphene citrate 252, 253, 267, 298
cohabitation 52, 55, 88
coital frequency 9, 11, 17–18, 171, 185, 189
adolescent 35, 37, 40
age and 77, 78, 85–7, 88, 201
constant 210, 222
controlling 217
daily 201, 216
decline 218–19; with age 81, 82
decreases 69, 75; with age 73
determinants 86–9
during menses 91
increasing 281
inter-coital intervals 199
low 187, 330
major determinant of conception 4
marital 35, 85–6, 212
marital duration and 86, 88, 213–14, 218–20, 222, 224, 348
maximum 357
measuring 94–5
non-marital 40, 212
number 200
overall 209
rate 10, 12, 15; heterogeneity in 211, 213
reducing 457
regular 345
risk factor 106
timing and 5, 32, 194–9, 202, 204
unusually high 345
variation/variance 222, 224

coitus 36, 85–95, 170, 214, 220–5
  coitus interruptus 449–50
  conditional risk of 214
  cycles of 90–4, 276, 281
  distribution throughout menstrual
    cycle 90–1, 92
  first 129
  loss of interest 94
  marital 85–6, 87
  number of partners 106, 128, 130, 164, 166
  outside marriage 33–4, 40, 42, 43, 44
  patterns 239, 357; woman's age and 198
  possible seasonal rhythms 90
  pre-marital 34, 40
  probability 33–6
  teenage 34
  times 288
  timing relative to ovulation 92, 194
  unprotected 107, 108, 127, 130, 209,
    210 n., 215, 273
  see also coital frequency; STDs
Collaborative Perinatal Project 329, 335,
    336–8, 339
Colombia 37
Columbia University 324
conception 32, 194, 217, 414
  assisted 5; infertility and 231–82
  chromosomally abnormal 294
  delays 17; between birth and next 346–7
  endocrine detection 316–25
  interval between marriage and 53, 345,
    346
  marker of 317
  monthly rates 349, 350, 357
  next 347–8
  optimal day for 233; 'best' 234–5
  probability 85, 86, 90, 415; *see also*
    fecundability
  products of 289
  recognized, probability of live birth 38–9
  risk of 204, 205, 348, 355, 415, 416;
    average 353; different days of the
    menstrual cycle 196; exposure to 186,
    273; failure 11, 12, 15–16, 17, 18; live
    birth rates 389
  stimulus of 318
  unsuccessful 80
  waiting time to 189–92, 202, 204, 223,
    345, 353–7; definition 347;
    expected 212, 224, 225; long 16;
    mean 56, 193, 213; nutritional status
    and 372, 374–8 *passim*
condoms 23, 43, 113, 273
congenital abnormalities 280, 281, 294
conization 302
consanguinity 232
contraception 70, 71, 130, 172, 204, 452
  adolescent 21, 23, 32, 36–7, 40, 43
  breastfeeding mothers 406, 429, 444

  cessation of 189, 190, 194, 273
  choices 113, 415
  differences in use of 12
  discontinuing 330
  failure rates 32, 43
  fertility following 5, 157–67
  histories 127
  hormonal 32, 416, 458
  increasing use 3
  intermittency of use 171
  married teenagers using 36–7
  never used 73, 74
  prevalence levels 13
  safe 406
  steroidal 406
  stopped 75
  see also barrier contraceptives; IUDs; oral
    contraception
Cook Islands 23
corpus luteum 316–17, 320, 397
  see also luteal phase/function
corticosteroids 280
cortisol 143
Costa Rica 4, 126–31
Cox proportional hazards model 331, 332
curettage 159, 300
cyclopia 291
Cyprus 23
cystic hygromas 293
cytogenetic abnormalities 288, 291, 293
cytomegalovirus 106

Dalkon Shield 113, 162, 164, 165, 166
DAMME (enkephalin analogue) 146, 147
deaths:
  ante-partum 294
  embryonic 211
  foetus in utero 290
  infant/child 51, 70, 346, 347;
    undetected 370
  intra-partum 171, 294
  neonatal 56, 294, 389, 310
  perinatal 294
  sub-clinical 216
dehydration 373
dehydro-epiandrosterone 143
Demographic and Health Surveys 82, 95
Denmark 108, 335, 392
dental assistants 332
developing countries 12, 13, 14, 50, 163
DHEW (Department of Health,
    Education, and Welfare) 243
diabetes mellitus 149, 299–300
diarrhoea 448, 451, 457
diethylstilbestrol 248, 310
diets 50, 139, 141, 373
  altered 142–3
dihydro-epiandrosterone sulphate 143, 144
dilatation and curettage 159

diseases:
  auto-immune 303–4
  cardiovascular 65
  hereditary 231, 232
  infectious 232
  life-threatening 309
  polycystic ovarian 263
  tubal 244
  venereal 14, 70, 81
  see also PID; STDs
Dobe !Kung 30, 136, 394
Dominican Republic 352
dopamine 146, 148, 404, 405, 406
Down's syndrome 296
doxycycline 303
drugs 280, 306
Duchenne muscular dystrophy 278
Duncan's multiple range test 258
duration of amenorrhoea 361–70, 433, 436,
    455
  duration of abstinence shorter than 8
  inconsistencies in data 6, 346, 348, 352–4,
    356
  nutritional status and 7, 375
  temporary 65
dysovulation 241

early pregnancy factor 317–18
Early Pregnancy Study 329, 336, 338–40
Edinburgh 443
education 88, 89, 128, 164, 337, 432
  age at menopause and 67
  and post-partum abstinence 450, 452
Egypt 392
El Salvador 35
embryos 293
  abnormal 279, 288
  cryopreservation of 241, 267
  early 220, 282, 288
  homozygous 306
  in vitro fertilized 288
  loss 38, 210, 211, 212, 220, 282
  multiple 251
  pre-implantation 269
  transfer 243, 244, 252, 266, 320;
      therapy 269
  viability of 280
endocervicitis 103
endocrine 142, 428, 429, 436, 438, 442
  detection of conception and early foetal
      loss 316–25
  research 60
  therapy 245
  see also anovulation; luteal phase/function
endogenous flora 104
endometriosis 240, 245–8, 335
endometritis 101, 102, 300
endometrium 104–5, 263–6, 288, 298–9, 303
  plasma cells within 102

poorly vascularized 309
thinning 301
Ureaplasma 302–3
endorphins 146, 147–8, 401
energy expenditure/output 51, 141
England 31, 73, 74, 108, 243
enkephalin analogue 146
environmental factors/hazards 282, 307–8,
    330, 332
erythema 102
Escherichia coli 232
Eskimo women 380
ethylene oxide 173, 307
Europe 67–8, 75, 104, 252, 288
  adolescent fertility 21–3, 31, 33
  age at menarche 50
EVMS (Eastern Virginia Medical
    School) 244–54 *passim*, 261
exercise 4–5, 50, 51, 136–49
  see also athletes
extended family 452

facultative anaerobes 113
fallopian tubes 103, 104, 288, 301
  blocked 329
  deformities 248
  ligations 324
  pus or exudate in area 102
  transport mechanisms 332
  see also tubal infertility
Family Planning Evaluation Project 223
famine 31, 139, 388
fatfold thickness 373, 374
fecundability 5, 6, 172, 281, 377, 428
  after menarche 21
  age patterns 80–1, 209–26
  apparent 211, 213, 217–21 *passim*, 223
  decline 80–1, 225
  determining 379
  effect of nutrition 415
  effective 32, 184, 186–7, 191, 193, 201
  estimates 79–80
  expected 223
  first month after return of 17
  gross and net 184
  heterogeneous 10, 211, 213, 214, 225
  homogeneous 212, 213, 214
  measuring 329–32
  models of 183–206, 214–16
  nutritional status and 380
  physiological and behavioural
      determinants 225
  and post-partum sterility 345–58
  and pregnancy outcome 271–84
  recognizable 184, 187–8, 189, 191, 194,
    197–8
  recognized 31, 37–8, 205
  reduced 329–40, 381, 388
  total 184, 194–5, 199, 201, 210, 217–18

fecundity 4, 67–9, 127, 216, 234–41, 428
Fédération CECOS 73–5, 210, 231–42
feeding episodes 383–90, 392, 393, 434
  see also bottle feeds; breastfeeding;
    supplementary foods
female circumcision 450
fertility 413, 457
  adolescent 21–64
  age at 4
  biological and behavioural factors 9–18
  breastfeeding and 391–407
  controlling 451
  declines in 73, 76–81, 279
  determinants 11–17, 456, 458
  effects on 5, 448–9; age 250–1
  exposure analysis 351–2
  following contraceptive use 5, 157–67
  impact of terminal abstinence 79
  important determinants 383
  male 81, 240, 241, 278
  marital 67–9, 79
  old-age 81
  physiological effect of lactation 457
  relative rates 69–70
fertilization 32, 38, 184, 198–9, 316–17,
    320
  probability 36–7, 235
  see also IVF
fever 302
fibroids 81
fimbrial ostia 112
Finland 145
foetal allograft 304
foetal loss 6, 171, 187, 188, 193, 201
  age and 82
  causes and frequency 285–341
  early 37, 38, 316–25
  increased risk 6
  pre-clinical 287–9
  probability 40
  spontaneous 81
  sub-clinical 217
  unrecognized 33
  wastage 51, 54–5, 61, 205
follicles 134, 249, 264, 392, 393
  developing 399
  growth 397, 400
  luteinenized unruptured 240
  maturation 259
  see also FSH; ultrasound
follicular phase 53, 93, 94, 287
  early 145, 146
  late 144
folliculogenesis 256
foods, *see* bottle feeds; breastfeeding;
    supplementary foods
formaldehyde 175, 307
France 34, 71, 191, 272–3, 446
  see also Fédération CECOS

FSH (follicle-stimulating hormone) 143,
    255–8, 320, 397–8, 402
  abnormality in 298
  increases in 141, 404, 405
  plus hMG plus hCG 253
  'pure' pituitary 263
  serum 145
  suppressed 391, 429

galactorrhoea 161
Gambia 384
gametes 269, 296, 297, 298
  ageing 199, 282
  over-ripe 81
gametogenesis 279
GEFCO study 271–2, 274–7, 279, 281, 282
genes 232, 269, 297, 306, 332–3, 335
  abnormalities/defects 288
  mutant 278, 294
  polymorphisms 305
Geneva 68
genital mycoplasmas 103, 105
genital tuberculosis 81
Georgetown University 428 n.
Germany 32
  see also Bavaria
gerontocratic societies 452
gestation 38, 44, 289–91, 298, 299, 300
  age 176, 334, 336, 337, 339
  early 303, 305
  ectopic 307
  first cycle 184
  full-term 10
  immune privilege of 269
  later in 293
  length 201
  various stages 287
Ghana 73, 74, 449, 451, 452
GLIM (General Linear Interactive
    Modelling) 417
glucuronides 92
glycosylateal haemoglobin 299
GnRH (gonadotrophin-releasing
    hormone) 144, 148, 258, 263, 397–401,
    405
  agonists 406
  early maturation 140
  gonadotrophin responses to 145
  pulsatile release 141, 397, 404, 407
gonadotrophins, *see* FSH; GnRH; hCG;
    hMG; LH
gonorrhoea 81, 108, 114, 115
  see also *Neisseria gonorrhoeae*
grandmotherhood 77, 78, 79
gravidity 310, 337
Greece 157
Guatemala 7, 34, 359, 361, 363, 379
  INCAP 383
Gumbel distribution 362

gynaecologists 233

haematological disorders 309
haemoglobin 299, 415
haemophilia 278
Haiti 447
haploidy 288, 291
hazard-model analysis 56, 348–53, 376–8, 380, 386–8, 414–17, 420, 431, 440, 442–3
hCG (human chorionic gonadotrophin) 211, 233, 255, 259–63, 265, 269, 338
  clomiphene citrate plus hMG plus 252, 253
  sensitive assays (urinary) 6, 38, 171, 287, 316–25, 336, 339
heavy labour/lifting 173, 176
heavy metals 173
Hegar dilator 302
height 58–60, 373, 374, 378
Helsinki 53
hepatitis 232
Herpes 232
  simplex 127, 129
heterozygotes 232, 297
Hindus 52, 77, 78
histocompatibility 304–6
historical populations 14, 73, 74, 75, 194
  see also Hutterites
HIV serology 232
hMG (human menopausal gonadotrophin) 252–65, 267
homosexual couples 232
Honduras 21
Hong Kong 23, 31
hormones 92, 137, 149, 175
  changes 145, 147
  disturbances 134
  glycoprotein 320
  imbalances 281, 329
  key 414
  pituitary 320
  regulation in IVF 243–69
  steroid 88, 318, 430
  thyroid-stimulating 144, 320
  thyrotrophin-releasing 145
  unique trophoblastic 269
  see also contraception; FSH; GnRH; hCG; LH; oestradiol; oestrogen; prolactin
horseshoe kidney 293
HPG (hypothalamic-pituitary-gonadal) axis 132, 140, 141, 148, 149
Hutterites 13, 68, 71, 186–7, 190, 191, 193, 305–6
hyperfertile women 237
hyperprolactinaemia 335, 402, 404
hyperthermia 233
hypogonadism 149
hypothalamus 147, 254, 332, 391, 398–400 *passim*, 413

adaptation 136
dopamine 405
opiate activity 148, 397, 401
opioid pathway 407
see also amenorrhoea; HPG axis
hypothermic phase 272
hypothyroidism 299
hypotropic trophoblasts 291
hysterectomy 288
hysterography 240
hysterosalpingograms 248
hysteroscopy 300

immunological factors 306
implantation 199, 279, 301, 304–5, 317, 320, 332, 336, 339
  embryos which abort between fertilization and 38
  inhospitable/unsupportive uterine environment 81, 298
  murine monosomies' failure to survive 291
  probability 185
  selection at, or immediately after 288
income 164
incomplete Mullerian fusion 300–1, 302
India 50, 55–6, 77–8, 139, 188, 384
  breastfeeding duration 368
  lactational amenorrhoea 361, 362, 363, 364
  see also Punjab
Indonesia 415
induced abortions 12, 32, 40, 44, 81, 157, 212
  previous 54
  risk of 38
infanticide 450
infections 279, 302–3
  ascending 106
  cervical 104, 105, 106, 108
  chlamydial 106, 108, 112
  chronic 309
  genital tract 102, 106, 115, 116
  gonococcal 106, 108
  intra-uterine, pre-existing 159
  new 107
  serological evidence of 126, 129, 131
  syphilis, previous 129
  tubal 102, 330
infecundability 170
  post-partum 6, 11, 12, 15, 352; and role of lactation 343–60
infecundity 75, 126, 128, 130
  history 129, 131
  lactational 352
  post-partum 433
  various countries 72
infertility 4, 75, 139, 233
  aetiological link between salpingitis and 108

and assisted conception 231–82
descriptive epidemiology 126–31
due to inadequate sperm of the male 249
gynaecological 241
immunological 249
intra-uterine devices and 164
lactational 391–406, 407, 416, 433
maintaining 394, 397
male 73, 232, 245–8
PID and 101–17
post-partum 7, 372–82
problems 335
reproductive impairments 170, 171, 172
STD-related 113–16
surgical 166
treatment for 330
see also tubal infertility
'inhibin' 263
injuries 137, 142
inseminations 32, 217
multiple 214
see also artificial insemination
intercourse, *see* coital frequency; coitus;
    sexual abstinence; sexual taboos
intrachorial haemorrhage 291
Inuit populations 139
IQ (intelligence quotient) 89
Iran 68
Irish men 81
IRMA (immuno-radiometric assay) 322, 324
irradiation 306–7
Islam 8, 450, 45
IUDs (intra-uterine devices) 32, 43, 89, 157,
    160, 308, 416
copper-containing 113, 164, 165, 166
Grafenberg 162
risks (PID and tubal infertility) 4, 5, 106,
    162–6, 167
IVF (*in vitro* fertilization) 5–6, 231, 233,
    239–69, 273–5, 279

Jamaica 34
Japan 23, 31, 86, 157, 385
Java 446–7
joggers 135, 137, 145
Johns Hopkins University 428 n., 430

Kaplan-Meier product-limit estimate 414
karyotypes 232, 288, 294, 307
Kenya 23, 57, 73, 74, 457
Kivu 449
Koranic tradition 450
kwashiorkor 448

La Lèche League women 385
labile tissues 373
lactation 348, 351, 357, 378, 379
duration 376
established 402

fertility-inhibiting effects 372
full absence of 347
prolonged 449
return of fecundity during 428
return of ovarian function during 428–44
role 6
suppression of LH release during 401
see also anovulation; infecundability;
    infecundity; infertility; lactational
    amenorrhoea
lactational amenorrhoea 8, 384, 391, 392,
    393, 402
abstinence and 456, 457
demographic research 359–70
effects of nutrition 405–6
first menstrual cycles following 399
and infertility 405
lactotrophes 391
Lancet 135
laparoscopy 101, 102, 244, 247, 248, 250
Lapp populations 139
Latin America 194, 347
lead 173, 175, 307
leiomyomas 301–2
lesions 161, 162, 240, 301
Lesotho 13, 73, 74
LH (luteinizing hormone) 4, 5, 7, 92–3, 134,
    141, 143–8, 253, 254–63 *passim*, 320–3,
    391, 397–407 *passim*, 429
Lippes Loop 164, 165, 166
Los Angeles County 39, 54
LUF (luteinenized unruptured follicle)
    syndrome 240
lupus:
anticoagulant 303, 309
erythematosis 291, 303, 309
luteal phase/function 53, 93, 94, 321, 430,
    438
abnormal 431, 437, 438
adequate 391, 429, 442
defects 5
deficiency 298–9
diminished 309
equivocal 437
inadequate 132, 134, 144, 391, 399
late 145, 318
normal 394, 396, 402, 431, 437
reinforced 266
short 33, 43, 80
see also progesterone
luteolysis 266
lymphocytes 305

malaria 81
Malawi 21
Malaysia 23, 34, 368, 414, 415
malformations 272, 274, 275, 276, 281, 300
Mali 7, 450
malnutrition 51, 52–3, 141, 373

chronic/severe 66, 134, 385
Manila 428–43
Mantel–Haenszel test 414
marasmus 448
marital duration 67, 69, 75, 187, 188, 346
 abstinence and 78
 coital frequency and 86, 88, 213–14,
  218–20, 222, 224, 348
Markov processes 362
marriage 55, 89–90, 189, 451, 452
 age at 10–12 *passim*, 15, 17, 76, 86, 345;
  and age at menarche 51, 52, 56, 60;
  first 187, 201; increase in 39
 births in the first year of 194
 coitus outside 33–4
 early 450
 interval between, and conception 53;
  first 60–1, 345, 346
 low rates, adolescents 34
 monogamous 453
 see also marital duration
masturbation 36
Matlab 31, 59, 352–7, 378–9, 385, 388
Meckel's syndrome 294
meiosis 278, 297, 295, 298
Melanesia 3
menarche 3, 65, 141, 164, 188, 394
 age at 23–31, 34, 38, 50–61, 67, 203, 337;
  decline 39; variation 21
 delayed 5, 132–4, 139, 140
 earlier 138–9
 fecundability after 21
 first birth and 52, 55–6
 interval from, to ovulation 33
 late 201
 later, strenuous exercise and 50
 probability of coitus after 36
Mengan's syndrome 278
menopause 278
 age at 4, 187, 203; and fecundity
  preceding 65–82
 early 201
 post- 65, 140
 premature 249
menses 52, 53, 105, 272, 287, 316–19 *passim*,
  334, 396, 413, 429–33 *passim*, 452
 abnormalities 159, 300
 absence 317
 anovulatory 433, 440
 cessation 65
 delayed 133, 134, 397
 expected 288
 first 351, 397, 417–20 *passim*, 433, 436–8,
  442
 frequency of coitus during 91
 intervals 356, 357, 376, 377, 380
 irregularity 81; predisposition to 143
 normal 160
 not resumed 377

onset 133, 140, 317, 321, 369, 431;
 determinants 50
 post-partum 6–7; second 416
 reduced frequency 149
 regular 137, 351
 response 370
 risk of 425
 see also menstrual cycle; resumption of
  menses
menstrual cycle 75, 184, 187, 234, 272, 330,
 402
 anovulatory 170
 distribution of coitus throughout 90–1, 92,
  94
 effects of exercise and nutrition 132–49
 first, following lactational
  amenorrhoea 399
 normal 397–8, 404
 onset 51, 57
 ovulatory 32–3, 205, 316
 PID symptoms within 104–5
 pre-ovulatory phase 393
 resumption 391, 397–8
Menstrual and Reproductive Survey 55
mentally ill women 308
mercury 173, 175
metabolic facilities 136
metabolites 318, 430
methotrexate 307
metoclopramide 148
Mexico 16, 31, 392, 443
micro-organisms 103, 302
milk, *see* lactation
Minnesota 330, 331
miscarriages 6, 39, 54, 177, 248, 386
MLE techniques 188–96 *passim*, 202
monogamy 128, 130, 453
monosomies 288, 289, 291, 292, 293, 294
 autosomal 289
Monte Carlo techniques 187, 362
Mormons 69
morbidity 4, 61, 157, 171
 see also diseases
mortality 4, 61, 157, 416
 intra-uterine 10–12 *passim*, 15–18 *passim*,
  201, 215, 217, 225
 see also deaths
mucosa 112
mullerian ducts 248, 300
 see also incomplete Mullerian fusion
multiparous women 108, 160, 305
muscle metabolism 137
musicians 51, 138
Muslims 31, 52, 77, 78, 90
myomectomy 300, 302
Mysore Population Study 77

naloxone 148
Narangwal 364, 365, 366

National Academy of Sciences 173
National Research Council 176
National Study of Family Growth (1982) 86
National Survey of Family Growth (1976) 43
Nature 91
NCHS (National Center for Health
    Statistics) 34, 43, 57
necrosis 301
Neisseria gonorrhoeae 102–5 *passim*, 108,
    113, 116, 163, 232
Nepal 30, 37, 79
Netherlands 34
neural tube defect 294
neurotic women 308
New Guinea 30, 52, 53, 66
New York City 335
New Zealand 23, 33
NFS (National Fertility Survey) 34, 86, 87,
    88
NICHD (National Institutes of Child Health
    and Development) 288, 290, 383 n.,
    428 n.
NIEHS (National Institute of Environmental
    Health Science) 322–4
Nigeria 78, 79, 447, 448, 450
NINCDS (National Institute of Neurological
    and Communicative Disorders and
    Stroke) 329 n., 335
nipple stimulation 413
nitrous oxide 173
non-Caucasian women 65
Normandy 68
North America 104
    see also Canada; United States
Norway 31, 38, 54, 68
Noyes criteria 264
nulliparous women 75, 108, 160, 164, 239
nursing mothers 330, 394, 417, 447, 451,
    454, 457
    and contraception 406
    resumed menses 379, 416
nutrition 4, 31, 67, 368, 429
    and fecundability 415
    and lactational amenorrhoea 405–6
    and menarche 3, 50–61
    and menstrual cycle 132–49
    and post-partum amenorrhoea 383–90
    and post-partum infertility 7, 372–82
    see also malnutrition; undernutrition

obesity 140, 141, 374, 385
obwosi 447
occupations 70, 88, 170, 432
    factors/hazards 174–6, 330, 332
Oceania 30
oedema 102, 293
oestradiol 143, 144, 262–4 *passim*, 397, 413,
    439
    serum 145, 254, 261

    see also pregnanediol
oestrogen 94, 141, 317, 318, 384, 399
    catechol 146, 148
    conversion of androgens to 140
    endogenous production 161
    exogenous administration 160
    metabolism 140
    negative feedback 398
    normal levels 167
    ovarian 393
    peripheral biological response 254
    serum 253
    substitute for 92
    substitution therapy with 250
    urinary 392, 402
oestrone 144, 145, 318, 319
Office of Technology Assessment 114
older women 5, 129, 239, 453
oligomenorrhoea 132, 135–6, 137, 167
oligospermia 237, 272
oncogenesis 269
oocytes 240, 250, 274, 279
    defective 263
    immature 268
    maturation 254, 258–9, 260, 261, 267, 281
    meiosis 260
    retrieval 252, 266
opiates 146, 147, 148, 397, 401
oral contraception 40, 43, 89, 157, 160–2,
    308
    breastfeeding mothers and 406
    discontinued 167
    duration of use 67
    effects 331; on coital distribution 92; on
        coital frequency 88
        high/low-progesterone 94
    PID and 106–7, 163,
    recent use 330
    tubal infertility and 113
organegenesis 302
osteoporosis 65, 149
ova 197, 198, 199, 316
    ageing 282
    blighted 291
    capture 112
    fertilized 317, 332, 324
    see also ovaries; ovulation; ovulatory cycle
ovaries 245, 318, 393
    activity: resumption 7, 391, 394–7;
        suppression 392–4, 404
    congenital absence 249
    cycles 210–11, 215; long 201
    failure 144
    follicular development 398
    function 53, 214; breastfeeding patterns
        and 429; return of, during
        lactation 428–44
    hormonal interactions of 332
    hypothalamic-pituitary regulation 149

inaccessibility 250
inactivity 406
liberation 250
methods of stimulation 251–3
steroid hormone metabolites 430
overhydration 373
ovulation 37, 81, 90–4 *passim*, 145, 185, 197,
    198, 316–17, 332, 432
  artificial insemination and 282
  breastfeeding and 8, 399, 400, 413, 416
  day of, determined 195
  delay in onset 385
  early 431, 441
  fecundability highest around time of 6
  first 351, 433, 437; prior to 436
  incipient 443
  induction 254
  late 322, 431, 441
  menses not preceded by 430
  normal 391
  pattern 240
  probability 32–3
  resumed 347, 348, 349, 394–7, 439–42
    passim, 455; delayed by sucking stimulus
    of breastfeeding 368
  risk of 440, 441, 443
  timing of 92, 194, 298, 430, 436, 437, 438
  whether menses predictive of 433
ovulatory cycle 33, 189, 287, 429, 437, 442
  first 438
  rapid onset 53
oxygen 104
oxytocin 406

Pakistan 34, 37
Pap smear 415
parous women 163
  see also multiparous women; nulliparous
    women; primiparous women
parturition 452
Pascal distribution 362
patrilocal/patrilinear exogamies 452
PCBs (polychlorinated biphenyls) 173, 175
Pearl Index 192
Pearson distribution 186, 190, 203
pelvis 59, 61, 415
  adhesions 157, 162, 167
  blocked 250
  see also PID
Pergonal 253
perineal orifices 300
peritoneal cavity 104, 105
peri-tubal scarring 112
Peru 60
pesticides 173, 175
phenylketonuria 309
pheromone effect 94
Philippines 7, 17, 33, 349–51, 352, 415
  see also Manila

physiology 199–201, 216–21, 225, 333, 414,
    457
PID (pelvic inflammatory disease) 158, 162,
    279, 330
  acute polymicrobial 104
  chlamydial/gonococcal 105, 106, 107
  and infertility 101–17
  polymicrobial nature of 102
  risk factors 106–7, 112–13; IUDs 4,
    162–6, 167
  silent 112, 114, 115, 117
  symptomatic 113
  upper genital tract 117
pill, *see* oral contraception
pituitary gland 7, 141, 161–2, 332, 391, 429
  see also endocrine
placenta 293, 298, 300, 306, 318, 391
  inadequate 60
  triploid 291
plasma 102, 143, 147, 391
Poisson distribution 216, 220, 222, 223, 417
Poland 23
polygamy 452, 453
polygyny 450
polyploidy 6, 288, 291–5
Population Association of America 91
Population Council 428 n.
porcine follicular fluid 263
post-partum amenorrhoea 187, 190, 201
  breastfeeding and 345, 383, 386, 389,
    413–26, 454, 457; selected countries 360
  determinants 378
  duration 192, 193, 349, 351, 356–70
    passim, 417–19, 456; extended 453;
    nutritional status and 372, 376, 377,
    379, 380, 381
pregnancy 74, 240, 266–7, 391
  apparent 322
  biochemical diagnosis 320
  complications 56
  detection 334, 339
  diagnosis 287
  dizygotic/monozygotic 280
  duration 345
  early 298, 316–22, 324
  echographical signs 233
  ectopic 157, 158, 248
  future 299
  immunological process responsible for
    maintaining 303
  length of 193
  losses 6; repeated 278
  maintenance 304
  multiple 69
  new 447
  outcomes 158, 170–8, 271–84
  planned 330, 332, 335
  positive hamster penetration test 245
  premature delivery 159

recognized 40, 199, 316, 333
recovery from 391–2
second 158, 159
subsequent 295
symptoms 317
termination 389; repeated 166; weight
  at 386, 387; *see also* abortions
tests 288
time to 330, 331, 332, 335, 337
transient or occult 318
viable 300
wastage 189
pregnanediol 318, 319, 391, 402, 439
glucuronide 396, 430
ovulation inferred from serum levels 32–3
substitute for progesterone 92
prematurity 157, 158, 159, 302
primiparous women 305
Princeton Fertility Study 189, 190, 191,
  194
progeria 278
progesterone 250, 263, 317, 320, 413
endogenous 92
insufficient luteal-phase increases 211
levels 145
luteal phase 265, 298–9, 391, 397
mid-luteal levels 134
oestradiol and 254
oestrogen and 318, 384
oral contraceptives 94
production 430
serum 264, 266
progestogen 406
prolactin 7, 143, 369, 384, 401–7 *passim*,
  413, 428
basal 145, 385, 395
plasma levels 391
responses 145, 148
serum 161
prolactinaemia 161, 162
see also hyperprolactinaemia
pronuclei 288
proteins 139, 320, 374, 448
chlamydial 105
C-reactive 102
placental 317, 318
pseudomolar degeneration 291
psychiatrists 233
psychological factors 308–9
psychological pathology 233
puberty 138, 139, 140–1
'catch-up' 134
delayed 132, 133
development 51, 57, 132, 144, 149
ovarian events 144
Puerto Rico 23
pulse frequency 146
punctures 240, 241
Punjab 65, 380

QUAC measurement 374
Quetelet's index 337

race 337
radiation 173, 176
radio-immunoassay 54, 317, 320, 321, 322
see also IRMA
religion 88, 89, 164
remarriage 187
repetitive abortions 296, 298–9, 300, 302,
  305, 308
explanation for 295
immunological perturbations leading
  to 306
reproduction 9–11
demographic and behavioural
  determinants 19–95
reproductive capacity: exercise-associated
  dysfunction 136–49; impairments 170;
  length of period 52; termination 69–76
resumption of menses 349, 353, 355, 359–61,
  374–5, 378–88 *passim*, 394–7, 455, 457
breastfeeding and 414, 415, 416, 428, 440
delayed: after oral contraceptives
  discontinued 167; after sucking stimulus
  of breastfeeding 368
early 6
likely 346
spotting and bleeding episodes confused
  with 351
stimulus 446
RETRO study 272–3, 274–5, 276, 279
Rhesus sensitization 303
rhythm method 32
runners 134, 135, 136
amenorrhoeic 137–8, 142, 143, 144, 145,
  148
Rwanda 30, 449

Saf-T-Coil 164, 165, 166
salpingectomies 248
salpingitis 105, 113
acute 163–4
aetiological link between infertility
  and 108
chlamydia 112
visually confirmed 101–2
SB6 assay 322, 323
Scandinavia 103
see also Denmark; Finland; Norway;
  Sweden
Schwangerschaftsprotein 1 (SP1) 318
Scotland 7, 392, 393
semen 232, 234, 236–8, 248, 447
cryopreserved 279, 282
oligoasthenospermic 240, 245
preservation 231–2
semiconductor manufacturing industry 173
Senegal 447, 450

sepsis (post-abortal) 81
sere 447
severe maternal illness 309
sexual abstinence 8, 9, 11, 18, 446–58
  age and 76, 78
sexual intercourse, *see* coital frequency;
  coitus
sexual taboos 446–52, 457
SHBG (serum hormone binding globulin)
  levels 140, 143
Singapore 23
skeletal measurements 373
skinfold thickness 142, 374
smoking status 67, 337
  see also cigarette smoking
social factors 3, 81–2
socio-cultural factors 76–80
socio-economic factors:
  conditions 39, 378, 429
  differentials 50
  indicators 379
  status 31, 373
solvents 173, 177
South Africa 31, 65, 139
spacing births, *see* birth intervals
Spain 31
sperm 94, 231, 446, 448, 452
  abnormalities 170
  actively motile 245
  age-related reduction in production 278
  capacitation 199
  donor, use in IVF 249
  healing power of 450
  mixing of women's blood and 458
spermatogenesis 81, 279
spermatozoa 106, 241–2, 282
spermicides 113, 308
spinnbarkheit 233, 235, 236, 241
spontaneous abortions 6, 38, 40, 44, 54, 55,
  272, 274–80 *passim*, 288, 299, 306–10
  passim, 335–40 *passim*
  chromosomal abnormalities 81, 279, 291–4
  cigarette smoking and 307
  early 198
  effect on fecundability 187
  late 191
  micro-organisms associated with 302, 303
  repetitive 298, 305
  risk 279, 282; increased 339
  subsequent pregnancies 158, 159
  VDUs and 176, 177
spousal separations 192
starvation 139
STDs (sexually transmitted diseases) 4, 126,
  131, 172
  pathology and epidemiology 101–17
  rapidly increasing incidence 157
  see also AIDS virus; venereal disease
sterility 67, 76, 188, 205

adolescent 3
age-specific prevalence 69, 70–6
  high levels 14
  male 89
  onset of 15, 17, 18, 70; age at 10, 11;
    early 16
  permanent 12
  post-partum 187; fecundability and 345–58
  premature 81
  secondary 189
steroidogenesis 254, 257, 397
steroids 141, 144, 280, 404
  ovarian 392
  placental 391
  urinary 318
stillbirths 280, 294, 310, 370, 386, 389
  and age at menarche 54, 61
  poor nutritional status and 55
streak gonads 249
stress 177
  emotional/psychological 50, 136, 137–8
  physical 50, 51, 134, 136, 137, 148;
    nutritional 139
sub-placental clotting 303
suckling episodes 7, 392–4, 395, 430
  duration 440, 441
  frequency 421–6, 433, 443
  suppressive effects 429
Sudan 73, 74
sulpiride 406
supplementary foods 7, 372, 380, 386, 389,
  413, 416, 419–21, 429–33 *passim*, 438–3
  passim, 454
  and early resumption of menstruation 384
  and suckling: duration 394, 395;
    frequency 425–6
suppositories 299
Sweden 34, 108, 113, 161, 163, 201
synechiae 159, 300
syphilis 81, 129
systemic lupus erythematosis 303

Taiwan 222, 223, 224, 226, 359, 379
temperature 102, 134, 235, 272, 277
  basal 32, 233, 248, 288, 429
'tender loving care' 308–9
teratogenicity 299
terminations, *see* abortions
testosterone 36, 94, 140, 145
tetracycline 303
tetraploidy 291, 292
Thailand 86, 392
thalidomide 280
thelarche 144
therapies:
  antibiotic 303
  clomiphene 161
  embryo transfer 269
  endocrinological/surgical 245

oestrogen/progesterone 250
  somatic cell gene 269
thinness 148
thrombocytopenia 318
thromboses 293, 303
thyroid abnormalities 299
time-varying covariates 352, 419–25
Togo 450, 451 452
tomograms 161
Toronto 385
toxic substances 170–8, 307, 308, 309, 335
training, *see* exercise
translocations:
  D/G 296
  Robertsonian 289, 295, 296
trauma 81, 308
Treponema pallidum 127
triploidy 291, 292, 294
trisomies 279, 280, 288, 291, 295, 309
  autosomal 293, 294; murine 289
trophoblasts 291, 320
tubal infertility 105, 107, 113, 115, 131, 167
  distal tubal obstruction 112, 114
  occlusion 108, 112, 116, 117, 279
  primary 164–6
  unilateral tubo-ovarian abscess 163
tumours 269
  benign 161, 162, 301
  hormone-dependent 149
Tunis 68
twinning rates 274, 275, 276, 280, 281

Uganda 450
ultrasound 250, 290, 293, 302, 393
  follicular 253, 254
umbilical cord 293
undernutrition 372, 373, 374
United Kingdom 34, 75
  Working Party on Amniocentesis
    (1978) 291
  see also England; Scotland
United Nations 21–3, 24, 35, 42, 77
  Fund for Population Activities
    (UNFPA) 447
United States 7, 170, 171, 201, 252, 278
  abortions 157, 166
  adolescents 23, 31, 33–5 *passim*, 38–9, 40;
    contraceptive use and failure rates 42–3;
    menarche 50, 52; statural growth 59
  age patterns of fecundability 210, 212,
    218, 223–4, 226
  dietary inadequacy 139
  frequency of coitus 86, 88, 90
  high prevalence of amenorrhoea 137
  menopause 66
  PID/STDs 103, 115, 116
  suckling 392, 394
  see also Baltimore; Boston; DHEW;
    EVMS; Hutterites; Los Angeles

County; National Academy of Sciences;
    National Research Council; NCHS; New
    York City; NFS; NIEHS; NICHD;
    NINCDS; Office of Technology
    Assessment; Princeton Fertility Study
University of Utah 321
urbanization 450
Ureaplasma urealyticum 302–3
urethra 106
urine 92–3, 94, 171, 317, 318, 320–4 *passim*
uterus 54, 103, 163, 300–1, 317
  abnormalities 81
  deformity 248
  tenderness 101
  see also endometrium

vagina 300, 303, 322, 406
vaginosis 103, 104
VDUs (visual display units) 176, 177, 308
venereal disease 14, 70, 81
  see also gonorrhoea; syphilis
Venezuela 21, 31
venipuncture 92
virulence factors 105–6
viruses 106, 232
  agents 173

war 31, 139
weight 373–4, 378–9, 384, 389, 432
  growth spurt in height and 53, 58–60, 140
  loss 141; self-induced 139
  pregnancy termination 386, 387
  see also birth-weights
WFS (World Fertility Survey) 4, 71–2, 73,
    126, 194, 347, 351
  abstinence 447, 449, 453, 454, 455
  adolescent fertility 27, 28, 33, 36
WHO (World Health Organization) 4, 25,
    27, 28, 29
  Task Force on the Diagnosis and
    Treatment of Infertility 107, 108
  Task Force on Oral Contraceptives 406
  Task Force on the Sequelae of
    Abortion 158, 159, 163
working conditions 176

X-rays 306–7

Yemen 13
Yoruba 78, 448–9, 450–1, 452, 453
younger women 112, 238, 239

Zaïre 394, 447, 452
Zimbabwe 92
zygotes 305
  see also heterozygotes

Index compiled by Frank Pert